AF566813

LUNG VASCULAR INJURY

LUNG BIOLOGY IN HEALTH AND DISEASE

Executive Editor

Claude Lenfant
Director, National Heart, Lung, and Blood Institute
National Institutes of Health
Bethesda, Maryland

1. Immunologic and Infectious Reactions in the Lung, *edited by Charles H. Kirkpatrick and Herbert Y. Reynolds*
2. The Biochemical Basis of Pulmonary Function, *edited by Ronald G. Crystal*
3. Bioengineering Aspects of the Lung, *edited by John B. West*
4. Metabolic Functions of the Lung, *edited by Y. S. Bakhle and John R. Vane*
5. Respiratory Defense Mechanisms (in two parts), *edited by Joseph D. Brain, Donald F. Proctor, and Lynne M. Reid*
6. Development of the Lung, *edited by W. Alan Hodson*
7. Lung Water and Solute Exchange, *edited by Norman C. Staub*
8. Extrapulmonary Manifestations of Respiratory Disease, *edited by Eugene Debs Robin*
9. Chronic Obstructive Pulmonary Disease, *edited by Thomas L. Petty*
10. Pathogenesis and Therapy of Lung Cancer, *edited by Curtis C. Harris*
11. Genetic Determinants of Pulmonary Disease, *edited by Stephen D. Litwin*
12. The Lung in the Transition Between Health and Disease, *edited by Peter T. Macklem and Solbert Permutt*
13. Evolution of Respiratory Processes: A Comparative Approach, *edited by Stephen C. Wood and Claude Lenfant*
14. Pulmonary Vascular Diseases, *edited by Kenneth M. Moser*
15. Physiology and Pharmacology of the Airways, *edited by Jay A. Nadel*
16. Diagnostic Techniques in Pulmonary Disease (in two parts), *edited by Marvin A. Sackner*
17. Regulation of Breathing (in two parts), *edited by Thomas F. Hornbein*
18. Occupational Lung Diseases: Research Approaches and Methods, *edited by Hans Weill and Margaret Turner-Warwick*
19. Immunopharmacology of the Lung, *edited by Harold H. Newball*
20. Sarcoidosis and Other Granulomatous Diseases of the Lung, *edited by Barry L. Fanburg*
21. Sleep and Breathing, *edited by Nicholas A. Saunders and Colin E. Sullivan*

22. *Pneumocystis carinii* Pneumonia: Pathogenesis, Diagnosis, and Treatment, *edited by Lowell S. Young*
23. Pulmonary Nuclear Medicine: Techniques in Diagnosis of Lung Disease, *edited by Harold L. Atkins*
24. Acute Respiratory Failure, *edited by Warren M. Zapol and Konrad J. Falke*
25. Gas Mixing and Distribution in the Lung, *edited by Ludwig A. Engel and Manuel Paiva*
26. High-Frequency Ventilation in Intensive Care and During Surgery, *edited by Graziano Carlon and William S. Howland*
27. Pulmonary Development: Transition from Intrauterine to Extrauterine Life, *edited by George H. Nelson*
28. Chronic Obstructive Pulmonary Disease: Second Edition, Revised and Expanded, *edited by Thomas L. Petty*
29. The Thorax (in two parts), *edited by Charis Roussos and Peter T. Macklem*
30. The Pleura in Health and Disease, *edited by Jacques Chrétien, Jean Bignon, and Albert Hirsch*
31. Drug Therapy for Asthma: Research and Clinical Practice, *edited by John W. Jenne and Shirley Murphy*
32. Pulmonary Endothelium in Health and Disease, *edited by Una S. Ryan*
33. The Airways: Neural Control in Health and Disease, *edited by Michael A. Kaliner and Peter J. Barnes*
34. Pathophysiology and Treatment of Inhalation Injuries, *edited by Jacob Loke*
35. Respiratory Function of the Upper Airway, *edited by Oommen P. Mathew and Giuseppe Sant'Ambrogio*
36. Chronic Obstructive Pulmonary Disease: A Behavioral Perspective, *edited by A. John McSweeny and Igor Grant*
37. Biology of Lung Cancer: Diagnosis and Treatment, *edited by Steven T. Rosen, James L. Mulshine, Frank Cuttitta, and Paul G. Abrams*
38. Pulmonary Vascular Physiology and Pathophysiology, *edited by E. Kenneth Weir and John T. Reeves*
39. Comparative Pulmonary Physiology: Current Concepts, *edited by Stephen C. Wood*
40. Respiratory Physiology: An Analytical Approach, *edited by H. K. Chang and Manuel Paiva*
41. Lung Cell Biology, *edited by Donald Massaro*
42. Heart–Lung Interactions in Health and Disease, *edited by Steven M. Scharf and Sharon S. Cassidy*
43. Clinical Epidemiology of Chronic Obstructive Pulmonary Disease, *edited by Michael J. Hensley and Nicholas A. Saunders*
44. Surgical Pathology of Lung Neoplasms, *edited by Alberto M. Marchevsky*
45. The Lung in Rheumatic Diseases, *edited by Grant W. Cannon and Guy A. Zimmerman*

46. Diagnostic Imaging of the Lung, *edited by Charles E. Putman*
47. Models of Lung Disease: Microscopy and Structural Methods, *edited by Joan Gil*
48. Electron Microscopy of the Lung, *edited by Dean E. Schraufnagel*
49. Asthma: Its Pathology and Treatment, *edited by Michael A. Kaliner, Peter J. Barnes, and Carl G. A. Persson*
50. Acute Respiratory Failure: Second Edition, *edited by Warren M. Zapol and Francois Lemaire*
51. Lung Disease in the Tropics, *edited by Om P. Sharma*
52. Exercise: Pulmonary Physiology and Pathophysiology, *edited by Brian J. Whipp and Karlman Wasserman*
53. Developmental Neurobiology of Breathing, *edited by Gabriel G. Haddad and Jay P. Farber*
54. Mediators of Pulmonary Inflammation, *edited by Michael A. Bray and Wayne H. Anderson*
55. The Airway Epithelium, *edited by Stephen G. Farmer and Douglas Hay*
56. Physiological Adaptations in Vertebrates: Respiration, Circulation, and Metabolism, *edited by Stephen C. Wood, Roy E. Weber, Alan R. Hargens, and Ronald W. Millard*
57. The Bronchial Circulation, *edited by John Butler*
58. Lung Cancer Differentiation: Implications for Diagnosis and Treatment, *edited by Samuel D. Bernal and Paul J. Hesketh*
59. Pulmonary Complications of Systemic Disease, *edited by John F. Murray*
60. Lung Vascular Injury: Molecular and Cellular Response, *edited by Arnold Johnson and Thomas J. Ferro*

ADDITIONAL VOLUMES IN PREPARATION

Cytokines of the Lung, *edited by Jason Kelley*

The Mast Cell in Health and Disease, *edited by Michael A. Kaliner and Dean Metcalfe*

Pulmonary Disease in the Elderly Patient, *edited by Donald A. Mahler*

LUNG VASCULAR INJURY

MOLECULAR AND CELLULAR RESPONSE

Edited by

Arnold Johnson

Thomas J. Ferro

Stratton Veterans Affairs Medical Center
and Albany Medical College
Albany, New York

Marcel Dekker, Inc. **New York • Basel • Hong Kong**

Library of Congress Cataloging-in-Publication Data

Lung vascular injury : molecular and cellular response / edited by
Arnold Johnson, Thomas J. Ferro.
p. cm. -- (Lung biology in health and disease ; v. 60)
Includes bibliographical references and indexes.
ISBN 0-8247-8718-8 (alk. paper)
1. Respiratory distress syndrome, Adult--Pathogenesis. 2. Lungs--Blood-vessels--Pathophysiology. 3. Respiratory distress syndrome, Adult--Molecular aspects. I. Johnson, Arnold. II. Ferro, Thomas J. III. Series.
[DNLM: 1. Lung--injuries. 2. Lung--physiopathology. WF 600 L96365]
RC776.R38L86 1992
616.2'407--dc20
DNLM/DLC
for Library of Congress 92-18425
CIP

This book is printed on acid-free paper.

Copyright © 1992 by Marcel Dekker, Inc. All Rights Reserved

Neither this book nor any part may be reproduced or transmitted in any form or by any means, electronic or mechanical, including photocopying, microfilming, and recording, or by any information storage and retrieval system, without permission in writing from the publisher.

Marcel Dekker, Inc.
270 Madison Avenue, New York, New York 10016

Current printing (last digit):
10 9 8 7 6 5 4 3 2 1

PRINTED IN THE UNITED STATES OF AMERICA

To the loving spirit of my mother
AJ

To mom and dad
TJF

INTRODUCTION

The adult respiratory distress syndrome (ARDS) has been a frequent topic in the series *Lung Biology in Health and Disease*, with Volumes 24 and 50 specifically devoted to this important area. Various aspects of ARDS have been touched on in several other volumes as well, and another new volume addressing ARDS is already in preparation. The current volume, *Lung Vascular Injury: Molecular and Cellular Response*, is one more step along the long and difficult path that will lead us to an understanding of this syndrome.

There are two converging reasons for the massive attention ARDS has been receiving. First, ever since this clinical syndrome was recognized in the 1950s, and its pathophysiology was defined in the 1960s, we have helplessly witnessed its tremendous morbidity and mortality. It is neither unfair nor overly critical to state that little progress has been made; both morbidity and mortality rates remain unacceptable. Thus, it is not surprising that there is great interest in basic and clinical research on this condition and in continuous assessment of the current state of knowledge.

The second reason is that research on ARDS is remarkably fruitful. Although no one yet is claiming success, all investigators know that opportunities for success are at hand. In 1986, a colleague and I wrote an editorial titled ''Physiology: is it time to cross the new frontier?''(1). We said ''Biomedical research has crossed into a new frontier where the emphasis is on such disciplines as molecular genetics, cell biology and immunochemistry. . . . Now is the time to raise questions of import to the physiologist: Has the field of physiology recognized this frontier . . . ?''

As we review the research findings on ARDS being published in 1992, there is no question that not only has the frontier been crossed but the territory beyond is being conquered with enthusiasm, and unbelievable discoveries are being made. This volume, edited by Drs. Arnold Johnson and Thomas J. Ferro, is like a travel guide into this new territory. Undoubtedly, our colleagues who in the 1950s and 1960s described the pathophysiology and the clinical manifestations of ARDS must marvel to see how much progress has been made in the field they opened.

In the conclusion of the editorial referred to earlier (1) we remarked: ''There can be no substitute for revitalizing the integrative approach of physiology, but it must be a comprehensive physiology that uses all the techniques and approaches of today.'' Drs. Johnson and Ferro have succeeded in bringing together distinguished investigators expert in ''the techniques and approaches of today,'' which they have applied to discovering the pathogenesis of lung vascular injury—the hallmark of ARDS. This is a first step toward the possible prevention of this syndrome, as the editors point out in their preface.

Claude Lenfant, M.D.
Bethesda, Maryland

Reference

1. Moskowitz, J. and Lenfant, C. (1986). *J. Appl Physiol.* 61:1609–1611.

PREFACE

According to Sir William Osler (1), progress in modern medicine proceeds in distinct phases. Progress begins with "a stage in which the clinical and anatomical features of disease [are] determined." In the second phase, the focus of attention becomes "the causes of disorders." Eventually, "the application of the knowledge for [disease] prevention" is achieved. Despite the great advances in medical technology that have occurred since the time of Osler, we believe that Osler's observations remain a valid philosophical framework for understanding the natural history of medical progress.

Where does the adult respiratory distress syndrome (ARDS) stand in Osler's scheme today? It appears as though we are well into the second phase, while still dealing with unresolved recognition and treatment issues. The first phase began with the recognition of the clinical entity in 1950 (2), although the name ARDS has been in use only since 1967 (3), and understanding of the relationship between ARDS and the multiple organ failure (MOF) syndrome has been achieved only in the past few years. Attempts to discover the cause of ARDS began more recently, once understanding of basic immunology and inflammation had advanced so that potential mechanisms of tissue injury could be identified. Phase two has progressed to the point that we can postulate a pathogenetic sequence in some detail for ARDS associated with sepsis. This sequence, which begins with bacterial endotoxin, includes specific inflammatory mediators, and ends with noncardiogenic pulmonary edema, may also apply at least partly to other forms of ARDS and to MOF.

This volume consists of eleven chapters dealing with specific cellular, biochemical, and molecular aspects of the pathogenesis of experimental lung vascular injury. Emphasis is placed on the intermediary factors, such as endotoxin-induced monokines and intracellular stimulus-response coupling mechanisms, including protein kinase C and cAMP. This volume is useful to those interested in the pathophysiology of lung disease: research scientists in the basic sciences, academic physicians (particularly those in the areas of pulmonary disease, pathology, and pharmacology), and anyone with a general interest in inflammation.

Detailed knowledge of the pathogenesis of experimental lung vascular injury may help us fill in the gap remaining from the first phase of study of ARDS (i.e. the lack of definitive therapy), and thus allow us to turn our attention to Osler's third phase, that of prevention.

Arnold Johnson
Thomas J. Ferro

References

1. Osler W. (1921). *The Evolution of Modern Medicine*. New Haven, Yale University Press, p. 221.

2. Jenkins M.T., Jones R.F., Wilson B., and Moyer C.A. (1950). Congestive atelectasis–a complication of the intravenous infusion of fluids. Ann Surg 132: 327–347.

3. Ashbaugh D.G., Bigelow D.B., Petty T.L., and Levine B.E. (1967). Acute respiratory distress in adults. Lancet 2: 319–323.

CONTRIBUTORS

Edward R. Block, M.D. Professor, Department of Medicine, University of Florida College of Medicine, and Associate Chief of Staff for Research, Veterans Affairs Medical Center, Gainesville, Florida

Franklin Cerasoli, Jr., Ph.D. Assistant Fellow, Department of Cellular Pharmacology, Sandoz Research Institute, East Hanover, New Jersey

Thomas J. Ferro, M.D. Chief, Pulmonary and Critical Care Section, Stratton Veterans Affairs Medical Center, and Associate Professor, Division of Pulmonary and Critical Care Medicine, Department of Medicine, Albany Medical College, Albany, New York

Joe G. N. Garcia, M.D. Calvin H. English Professor of Medicine, Physiology, and Biophysics, Department of Medicine, Indiana University School of Medicine, Indianapolis, Indiana

Alasdair M. Gilfillan, Ph.D. Associate Research Investigator, Department of Pharmacology, Hoffmann-La Roche, Nutley, New Jersey

G. H. Gurtner, M.D. Professor of Medicine and Physiology, and Director, Division of Pulmonary and Critical Care Medicine, Department of Medicine, New York Medical College, Valhalla, New York

C. Michael Hart, M.D. Assistant Professor of Medicine, Division of Pulmonary and Critical Care Medicine, Indiana University Medical Center, Indianapolis, Indiana

Paul J. Higgins, Ph.D. Associate Professor, Department of Microbiology, Immunology, and Molecular Genetics, Albany Medical College, Albany, New York

Arnold Johnson, Ph.D. Research Scientist, Research Service, Stratton Veterans Affairs Medical Center, and Associate Professor, Division of Molecular and Cellular Medicine, Department of Medicine and Department of Physiology and Cell Biology, Albany Medical College, Albany, New York

John E. Kaplan, Ph.D. Professor, Department of Physiology and Cell Biology, Albany Medical College, Albany, New York

A. Knoblauch, M.D. Director, Division of Pulmonary Medicine, Department of Medicine, Kantonsspital St. Gallen, St. Gallen, Switzerland

Steven L. Kunkel, Ph.D. Professor, Department of Pathology, University of Michigan Medical School, Ann Arbor, Michigan

Andrew P. Metinko, M.D. Division of Pulmonary and Critical Care Medicine, Department of Medicine, University of Michigan Medical Center, Ann Arbor, Michigan

Viswanathan Natarajan, Ph.D. Assistant Professor, Department of Medicine and Biochemistry, Indiana University School of Medicine, Indianapolis, Indiana

C. Subah Packer, Ph.D. Assistant Professor, Department of Physiology and Biophysics, Indiana University School of Medicine, Indianapolis, Indiana

Patricia G. Phillips, Ph.D. Research Scientist, Stratton Veterans Affairs Medical Center, and Assistant Professor, Albany Medical College, Albany, New York

Rodney A. Rhoades, Ph.D. Professor and Chairman, Department of Physiology and Biophysics, Indiana University School of Medicine, Indianapolis, Indiana

A. M. Sciuto, Ph.D. Physiologist, U.S. Army Medical Research Institute of Chemical Defense, Aberdeen Proving Grounds, Maryland

William M. Selig, Ph.D. Associate Research Investigator, Department of Bronchopulmonary and Gastrointestinal Research, Hoffmann-La Roche, Nutley, New Jersey

Theodore Standiford, M.D. Division of Pulmonary and Critical Care Medicine, Department of Internal Medicine, University of Michigan Medical Center, Ann Arbor, Michigan

Robert M. Streiter, M.D. Division of Pulmonary and Critical Care Medicine, University of Michigan Medical Center, Ann Arbor, Michigan

Min-Fu Tsan, Ph.D. Associate Chief of Staff for Research and Development, Stratton Veterans Affairs Medical Center, and Professor of Physiology and Cell Biology and Professor of Medicine, Albany Medical College, Albany, New York

Catherine M. Venturini, Ph.D. Postdoctoral Fellow, Wellcome Research Laboratories, Beckenham, Kent, England

Carl W. White, M.D. Associate Staff Physician and Associate Professor, Department of Pediatrics, National Jewish Center for Immunology and Respiratory Medicine, University of Colorado Health Sciences Center, Denver, Colorado

CONTENTS

Introduction Claude Lenfant *v*

Preface *vii*

Contributors *ix*

1. Mechanisms of Transmembrane Signal Transduction and Activation of Phospholipases in Vascular Endothelium: Implications for Lung Inflammation **1**

Joe G. N. Garcia and Viswanathan Natarajan

I. Introduction: Endothelial Cell Activation and Dysfunction 1
II. Role of Guanine Nucleotide Regulatory Proteins in Cellular Activation 3
III. Regulation of Phospholipase C Activity and Ca^{2+} Mobilization 7
IV. Protein Kinase C and Signal Transduction 11
V. Phospholipase A_2 (PLA_2) and Signal Transduction 16
VI. Phospholipase D and Signal Transduction 19
VII. Transmembrane Signaling After Thrombin Receptor Occupancy 29

VIII. Regulation of Thrombin-Induced PGI_2 Synthesis 36
IX. Regulation of ∝-Thrombin-Induced Endothelial Cell Barrier Dysfunction 40
X. Oxidant-Induced Activation of Phospholipases and Modulation of Signal Transduction 46
XI. Summary 50
References 53

2. Lung Injury and Edema Associated with the Activation of Protein Kinase C **67**

Arnold Johnson and Thomas J. Ferro

I. Introduction 67
II. Mechanisms of Stimulus-Response Coupling Mediated by PKC Activation 67
III. Activators and Inhibitors of PKC 69
IV. Effects of PKC Activation at the Cellular Level 69
V. Effects of Pulmonary PKC Activation 76
VI. Summary 85
References 87

3. The Role of cAMP in the Regulation of Pulmonary Vascular Permeability **99**

G. H. Gurtner, A. M. Sciuto, and A. Knoblauch

I. Introduction 99
II. Effects of cAMP in Acute Lung Injury 100
III. Effects of Drugs That Increase cGMP in Acute Lung Injury 101
IV. Temporal Nature of cAMP-Related Protection 101
V. Effects of cAMP on the Permeability of Endothelial Cell Monolayers 102
VI. Effects of cAMP on Mediator Production 103
VII. Cyclic AMP and the Immune System 106
VIII. Mechanisms of Action of cAMP and cGMP on Vascular Permeability and Vasomotor Tone 107
IX. Possible Therapeutic Strategy for the Use of Drugs That Increase cAMP in Acute Lung Injury 108
References 108

4. Cytoarchitectural Aspects of Endothelial Barrier Function in Response to Oxidants and Inflammatory Mediators **113**

Patricia G. Phillips and Min-Fu Tsan

I. Introduction 113
II. Structure of Endothelial Tight Junctions 114
III. Actin Microfilament System in Endothelial Cells: General Considerations 116
IV. Functional Links Between the Cytoskeleton and Tight Junctions 118
V. Unifying Concepts 126
VI. Future Directions 129
VII. Summary 129
References 130

5. Modification of Lipid Composition to Reduce Susceptibility of Vascular Endothelial Cells to Oxidant Injury: A Novel Defense Strategy **137**

C. Michael Hart and Edward R. Block

I. Introduction 137
II. Background 139
III. Experimental Protocol 142
IV. Experimental Results 142
V. Summary and Conclusions 166
VI. Future Directions 167
References 168

6. Induced Expression of p52(PAI-1) in the Cellular Response to Hyperoxia: Common Changes in Gene Expression Elicited by Growth Factors and Hyperoxic Stress **175**

Paul J. Higgins

I. Pulmonary Tissue Response to Hyperoxia 175
II. Analysis of Hyperoxia-Associated Changes in Cellular Gene Expression 176
III. p52 is Plasminogen Activator Inhibitor Type 1 180
IV. Potential Molecular Mechanisms Underlying Control of ECM-Regulating Gene Expression by Growth Factors and Hyperoxic Stress 183
V. Conclusions 185
References 186

7. Molecular Mechanisms of Cytokine-Induced Tolerance to Acute Oxidant Lung Injury **191**

Carl W. White

I. Introduction 191
II. Endotoxin-Induced Tolerance to Hyperoxia and Copper,Zinc Superoxide Dismutase 193
III. Cytokine-Induced Tolerance to Hyperoxia 194
IV. Role of Manganese SOD in Cytokine-Induced Tolerance to Oxidants 196
V. Potential Effects of Cytokines on Oxidant Production 199
VI. Potential Role of Arachidonate Metabolites and Other Inflammatory Mediators in Cytokine-Induced Oxidant Tolerance 200
VII. Summary 201
References 203

8. Endothelial Cell-Derived Novel Chemotactic Cytokines **213**

Steven L. Kunkel, Theodore Standiford, Andrew P. Metinko, and Robert M. Streiter

I. Introduction 213
II. Initiation of Cell Movement 214
III. Chemotactic Cytokines: Interleukin-8/Neutrophil Activating Protein (IL-8) and Monocyte Chemotactic Protein (MCP) 217
IV. Interleukin-8 Gene Expression by Endothelial Cells 218
V. Monocyte Chemotactic Protein (MCP) Expression by Endothelial Cells 222
References 224

9. Impaired Pulmonary Vascular Smooth Muscle Function in Lung Injury **227**

C. Subah Packer and Rodney A. Rhoades

I. Introduction 227
II. Chronic Hypoxia-Induced Pulmonary Hypertension 228
III. Hyperoxia-Induced Pulmonary Hypertension 237
IV. Reactive Oxygen Species–Mediated Injury 238

V. Ischemia-Reperfusion 249
VI. Neutrophil Injury 252
References 256

10. Eosinophils, Mast Cells, and Basophils: Cellular Mechanisms Contributing to Lung Microvascular Injury 263

Franklin Cerasoli, Jr., Alasdair M. Gilfillan, and William M. Selig

I. Introduction 263
II. Location, Morphology, and Function of Eosinophils, Basophils, and Mast Cells 264
III. Signal Transduction Mechanisms in Eosinophils, Mast Cells, and Basophils 269
IV. Interrelationship Between Eosinophils, Mast Cells, and Basophils 273
V. Contribution of Eosinophils, Mast Cells, and Basophils to Lung Microvascular Injury 276
VI. Conclusions 289
References 290

11. Thrombin-Induced Platelet Adhesion to the Pulmonary Vasculature 309

Catherine M. Venturini and John E. Kaplan

I. Introduction 309
II. Pathophysiology of Pulmonary Thrombosis 310
III. Thrombin-Induced Platelet Adhesion to Pulmonary Endothelium 311
IV. Conclusion 320
References 321

Author Index *329*
Subject Index *365*

LUNG VASCULAR INJURY

1

Mechanisms of Transmembrane Signal Transduction and Activation of Phospholipases in Vascular Endothelium: Implications for Lung Inflammation

JOE G. N. GARCIA and VISWANATHAN NATARAJAN

Indiana University School of Medicine
Indianapolis, Indiana

I. Introduction: Endothelial Cell Activation and Dysfunction

The vascular endothelium is uniquely located to participate actively in the induction of inflammatory processes. The disruption of endothelial cell integrity profoundly alters vascular function, resulting in the loss of a selective barrier to plasma macromolecules, the initiation of coagulation, and tissue ischemia. In the lung, for example, pulmonary artery endothelial cells regulate both vascular permeability and tone, and endothelial cell dysfunction leads to a variety of lung disorders, such as the adult respiratory distress syndrome, hypoxemic respiratory failure, and pulmonary hypertension.

The maintenance of a nonthrombogenic surface and preservation of vascular barrier function are dynamic endothelial cell processes, and in recent years the high metabolic activity of endothelial cells has been documented. The endothelium is an initial and primary target of vascular proteins, and an exhaustive list of diverse endothelial cell functions has been recognized as being modulated by endothelial cell interaction with circulating hormones, cytokines, and inflammatory mediators. In prior years, a great deal of attention was focused on agents that were overtly cytotoxic to endothelial cells. Alterations in in vivo or in vitro endothelial cell function were observed in a variety of models of drug- or protease-mediated endothelial cell cytotoxicity. In one model, injury is mediated by toxic oxygen radicals either added directly to cultured endothelium, generated by leukocyte activation, or produced by alterations in ambient oxygen concentrations. However, based on the morphologic observation that extensive areas of denuded endothelium are never found in organs damaged by the aforementioned agents, as well as the finding that endothelial cell viability is relatively well maintained until superphysiological concentration of the injurious agents are utilized, the concept of endothelial cell activation and dysfunction has emerged, and attention is now focused on mechanisms of intracellular regulation, rather than injury, in the initiation and maintenance of pathogenic vascular syndromes.

There is now abundant evidence that the regulation of cellular activation involves intricate and well-integrated signals that are received by the cell and transduced into cellular responses indicative of activation. Endothelial cells respond to their environment through their cell-surface receptors, which bind specific ligands, generating a signal that is transduced into a cellular metabolic function by the action of second messenger molecules generated as the result of the activation of membrane phospholipases. Phospholipases are essential effector molecules that catalyze the hydrolysis of membrane phospholipids and are classified according to the bond cleaved in a phospholipid. The important membrane phospholipases involved in transmembrane signaling include phospholipase A_2 (PLA_2; EC 3.1.1.4), which selectively removes fatty acids from the sn-2 position of the phospholipid; phospholipase C (PLC; EC 3.1.4.3), which cleaves the bond between glycerol and a phosphate; and phospholipase D (PLD; EC 3.1.4.4), which hydrolyzes the amino alcohol moiety from a phospholipid (Fig. 1).

In this chapter we focus on the transmembrane signaling events involved in receptor- and non-receptor-mediated activation of these three important membrane phospholipases in cultured endothelium. Although there are numerous endothelial cell functional responses that are suitable for examination of stimulus–coupling regulatory pathways, we have chosen to concentrate on the regulation of two important indices of endothelial cell activation: prostaglandin synthesis and barrier dysfunction. Specific attention is directed to the role of phospholipase-generated second messengers in accomplishing these key endothelial cell events. The signal transducing events that follow occupation of the receptor specific for the bioregulatory coagulant protease thrombin are addressed in greatest detail as they provide a useful paradigm by which to analyze receptor-mediated endothelial cell activation. In addition, since conditions of oxidant stress exist in a number of inflammatory lung and vascular syndromes, the effect of oxidants on endothelial cell activation pathways is also discussed.

Finally, endothelial cells from different species, distinct in their response to specific inflammatory stimuli and physiologic and biochemical differences, have been documented to exist between endothelial cells derived from large ves-

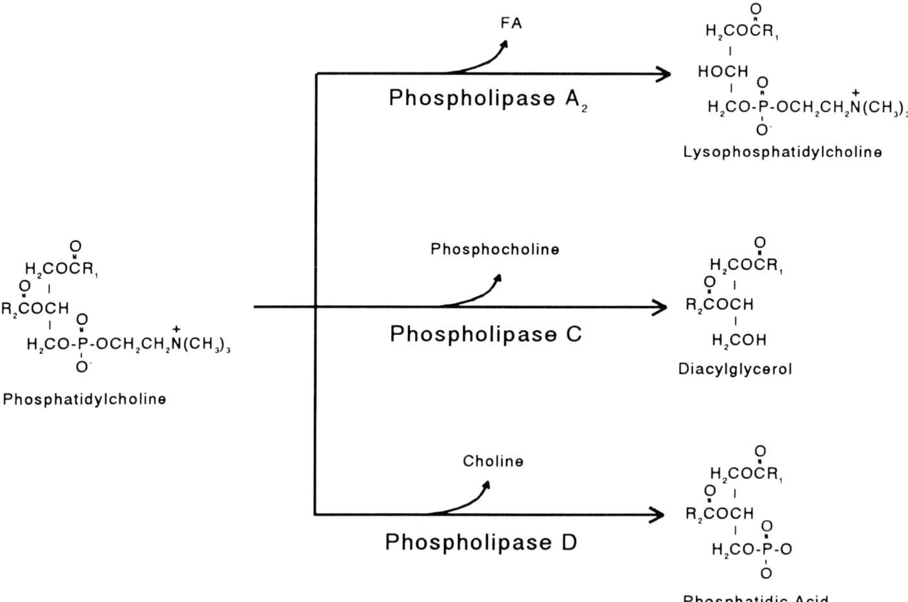

Figure 1 Action of phospholipases on phosphatidylcholine. R_1 represents saturated and monounsaturated fatty acids (FA); R_2 represents polyunsaturated fatty acids such as arachidonic acid.

sels as contrasted with those obtained from the microvasculature. In this chapter we report on transmembrane signaling responses of endothelial cells obtained from the bovine pulmonary artery and human umbilical vein, although studies performed with endothelium derived from other sites (aorta) and species (porcine) are also reported where appropriate.

II. Role of Guanine Nucleotide Regulatory Proteins in Cellular Activation

A variety of agonists that bind to their specific receptors are coupled to subsequent effector enzymes via guanine nucleotide (GTP)-binding regulatory proteins, or G proteins, which transmit signals across the cell membrane into the cell interior (Gilman, 1987). G proteins are involved in communication of a vast array of diverse extracellular signals, varying from hormones and physiologic agonists to carcinogens, and participate in visual regulation, operation of ion channels, hematopoiesis regulation, and the host defense mechanism of leukocytes (Gilman, 1987; Barbacid, 1987; Rizzo et al., 1990). More important, they are involved directly in regulation of the biosynthesis of second messengers which perform a transduction function in accomplishing cellular activation.

The GTP-binding proteins are a family of membrane-bound heterotrimeric proteins composed of α, β, γ subunits, with the α subunit typically migrating at a molecular weight between 39 and 52 kD. The β subunit generally corresponds to one or another of closely related 35- and 36-kD proteins, and the γ subunit is a low-molecular-weight protein ranging from 6 to 10 kD. The α subunit of each G protein binds either GTP or GDP, or their nonhydrolyzable analogs GDPβS (guanosine 5′-*O*-(2-thio) diphosphate) and GTPγS (guanosine 5′-*O*-(3-thio) triphosphate) via a single high-affinity binding site. In addition, the α subunit possesses GTPase activity that is critical to the regulation of this coupling protein. The interaction of the occupied receptor with a heterotrimeric G protein induces dissociation of the α subunit with release of the β/γ subunits (Gilman, 1987).

The best characterized receptor/G protein/effector coupling system is the G protein system, originally described as regulating adenylyl cyclase activity (Gilman, 1984). Occupancy of the β adrenergic receptor initiates activation of the G protein, G_s, stimulating adenylate cyclase activity and resulting in the production of cyclic adenosine 3′5′-monophosphate (cAMP). In contrast, binding of the specific α adrenergic receptor coupled to a distinct G protein, G_i, causes inhibition of adenylate cyclase activity and therefore lowers cAMP production. Additional heterotrimeric structured G proteins, G_o and G_z, have been identified. Methods employed to assess the role of G proteins in the specific functional responses of intact cells have relied on the use of specific G protein activators, G protein inhibitors, or bacterial toxins which via their intrinsic ADP-ribosyltransferase activity either augment or inhibit a given G protein–regulated response. The various α subunits within the family of G proteins contain the site specifically ADP-ribosylated by cholera toxin (α_s), by pertussis toxin (α_i, α_o), by both toxins (α_t), or unaffected by toxin-induced ADP ribosylation (α_z) (Gilman, 1984, 1987). For pertussis toxin, nicotinamide adenine dinucleotide (NAD)-dependent ADP ribosylation occurs on a cysteine residue, whereas cholera toxin–catalyzed ADP ribosylation occurs on an arginine residue. Several species of $G_s\alpha$ and $G_i\alpha$ have been described. For $G_{i\alpha}$, three distinct proteins have been identified, which are about 90% identical, are localized in specific tissues, and are referred to as $G_{i\alpha 1}$, $G_{i\alpha 2}$, and $G_{i\alpha 3}$ (Carlson et al., 1989).

Although bacterial toxins are clearly useful probes by which to examine the contribution of G proteins to subsequent cellular functions, the utility of bacterial toxins in the exploration of G protein involvement in stimulus/coupling responses is limited by the observation that many G proteins described to date are unaffected by these toxins. Therefore, another method by which to assess the functional consequences of G protein activation is to add the G protein activator GTP (or its nonhydrolyzable form GTPγS) to permeabilized cells or to plasma membrane preparations. Permeabilization is required, as guanine nucleotides do not readily cross intact cell membranes (Cockcroft and Gomperts, 1985). The G protein inhibitor GDPβS can similarly be introduced into cells or utilized in membranes to inhibit agonist-induced G protein–coupled responses. Finally, another extremely useful approach which assesses G protein participation involves exposure of cells to fluoride ion (fluoroaluminates), a nonspecific G protein activator (Allende, 1988). Fluoride is particularly useful in intact cells, as the fluoride ion readily crosses the plasma membrane to bind to GDP contained in the α subunit of the heterotrimeric G protein. Binding to GDP by fluoride in this fashion conveys upon GDP the physicochemical properties of GTP, thus initiating G protein dissociation (Bigay et al., 1985).

A. Bacterial Toxin Substrates in Endothelium

G proteins in human umbilical vein and bovine pulmonary artery endothelial cells have been characterized based on their ability to be ADP ribosylated by bacterial toxins, and the membrane proteins from these cells appear to have similar [^{32}P]ADP ribosylation profiles. Shown in Fig. 2 is the spectrum of substrates for bacterial toxin–mediated ADP ribosylation in bovine pulmonary artery endothelium homogenates. In human (Garcia et al., 1990, 1991a, 1992a), bovine (Voyno-Yasenetskaya et al., 1989a,b), and porcine endothelium (Lambert et al., 1986) pertussis toxin catalyzes the ADP ribosylation of a 40- to 41-kD membrane protein which is immunologically related to other $G_{i\alpha}$ subunits (Garcia et al., 1990), especially $G_{i\alpha 2}$ and $G_{i\alpha 3}$ (Voyno-Yasenetskaya et al., 1989b). In human and bovine endothelium, cholera toxin induced the ADP ribosylation of 39-, 45-, and 52-kD proteins which were confirmed immunologically to be $G_{s\alpha}$-related proteins and probably represents alternatively spliced $G_{s\alpha}$ proteins (Fig. 2). A family of low-molecular-weight G proteins have been described, with several possessing GTPase activity, and may be related to the ras family of GTP-binding proteins (Yamamoto et al., 1989). Although the role of small G proteins in endothelial cell signal transduction is incompletely understood, they have been reported to couple specific receptors, particularly growth factor receptors, to effectors such as phosphatidylinositol-specific PLC. The neurotoxin botulinum C catalyzes the ADP ribosylation of a substrate which is a small G protein containing high-affinity guanine nucleotide-binding sites. In contrast to pertussis and cholera, botulinum C catalyzed the ADP ribosylation in both bovine and human endothelium of a distinct 21-kD substrate (Fig. 2), although a doublet of

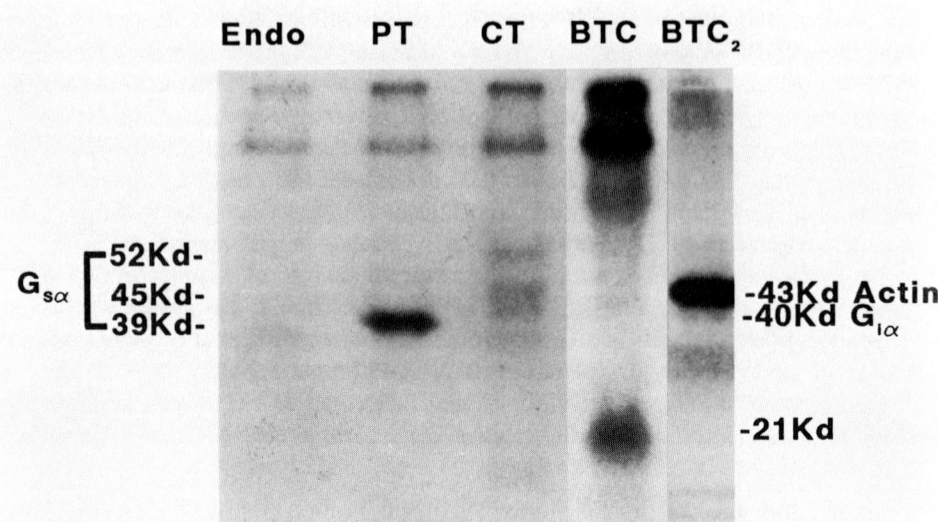

Figure 2 Bacterial toxin–catalyzed incorporation of [^{32}P]NAD into human endothelial cell homogenates. ADP ribosylation of human umbilical vein endothelial cell homogenates was carried out as described previously (Garcia et al., 1990, 1991a) by SDS-polyacrylamide electrophoresis and autoradiography. Lane 1 represents the autoradiogram of [^{32}P]NAD ADP ribosylation of control homogenates (without toxins), demonstrating minimal endogenous ribosylation. Lane 2 is the same as lane 1, with the exception of the addition of pertussis toxin (PT) (1 μg/mL) to the ADP-ribosylation media. There is marked pertussis toxin–catalyzed ADP ribosylation of a 40-kD protein ($G_{i\alpha}$), as we have described previously (Garcia et al., 1990). Lane 3 represents the cholera toxin (CT) (50 μg/mL)–catalyzed ADP ribosylation of 39-, 45-, 52-kD toxin substrates ($G_{s\alpha}$). In lane 4 the 21-kD botulinum C (BTC) substrate (5 μg/mL) is depicted. Lane 5 demonstrates botulinum C_{2a}-(BTC_2)-induced ADP ribosylation of endothelial cell actin.

24- to 26-kDa proteins have been described as a ADP-ribosylation substrate for the C_3 component of botulinum toxin (Voyno-Yasenetskaya et al., 1989b). Incubation of human or bovine endothelial cell membranes with the botulinum D toxin was a very poor stimulus for ADP ribosylation, although this is reported to occur readily in other tissues (Ohashi and Narumiya, 1987). Finally, botulinum $C_{2\alpha}$ toxins catalyze the ADP ribosylation of actin in intact cells, in isolated β/γ actin in its monomeric G form, but not in polymerized F actin, thereby reducing the ability of actin to polymerize (Aktories et al., 1986). Figure 2 shows botulinum $C_{2\alpha}$ to catalyze readily the ADP ribosylation of actin in bovine pulmonary artery endothelial cell homogenates.

III. Regulation of Phospholipase C Activity and Ca^{2+} Mobilization

An impressive number of cellular responses are linked to increases in the intracellular calcium [Ca_i^{2+}], and therefore the regulation of cytosolic Ca_i^{2+} is of fundamental importance to the transduction of cell activation. Although the relationship between Ca^{2+} mobilization and phosphoinositide metabolism was first noted in the 1950s (Hokin and Hokin, 1953), the molecular basis of this link has only recently been appreciated and an array of cellular responses have now been determined to be initiated by receptor-mediated activation of a phosphoinositol-specific phospholipase C (PI-PLC). The activation of PI-PLC catalyzes the hydrolysis of phosphatidylinositol 4,5-bisphosphate (PIP_2), resulting in the generation of the short-lived but critical second messengers inositol 1,4,5-trisphosphate (IP_3) and diacylglycerol (DAG). Whereas DAG acts by stimulating protein kinase C (PKC), IP_3 is generally accepted as directly regulating [Ca_i^{2+}] by mobilizing the release of Ca^{2+} from internal stores and indirectly by stimulating Ca^{2+} entry, possibly in concert with its phosphorylated metabolite inositol tetrakisphosphate (IP_4) (Berridge and Irvine, 1984). The final consequence of PI-PLC activation is an increase in [Ca_i^{2+}] from 80 to 120 n*M* to 500 to 1000 n*M*. These reactions form the foundation of a widespread stimulus–response transduction mechanism which is now recognized as regulating diverse cellular processes, such as metabolism, secretion, contraction, and proliferation.

Multiple isoenzyme forms of membrane-associated and cytosolic PI-PLC have been described which exhibit specificity for the polar head group hydrolyzed. Mammalian PI-PLC will hydrolyze all three phosphoinositides: PI, PIP, and PIP_2. The pH optima for PI-PLC activity falls into two ranges, 5.0 to 5.5 and 6.5 to 7.0 (Crooke and Bennett, 1989). With PIP_2 as the substrate, the ideal [Ca^{2+}] for PLC activity ranges from 10 to 100 μ*M*, whereas with PI as the substrate, the ideal [Ca^{2+}] is 1 to 2 m*M*. Multiple forms of PLC have been purified from a variety of tissues and the amino acid sequence has been determined for PLC of molecular sizes of 56, 86, 138, and 148 kD. Three broad molecular weight classes for the PI-PLC isoenzymes exist: 60 to 70, 85 to 88, and 143 to 154 kD (Crooke and Bennett, 1989). The functions of the isoenzymes are unclear, as are the extent that they are coupled to specific receptors.

There is abundant evidence that a G protein (G_p—GTP-binding protein coupled to phosphoinositol-specific phospholipase C) plays an essential transducing role in the coupling of receptors for Ca^{2+}-mobilizing hormones to PI-specific PLC in various cell types (Cockroft and Gomperts, 1985; Gilman, 1987). There are now several reports of partial purification and cloning of G_p, which regulates PI-PLC (Taylor et al., 1990a; Shaw and Exton, 1991). G_p in some tissues may be similar or identical to G_i, as investigators have implicated G_i in the modulation of PI-PLC in those cases where pertussis toxin inhibits the agonist-induced stimulation of PI-PLC (Carlson et al., 1989). G_z has also been postulated as a mediator for activation of PI-PLC through a pertussis toxin–insensitive pathway (Carlson et al., 1989), and a recent publication indicates that G_o is involved directly in the regulation of PI-PLC (Moriarty et al., 1990). Recently, in a cell-free membrane system, ras proteins were determined to stimulate PI-PLC activity (Cockcroft and Bar-Saci, 1990).

A. PI-PLC and Ca^{2+} Mobilization in Endothelium

Elevation in cytosolic free Ca^{2+} is a feature of endothelial cell activation following stimulation with many agonists, including ATP (Luckoff and Busse, 1986; Hallam and Pearson, 1986; Pirotton et al., 1987a; Forsberg et al., 1987), bradykinin (Lambert et al., 1986), histamine (Rotrosen and Gallin, 1986; Lo and Fan, 1987; Resink et al., 1987; Halldorsson et al., 1988; Pollock et al., 1988), and thrombin (Jaffe et al., 1987; Brock and Capasso, 1988; Halldorsson et al., 1988; Pollock et al., 1988), and is linked to PLC-mediated PIP_2 hydrolysis. It is unlikely that these agonists activate voltage-operated Ca^{2+} channels since these channels do not appear to be present in endothelial cells (Colden-Stanfield et al., 1987; Jacob, 1990). Ca_i^{2+} increases occur in temporal fashion following PLC-mediated IP_3 generation, and IP_3 appears to be responsible for the mobilization of intracellular Ca^{2+}. In addition, neither Ca^{2+} channel blockers nor Ca_E^{2+} (extracellular calcium) chelation abolishes the bradykinin-mediated phosphoinositide and Ca^{2+}-mobilizing response (Lambert et al., 1986). Receptor occupancy is required for PLC activation, as Ca^{2+} ionophores such as A23187 do not induce IP_3 formation in bovine (Lambert et al., 1986) or in human endothelium (Halldorsson et al., 1988; Derian and Moskowitz, 1986), although the effect of A23187 in other endothelial cells, such as porcine (Moscat et al., 1987b), may be very different. The species-receptor dynamics are important for determining the level of agonist-stimulated, PI-PLC-mediated PIP_2 hydrolysis. For example, bradykinin is a potent stimulus for IP_3 formation in bovine pulmonary artery (Voyno-Yasenetskaya et al., 1989a), aortic (Bartha et al., 1989), and cerebral microvascular endothelium, as well as in porcine aortic endothelium (Lambert et al., 1986) but is only marginally effective, if at all, in human umbilical vein endothelium (Bartha et al., 1989).

B. Protein Regulation of Endothelial Cell PI-PLC

Several lines of evidence indicate that GTP-binding proteins (G proteins) in endothelial cell membranes are involved in the activation of PI-PLC and Ca^{2+} mobilization by receptor-mediated agonists such as histamine (Brock et al.,

1988; Carson et al., 1989; Voyno-Yasenetskaya et al., 1989b), bradykinin (Lambert et al., 1986; Voyno-Yasenetskaya et al., 1989a), and thrombin (Garcia et al., 1990, 1991a, 1992a,b,c). Phosphoinositide (PI) turnover during histamine or bradykinin treatment in permeabilized endothelial cells is potentiated by GTPγS, an activator of G protein and agonist-induced IP_3 formation depressed by GDPβS, an inhibitor of G protein (Voyno-Yasenetskaya et al., 1989a,b). The addition of the nonhydrolyzable analog GTPγS, a recognized G protein activator, to permeabilized human endothelium (Brock et al., 1988) or to radiolabeled HUVEC membranes (Fig. 3) produces an increase in the level of inositol phosphates consistent with G protein regulation of PI-PLC (Garcia et al., 1991a). Additional evidence of PI-PLC regulation by G proteins is derived from studies

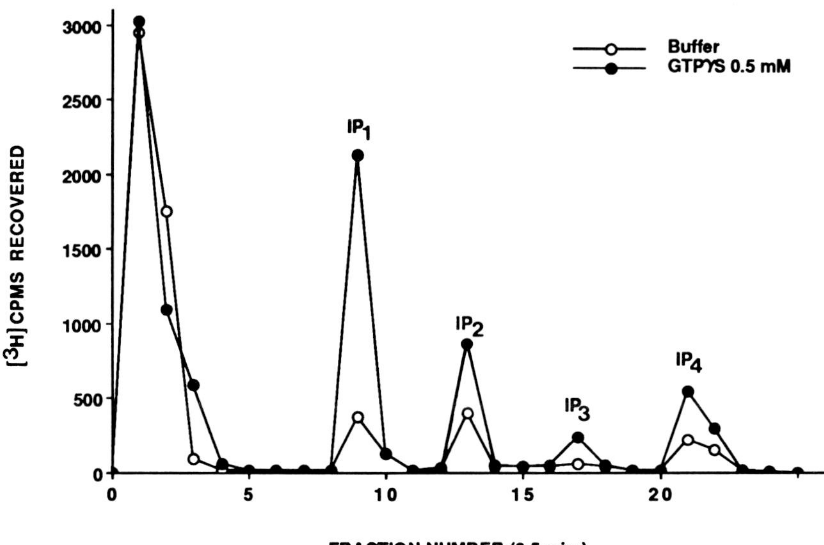

Figure 3 HPLC analysis of [^{3}H]-labeled water-soluble material from GTPγS- stimulated HUVEC microsomal membranes. HUVEC monolayers were treated with [^{3}H]2-myoinositol (10 μCi/mL). Scraped and microsomal membranes were prepared as described previously (Garcia et al., 1991a). Shown is a representative chromatogram of [^{3}H]-2-myoinositol recovered as water-soluble inositol phosphates in cpm by high-pressure liquid chromatography in radiolabeled HUVEC microsomal membranes. Equal aliquots of membranes were challenged for 10 min with either buffer (open circles) or GTPγS (0.5 m*M*) (closed circles). The water-soluble cellular extracts were subjected to HPLC on 0 to 100% gradient of 0.5 *M* NaH_2PO_4, pH, 2.7 with 99% formate, as described previously (Taylor et al., 1990b). The elution of internal standards of IP_1, IP_2, IP_3 (1,4,5-inositol trisphosphate), and IP_4 (1,3,4, 5-tetrakisinositol phosphate) are indicated. Fractions were collected every 0.5 min. (From Garcia et al., 1991a.)

using the G protein activator sodium fluoride (NaF) or fluoroaluminates (AlF_4^-) in intact cells. Fluoride stimulates rapid PIP_2 hydrolysis (Garcia et al., 1991a) in association with the appearance of the PIP_2 hydrolysis products DAG and IP_3, as well as an increase in cytosolic Ca^{2+} (Fig. 4). Fluoride-stimulated PI-PLC activity, DAG production, and Ca_i^{2+} mobilization is independent of Ca_E^{2+} availability (Garcia et al., 1991a).

G proteins involved in receptor-dependent regulation of PI-PLC can often be distinguished by their different sensitivities to bacterial toxins. In neutrophils, macrophages, and foam cells, hormone-dependent stimulation of PI-PLC occurs through a pertussis-sensitive G protein (Gilman, 1987), whereas in hepatocytes and 3T3 fibroblasts, the G protein responsible for coupling is insensitive to pertussis toxin (Murayama and Ui, 1985; Gilman, 1987). In bovine endothelial cells, pertussis toxin inhibits ATP-induced inositol phosphate generation and Ca^{2+} mobilization (Pirotton et al., 1987b; Kitazono, et al., 1989) and histamine-dependent activation of PI turnover in human cells (Voyno-Yasenetskaya et al., 1989b). In contrast, bradykinin-dependent PI-PLC activation in human, porcine, and bovine endothelium was insensitive to pertussis toxin (Voyno-Yasenetskaya et al, 1989b; Lambert et al., 1986). In one report, botulinum toxin C (C_2 and C_3

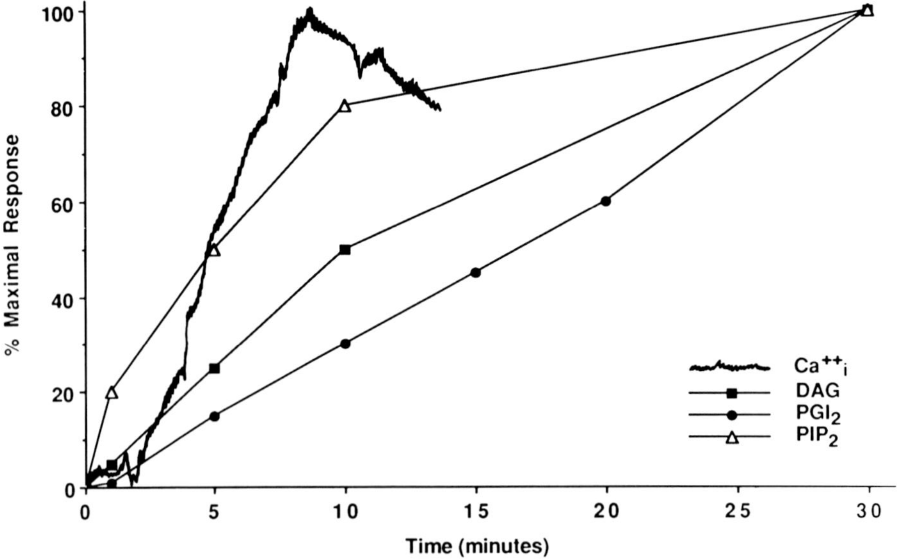

Figure 4 Temporal relationship between the various NaF-mediated endothelial cell signaling pathways. Depicted is the kinetics and sequential nature of NaF-mediated PIP_2 hydrolysis, DAG formation, and Ca^{2+} mobilization (shown as the percent of the maximal response). (Reprinted with permission from Garcia, 1991a.)

components) blocked bradykinin-dependent PI turnover but did not affect the histamine-stimulated PI turnover in human endothelium (Voyno-Yasenetskaya et al., 1989b). These studies suggest that in bovine and human endothelium, ATP, histamine, and bradykinin receptors activate PI turnover via distinct G proteins. Differences between the time courses of agonist-dependent accumulation of inositol phosphates may also point to differences in either the extent of coupling of ATP, histamine, and bradykinin receptors to PI-PLC, to different mechanisms of coupling between these receptors and PI-PLC or to receptor coupling to distinct PI-PLC isoenzymes. The inhibition of the bradykinin-dependent stimulation of PI turnover by botulinum C toxin may depend on ADP ribosylation of low-molecular-mass G proteins as well as actin depolymerization if bradykinin-stimulated PLC is associated with actin filaments, as is suggested in specific agonist-induced platelet responses (Siess et al., 1982).

IV. Protein Kinase C and Signal Transduction

A second messenger system that has received a great deal of attention is that which activates protein kinase C (PKC), a Ca^{2+}-phospholipid-dependent kinase. Protein kinase C is activated by the PI-PLC-mediated production of the intracellular second messenger, diacylglycerol (DAG), and the prior activation of PKC in intact cells results in profound alterations of receptor-mediated responses, thereby implicating PKC activation as an important participant in transmembrane signal transduction (Nishizuka, 1986). Binding of the regulatory domain of PKC by DAG lowers the PKC requirements for Ca^{2+}, thus increasing PKC enzymatic activity and promoting translocation of the enzyme from the cytosol to the plasma membrane (Nishizuka, 1986). Although PKC is capable of phosphorylating a variety of cellular substrates in vitro (Nishizuka, 1986), the exact identification of the physiologically relevant substrates for PKC has not been completely accomplished, nor is it clear how protein phosphorylation is linked to the mechanism of cell activation.

Phorbol esters like phorbol myristate acetate (PMA), are DAG analogs that activate PKC, and were first shown to block IP formation in brain slices. Several reports have subsequently described inhibitory effects of PKC activators on receptor-mediated responses in many tissues. In platelets, for example, PKC inhibits agonist-induced phosphoinositide turnover (Krishnamurthi et al., 1989), increases in Ca_i^{2+}, arachidonate (AA) mobilization, and granule secretion (Akiba et al., 1989), implicating PKC in the termination of platelet signal transduction. Similar to the G protein–coupled regulation of cellular stimulus–responses, PKC appears to be a key modulator of endothelial cell signal transduction pathways. PKC activity has been identified in cultured endothelial cells, and profound regulatory effects of PKC on cAMP production (Newman et al., 1989), serotonin transport (Myers et al., 1989), and the Na^+/H^+ exchanger have been reported (Kitazono et al., 1989).

A. PKC Activation in Cultured Endothelium

The duration of exposure to PKC activators dictates subsequent PKC alteration of signal transduction pathways involved in specific phospholipase activities in human endothelium (Halldorsson et al., 1988). The PKC activator PMA was used to accomplish PKC activation. Dose- and time-dependent PKC activation and translocation was induced by PMA in human endothelium (Fig. 5A and B) (Garcia et al., 1992c), with similar results observed in bovine pulmonary artery endothelium (Stasek et al., 1992a,b). PMA produced a dose-dependent stimulation of PKC translocation from the cytosol to the membrane compartment (Fig.

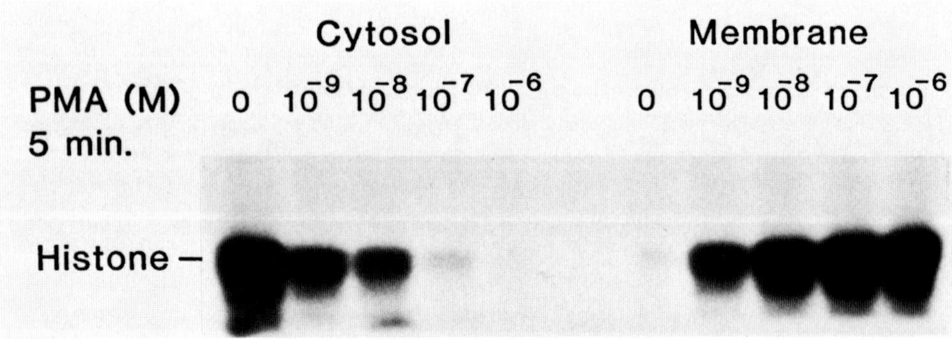

A

Figure 5 PMA-induced protein kinase C (PKC) activation and translocation from cytosolic to membrane compartments. (A) Confluent HUVEC monolayers were treated with varying concentrations of PMA for 5 min and the cytosolic and membrane fractions assayed for PKC activity by phosphorylation of histone-1 detected by SDS-PAGE and autoradiography as described previously (Garcia et al., 1992c,d). PMA-induced PKC activity and translocation was dose dependent with near-maximal PKC activity observed with 100 n*M* PMA. (B) In experiments similar to (A), buffer or 100 n*M* PMA were added to the HUVEC monolayers and at specified times the cytosolic and membrane fractions retrieved and PKC activity determined. PMA-induced PKC translocation of activity was rapid and nearly complete by 5 min. (C) PKC translocation from the cytosol to the membrane induced by α-thrombin and NaF. Confluent HUVEC monolayers were treated with buffer, 10 n*M* α-thrombin, or 20 m*M* NaF for specified intervals and cytosolic or membrane PKC-containing fractions used to phosphorylate fractions used to phosphorylate histone 1. Both α-thrombin and NaF induce rapid PKC translocation. (Panel (C) reprinted with permission from Stasek and Garcia, 1992b.)

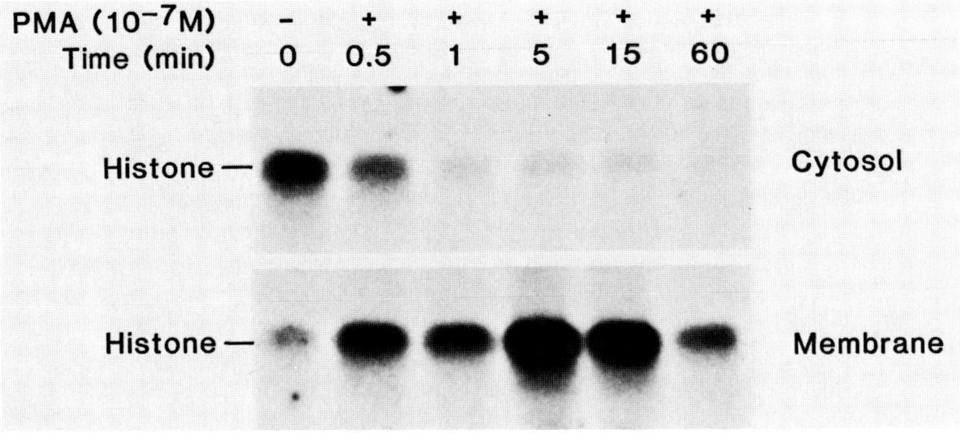

B

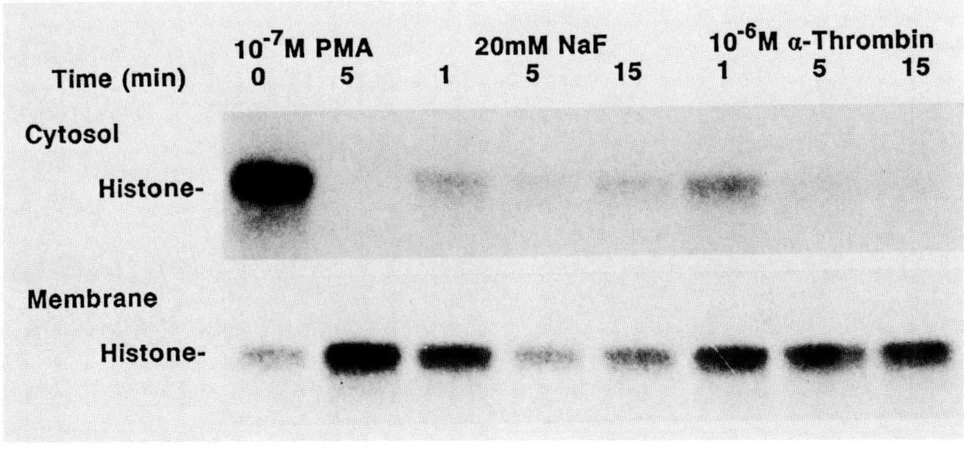

C

5A) which correlated with specific H1 histone phosphorylation activity. Activation was rapid, beginning at 30 s, and was essentially maximal by 5 min (Fig. 5B). As mentioned above, a number of mediators, such as bradykinin, ATP, and histamine, induce the formation of DAG, at least in part via the activation of a PI-specific PLC. The physiologic relevance of PKC activation was demonstrated by experiments which showed that receptor-mediated endothelial cell activation with α-thrombin, or direct G protein activation with sodium fluoride (NaF), like PMA, induces rapid PKC translocation (Fig. 5C) (Garcia et al., 1992c, Stasek and Garcia, 1992b.)

B. PKC Regulation of PLC Activation and Ca^{2+} Mobilization

PMA pretreatment inhibits subsequent bradykinin-, histamine-, and ATP-stimulated mobilization of Ca_i^{2+} (Halldorsson et al., 1988; Magnusson et al., 1989; Brock and Capasso, 1988). Whereas PMA alone produces less than a 1% change in [Ca_i^{2+}] over 30 min, brief (5 min) PMA (100 n*M*) pretreatment markedly attenuated α-thrombin-induced increases in aequorin luminescence and produced significant (≈ 50%) inhibition of the 20 m*M* NaF-mediated Ca^{2+} mobilizing response (Fig. 6), while aequorin luminescence evoked by Ca^{2+} ionophore A23187 was essentially unaltered (Garcia et al., 1991a, 1992c). It is now well accepted that one mechanism by which PKC inhibits agonist-induced Ca^{2+} mobilization is via downregulation of PI-PLC activities. Phorbol-mediated PKC activation produces inhibition of agonist-induced or NaF-mediated endothelial cell inositol phosphate formation (Brock and Capasso, 1988; Halldorsson et al., 1988; Carter et al., 1989a; Garcia et al. 1992c), suggesting that PKC inhibitory effects occur at a site that is distal to the occupied receptor. Whether PKC di-

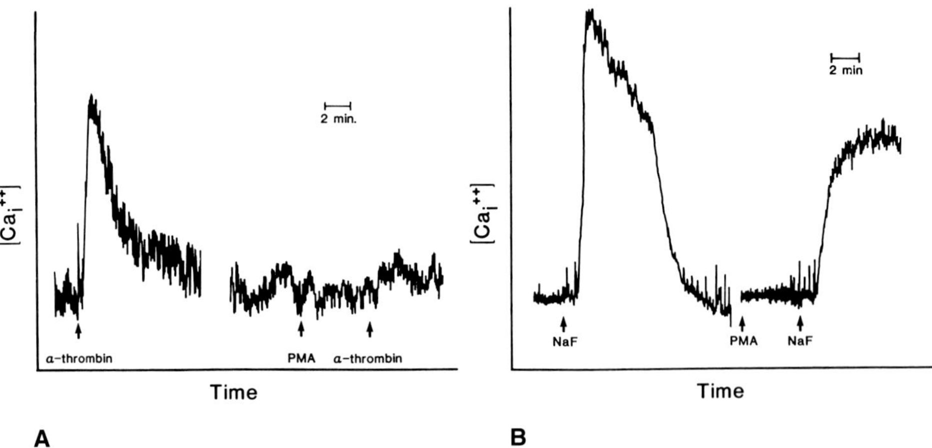

Figure 6 Effect of PKC activity on α-thrombin- and NaF-stimulated aequorin luminescence in human endothelium. Human endothelial cells loaded with aequorin were embedded in agarose threads as we have described (Garcia et al., 1991a). (A) Representative changes in aequorin luminescence by 10 n*M* α-thrombin in the presence of 1.2 m*M* Ca^{2+} with or without 5 min pretreatment with 100 n*M* PMA; (B) 20 m*M* NaF-induced aequorin luminescence determined in the presence of 1.2 m*M* Ca^{2+} with or without prior 100 n*M* PMA pretreatment (5 min). (Reprinted with permission from Garcia et al., 1992c.)

rectly modulates PLC enzymatic activity or exerts its regulatory effect on $[Ca_i^{2+}]$ via inhibition of G_p, the putative GTP-binding protein coupled to PLC, has been unclear. PMA, as well as exogenously purified PKC, inhibits guanine nucleotide–induced PLC activation in astrocytoma membranes (Orellana et al., 1987), in platelets (Zavoico et al., 1985), in fluoride-stimulated hepatocytes (Blackmore and Exton, 1986), and in GTPγS-stimulated permeabilized fibroblasts (Muldoon et al., 1987). A second potential site of PKC modulation of G_p includes PKC potentiation of GTPase activity (Krishnamurthi et al., 1989). Protein kinase C is known to interact with GTP-binding proteins in cellular membranes, and to suppress the inhibitory effects of G_i on adenylate cyclase activity, possibly by phosphorylation of the $G_i\alpha$ subunit (Katada et al., 1985; Crouch and Lapetina, 1988a). In addition to PLC inhibition, PKC probably alters intracellular Ca^{2+} concentrations via effects at sites that are distal to PLC activity as well. PKC activates a 5′-monoesterase specific for IP_3 degradation (Connolly et al., 1986), and staurosporine, a PKC inhibitor, increases IP_3 and IP_4 levels in human platelets (King and Rittenhouse, 1989) and human endothelium (Garcia et al., 1992c), suggesting PKC regulation of IP_3 degradative pathways. A potential effect of PKC on IP_3-specific phosphatase activity in endothelium has not been addressed specifically. PKC may also produce alterations in $[Ca_i^{2+}]$ via PKC-modulated activation of Ca^{2+} extrusion pathways as described in several cell types (Shearman et al., 1989). Although human endothelial cells are perceived as lacking voltage-operated Ca^{2+} channels (Colden-Stanfield et al., 1987; Jacob, 1990), PMA has been noted to alter a PKC-sensitive Na^+–Ca^{2+} exchanger, leading to enhanced Ca^{2+} extrusion (Shearman et al., 1989; Dominguez et al., 1989). In human endothelium, alterations in $[Na^+]_E$, however, failed to produce significant changes in aequorin luminescence, regardless of Ca^{2+} availability, (<5 n*M* change in $[Ca_i^{2+}]$), suggesting that human endothelium does not possess a functional Na^+–Ca^{2+} exchanger (Garcia et al., 1992c). Although PKC promotes Ca^{2+} extrusion from the cytosolic compartment in several cell types (Shearman et al., 1989), the absence of both voltage-operated Ca^{2+} channels (Jacob, 1990) and a functional Na^+–Ca^{2+} exchanger in human endothelium (Garcia et al., 1992c) argue against PKC-mediated alterations of Ca^{2+} influx as an important contributor to PKC's inhibitory action on $[Ca_i^{2+}]$ increases after agonist stimulation. As PMA alone did not alter basal aequorin luminescence, PKC alteration of Ca^{2+} extrusion mechanisms is unlikely to contribute significantly to the PMA-mediated attenuation of agonist-induced $[Ca_i^{2+}]$ increases, and PKC downregulation of PLC activity represents the major mechanism by which brief PMA pretreatment inhibits agonist-stimulated Ca_i^{2+} increases (Halldorsson et al., 1988; Brock and Capasso, 1988; Carter et al., 1989a).

V. Phospholipase A2 (PLA2) and Signal Transduction

PLA_2s are a family of enzymes that catalyze the release of sn-2 fatty acids from membrane phospholipids and are widespread throughout eukaryotic cells. PLA_2s exist in both membrane-associated and soluble forms, are generally of low molecular weight (12 to 15 kD), and are extremely stable to heat and acid treatment—important attributes for an enzyme that is involved in phospholipid degradation.

A. PLA_2 Activity in Endothelium

Although Ca^{2+}-independent PLA_2s exist (Martin and Wysolmerski, 1987), most PLA_2 enzymes require Ca^{2+} ions for full activity (Van Den Bosch, 1980), and in the presence of elevated cytosolic Ca^{2+}, PLA_2 is activated to split phospholipids into lysophospholipid and fatty acid (Fig. 1). Phosphatidylcholine represents the major substrate for the PLA_2 activity that leads to prostanoid production; however, other phospholipids may also be substrates for arachidonate (AA)-releasing PLA_2 activity. The existence of two pathways for AA release from phosphatidylinositol has been reported in endothelial cells: a phospholipase A_1–lysophospholipase pathway that is Ca^{2+} independent and a phospholipase C–diacylglycerol lipase pathway that is Ca^{2+} dependent (Martin and Wysolmerski, 1987).

Arachidonate liberated by PLA_2 is available for subsequent metabolism to a variety of bioactive products. The primary arachidonate metabolite produced by cultured human endothelial cells is PGI_2 (Weksler et al., 1978), with additional prostaglandins such as PGD_2, PGE_2, $PGF_{2\alpha}$, thromboxane, and dihydroperoxyacids such as 5- and 15-HETES produced in smaller quantities (Hong, 1980; Johnson et al., 1985; Goldsmith and Needleman, 1982). The liberated arachidonate is sequentially converted to PGG_2 and PGH_2 by the cyclooxygenase enzyme and PGH_2 is subsequently metabolized to PGI_2 (prostacyclin) by prostacyclin synthetase (Marcus, 1978). PGI_2 is a potent vasodilator and inhibitor of platelet aggregation and a principal participant in maintaining vascular tone and vessel patency. Marked disruption of endothelial cell prostaglandin synthesis is observed in arteriosclerotic or diabetic vessels, implicating a pathogenetic role for PGI_2 synthesis in vascular disease (Weksler, 1984).

B. PLC and Ca^{2+} Regulation of PLA_2 in Endothelium

Although PLA_2 activity is the rate-limiting step in the agonist-stimulated synthesis of prostanoids in endothelium, the regulation of PLA_2 in endothelium is incompletely understood. Based on a very close temporal relationship between receptor occupancy, PI-PLC activity, IP_3 production, [Ca_i^{2+}] increases, PLA_2 activity, and PGI_2 synthesis, the tight linking of [Ca_i^{2+}] to PLA_2 activity as the major determining factor in the PGI_2 production after receptor activation has been proposed (Hong and Deykin, 1982; Hong et al., 1985; Forsberg et al., 1987; Jaffe et al., 1987; Halldorsson et al., 1988; Pollock et al., 1988; Hallam et al., 1988; Garcia et al., 1991a). Although it has been widely accepted that Ca^{2+} mobilization—a consequence of PI-PLC activation—is a prerequisite for the activation of PLA_2 in cultured endothelium, there are indications that PLA_2 is not under the control of the prevailing Ca^{2+} level in intact cells other than endothelium (Crouch and Lapetina, 1988b). In the platelet, for example, the ability of α-thrombin to induce the release of Ca^{2+} stores does not parallel the liberation of arachidonic acid (Crouch and Lapetina, 1988b), suggesting that PI-PLC activation and PLA_2 activation are separate events in platelet activation. Apparent dissociation of receptor-mediated activation of PLC and Ca^{2+} mobilization from PLA_2 activities has been noted in several cell lines (Burch et al., 1986; Crouch and Lapetina, 1988b; Pollock et al., 1986). Nevertheless, the sequential nature of PLC-PLA_2 activation after agonist challenge in endothelium has been generally accepted, with [Ca_i^{2+}] increases both a necessary and a sufficient signal for endothelial cell PGI2 synthesis (Hallam et al., 1988). When Ca_i^{2+} chelators such as TMB-8 or BAPTA [1,2-bis(2-aminophenoxy)ethane-*N*, *N*, *N′N′*-tetraacetic acid] are utilized to attenuate [Ca_i^{2+}] agonist-induced PGI_2 synthesis is markedly inhibited (Jaffe et al., 1987; Garcia et al., 1992c).

C. PKC Regulation of PLA_2 in Endothelium

The contribution of PKC to endothelial cell PLA_2 pathways has been investigated (Halldorsson et al., 1988; Carter et al., 1989a). Treatment with phorbol esters or synthetic DAG prior to cellular stimulation produced complex effects on endothelial cell PGI_2 synthesis which were dependent on [Ca_E^{2+}], agonist concentration, and both the dose and duration of phorbol ester pretreatment. In general, however, PKC activation dramatically potentiates the level of PGI_2 formed after agonist stimulation (Demolle and Boeynaems, 1988; Halldorsson et al., 1988; Jeremy and Dandona, 1988; Carter et al., 1989a). PMA alone is known to induce PGI_2 synthesis after prolonged exposure (Demolle and Boeynaems, 1988). However, maximum concentrations of PMA (1 μ*M*) failed to induce an increase in PGI_2 synthesis when analyzed for up to 60 min in the absence of additional cell stimulation (Garcia et al., 1992c). Protein kinase C activity is a critical regulator of PLA_2 activity, as the requirement for increases in [Ca_i^{2+}]) can be partially bypassed by prior activation of PKC (Garcia et al., 1992c). This proposed important regulatory role of PKC in PLA_2 activity is based on the demonstration that (1) although agonist and NaF-mediated rises in [Ca_i^{2+}]) are significantly reduced by PMA pretreatment, AA release and PGI_2 synthesis are augmented by prior PKC activation; (2) whereas Ca_i^{2+} chelation with agents such as BAPTA inhibits agonist-stimulated AA-releasing activity, PMA-mediated PKC translocation is not inhibited; (3) PMA pretreatment potentiates PGI_2 synthesis even in the presence of BAPTA inhibition of $[Ca_i^{2+}]$; and (4) agonist stimulation of PLA_2 activity and PGI_2 synthesis is dramatically sensitive to PKC inhibition with either staurosporine or PKC downregulation with chronic PMA exposure (Zavoico et al., 1990; Garcia et al., 1992c). This sensitivity occurs despite an upregulatory effect of staurosporine or PKC downregulation on inositol phosphate levels after agonist stimulation (Demolle and Boeynaems, 1988; Halldorsson et al., 1988; Carter et al., 1989; Magnusson et al., 1989; Zavoica et al., 1990; Garcia et al., 1992c).

Although the exact site of PKC effects in endothelial cell desensitization involving PGI_2 synthesis is unidentified, PKC has been implicated via mechanisms that include receptor phosphorylation, receptor inactivation, phosphorylation of G proteins, and/or activation of inositol phosphate kinase systems (Connolly et al., 1986; King and Rittenhouse, 1989). Although there are indirect data which suggest that PKC may augment PLA_2 activity by lowering its requirement for cytosolic Ca^{2+} (Garcia et al., 1992c), PKC may also enhance PLA_2 activity via a reduction in the activity of antiphospholipase A_2 proteins, known collectively as lipocortins (Hirata et al., 1981), or by activation of the Na^+/H^+ antiporter (Kitazono et al., 1989), as most non-liposomal PLA_2s are maximally active at an alkaline pH. PKC may also directly modulate a G protein that couples receptors directly to phospholipase A_2, as described in other tissues (Okano et al., 1987; Kajiyama et al., 1989), in a manner that is independent of PLC, inositol phosphate generation, and thus of intracellular Ca^{2+} release. Both GTPγS (Garcia et al., 1990) and NaF (Garcia et al., 1991a) increase AA release and PGI_2 synthesis in human endothelium consistent with G protein regulation of PLA_2 (Fig. 7). However, whether this effect is due to an interaction with G_{PLA2} or G_{PLC} is unclear. As porcine, bovine, and human endothelial PLC, PLA_2, and PGI_2 activities stimulated by receptor-mediated agonists are variably inhibited by pertussis toxin, the existence of a distinct PKC-modulated G protein linked to PLA_2 (G_{PLA2}) remains speculative. Even if G_{PLA2} does exist, PKC-mediated activation of G_{PLA2} would appear an unlikely mechanism of PKC upregulation of PGI_2 synthesis in human endothelium, as either PKC inhibition with staurosporine or downregulation of PKC activity with chronic PMA treatment (Fig. 8) attenuated the AA release and PGI_2 synthesis induced by Ca^{2+} ionophore A23187, as well as NaF and α-thrombin, suggesting a non-G-protein-mediated mechanism of PKC modulation of PLA_2 (Garcia et al., 1992b,c). A final mechanism of PKC regulation of PGI_2 synthesis may occur by alteration of lysophosphatidylcholine

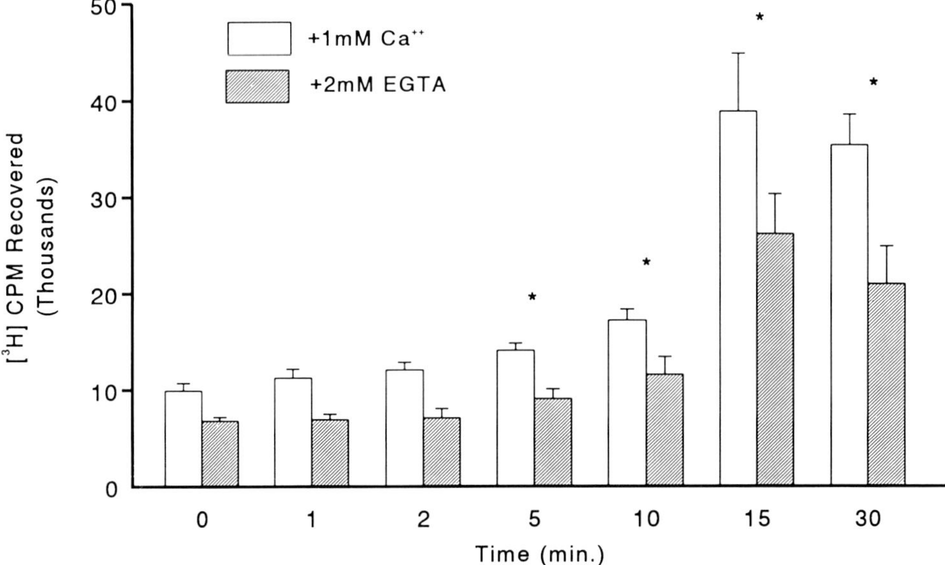

Figure 7 Extracellular release of [^{3}H]arachidonate and metabolites by sodium fluoride. HUVEC monolayers were labeled with [^{3}H]arachidonate 1 μCi/mL for 24 h and the labeled medium removed and the monolayers washed twice and replaced with buffer containing either 20 m*M* NaCl or 20 m*M* NaF. Cells were stimulated with NaCl or NaF in the presence of either 2 m*M* $CaCl_2$ or 2 m*M* EGTA. Results represent cpm of [^{3}H]arachidonate or [^{3}H]arachidonate metabolites recovered in the cell supernatants by bovine serum albumin trapping at the specified times. Shown is a representative experiment performed in triplicate at each time point ($n = 5$), $\bar{x} \pm SD$, $*p < 0.05$ versus NaCl control. All the cpm values derived from NaCl-stimulated monolayers were within 20% of the 0-min value.

acyltransferase activity, resulting in increased AA availability for PGI_2 synthesis (Kanzaki et al., 1989).

VI. Phospholipase D and Signal Transduction

Although the widely accepted and established pathway for generation of diacylglycerol (DAG) in endothelial cells is via receptor-mediated hydrolysis of PIP_2 by PI-PLC, production of DAG from phospholipids other than PIP_2 has received increased attention, as PLC-catalyzed breakdown of PIP_2 cannot account for all DAG accumulation (Billah and Anthes, 1990; Exton, 1990). Mounting evidence indicates that other important mechanisms for DAG generation

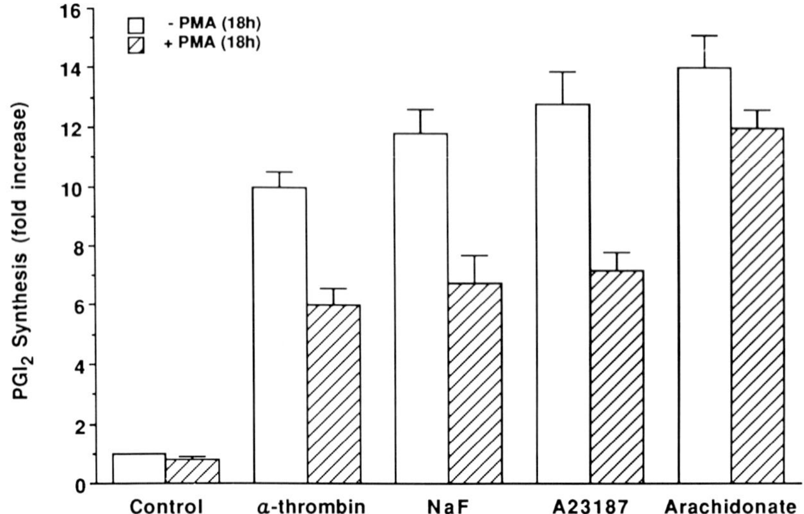

Figure 8 Effect of chronic PMA exposure on PKC activity and PGI_2 synthesis. HUVEC monolayers in T 75-cm_2 flasks or 24-well plates were treated with either buffer or PMA 100 n*M* for 18 h, which results in profound downregulation of PKC activity (Garcia et al., 1991d). PKC downregulation produced by chronic PMA exposure significantly attenuated PGI_2 synthesis produced by α-thrombin, NaF, and A23187 but not arachidonate.

must therefore exist and include (1) the hydrolysis of triacylglycerol catalyzed by lipase, (2) PLC-catalyzed breakdown of phospholipids, and/or (3) phospholipase D (PLD)-mediated generation of phosphatidic acid (PA) (Fig. 1) which is dephosphorylated by phosphatidic acid phosphatase (PAPase).

Phospholipase D hydrolyzes phospholipids, releasing PA and a water-soluble polar head group (e.g., choline, ethanolamine, inositol, serine, or glycerol) (Fig. 1; Heller, 1978). In addition to hydrolytic activity, the enzyme also exhibits transphosphatidylation activity in the presence of short-chain primary alcohols (Kobayashi and Kanfer, 1987). Phospholipase D activity was initially reported in plants, subsequently identified in bacteria and mammalian tissues, and later demonstrated in homogenates and membrane fractions from the liver (Bocckino et al., 1987), HL-60 cells (Kiss and Anderson, 1989; Anthes et al., 1989), spermatozoa (Domino et al., 1989), rat brain (Chalifa et al., 1990) rat sciatic nerve (Chattopadhyay et al., 1991), human neutrophils (Gelas et al., 1989), and endothelial cells and lung tissue (Martin, 1988). Partial purification of PLD has been achieved in particulate fractions from rat brain (Takai and Kanfer, 1979) and human eosinophils (Kater et al., 1976). While phosphatidylcholine (PC) is the preferred substrate for mammalian and nonmammalian PLD, other phospholipids, such as PI, phosphatidylethanolamine (PE), and *N*-acyl phosphatidylethanolamine (*N*-acyl PE), are also degraded under certain conditions. A membrane-bound PLD active toward *N*-acyl PE has been demonstrated on canine myocardium (Schmid et al., 1983) and in rat (Natarajan et al., 1986) and canine brain (Natarajan et al., 1984). There is also evidence for the presence of PI-specific PLD in human neutrophils (Balsinde et al., 1988) and a PLD that hydrolyzes the glycophosphatidylinositol anchor of cell surface proteins in plasma (Davitz et al., 1989; Huang et al., 1990).

A. PLD Activity in Endothelium

In endothelial cells there is compelling evidence for the activation of PLD in response to agonists, and this pathway probably represents an important mechanism for signal transduction (Garcia et al., 1992a). The presence of PLD activity in bovine endothelial cells was demonstrated in a 15,000*g* particulate fraction using exogenous 1-oleyl-2-[^{3}H]oleyl PC and phosphatidyl-[^{3}H] choline (Martin, 1988). The activity was optimal at pH 7.0 and was dependent on the presence of EDTA and Triton X-100. The endothelial cell–derived enzyme was active toward PC and did not hydrolyze PE, PI, or sphingomyelin. Human endothelial cell–free preparations exhibited PLD activity with exogenous 1-palmitoyl-2-[1-^{14}C]oleyl PC as substrates. Similar to bovine endothelial cell PLD preparations, human PLD hydrolysis of PC was stimulated by Triton X-100, whereas high [Ca^{2+}] were inhibitory (V. Natarajan and J. G. N. Garcia, unpublished observation).

Agonist-induced endothelial cell PLD activation has been studied using a variety of isotopes, such as radiolabeled orthophosphate, choline, fatty acid, and glycerol (Martin and Michaelis, 1988, 1989; Martin et al., 1989; Huang and Cabot, 1990; Natarajan and Garcia, 1992; Garcia et al., 1992a). Endothelial cells from bovine pulmonary artery (BPAE) (Table 1) and human umbilical vein (HUVEC) prelabeled with either [^{32}P]orthophosphate or [^{3}H]myristic acid exhibited sustained accumulation of [^{32}P] or [^{3}H]PEt (phosphatidylethanol) after stimulation with a number of agonists. The formation of labeled PEt is an unambiguous index of PLD activity and is dependent on addition of agonists and cell activation, as PEt does not accumulate in nonstimulated cells even in the presence of ethanol (Natarajan and Garcia, 1992). The formation of PEt was linear up to 0.75% of ethanol and up to 1 h of incubation without cytotoxic effects. The possibility of PEt formation by a base-exchange mechanism was excluded by demonstrating the formation of [^{32}P]phosphatidylglycerol in the presence of glycerol (Natarajan and Garcia, 1992).

While [^{32}P]orthophosphate labeling studies do not define the substrate for PLD-catalyzed PA and PEt formation, [^{3}H]myristic acid and [^{3}H]choline labeling

Table 1 Activation of Bovine Endothelial Cell Phospholipase D by Agonists[a]

Agonist	Concentration (μM)	[^{32}P]PEt (dpm/dish)	^{3}[H]PEt (dpm/dish)
None	—	36 ± 18	89 ± 16
Bradykinin	1	406 ± 26	638 ± 46
Histamine	100	198 ± 46	277 ± 39
Vasopressin	1	177 ± 22	256 ± 54
α-Thrombin	1	233 ± 39	332 ± 35
ATP	100	621 ± 27	785 ± 95

[a]BPAEC were prelabeled with [^{32}P]orthophosphate (30 μCi/dish) or [^{3}H]myristic acid (2 μCi/dish) for 24 h. Washed cells were stimulated with agonist for 5 min in the presence of 0.5% ethanol, lipids were extracted, and phosphatidylethanol was separated by TLC on silica gel using chloroform/methanol/NH_4OH (80:20:2 by OOH) on the solvent system. Autoradiography was performed and radioactivity was determined by liquid scintillation spectrometry. Labeling of lipids were as follows: For [^{32}P]orthophosphate, total incorporation/dish (8×10^5 cells) = 532,902 ± 2966 dpm and into phospholipids (% total)—choline phospholipids, 47.5; ethanolamine phospholipids, 26.3; serine phospholipids, 6.6; phosphatidylinositol, 5.8; sphingomyelin, 9.8; cardiolipin, 3.4; bis(monoacyl)glycerophosphate, 0.1; and nonpolar lipids, 16.1. Data represent mean ± SD of triplicate determinations from two independent experiments. Choline phospholipids contain 95% diacyl and 5% alkylacyl species, while ethanolamine phospholipids contain 70% alkenylacyl, 25% diacyl, and 5% alkylacyl species.

suggest that PC is the preferred substrate for PLD in intact endothelial cells (Martin and Michaelis, 1989). Phosphodiesteric cleavage of PC by PLD in agonist-stimulated endothelium is similar to PLD-catalyzed hydrolysis of PC in many other mammalian cells (Billah and Anthes, 1990). In BPAEC prelabeled with [^{14}C]myristic acid, ATP stimulated a rapid but transient increase in [^{14}C] PA followed by accumulation of [^{14}C]DAG. The formation of [^{14}C]PA and DAG were associated with a loss of label from PC but not from PI (Martin and Michaelis, 1989). Recent studies in BPAEC using [^{32}P]-labeled lyso PC and PC clearly demonstrated that both ATP and bradykinin stimulated formation of [^{32}P]PA and [^{32}P]PEt confirming the role of PC as a precursor for receptor-mediated PLD activation (V. Natarajan and J. G. N. Garcia, unpublished observation). The role of ethanolamine phosphoglycerides as a precursor for agonist- or TPA-induced PLD activity is yet to be clearly established for endothelial cells but has been reported in cell systems such as NIH 3T3 fibroblasts, BHK cells, HL-60 (Kiss and Anderson, 1989), and rat mesengial cells (Kester et al., 1989).

Although cellular regulation of receptor-linked activation of PLD has been investigated in detail in several cell types (Billah and Anthes, 1990; Exton, 1990) there is little known regarding PLD regulation in endothelial cells. Based on information from a variety of mammalian cells, PLD activation may involve several regulatory cellular components, including protein kinase C, G proteins, and Ca^{2+}/calmodulin. The mechanism(s) of activation of PLD seems to depend on the cell type studied, and endothelial cells offer an unique challenge in understanding the mechanism(s) of PLD activation.

B. Protein Kinase C Regulation of Endothelial Cell PLD Activity

In addition to agonist-induced PLD activation (Table 1), tumor-promoting phorbol esters and exogenous cell-permeant DAGs promote [^{32}P]PEt accumulation (Garcia et al., 1992a). In both bovine and human endothelium prelabeled with [^{32}P]orthophosphate or [^{3}H]myristic acid, 12-O-tetradecanoylphorbol-13-acetate (TPA) stimulated a five- to eightfold increase in PEt, which occurred in a time- and dose-dependent manner (Natarajan and Garcia, 1992; Garcia et al., 1992a). The possibility that the effect of TPA on PEt accumulation is through activation of PKC was investigated using (1) active and inactive phorbol derivatives, (2) cell-permeant DAGs that mimic TPA, (3) inhibitors of PKC, and (4) down-regulation of PKC by prolonged treatment with TPA. In contrast to TPA, 4-α-phorbol-12,13-didecanoate and 4-β-phorbol, which cannot activate PKC, failed to stimulate PLD activation, as evidenced by PEt accumulation (Fig. 9). Stimulation of PEt formation was mimicked by 1-oleoyl-2-acetylglycerol and 1,2-dioc-

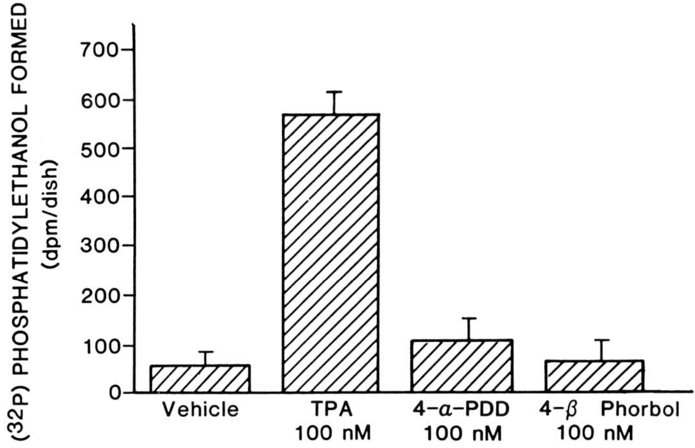

Figure 9 Effect of TPA and phorbol derivatives on [^{32}P]PEt formation. BPAEC were prelabeled with [^{32}P]orthophosphate (28 μCi/35 mm dish) for 18 h and challenged with TPA and other phorbol derivatives (dissolved in Me_2SO) and diluted in buffer containing $CaCl_2$ and 0.75% ethanol for 15 min. The concentration of Me_2SO in all incubations was 0.02%. Lipids were extracted under acidic conditions, the [^{32}P]PEt separated, and was quantified by TLC. Results are expressed as mean ± SD of triplicate determinations.

tanoyl-*sn*-glycerol. The effect of TPA on PEt accumulation was inhibited by PKC inhibitors staurosporine (10 μ*M*, 95% inhibition) and sphingosine (10 μ*M*, 50% inhibition) (Natarajan and Garcia, 1992). Phosphatidylethanol formation was also completely abolished by downregulation of PKC accomplished by long-term treatment (18 h) of BPAEC with 100 to 200 n*M* TPA (Garcia et al., 1992a). These results in bovine and human endothelium were the first to demonstrate that PEt biosynthesis catalyzed by PLD was dependent on the activation of endothelial cell PKC. Human umbilical vein endothelial cells exhibited a similar response to TPA and inhibitors of PKC on PEt formation (Garcia et al., 1992a).

All agonists that induce the accumulation of PEt via PLD activation also stimulate PLC-mediated breakdown of PIP_2, generating DAG and IP_3. Thus increases in PKC activation and Ca^{2+} levels due to the PLC-PIP_2 pathway may be a necessary step for agonist-induced PLD activation in endothelial cells. The relative contribution of PKC activation to endothelial cell PLD stimulation was addressed by using the PKC inhibitor staurosporine and downregulation of PKC by prolonged treatment with TPA (Natarajan and Garcia, 1990a,b, Garcia et al., 1992a). While TPA-induced PLD activation appears to be inhibited completely

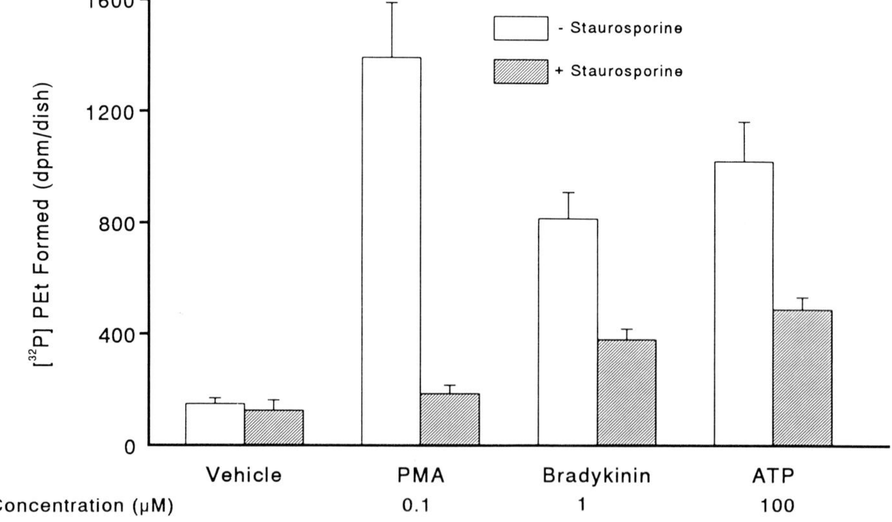

Figure 10 Effect of staurosporine on PLD activation. BPAEC were prelabeled with [32P]orthophosphate (28 mCi/dish) for 18 h, washed three times, and incubated with staurosporine (10 mM). After 15 min, the cells were washed again and stimulated with PMA, bradykinin, or ATP in the presence of 0.5% ethanol for 5 min. Lipids were extracted and [32P]phosphatidylethanol separated by TLC. Values are expressed as mean ± SEM of three independent experiments in triplicate.

by either staurosporine or PKC downregulation, ATP- or bradykinin-mediated PLD activation appears to be only partially inhibited (about 70% inhibition) (Fig. 10). This strongly suggests in BPAEC that (1) the majority of ATP- and bradykinin-mediated PLD activation occurs via receptor-mediated, PLC-derived DAG generation with sequential activation of PKC and PLD, and (2) approximately 30 to 40% of ATP- and bradykinin-induced PLD activation is independent of PKC activation and may involve direct coupling of the receptor to PLD via a GTP-binding protein (G_{PLD}). Our studies differ from those of Martin et al. (1989), who reported that downregulation of PKC completely abolished bradykinin-induced PLD activation in BPAEC. This discrepancy could be due to differences in the labeled precursor used to detect PLD activation.

C. Ca^{2+} Regulation of PLD Activity

Although hydrolysis of exogenously labeled PC by PLD-containing BPAEC membrane preparations occurs in the presence of EGTA or EDTA (Martin, 1988), there is evidence that agonist-mediated activation of PLD requires the presence of Ca_E^{2+} influx across the endothelial cell plasma membrane. The role of Ca^{2+} mobilization in the activation of PLD was evaluated using Ca^{2+} ionophores A23187 and ionomycin and Ca^{2+} chelators EGTA and BAPTA. In the presence of 1.0 m*M* Ca_E^{2+}, A23187 or ionomycin activated PLD (eight- to 10-fold), and this activation was comparable to agonist-induced or TPA-mediated PLD stimulation (Natarajan and Garcia, 1992; Garcia et al., 1992a). The addition of EGTA to chelate Ca_E^{2+} blocked [^{32}P]PEt accumulation in response to bradykinin, ATP, A23187, or ionomycin but not to TPA. Huang and Cabot (1990) similarly observed TPA-induced [^{3}H]PEt formation to occur irrespective of the presence of Ca_E^{2+} in the culture medium. However, as compared to almost total suppression of Ca^{2+} ionophore–mediated [^{32}P]PEt formation, EGTA attenuated only 50% of the PLD activity elicited either by bradykinin or ATP (Natarajan and Garcia, 1992). The effect of both A23187 and ionomycin was Ca^{2+} dependent and was not due to cellular damage as assessed by the absence of [^{3}H]2-deoxyglucose release. The requirement of intracellular Ca^{2+} for PLD activation was further demonstrated using cell-permeant acetoxymethyl ester of BAPTA. BAPTA lowered the basal level of free intracellular Ca^{2+} in BPAEC by about 50% (resting [Ca_i^{2+}] = 107 + 17 n*M*; after BAPTA treatment [Ca_i^{2+}] = 58 ± 7 n*M*) (Garcia et al., 1992c). Pretreatment of BPAEC with BAPTA (25 μ*M*, 30 min) significantly reduced both [^{32}P]PEt and [^{32}P]PA formation in response to bradykinin and ionomycin (Natarajan and Garcia, 1992). However, BAPTA pretreatment lowered TPA-induced formation of [^{32}P]PA and PEt by about 50% compared to control cells. BAPTA treatment by itself had no effect on the formation of [^{32}P]PEt or [^{32}P]PA in BPAEC (Natarajan and Garcia, 1992).

Table 2 In Vitro Activation of Bovine Endothelial Membrane PLD by GTPγS[a]

Addition	[^{32}P]Phosphatidylethanol formed (dpm/mg protein/h)	Activity (% control)
None	2457 ± 175	100
GTPγS (250 μ*M*)	4884 ± 242	199
GTPγS (250 μ*M*) and EGTA (m*M*)	1972 ± 110	80
GDPβS (250 μ*M*)	2597 ± 97	105

[a]Isolated [^{32}P]-labeled 100,000g BPAE cell membranes (100 μg protein) were incubated at 37°C for 1 h in a final volume of 0.4 mL containing 100 m*M* MES buffer pH 6.0, 1% ethanol, 1 m*M* $CaCl_2$, and 10 m*M* $MgCl_2$. $CaCl_2$ was omitted from EGTA experiments. PEt was separated by TLC on precoated silica gel G plates developed in $CHCl_3/CH_3OH/NH_4OH$ (80:20:2 by volume). Values are mean from representative experiment done in triplicate. 100 μg of protein contained 42.3 × 10^4 dpm.

D. GTP-Binding Protein(s) in Regulation of PLD Activation

Martin and Michaelis (1989) were the first to demonstrate an involvement of a G protein in the activation of PLD in BPAEC. In saponin-permeabilized BPAEC prelabeled with [^{3}H] choline, ATP and GTPγS stimulated release of [^{3}H]choline but not [^{3}H]phosphocholine, suggesting that breakdown of PC by ATP and GTPγS was due to the activation of PLD and involves a GTP-binding protein. The effects of ATP and GTPγS were synergistic at low GTPγS concentrations. A role for G protein in the activation of PLD in [^{32}P]BPAEC was confirmed in our laboratory using GTPγS, GDPβS, and GTP (Natarajan and Garcia, 1990a). GTPγS (10μ*M*) but not GDPβS (10 μ*M*) stimulated PLD activity in saponin-permeabilized BPAECs. To gain further insight into the role of G proteins in PLD activation, PLD activity was examined in [^{32}P]-labeled membranes from BPAEC. In the presence of Ca^{2+}, GTPγS (250 μ*M*) induced [^{32}P]PEt production in the presence of 0.5% ethanol (Table 2). However, when either EGTA was present in excess of Ca^{2+}, or Ca^{2+} was omitted, GTPγS did not stimulate [^{32}P]PEt production. As compared to GTPγS, GDPβS (250 μ*M*) had no direct effect on PLD activity. These in vitro data demonstrate that cell-free preparations from BPAEC contain PLD activity that requires Ca^{2+} for GTP activation.

Fluoroaluminate, another nonspecific activator of GTP-binding protein, also stimulated PLD activity as quantified by accumulation of [^{32}P] and [^{3}H]PEt in BPAEC (Fig. 11) in HUVEC monolayers (Natarajan and Garcia, 1990a,b). However, the data based on GTPγS and AlF_4^- do not establish that G proteins (G_{PLD}) are coupled directly to the effector PLD enzyme in endothelial cells, as activation of PLD could have resulted from the indirect effect of G protein activation, such as GTPγS and AlF_4^- activation of endothelial cell PI-PLC, result-

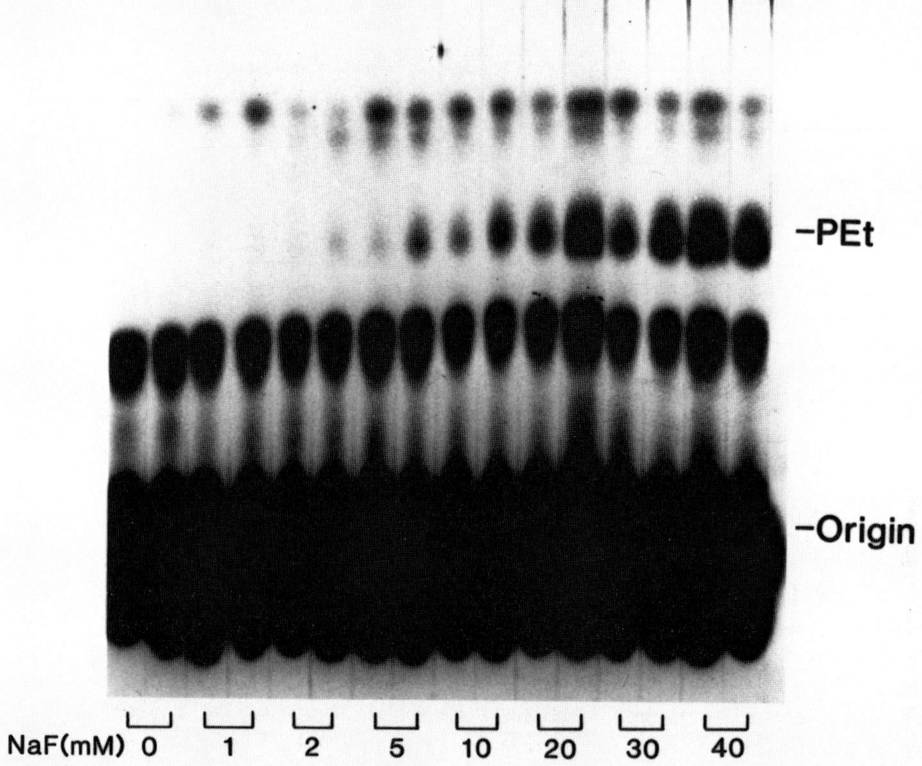

Figure 11 AlF_4^- -induced [^{32}P]PEt production in bovine pulmonary artery endothelial cells. Endothelial cells were prelabeled with [^{32}P]orthophosphate (30 μCi/ dish) for 18 h. The cells were washed and then incubated with vehicle or varying concentrations of AlF_4^- for 30 min in the presence of 0.5% ethanol. Depicted is an autoradiograph of [^{32}P]PEt formed with varying concentrations of NaF. [^{32}P]PEt was separated by TLC as described in Table 1.

ing in the generation of DAG and PKC activation. Recent work carried out in our laboratory (V. Natarajan and J. G. N. Garcia, manuscript in preparation) on GTPγS and AlF_4^- induced PLD activation in BPAEC and HUVEC in conjunction with staurosporine and PKC downregulation distinguished between the two possible mechanisms for G protein–mediated PLD activation. Neither PKC inhibition with staurosporine (10 μ*M*) nor downregulation of PKC by prolonged treatment with TPA (18 h, 100 n*M*) inhibited AlF_4^- induced stimulation (Table 3), demonstrating for the first time that the endothelial cell PLD enzyme may be coupled directly to GPLD. (Garcia et al., 1992a.)

Table 3 Effect of Staurosporine on TPA- and AlF_4^--Induced Phosphatidlethanol Formation[a]

Pretreatment	Treatment	[^{32}P]PEt formed CPM/dish	% Activity
Vehicle	Vehicle	78 ± 22	100
Vehicle	AlF_4^-	277 ± 90	355
Vehicle	TPA	262 ± 17	335
Staurosporine	Vehicle	76 ± 13	100
Staurosporine	TPA	85 ± 15	5
Staurosporine	AlF_4^-	322 ± 55	454

[a]BPAEC prelabeled with [^{32}P]orthophosphate (23 μCi/dish) for 24 h was washed and treated with staurosporine (10 μ*M*) or 0.1% DMSO for 15 min followed by stimulation with AlF_4^- (NaF, 20 m*M*; $AlCl_3$, 10 μ*M*) or TPA (100 n*M*) for 30 min in the presence of 0.5% ethanol. Data are the average ± SD of triplicate determinations.

E. Phosphatidic Acid Directly Activates Endothelial Cell Protein Kinase C

Recent studies in our laboratory (Stasek et al., 1991) suggest that an additional second-messenger function of PLD-generated PA may be the direct activation of endothelial cell PKC independently of DAG (Fig. 12). Specifically, PKC activa-

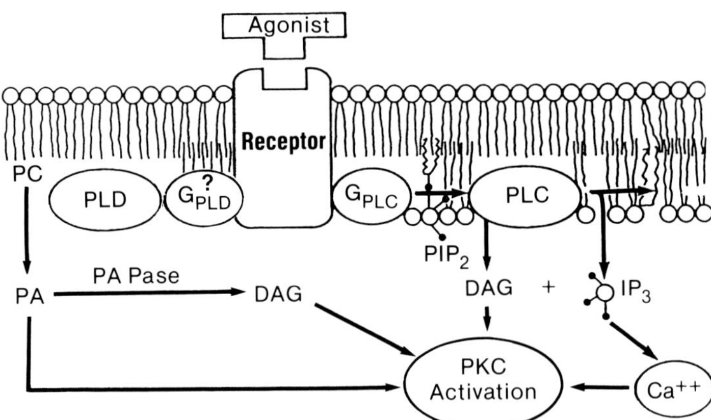

Figure 12 Activation of PKC through PLC and PLD pathways. The scheme indicates that occupancy of the receptor by an agonist results in the activation of PLC and PLD, most likely involving G_{PLC} and G_{PLD}. In addition to direct activation of PLD by G_{PLD}, DAG generation via PLC pathway activates PKC, which can activate PLD. PLD activation generates PA, which activates PKC directly without DAG. Thus PLD by-products can stimulate PKC directly without a PLC pathway, and this may represent an alternative mechanism of endothelial cell PKC stimulation.

tion induced by dioleoylglycerol (40 μ*M*) produced 6.4 pmol of $\gamma[^{32}P]$ATP incorporation/μg PKC/per minute (100%) as compared to 1.5 pmol/μg/per minute (23%) obtained with dioleoyl, 1-stearyl 2-arachidoyl, or egg yolk PA. De novo DAG formation from PA by PAPase was excluded by carrying out the assays with $[^{14}C]$dioleoyl PA followed by TLC assessment of $[^{14}C]$DAG formed. PKC preparations from endothelial cells under the assay conditions employed did not hydrolyze $[^{14}C]$PA to DAG, confirming that PA had the capability to activate PKC independently of DAG in the presence of Ca^{2+} and phosphatidylserine.

VII. Transmembrane Signaling After Thrombin Receptor Occupancy

To link the PI-PLC, PLA_2, PLD, and PKC activities to functional endothelial cell responses, we have focused on one specific receptor-mediated agonist, α-thrombin. The response of the endothelium to thrombin is diverse, with thrombin stimulating the release of substances that exert effects on both vascular tone and vascular permeability. Thrombin binds to high- and low-affinity endothelial cell-surface receptors (Awbrey et al., 1979; Lollar and Owen, 1980a,b), augments endothelial cell proliferation (Gospodarowicz et al., 1978), enhances the synthesis of platelet-activating factor (Camussi et al., 1983; Prescott et al., 1984), enhances expression of tissue factor on the cell surface (Galdal et al., 1985), and increases transcription and release of platelet-derived growth factor (DiCorleto and Bowen-Pope, 1983; Harlan et al., 1986), release of tissue plasminogen activator (Levin et al., 1984) and its inhibitor (Gelehrter and Sznycer-Laszuk, 1986), and release of factor VIII and von Willebrand factor from vascular endothelium (Levine et al., 1982).

A. Thrombin-Receptor Dynamics in Endothelium

The interaction between thrombin and its specific receptor in cultured human or bovine endothelial cells is a rapid, reversible, and saturable (Awbrey et al., 1979; Lollar et al., 1980), and the receptors have been characterized as containing a limited number of distinct high-affinity states (kD ≈ 0.1 n*M* for human endothelium and 0.5 n*M* for bovine endothelium). In addition to these high-affinity sites, more numerous low-affinity sites with kD values of about 10 and 50 n*M* have been identified on human and bovine endothelium, respectively (Awbrey et al., 1979; Lollar et al., 1980; Parkinson et al., 1990). The difference in thrombin-receptor dissociation constraints between the two species appears to be important in determining the potency of thrombin's effects on AA metabolism, with thrombin-stimulated bovine endothelium producing markedly reduced levels of prostaglandins over those of similarly challenged human endothelium.

One high-affinity thrombin-binding site on the endothelial cell surface (possibly the sole high-affinity site) is the surface glycoprotein thrombomodulin (Esmon and Owen, 1981). Recent work has further identified that the glycosoamino-glycan chain attachment of the thrombomodulin molecule appears to be critical for α-thrombin binding to thrombomodulin (Parkinson et al., 1990). Substantial evidence, however, suggests that it is not the high-affinity binding site (i.e., thrombomodulin) but a low-affinity binding site that is the thrombin receptor which is functionally coupled to PGI_2 synthesis (Horie et al., 1990; Lollar and Owen, 1980b).

B. Use of Modified Thrombins in Endothelial Cell Signaling

The native α-thrombin enzyme contains several distinct topographic regions, including the active catalytic site, the anionic-binding exosite, and the fibrinogen recognition site (Fenton, 1988). Because of the complex ways in which thrombin interacts with endothelial cells, it has been difficult to assign cause-and-effect relationships to thrombin's cellular interactions and the observed biological responses, such as the two thrombin-mediated responses discussed in this chapter, PGI_2 synthesis, and barrier dysfunction. In this regard, modified forms of thrombin have been useful tools in dissecting the complex interactions between thrombin and endothelial cells.

The high-affinity thrombin binding site on endothelium is active-site independent, as a catalytically-inactive thrombin preparation, DIP-α-thrombin, binds to the same site with an affinity similar to that of native α-thrombin (Awbrey et al., 1979; Lollar and Owen, 1980a). If transmembrane signal generation is active-site dependent, catalytic cleavage of a plasma membrane substrate may be involved, with one possible substrate being the thrombin "receptor." In this regard, thrombin-stimulated fibroblast proliferation involves proteolysis of its cell-surface receptor (Glenn and Cunningham, 1979; Glenn et al., 1980; Carney et al., 1986). Alternatively, there may be an active-site-dependent receptor for thrombin which is different from the receptor that binds both DIP-α-thrombin and active α-thrombin. However, this receptor must be of low binding affinity or may be present in such low numbers as to explain the difficulty in distinguishing it from "nonspecific" binding. The catalytic action of α-thrombin might also be directed toward G_p, with either direct proteolysis of the α subunit of this GTP-binding protein or thrombin-mediated activation of an endogenous protease causing a proteolytic modification of G_p.

Thrombin-induced endothelial cell activation requires the presence of proteolytic activity, as DIP-thrombin does not induce PGI_2 synthesis (Table 4) (Jaffe et al., 1987; Garcia et al., 1990) or barrier dysfunction (Aschner et al., 1990; Garcia et al., 1992b; Patterson et al., 1992). The addition of catalytically inactive DIP/α-thrombin to block high-affinity binding sites, however, blunts the effects of α-thrombin, suggesting that high-affinity binding by α-thrombin facilitates contact between the active serine site and its substrate (Aschner et al., 1990) and that the region of the thrombin molecule involved in high-affinity binding is close to the active serine site (Carney et al., 1984). High-affinity binding may accelerate the active-site reaction by facilitating contact between the active site and its substrate or by conferring a conformational change on the receptor which enhances affinity of the enzyme for its substrate. Another thrombin preparation, γ-thrombin, which is catalytically active but without clotting activity, activates endothelium but does so less efficiently than α-thrombin (Garcia et al., 1990; Aschner et al., 1990) due to its inability to bind to high-affinity sites.

C. Thrombin-Induced PLC Activity and Ca_i^{2+} Mobilization

Like a variety of hormones and inflammatory mediators that induce endothelial cell activation, thrombin causes an increase in intracellular Ca^{2+}, $[Ca_i^{2+}]$. Using the photoprotein Ca^{2+} probe aequorin or fluorescent indicator probes such as Quin 2, Indo-1, and Fura-2, α-thrombin has been found to be a rapid and potent stimulus for increases in levels of cytosolic Ca^{2+} in cultured human umbilical vein and pulmonary artery endothelium (Jaffe et al., 1987; Brock et al., 1988a; Hallam et al., 1988; Garcia et al., 1990, 1991a, 1992c) as well as in bovine pulmonary artery endothelium (Lum et al., 1989; Goligorski et al., 1989).

As the vast majority of thrombin effects on cultured endothelium appear to involve a second-messenger action of Ca_i^{2+}, a key stimulus–coupling event, and one of the earliest measurable reaction in the cascade of events that follow thrombin-mediated cell activation, is its potent activation of PI-PLC-mediated PIP_2 hydrolysis in human and porcine endothelium (Hong and Deykin, 1982; Moscat et al., 1987b; Jaffe et al., 1987; Brock and Capasso, 1988; Halldorsson et al., 1988; Lampugnani et al., 1989; Carter et al., 1989b), in bovine pulmonary microvascular endothelial cells (Garcia et al., 1992b), but not in bovine aortic endothelial cells (Jaffe et al., 1987) or in microvascular endothelial cells obtained from human omentum (Carter et al., 1989b). Thrombin stimulation of phosphoinositide turnover in endothelial cells is dependent on the thrombin dose (Lampugnani et al., 1989) as well as the presence of an active catalytic site. Both α- and γ-thrombin activate PLC, resulting in IP_3 generation, whereas DIP-α-thrombin and active site–inhibited PPACK-α-thrombin do not increase IP_3 or $[Ca_i^{2+}]$ in HUVEC (Jaffe et al., 1987; Brock and Capasso, 1988), indicating that for the induction of PLC activities, the proteolytic activity of thrombin is a strict requirement.

The initial component of the thrombin-stimulated Ca^{2+} response results from rapid mobilization of Ca^{2+} from intracellular pools, as this component is insensitive to [Ca_E^{2+}] and is consistent with thrombin-induced PLC-mediated PIP_2 hydrolysis. The second phase is a sustained increase in $[Ca^{2+}]_i$ via [Ca_E^{2+}] influx, as it correlates well with the time course of $^{45}Ca^{2+}$ uptake and is abolished by a Ca^{2+}-free medium (Lum et al., 1989; Goligorski et al., 1989). The overall increase in HUVEC cytosolic Ca^{2+}, however, is derived primarily from endogenous Ca^{2+} stores, as the removal of [Ca_E^{2+}] attenuates but does not abolish the early increase in [Ca_i^{2+}] (Garcia et al., 1991a, 1992b).

Arachidonate metabolites produced as the result of PLC-Ca^{2+} activation of PLA_2 may also participate in determining the magnitude of the thrombin-stimulated Ca^{2+} response. Microinjection of PIP_2-specific PLC, IP_3, or Ca^{2+} causes an immediate Ca_i^{2+} increase but is not followed by the sustained Ca^{2+} elevation characteristic of α-thrombin. Only microinjection of PLA_2 or coinjection of PLA_2 with PIP_2-specific PLC resulted in sustained thrombin-induced increases in Ca_i^{2+}. These results are most consistent with sequential thrombin–mediated activation of PLC and PLA_2 but do not exclude dual coupling of the thrombin receptor to GTP-binding proteins linked to PLC and PLA_2 or activation of two types of thrombin receptors with different coupling pathways.

D. Protein Kinase C and G Protein Regulation of Thrombin-Stimulated PLC and Ca^{2+} Activities

We have implicated GTP-binding protein participation in the regulation of α-thrombin- and NaF-induced PLC activation and Ca^{2+} mobilization (Garcia et al., 1990, 1991a). Activation of Gp by either α-thrombin or NaF resulted in PI-PLC-mediated phosphoinositide hydrolysis, the generation of DAG and IP_3, and luminescence of the photoprotein aequorin indicative of Ca^{2+} mobilization from endogenous pools (Garcia et al., 1991a, 1992c; Brock et al., 1988b; Magnusson et al., 1989). The α-thrombin-stimulated DAG production is rapid, occurring within 15 s (Brock et al., 1988b), whereas NaF-induced DAG formation is more delayed, at more than 2 min (Garcia et al., 1991a).

The G protein inhibitor GDPβS markedly attenuated both α-thrombin- and NaF-induced Ca_i^{2+} increases in aequorin-loaded human endothelium, but did not inhibit the increase in $[Ca^{2+}]_i$ produced by ionophore A23187 consistent with Gp regulation of PI-specific phospholipase C activity and Ca^{2+} mobilization in these cells (Fig. 13) (Garcia et al., 1991a). These results are consistent with the results of Brock and Capasso (1989), who found GTPgS to augment α-thrombin-induced inositol phosphate generation and indicate G_p modulation of Ca_i^{2+} via an effect on PLC. As reported above (Fig. 5C), the increase in DAG by α–thrombin and NaF correlates with rapid time-dependent translocation of protein kinase C activity from the cytosolic to membrane compartments as assessed by phos-

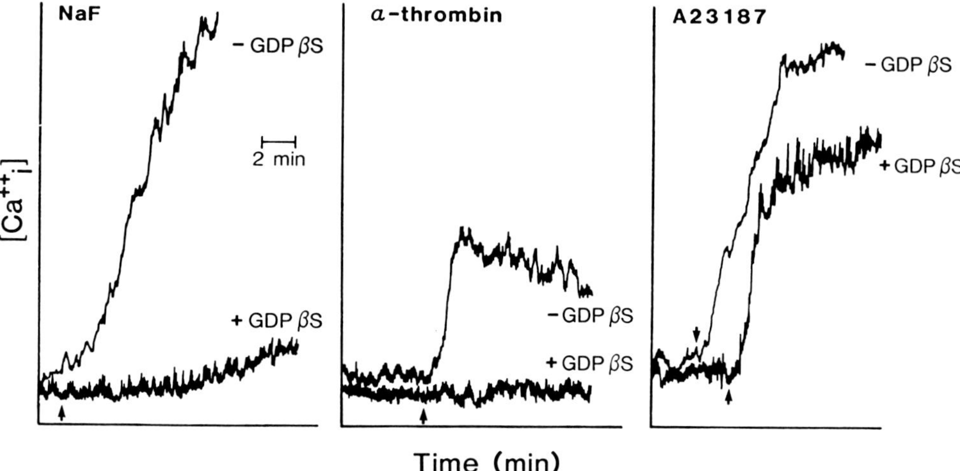

Figure 13 Effect of GDPβS on thrombin- and NaF-induced aequorin luminescence. HUVEC monolayers were scrape-loaded with either buffer or GDPβS (0.5 m*M*) prior to aequorin loading. Depicted are 20 m*M* NaF-, 10 n*M* α-thrombin-, and 1 μ*M* A23187-induced aequorin luminescence determined in the presence of 1.2 m*M* Ca^{2+} with or without prior loading with GDPβS. (From Garcia et al., 1991a.)

phorylation of histone-1 (Garcia et al., 1992c, Stasek and Garcia 1992). Pretreatment with stimuli that activate PKC, such as PMA, mezerein, and *sn*-1,2-dioctanylglycerol, attenuate thrombin-induced increases in the concentration of intracellular cytosolic $Ca^{2+,}$ as well as IP_3 formation (Brock and Capasso, 1988; Garcia et al., 1992c). As shown in Figs. 7 and 8, PKC participates in a central fashion in the regulation of both Ca_i^{2+} responses and PLA_2 activities in HUVEC, with PLC activation resulting in the inhibition of α–thrombin- and NaF-induced inositol phosphate increases and attenuation of both α-thrombin- and NaF-activated increases in Ca_i^{2+} (Garcia et al., 1991a, 1992c). Ca^{2+} mobilization induced by ionophore A23187 was not affected by PKC preactivation, suggesting PKC-dependent negative-feedback inhibition of PI-specific PLC.

E. Regulation of Thrombin-Induced PLD Activity

Similar to bradykinin and ATP in bovine endothelium, α-thrombin (10 n*M*) stimulates a six- to eightfold increase in [^{32}P]PEt in human endothelium, indicative of potent PLD activation (Garcia et al., 1992a). Treatment of [^{32}P]HUVEC monolayers with modified forms of thrombin indicate that as with other thrombin-stimulated responses, the catalytic site of α-thrombin is necessary for PLD activation (Fig. 14) (Garcia and Natarajan, 1990; Garcia et al., 1992a). DIP–α-thrombin, which exhibits the fibrinogen recognition site but which is estrolytically inactive, failed to elicit an increase in PEt formation up to 1 μ*M*. γ-Thrombin lacking fibrinogen recognition activity but retaining about 70% of its esterolytic activity at 10 n*M* had no effect on PLD activity, whereas 1 μ*M* γ-thrombin (100-fold increase)-induced PLD activation, which approached 50% of the 10 n*M* α-thrombin response. ζ-Thrombin possessing fibrinogenic and esterolytic activities, but which is thermally less stable than α-thrombin, at equimolar concentration produced approximately 60% of α-thrombin-mediated PEt accumulation (Fig. 14). These data strongly suggest that an active catalytic site with resultant enzymatic activity is essential for thrombin stimulation of PLD activity in HUVEC.

The role of Ca^{2+} flux in thrombin-stimulated human PLD activation was investigated and PEt formation was enhanced significantly by Ca^{2+} ionophores

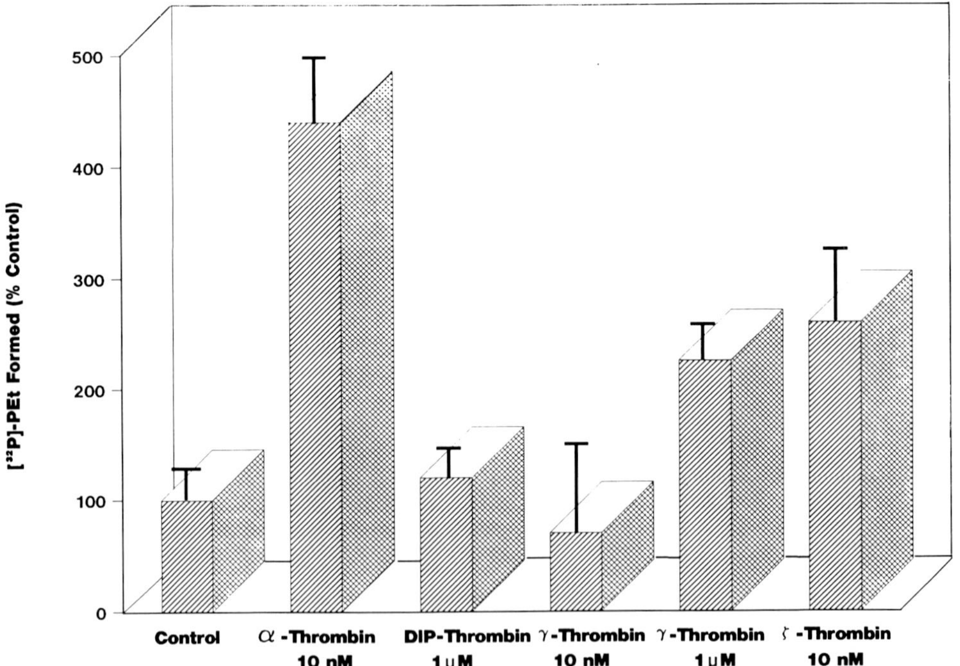

Figure 14 Effect of modified thrombins on HUVEC PLD activity. Radiolabeled HUVEC monolayers were challenged with α-thrombin and modified thrombin preparations at the stated concentrations for 5 min in the presence of 0.5% ethanol. Cellular lipids were extracted, and levels of [^{32}P]PEt determined. Results represent mean ± SD of dishes performed in triplicate. (From Garcia et al., 1992a.)

A23187 and ionomycin (1 μ*M*, three- to fourfold increase). α-Thrombin-stimulated PEt formation was abolished (>90% inhibition) by chelation of Ca_i^{2+} with BAPTA-AM (25 μ*M*, 30 min) but was only mildly attenuated (30% inhibition) by removal of Ca_i^{2+} with EGTA (5 m*M*) (Garcia et al., 1992a). Protein kinase C also participates in a central fashion in thrombin-stimulated PLD activation, as the PKC inhibitor staurosporine reduced α–thrombin-induced PEt formation in a dose-dependent manner (10 μ*M* 78% inhibition) and PKC downregulation with chronic PMA treatment (19 h) also resulted in marked inhibition of α-thrombin-induced PEt formation (Garcia et al., 1992a). Neither pertussis nor botulinum C bacterial toxin pretreatment significantly altered the α-thrombin-induced PLD response. In contrast, however, similar pretreatment with cholera toxin (1 mg/mL, 60 min) consistently augmented a-thrombin-stimulated PLD activity by

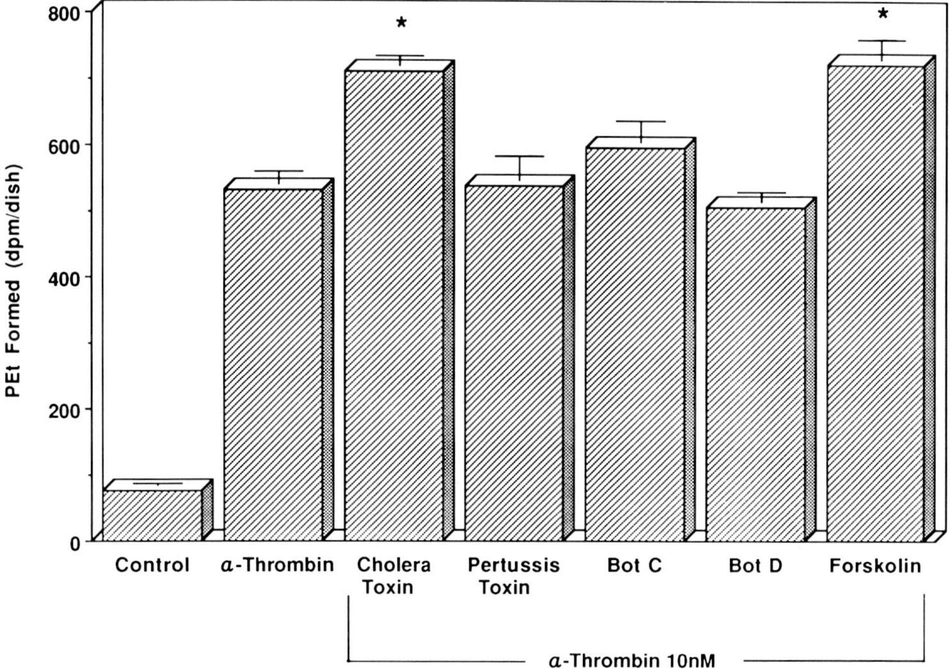

Figure 15 Radiolabeled HUVEC monolayers were challenged with buffer or 10 n*M* α-thrombin in the presence or absence of prior treatment (1 μg/mL, 60 min) with cholera, pertussis, or botulinum C and D toxins. After 5 min of α-thrombin challenge, the reaction was terminated and levels of [^{32}P]PEt quantified. Treatment with these toxins did not alter basal PLD activity, whereas cholera toxin pretreatment significantly potentiated the thrombin-stimulated PLD response.

50 to 90% (Fig. 15). Because comparable results were observed with agents that increase cAMP, such as forskolin, 8-bromo cAMP, or dibutyryl cAMP, these studies demonstrate that a-thrombin is a potent stimulus for human PLD-mediated PA formation and that cyclic adenosine nucleotides modulate agonist-induced cellular PLD activity (Garcia, 1992a). Thrombin-stimulated PA formation and subsequent DAG production catalyzed by PLD represents an important and heretoforth unrecognized pathway in thrombin-induced signal transduction in human endothelium.

VIII. Regulation of Thrombin-Induced PGI_2 Synthesis

Thrombin is an excellent stimulus for PLA_2 activity and prostacyclin (PGI_2) synthesis by cultured human umbilical vein endothelium (HUVEC), whereas bovine aortic endothelium and human foreskin microvascular endothelium are unresponsive. As with other agonists, AA release by PLC hydrolysis of PC to lyso-PC catalyzed by PLA_2 is the rate-limiting step involved in thrombin-induced endothelial cell PGI_2 synthesis (Hong and Deykin, 1982; Hong et al., 1985). Additional, albeit smaller pools of AA are derived from DAG lipase action on

Table 4 Effect of Modified Thrombins on HUVEC PGI_2 Synthesis[a]

Agent	Concentration (μM)	6-keto $PGF_{1\alpha}$
α-Thrombin		
(n = 6)	1	10.2 ± 0.2
(n = 10)	0.01	8.1 ± 0.6
(n = 6)	0.0001	0.8 ± 0.2
γ-Thrombin		
(n = 6)	1	5.4 ± 0.3
(n = 6)	0.1	0.8 ± 0.1
DIP-α-thrombin		
(n = 6)	1	1.1 ± 0.3
(n = 6)	0.1	1.0 ± 0.1
Histamine		
(n = 8)	10	5.6 ± 0.3
Arachidonate		
(n = 4)	5	11.6 ± 0.5

[a]PGI_2 levels are expressed as the x-fold increase in levels of 6-keto $PGF_{1\alpha}$ over buffer-treated HUVEC monolayers. Confluent HUVEC monolayers were challenged with α-thrombin, γ-thrombin, and DIP-thrombin at the concentration depicted and aliquots of cell-free supernatants removed at 10 min. Rapid increases in 6-keto $PGF_{1\alpha}$ were observed with 10 nM α-thrombin, whereas proteolytically inactive DIP-thrombin (1 μM) did not increase levels of the PGI_2 metabolite. γ-Thrombin produced significant levels of PGI_2 but required a 100-fold greater concentration that than of α-thrombin.
Source: Adapted from Garcia et al., 1990.

DAG produced by either PI-PLC- or PLD-mediated PA generation and subsequent PA conversion to DAG by PAPase. Both pathways are functional in cultured human endothelial cells with approximately two-thirds of the AA released in thrombin-stimulated HUVEC being derived via the deacylating action of PLA_2 on membrane phospholipids. Results from kinetic experiments from several laboratories suggest a sequential association between thrombin-mediated hydrolysis of phosphoinositides and the ultimate generation of prostaglandins (Jaffe et al., 1987, Halldorsson et al., 1988). Thus thrombin-induced PGI_2 synthesis involves the sequential action of two Ca^{2+}-dependent phospholipases, PLC and PLA_2. The mobilization of Ca^{2+} probably occurs as a result of thrombin effects on phosphoinositide metabolism by PLC and the transient generation of IP_3, events that precede the release of AA by PLA_2 and the secretion of PGI_2.

We have monitored the generation of PGI_2 in HUVEC monolayers by RIA of 6-keto $PGF_{1\alpha}$ and dose-dependent increases observed within human α- and γ-thrombins, histamine, or arachidonate (Table 4) (Garcia et al., 1990). Native α-thrombin stimulation of PGI_2 synthesis is rapid and 10 n*M* α-thrombin produces near-maximal levels of 6-keto $PGF_{1\alpha}$, approximating responses with 1 μM γ-thrombin, 5 μM arachidonate, or 10 μM histamine. Catalytically inactive DIP-α-thrombin did not stimulate PGI_2 release (Table 4), suggesting that as with PLC and PLD activities, proteolytic activity is required for thrombin-stimulated PLA_2 activity and subsequent PGI_2 synthesis. As expected, repeated stimulation of human umbilical vein endothelial cells with α-thrombin results in desensitization to further PGI_2 production consistent with a receptor-mediated mechanism for PGI_2 synthesis (Halldorsson et al., 1988). As with other agonists described earlier, neither α-thrombin nor NaF-stimulated PGI_2 release is totally dependent on the availability of extracellular Ca^{2+} (Garcia et al., 1990, 1991a). The level of $[Ca_i^{2+}]$ is critical to thrombin effects, as the addition of Ca_i^{2+} chelators such as TMB-8 (Jaffe et al., 1987) or BAPTA (Garcia et al., 1992c) abolishes α-thrombin-induced PGI_2 synthesis.

A. G Protein Regulation of Thrombin-Stimulated PGI_2 Synthesis

The contribution of G proteins in human endothelial cell membranes to the regulation of thrombin-induced PGI_2 synthesis has also been explored (Garcia et al., 1990, 1991a; Magnusson et al., 1989). The participation of G proteins in the generation of PGI_2 was implicated by experiments wherein the addition of the known G protein activators NaF and GTPγS to intact and digitonin-permeabilized monolayers, respectively, results in time- and dose-dependent increase in the levels of 6-keto $PGF_{1\alpha}$ over control values (Garcia et al., 1990, 1991a). The involvement of G proteins in regulating thrombin-induced Ca^{2+} mobilization and prostaglandin synthesis has been further demonstrated in studies using the G protein inhibitor GDPβS. Pretreatment of HUVEC monolayers with the GDPβS (15 to 120 min exposure) does not significantly alter spontaneous PGI_2 synthesis (<5% inhibition all doses tested, 0.05 to 5 m*M*). However, there is marked dose-dependent attenuation of α-thrombin-stimulated PGI_2 responses in permeabilized cells pretreated with GDPβS for 1 h (Garcia et al., 1990).

As these studies suggested that thrombin-induced Ca^{2+} mobilization and PGI_2 synthesis in human endothelium is regulated by GTP-binding proteins, attempts were made to further characterize the G protein, G_p, which is functionally coupled to thrombin-stimulated PLC activity. In HUVEC monolayers thrombin decreased the availability of a GTP-binding protein substrate susceptible to ADP ribosylation by pertussis toxin (Garcia et al., 1990) (Fig. 2). Preincubation with either cholera toxin or pertussis toxin (1 μg/mL, 60 min), however, failed to block either thrombin-induced PLC activity, IP_3 formation, Ca^{2+} mobilization (Brock and Capasso, 1989; Garcia et al., 1991a, 1992a,c), or PGI_2 synthesis (Garcia et al., 1990, 1992b; Patterson et al., 1992b). Low-molecular-weight GTP binding proteins play important roles in the regulation of various cell functions, including cell transformation, proliferation, and differentiation (Yamamoto et al., 1989). We examined whether botulinum C p21 substrates (Fig. 2) were involved in thrombin-induced transmembrane signaling. Thrombin-challenged HUVEC monolayers pretreated with botulinum C (5 μg/mL) for 2 h generated levels of IP_3 comparable to untreated monolayers, suggesting that like pertussis and cholera toxins, botulinum C does not affect α-thrombin-induced PLD activity (Dukes et al., 1991). However, botulinum C alone appeared to increase IP production in a time-dependent manner, suggesting that rho p21 may modulate PLC activity. Together, these studies suggest that bacterial toxin-insensitive G proteins are involved in transducing signals from the thrombin receptor to its intracellular targets, which result in prostaglandin synthesis.

The evidence to date for G protein regulation of thrombin-mediated PLC activity does not exclude the possibility of a distinct G protein directly regulating PLA_2 activity. Because PLA_2, like PLC, is a Ca^{2+}-requiring enzyme, and GTP-binding proteins appear to activate PLC by reducing the Ca^{2+} requirement of this enzyme (Smith et al., 1986), G proteins have also been suggested to couple receptors directly linked to PLA_2 (Okano et al. 1987; Kajiyama et al., 1989; Nakashima et al., 1988) independent of PLC, inositol phosphate generation, and thus intracellular Ca^{2+} release. Jelsema and Axelrod (1987) have shown that the β-γ subunit dimer of G proteins is capable of activating PLA_2 in retinal rod outer segments supporting a link between the receptor and phospholipase A_2 by GTP-binding proteins in specific cellular systems. As neither HUVEC phospholipase C activity, PLA_2 activity, nor PGI_2 synthesis stimulated by either NaF or thrombin is inhibited by bacterial toxins (pertussis, cholera, botulinum C) (Garcia et al., 1990, 1991b; Dukes et al., 1991; Patterson et al., 1992b), the existence of a distinct G protein directly linking the occupied thrombin receptor to PLA_2 (G_{PLA2}) in human endothelium remains speculative.

B. Protein Kinase C Regulation of Thrombin-Induced Endothelial Cell PGI_2 Synthesis

Recent studies have addressed the role of PKC activation in human endothelial cell PLC, PLA_2, and PLD, as well as in Ca^{2+} mobilization, a response that is functionally coupled to the production of PGI_2. As shown in Fig. 5, PMA, α-thrombin, and NaF, a direct G protein activator, produced a rapid and time-dependent translocation of PKC from the cytosol to the membrane (Garcia et al., 1992c; Stasek et al., 1992a,b). Although PKC appears to reduce $[Ca_i^{2+}]$ after thrombin or NaF (Fig. 6), thrombin- or NaF-stimulated PLA_2 activity, AA release, and PGI_2 synthesis in PMA-pretreated cultured human endothelial cells was potentiated, and the enhanced PGI_2 synthesis produced by A23187, NaF, and α-thrombin was dependent on the dose of PMA (Garcia et al., 1992c). The thrombin-stimulated production of PGI_2 was further implicated as a PKC-dependent event by studies involving either staurosporine, a potent protein kinase C inhibitor, or downregulation of protein kinase C activity by prolonged (18 h)

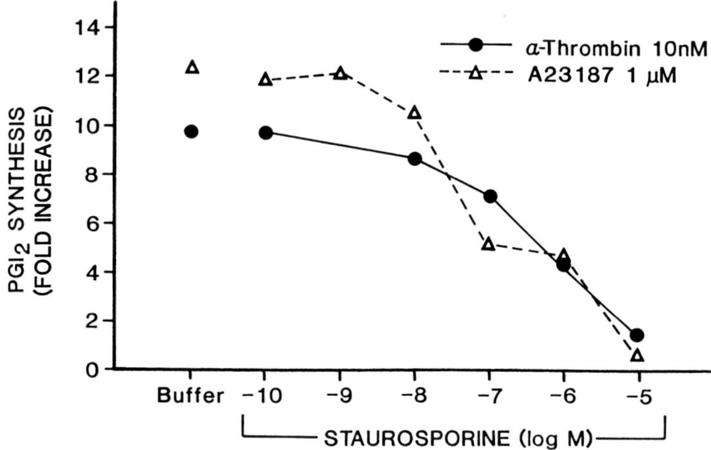

Figure 16 Effect of staurosporine on agonist-stimulated PGI_2 synthesis. Having established the range of PKC inhibition by staurosporine, HUVEC monolayers in 24-well plates were treated with either buffer or staurosporine (15 min, 1 μ*M*) prior to agonist challenge. Noted is the profound inhibition of agonist-stimulated PGI_2 synthesis by staurosporine. Similar staurosporine pretreatment had only a marginal effect on arachidonate-stimulated PGI_2 synthesis.

treatment with PMA (Garcia et al., 1992c). Staurosporine, at concentrations that inhibit PKC-induced phosphorylation of histone-1, augments α-thrombin- or NaF-induced production of inositol phosphates but markedly inhibits α-thrombin-, NaF-, and A23187-induced PGI_2 synthesis (Fig. 16) (Garcia et al., 1992c). The downregulation of PKC activity by prolonged PMA treatment produces similar inhibition of PGI_2 synthesis by these agonists (about 50% inhibition) (Garcia et al., 1992c). Neither staurosporine nor PKC downregulation attenuates agonist-induced Ca^{2+} mobilization, nor does it alter PGI_2 synthesis after exogenous AA (Carter et al., 1989a; Garcia et al., 1992c). This modulation of PGI_2 production by PKC may involve a reduction in the Ca^{2+} requirements for activation of PLA_2, or alternatively, PKC may directly modulate PLA_2 and hence AA release via a mechanism that is independent of PLA_2's Ca^{2+} requirements. To explore these findings further, HUVEC monolayers were pretreated with the intracellular Ca^{2+} chelator BAPTA to chelate cytosolic free Ca^{2+}. Pretreatment with BAPTA as its acetoxymethyl ester (BAPTA-AM) (25 μ*M* for 30 min) produced approximately 50% quenching of basal aequorin luminescence, and dose-dependently inhibited agonist-stimulated PGI_2 synthesis (Garcia et al., 1992b,c). BAPTA-AM treatment of HUVEC monolayers, however, did not inhibit PKC translocation and activation induced by PMA, and for each level of BAPTA-mediated inhibition of PGI_2 synthesis, HUVEC monolayers treated with PMA 100 n*M* prior to BAPTA pretreatment were observed to demonstrate a reduction in the BAPTA-induced attenuation of PGI_2 synthesis (Garcia et al., 1992b,c). These results indicate that thrombin-stimulated PLA_2 activity occurs in a manner that remains dependent on cytosolic Ca^{2+} concentrations. Furthermore, these findings indirectly suggest that PKC-mediated increase of PLA_2 activity may occur by lowering PLA_2 [Ca^{2+}] requirements for enhanced enzymatic activity. The exact site of PKC effects on thrombin-induced endothelial cell prostaglandin responses is not yet delineated; however, as PMA inhibits both thrombin and NaF-induced Ca^{2+} increases, the site of PKC regulation appears to be distal to the occupancy of the thrombin receptor (Brock and Capasso, 1988; Garcia et al., 1992c).

IX. Regulation of α-Thrombin-Induced Endothelial Cell Barrier Dysfunction

Inflammatory mediators such as histamine and thrombin cause an increase in lung weight gain and enhance macromolecule flux across endothelial cell monolayers (Rotrosen and Gallin, 1986; Garcia et al., 1986). α-Thrombin causes concentration-dependent and reversible increases in endothelial permeability across bovine pulmonary artery endothelial cells as measured by the clearance rate of either [^{125}I]albumin (Garcia et al., 1986) or Evans Blue dye–labeled albumin (Patterson et al., 1992a) as well as across monolayers of bovine pulmonary microvessel endothelial cells (Aschner et al., 1990). The effect of thrombin is rapid, occurring within minutes and is reversible within 15 min after washing away the thrombin from the monolayer (Garcia et al., 1986, 1992b). As with the PGI_2 synthesis, occupancy of the thrombin receptor alone is insufficient for activation of the transmembrane events that trigger the increase in permeability (Aschner et al., 1990). DIP-α-thrombin in micromolar concentrations is unable to increase albumin permeability (Aschner et al., 1990). In contrast to DIP-α-thrombin, γ-thrombin does not compete for high-affinity binding sites (Glenn and Cunningham, 1979; Carney et al., 1986); it has an intact serine active site and consistently increased monolayer permeability (Garcia et al., 1986, 1992b), although on an equimolar basis, the response is less than with α-thrombin (Aschner et al., 1990). Alpha- or γ-thrombin preparations inactivated by exposure to the specific thrombin inhibitor hirudin (Patterson et al., 1992a) or D-PPACK (Garcia, 1992b) do not increase endothelial cell permeability, suggesting that again, as with other functional responses induced by α-thrombin, a functional catalytic site is essential for the permeability increase.

A. Ca_i^{2+} Regulation of Thrombin-Induced Barrier Dysfunction

The availability of Ca_E^{2+} appears to be crucial in the regulation of endothelial permeability, as removal of extracellular Ca^{2+} with EGTA or with lanthanum chloride, which competes for Ca^{2+} entry, diminished the α-thrombin-induced increase in bovine endothelial cell permeability (Lum et al., 1989). An increase in Ca_i^{2+} is also critical to α-thrombin-stimulated barrier dysfunction, as chelation of cytosolic Ca^{2+} with Quin 2 produced dose-dependent reduction in the α-thrombin-induced permeability response (Lum et al., 1989).

The mechanism by which thrombin-stimulated increases in [Ca_i^{2+}] produce enhanced endothelial cell permeability are probably related to Ca^{2+} effects on the endothelial cell cytoskeleton and contractile apparatus, via activation of Ca^{2+}-dependent enzymes such as myosin light-chain kinase (Wysolmerski and Lagunoff, 1990). The actin–myosin cytoskeleton plays a critical structural and mechanical role in maintaining the integrity of the endothelial cell monolayer and is sensitive to micromolar concentrations of Ca^{2+}. Thrombin alters the actin filaments that organize and stabilize junctional proteins and induces the reversible loss of peripheral actin bands, an increase in the number and thickness of stress fibers, and formation of interendothelial cell ''gaps'' (Garcia et al., 1986). Furthermore, treatment of bovine pulmonary artery endothelial cells with NBD-phallacidin, which is rapidly incorporated into cells and stabilizes actin filaments, prevents the thrombin-induced increase in permeability (Phillips et al.,

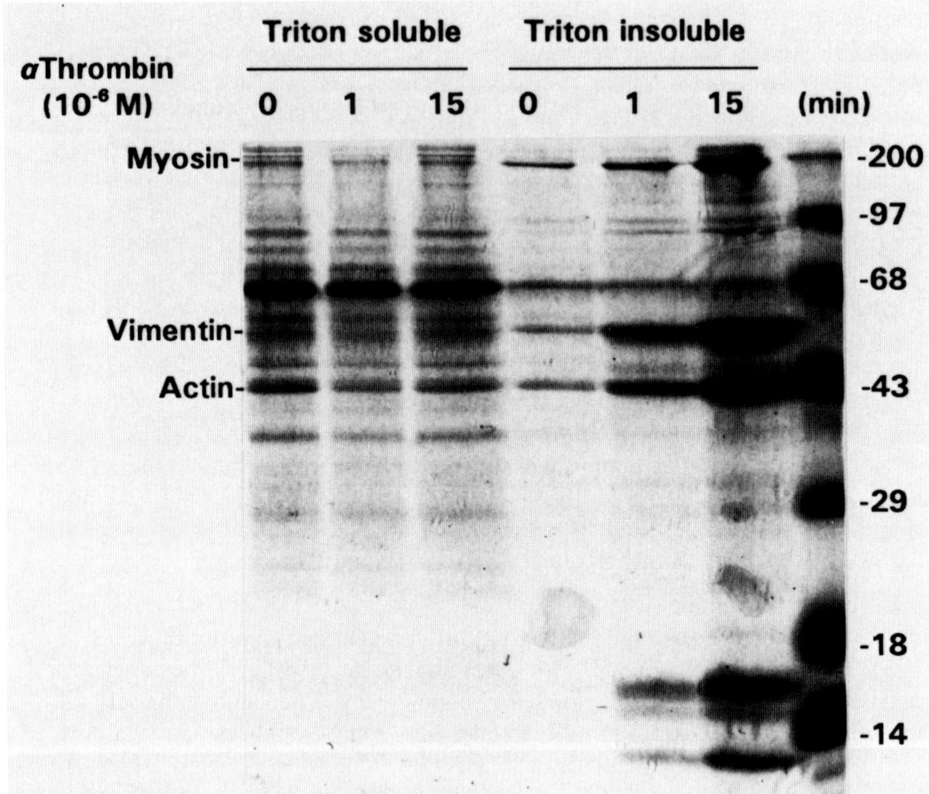

Figure 17 Cytoskeletal protein redistribution in response to α-thrombin stimulation in BPAEC monolayers. Confluent BPAEC monolayers in 75-cm_2 tissue culture flasks were stimulated with 10_{-6} *M* α-thrombin for the specified time periods, followed by detergent solubilization of cellular proteins with 1% Triton X-100. Triton-soluble and Triton-insoluble cellular protein fractions were then solubilized with SDS sample buffer and analyzed by SDS-PAGE, followed by protein staining with Coomassie Brilliant Blue. Redistribution of several cytoskeletal proteins from Triton-soluble to Triton-insoluble fractions is observed, including myosin heavy chain, vimentin, and actin, the identities of which were confirmed by Western blot analysis.

induces rapid and prominent redistribution of several cytoskeletal proteins, including actin and myosin from Triton-soluble fraction to the Triton-insoluble fraction, indicative of actomyosin filament formation and activation of the contractile apparatus (Fig. 17) (Stasek et al., 1992a,b). Together, these studies strongly suggest that thrombin-stimulated endothelial cell contraction is causally related to subsequent barrier dysfunction.

B. PKC Regulation of Thrombin-Induced Barrier Dysfunction

There is now accumulating evidence that one mechanism by which increased $[Ca^{2+}]_i$ may increase permeability is by activation of Ca^{2+}-dependent PKC. Dose-dependent increases in albumin clearance rates occur in bovine pulmonary artery endothelial cells exposed to PMA, and more important, inhibition of endothelial PKC with H7 significantly reduces the permeability-increasing effects of α-thrombin (Lynch et al., 1990; Stasek et al., 1992a). This was temporally associated with light-microscopic evidence of PMA-mediated endothelial cell contraction (Antonov et al., 1986; Stasek et al., 1992a,b). PKC activation results in phosphorylation of cytoskeletal proteins in several tissues (Stasek et al., 1992a,b; Lynch et al., 1990; Werth et al., 1983; Wysolmerski and Lagunoff, 1990), including α-thrombin-challenged endothelium (Stasek et al., 1992a) leading to changes in endothelial cell shape and altered cell–cell contact (Garcia et al., 1986; Stasek et al., 1992b). For example, PKC mediates the phosphorylation of the actin- and calmodulin-binding protein $caldesmon_{77}$ and the intermediate filament protein vimentin, two specific cytoskeletal proteins present in vascular endothelium (Stasek et al., 1992a). The addition of threonine–sepharose chromatographically purified BPAEC PKC to unstimulated BPAEC homogenates, purified bovine platelet caldesmon ($caldesmon_{77}$), or purified smooth muscle caldesmon ($caldesmon_{150}$) produced marked caldesmon phosphorylation (Stasek et al., 1992a). Furthermore, $caldesmon_{77}$ and vimentin phosphorylation were observed in intact $[^{32}P]$ BPAEC monolayers stimulated with either PMA or α-thrombin, as detected by immunoprecipitation, immunoaffinity column chromatography, and affinity purification techniques (Fig. 18A and B) (Stasek et al., 1992a). These results demonstrate that thrombin- or PMA-stimulated PKC activity results in cytoskeletal protein phosphorylation in BPAEC monolayers, an event that is functionally linked to agonist-mediated endothelial cell contraction and resultant barrier dysfunction.

C. G Protein Regulation of Thrombin-Induced Barrier Dysfunction

We have recently investigated the role of G proteins in regulation of endothelial cell barrier function by assessing the effect of cholera toxin on human and bovine endothelial cell permeability properties. Pretreatment of either human or bovine monolayers with cholera toxin (1 μg/mL, 60 min), a dose and time that results in $G_{s\alpha}$ ADP ribosylation (Fig. 2), reduced basal transmonolayer flux of

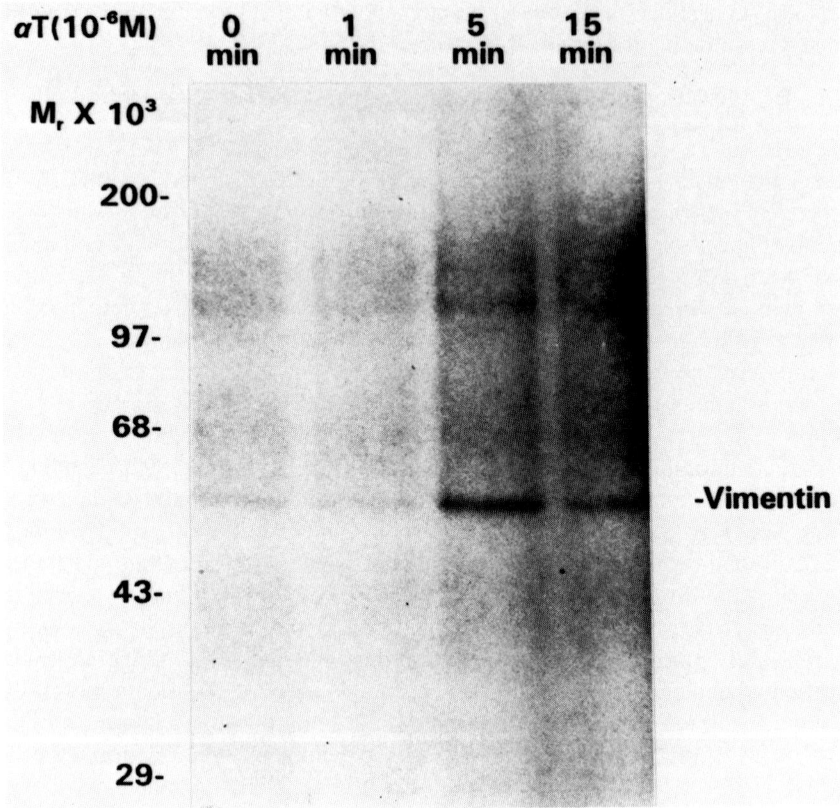

A

Figure 18 Agonist-induced vimentin phosphorylation in [^{32}P]-labeled BPAEC as detected by immunoprecipitation. Confluent BPAEC monolayers were labeled with [^{32}P]orthophosphate for 2 h (0.25 mCi/flask), followed by stimulation with 10^{-6} *M* α-thrombin or 10^{-7} *M* PMA for the time periods specified. Cellular proteins were SDS-solubilized, and vimentin was immunoprecipitated using anti-vimentin antibody. Isolated vimentin fractions were analyzed by SDS-PAGE, followed by immuno- blotting with anti-vimentin antibody, and subjected to autoradiography. Both α-thrombin (A) and PMA (B) induced a rapid, time-dependent increase in vimentin phosphorylation in intact BPAEC.

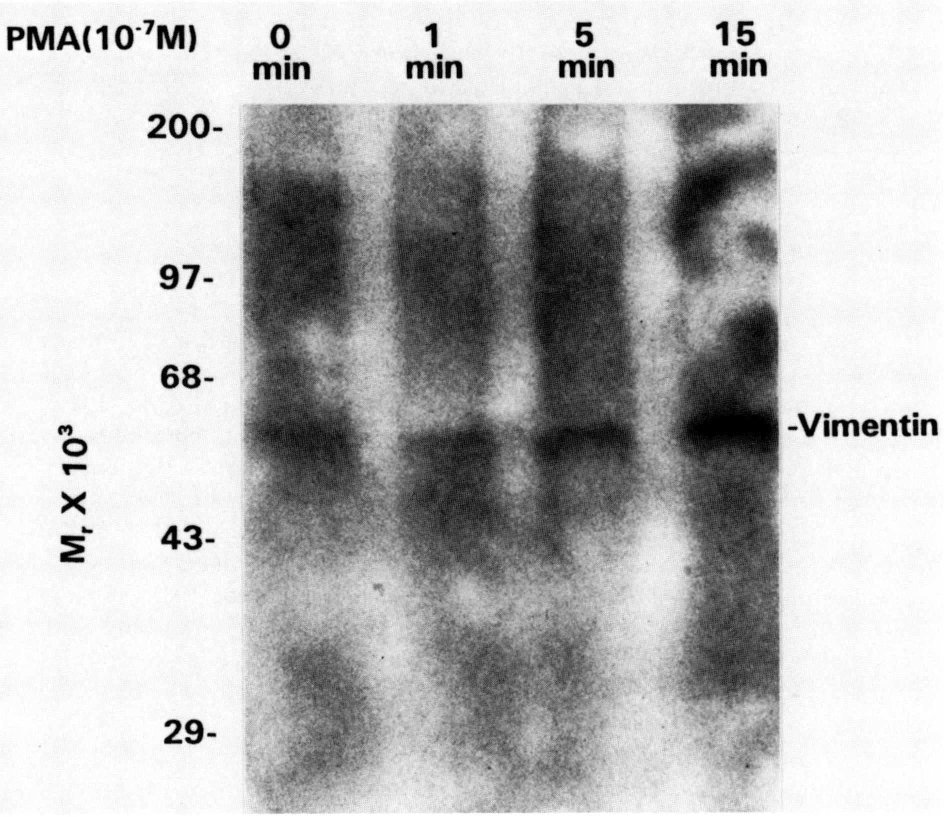

Evans Blue albumin across confluent monolayers grown on polycarbonate filters and also significantly attenuated α-thrombin-mediated increases in Evan's blue albumin flux (Garcia et al., 1991e; Patterson et al., 1992b). Pretreatment with cholera toxin also markedly attenuated thrombin-induced endothelial cell gap formation assessed by light microscopy, consistent with inhibition of thrombin-induced activation of the contractile apparatus. Cholera toxin produced significant dose- and time-dependent increases in cyclic AMP (10-fold increase at 30 min) (Garcia et al., 1991e; Patterson et al., 1992b), suggesting G_s-mediated adenylyl cyclase stimulation. Because cyclic AMP–dependent protein kinase

(PKA) is the only known target for cAMP, these studies indicate that G_s, via PKA activation, modulates thrombin-induced endothelial cell contraction and that barrier dysfunction and PKA-mediated relaxation may be critical to the maintenance of barrier function (Stelzner et al., 1989; Patterson et al., 1992b).

X. Oxidant-Induced Activation of Phospholipases and Modulation of Signal Transduction

Oxidants such as hydrogen peroxide (H_2O_2), superoxide anion ($O_2^{\bullet -}$) and hydroxyl radical (OH•) have been implicated in the pathophysiology of several forms of lung injury (Brigham, 1986; Cross, 1987; Heffner and Repine, 1989). These reactive species are normal constituents in the lung, and other cells and are present in very small amounts. Transformation of these reactive oxygen species to less active molecules by enzymatic and nonenzymatic mechanisms protects the cell from injury. An overload of active oxygen species results in oxidative modification of cellular lipids, proteins, carbohydrates, and nucleic acids, leading to cell injury and ultimate cell death (Trotta et al., 1981; Jornot et al., 1987). Within the lung, endothelial cells are in close proximity with neutrophils, monocytes and platelets that produce the reactive oxygen species when stimulated (Weiss et al., 1981). Oxidant-induced injury to the endothelium is therefore an important mechanism of vascular damage, and oxidants have been implicated in endothelial cell injury (Heffner and Repine, 1989), increased vascular permeability (Callahan and Garcia, 1987; Shasby et al., 1985; Garcia et al., 1986, 1988), thrombogenicity (Crapo et al., 1980), and pulmonary edema (Johnson et al., 1989).

The mechanisms by which oxidants alter endothelial cell function are not well understood but probably involve, at least in part, the modulation of phospholipase activities, resulting in altered signaling pathways. Exposure to oxidants causes several metabolic alterations, including permeability changes (Johnson et al., 1989; Shasby et al., 1985), activation of glutathione-redox cycle (Harlan et al., 1984), elevation of intracellular Ca^{2+} (Elliot et al., 1989), depletion of ATP and other high-energy phosphates (Andreoli, 1989), release of fatty acids, and increased prostanoid synthesis (Harlan and Callahan, 1984; Chakraborti et al., 1989). Oxidative stress causes membrane damage, which is often accompanied by hydrolysis of membrane lipids with accumulation of fatty acids and lysophospholipids. The release of free fatty acid and lysophospholipid suggest activation of phospholipase A_1 or A_2 (Harlan and Callahan, 1984; Chakraborti et al., 1989), while accumulation of DAG may be due to activation of PLC (Shasby et al., 1988).

A. Oxidant-Mediated Modulation of PLA_2 and Altered Prostaglandin Synthesis

Exposure of endothelial cells to oxidants such as H_2O_2 or *tert*-butylhydroperoxide (*t*-buOOH) increases synthesis of arachidonic acid metabolites. Increased PGI_2 synthesis was observed after exposure to H_2O_2 in endothelial cells from bovine pulmonary artery (Harlan and Callahan, 1984; Lewis et al., 1988; Chakraborti et al., 1989), bovine and porcine aorta (Ager and Gordon, 1984; Harlan and Callahan, 1984), and human umbilical vein (Harlan and Callahan, 1984; Lewis et al., 1988). In addition to PGI_2, increased prostaglandin E_2 (PGE_2) and 15-hydroxyeicosatetraenoic acid production was observed in bovine coronary artery endothelial cells (Callahan and Garcia, 1987). Similarly, exposure of bovine pulmonary artery endothelial cell to *t*-buOOH caused a dose-dependent increase in the release of [^{14}C]-labeled arachidonic acid and cyclooxygenase products such as thromboxane, PGE_2, PGD_2, and PGI_2 (Chakraborti et al., 1989). In contrast to the above-mentioned studies on oxidant-induced PGI_2 synthesis, Whorton et al. (1985) reported H_2O_2-mediated inhibition of PGI_2 synthesis to exogenous AA in cultured porcine aorta endothelial cells. In addition to H_2O_2, the superoxide-generating system, xanthine plus xanthine oxidase, also produced a similar inhibition of PGI_2 formation (Whorton et al., 1985). The inhibition of PGI_2 formation was attributed to H_2O_2 inhibition of cyclooxygenase activity exclusively without measurable effects on PGI_2 synthase or PLA_2 activities. A similar inhibition of PGI_2 and platelet activation factor synthesis in H_2O_2-treated human umbilical endothelial cells by thrombin has been observed (Vercellotti et al., 1990). In experiments using isolated rabbit lung, infusion of *t*-buOOH not only increased synthesis of cyclooxygenase-derived products thromboxane and prostacyclin but also elevated the levels of lipooxygenase-derived products leukotriene B_4, C_4, D_4, and E_4 (Farrukh et al., 1988). The physiological role of cyclooxygenase and lipooxygenase mediators in oxidant lung injury appears to be responsible for pulmonary vasoconstriction (Gurtner et al., 1983) and increase in vascular permeability (Tate et al., 1982).

The stimulation of prostaglandin production in endothelial cells due to oxidants could involve either (1) an increase in PLA_2 activity, (2) an increase in the conversion of released arachidonic acid to prostaglandins, and (3) increased availability of arachidonic acid for prostaglandin synthesis due to inhibition of reacylation of arachidonic acid to lyso PC catalyzed by acyltransferase. Although there is indirect evidence for the activation of PLA_2, cyclooxygenase, and lipooxygenase enzymes in endothelial cells (Harlan and Callahan, 1984; Chakrobarti et al., 1989), and perfused tissue (Farrukh et al., 1988) after exposure to oxidants, further studies are necessary to establish the mechanism(s) of increased prostaglandin synthesis.

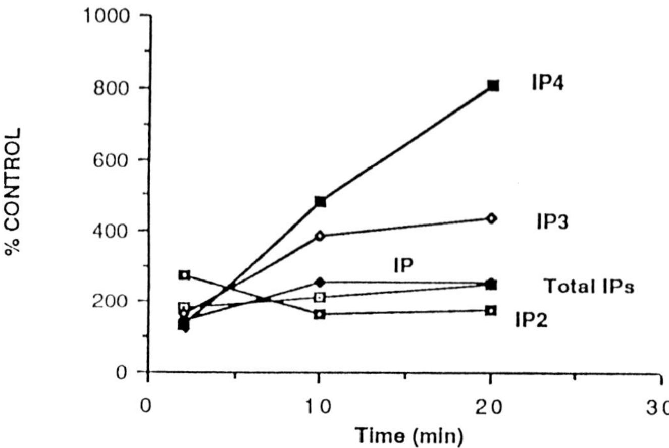

Figure 19 Effect of H_2O_2 on inositol phosphate release. Bovine pulmonary artery endothelial cells (2×10^6 cells/dish) were prelabeled with [^{3}H] inositol (5 μCi/flask) for 48 h. The monolayers were exposed to H_2O_2 (1 m*M*) in HEPES/glucose buffer containing 20 m*M* LiCl for 2, 10, and 20 min and inositol phosphates were extracted and determined by HPLC (Taylor et al., 1990b).

B. Oxidant-Mediated Activation of PLC

As discussed previously, agonist-induced, G_{PLC}-mediated, and PLC-catalyzed hydrolysis of PIP_2 represents an important signaling pathway in endothelial cells for the increase in intracellular free Ca^{2+} and activation of PKC. Recently, not only agonists, but also oxidants such as H_2O_2 and linoleic acid hydroperoxide (LOOH), have been noted to alter generation of water-soluble inositol phosphates. Shasby et al. (1988) showed H_2O_2 not only accelerated the release of AA but also the accumulation of lysophosphatidylinositol, DAG, and inositol phosphates in porcine pulmonary artery endothelial cells, suggesting oxidant-mediated activation of phospholipase A_1 or A_2 and PLC (Shasby et al., 1988). While only total inositol phosphates were measured in the foregoing studies, we have recently assessed changes in the levels of inositol tetrakisphosphate (IP_4), inositol trisphosphate (IP_3), inositol bisphosphate (IP_2), and inositol phosphate (IP) in [^{3}H]inositol-labeled bovine pulmonary artery endothelial cells exposed to 1 m*M* H_2O_2 (Fig. 19). Analysis of the aqueous/methanol phase of the lipid extract by HPLC revealed that H_2O_2 treatment for 2, 10, and 20 min increased the level of inositol phosphates recovered with maximal increases observed with IP_4 and IP_3 (V. Natarajan and J. G. N. Garcia, manuscript under preparation), although this appears to confirm an earlier report (Shasby et al., 1988) that increased accumulation of IP_3 after exposure to H_2O_2 is due to activation of PLC

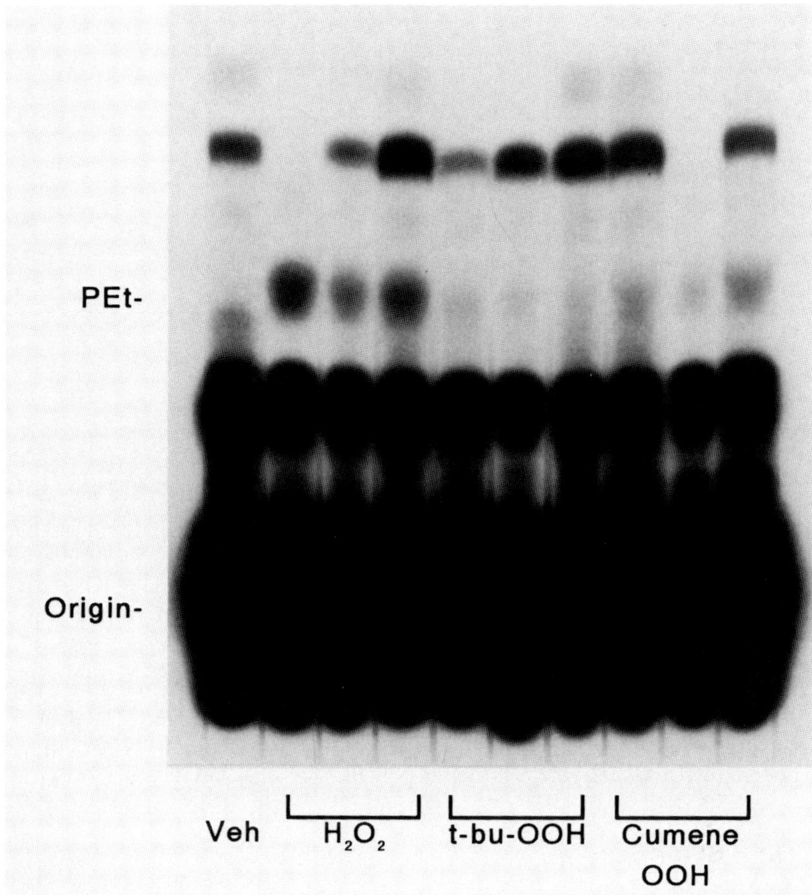

Figure 20 Localization of oxidant-induced accumulation of [^{32}P]PEt in BPAEC by autoradiography. BPAEC were prelabeled with [^{32}P]ortho phosphate (30 μCi/35-mm dish) for 24 h and were exposed to H_2O_2 (1 m*M*) or *tert*-butyl hydroperoxide (t-buOOH, 0.4 m*M*) or cumene hydroperoxide (CMOOH, 0.4 m*M*) for 90 min in 10 m*M* HEPES/150 m*M* NaCl/5.5 m*M* glucose/2 m*M* $MgCl_2$/2 m*M* EGTA (pH 7.4) containing 0.5% (85 m*M*) ethanol. Lipids were extracted under acidic conditions and [^{32}P]PEt was separated by TLC as described in Table 1.

in porcine endothelium. Pretreatment of human umbilical vein endothelial cells with varying levels of H_2O_2 (10^{-4} to 10^{-6} *M*) blocked the subsequent production of IP_3 in response to thrombin and histamine (Vercellotti et al., 1990). Further studies are required to more fully elucidate oxidant-stimulated PLC activities.

Table 5 Effect of H_2O_2, Linoleic Acid Hydroperoxide, and Iron on PLD Activation[a]

Addition	[^{32}P]PEt formed	% Control
Control	128 ± 24	100
H_2O_2 (1 m*M*)	544 ± 46*	425
LOOH (0.1 m*M*)	567 ± 31*	443
LOOH (0.4 m*M*)	793 ± 37*	620
H_2O_2 (1 m*M*) + $FeCl_2$ (100 μ*M*)	719 ± 40*	678
Con + $FeCl_2$ (100 μ*M*)	120 ± 26	100

[a]BPAECs were prelabeled with [^{32}P]orthophosphate (25 μCi/dish) for 24 h. Labeled cells were treated for 60 min with buffer or buffer-containing agents.
*Significantly different from control: $p < 0.005$.

C. Oxidant-Mediated Activation of PLD

Activation of PLD in response to external stimuli represents an important pathway in the generation of PA and DAG in endothelial cells. Experiments carried out with [^{32}P]orthophosphate-labeled bovine pulmonary artery endothelial cells incubated with H_2O_2, *t*-buOOH, and cumene hydroperoxide (CMOOH) revealed formation of phosphatidylethanol in the presence of ethanol due to activation of PLD (Fig. 20). In addition to H_2O_2, *t*-buOOH, CMOOH, and linoleic acid hydroperoxide (LOOH) also activated PLD (Table 5). The addition of $FeCl_2$ (100 μ*M*) also potentiated H_2O_2-induced [^{32}P]PEt formation (Table 5). These data demonstrate for the first time that H_2O_2 and other oxidants, including fatty acid hydroperoxides, can activate edothelial cell PLD (Natarajan et al., 1991).

XI. Summary

The regulation of endothelial cell stimulus–coupling events that lead to activation of membrane phospholipases is complex and involves PKC, G proteins(s), and elevation of intracellular Ca^{2+}. It is clear that binding of a wide variety of agonists, such as thrombin, bradykinin, histamine, ATP, and others, activate phospholipase A_2, C, and D activities in human umbilical vein and bovine pulmonary artery endothelial cells (Fig. 21). The sequence of activation of these phospholipases to an external stimulus is not well delineated but probably varies depending on the concentration, time of exposure, and source of the endothelial cells. An initial and critical event in endothelial cell activation is the PI-PLC-mediated breakdown of PIP_2, generating DAG and IP_3. Diacylglycerol and IP_3 act as intracellular second messengers in the interior of endothelial cell, thereby producing activation of PKC and raising intracellular Ca^{2+} concentrations, respectively. The increase in cytosolic free Ca^{2+} precedes PLA_2 and possibly PLD activity and governs the subsequent release of vasoactive molecules such

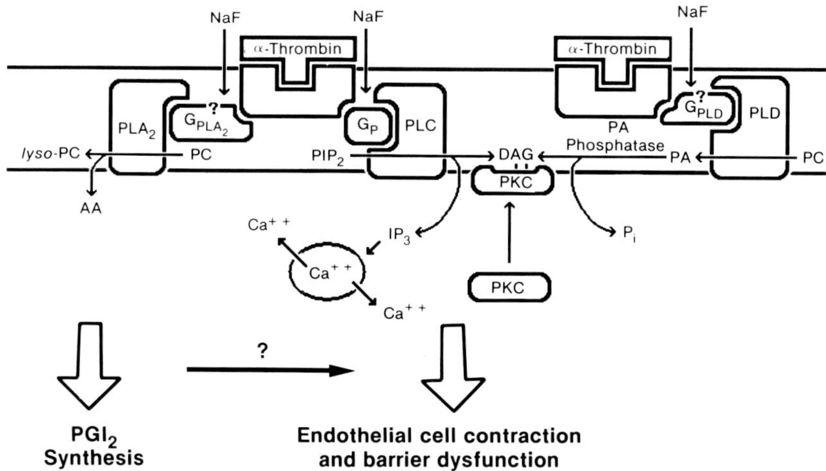

Figure 21 Potential pathways of endothelial cell activation by thrombin. The schema indicates that three membrane phospholipases are now recognized to be activated by occupancy of the thrombin receptor by proteolytically active thrombin. Interaction of thrombin with endothelial cell receptor(s) causes activation of PLC initially, with subsequent PLA_2, and PLD activation, resulting in generation of second messengers, which leads to endothelial cell contraction and alteration of barrier function as well as PGI_2 synthesis. Human endothelial cell PLC activation in response to thrombin stimulation involves receptor–G protein (G_P) interaction, resulting in PI-PLC-catalyzed hydrolysis of PIP_2 and subsequent production of DAG and IP_3. Activation of PKC directly stimulates PLD, which hydrolyzes membrane phospholipids, including PC, generating phosphatidic acid (PA). An increase in Ca_i^{2+} is essential to thrombin-induced PLD activity as well as PLA_2 activity, which results in arachidonate (AA) release and PGI_2 synthesis. Potentially, PA functions as an intracellular second messenger or is hydrolyzed by PA phosphatase to DAG, producing sustained activation of PKC. Thrombin-mediated PLD and/or PLA_2 activation may involve direct coupling of the enzyme to the receptor through a specific G protein (G_{PLD} or G_{PLA2}), but this is speculative.

as EDRF, prostacyclin, and other substances. Activation of PLA_2 and PLD in response to an agonist is therefore probably secondary to stimulation of PIP_2 specific PLC activity. Activation of PKC represents an important regulatory control in signal transduction in endothelial cells. PKC activation exerts multiple effects on agonist-induced modulation of phospholipases via negative-feedback inhibition of PLC and positive regulation of PLA_2 and PLD. PKC may be regulating AA release and subsequent PGI_2 synthesis possibly by lowering Ca^{2+} requirements for PLA_2 activity. In addition to PLA_2, PKC activation in endothelial cells exhibit a positive-feedback regulation of PLD stimulation and 70% of PLD activity is modulated by PKC in bovine endothelial cells.

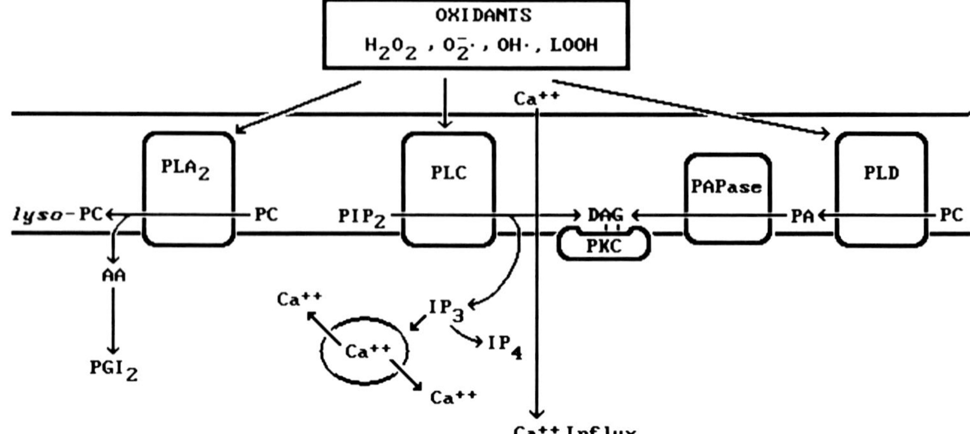

Figure 22 Oxidant-induced activation of phospholipases and generation of second messengers in endothelial cells. The schema indicates that phospholipases A_2, C, and D are activated by exposure of endothelial cells to hydrogen peroxide (H_2O_2), systems that generate superoxide anion radical ($O_2^{\bar{\bullet}}$) or hydroxyl radical (OH•) or fatty acid hydroperoxide (LOOH, linoleic acid hydroperoxide). The mechanism(s) of oxidant-induced activation of PLA_2, PLC, and PLD are not well understood, but phospholipase activation can generate second messengers. Activation of PLA_2 generates arachidonic acid (AA), which is further metabolized to oxygenated derivatives of AA by cyclooxygenase or lipoxygenase or cytochrome P_{450}–mediated enzyme. Stimulation of PLC can generate DAG and IP_3, which activates PKC and mobilize intracellular Ca^{2+}. Oxidants also stimulate PLD, resulting in the generation of phosphatidic acid (PA). PA thus generated can activate PKC directly or can be acted upon by PAPase to generate DAG independent of PLC pathway. Oxidants can also elevate intracellular Ca^{2+} by modulating the Ca^{2+} channels.

The physiologic role for PLD activation in endothelial cell signal transduction is not clear, but phosphatidic acid and lysophosphatidic acid generated by PLD may have second-messenger functions. Both PA and LPA have been reported to cause Ca^{2+} mobilization when added exogenously in various cell types (Putney et al., 1989; Moolenaar et al., 1986a; Kroll et al., 1989; Jalink et al., 1990) cause contraction of smooth muscle cells, inhibit adenylate cyclase (Muryama and Ui, 1985, 1987; Clark et al., 1980), and stimulate DNA synthesis and cell division in fibroblasts (Moolenaar et al., 1986b; Knauss et al., 1990). PLD activation and subsequent generation of PA has been functionally linked to activation of NADPH oxidase and superoxide anion generation in human neutrophils (Bonser et al., 1989; Rossi et al., 1990). Another potential function of PLD is the ability of the cell to generate DAG for a much prolonged period of time and thus bring about sustained activation of PKC, which may be a critical event for long-term responses such as cell proliferation. Further, PA and DAG generated through PAPase (Martin, 1988) may serve as a source of AA for eicosanoid synthesis (Lapetina et al., 1981).

It is evident that not only agonists like thrombin, but also oxidants such as H_2O_2, activate endothelial cell phospholipases independent of receptor/stimulus coupling. H_2O_2 and other oxidants, such as fatty acid hydroperoxide, induce activation of PLC, PLA_2, and PLD activities in endothelial cells (Fig. 22). The exact mechanism of oxidant-mediated activation of the phospholipases is not known, but their modulation can alter signal transduction pathways and barrier function. Regulation of phospholipases A_2, C, and D and the potential interaction between three different signaling pathways in endothelial cells needs further studies to better understand endothelial function in response to external stimuli.

Acknowledgments

The authors gratefully acknowledge the expert secretarial assistance of Shanna Dodd, and the contributions of Carolyn E. Patterson, Randal E. Dukes, R. Bruce Roehm, Paula L. Garcia, and Lakshmi Natarajan. Supported by Grants HL-02312 and HL-44746 (J.G.N.G.), from the NIH Heart, Lung, and Blood Institute, the Veteran's Administration Medical Research Service (J.G.N.G.), the American Heart Association–Indiana Affiliate (J.G.N.G.), and a Biomedical Research Support Grant from Indiana University School of Medicine (V.N.), and an American Lung Association Award (V.N.).

References

Ager, A., and Gordon, J. L. (1984). Differential effects of hydrogen peroxide on indices of endothelial cell function. *J. Exp. Med.* **159:**592.

Akiba, S., Sato, T., and Fujii, T. (1989). Differential effects of phorbol 12-myristate 13-acetate on GTPγS-induced diacylglycerol formation and arachidonate acid liberation in saponin-permeabilized rabbit platelets. *Thromb. Res.* **53:**503.

Aktories, R., Barmann, M., Ohishi, I., Tsuyama, S., Jakobs, K. H., and Habermann, E. (1986). Botulinum C2 toxin ADP-ribosylates actin. *Nature* **322:**390.

Allende, J. E. (1988). GTP-macromolecular interactions: The common features of different systems. *FASEB J.* **2:**2356.

Andreoli, S. P. (1989). Mechanisms of endothelial cell ATP deposits after oxidant injury. *Pediatr. Res.* **25:**97.

Anthes, J. C., Eckel, S., Siegel, M. I., Egan, R. W., and Bilah, M. M. (1989). Phospholipase D in homogenates from HL-60 granulocytes: Implications of calcium and G protein control. *Biochem. Biophys. Res. Commun.* **163:**657.

Antonov, A. S., Lukashev, M. E., Romanov, Y. A., Tkachuk, V. A., Repin, V. S., and

Smirnov, V. N. (1986). Morphological alterations in endothelial cells from human aorta and umbilical vein induced by forskolin and phorbol 12-myristate 13-acetate: A synergistic action of adenylate cyclase and protein kinase C activators. *Proc. Natl. Acad. Sci. USA* **83:**9704.

Aschner, J. L., Lennon, J. M., Fenton, J. W., Aschner, M., and Malik, A. B. (1990). Enzymatic activity is necessary for thrombin-mediated increase in endothelial permeability. *Am. J. Physiol.* **259**:L270–275.

Awbry, B. J., Hoak, J. C., and Owen, W. G. (1979). Binding of human thrombin to cultured human endothelial cells. *J. Biol. Chem.* **254:**4092.

Balsinde, J., Diez, E., and Mollinedo, F. (1988). Phosphatidyinositol specific phospholipase D: A pathway for generation of a second messenger. *Biochem. Biophys. Res. Commun.* **154:**502.

Barbacid, M. (1987). Ras genes. *Annu. Rev. Biochem.* **56:**779.

Bartha, K., Muller-Peddinghaus, R., and VanRooijen, L. A. A. (1989). Bradykinin and thrombin effects on polyphosphoinositide hydrolysis and prostacyclin production in endothelial cells. *Biochem. J.* **263:**149.

Berridge, M. J., and Irvine, R. F. (1984). Inositol trisphosphate, a novel second messenger in cellular signal transduction. *Nature* **308:**693.

Bigay, J., Deterrs, P., Pfister, C., and Chabre, M. (1985). Fluoroaluminates activate transducin-GDP by mimicking the γ phosphate of GTP in its binding site. *FEBS Lett.* **191:**181.

Billah, M. M., and Anthes, J. C. (1990). The regulations and cellular functions of phosphatidylcholine hydrolysis. *Biochem. J.* **269:**281.

Blackmore, P. F., and Exton, J. F. (1986). Studies on the hepatic calcium activity of aluminum fluoride and glucagon. *J. Biol. Chem.* **261:**11056.

Bocckino, S. B., Wilson, P. B., and Exton, J. H. (1987). Ca^{2+}-mobilizing hormones elicit phosphatidylethanol accumulation via phospholipase D activation. *FEBS Lett.* **255:**201.

Bonser, R. W., Thompson, N. T., Randall, R. W., and Garland, L. G. (1989). Phospholipase D activation is functionally linked to superoxide generation in the human neutrophil. *Biochem. J.* **264:**617.

Brigham, K. L. (1986). Role of free radicals in lung injury. *Chest* **89:**859.

Brock, T. A., and Capasso, E. A. (1988). Thrombin and histamine activate phospholipase C in human endothelial cells via a phorbol ester–sensitive pathway. *J. Cell. Physiol.* **136:**54.

Brock, T. A., and Capasso, E. L. (1989). GTPγS increases thrombin-mediated inositol trisphosphate accumulation in permeabilized human endothelial cells. *Am. Rev. Respir. Dis.* **140:**1121.

Brock, T. A., Dennis, P. A., Griendling, K. K., Diehl, T. S., and Davies, P. F. (1988). GTPγS loading of endothelial cells stimulated phospholipase C and uncoupled ATP receptors. *Am. J. Physiol.* **225:**667.

Burch, R. M., Luini, A., and Axelrod, J. (1986). Phospholipase A_2 and phospholipase C are activated by distinct GTP-binding proteins in response to α_1-adrenergic stimulation in FRTL5 thyroid cells. *Proc. Natl. Acad. Sci. USA* **83:**7201.

Callahan, K. S., and Garcia, J. G. N. (1987). Effects of hyperoxic exposure on cultured bovine coronary artery endothelium (BCAs). *Circ. Res.* **76:**54.

Camussi, G., Aglietta, M., Malavasi, F., Tetta, C., Piacibello, W., Sanavio, F., and Bussolino, F. (1983). The release of platelet-activating factor from human endothelial cells in culture. *J. Immunol.* **131:**2397.

Carlson, K. E., Brass, L. F., and Manning, D. R. (1989). Thrombin and phorbol esters cause the selective phosphorylation of a G-protein other than G_i in human platelets. *J. Biol. Chem.* **264:**13298.

Carney, D. H., Stiernberg, J., and Fenton, J. W. (1984). Initiation of proliferative events by human a-thrombin requires both receptor binding and enzymic activity. *J. Cell. Biochem.* **256:**181.

Carney, D. H., Herbosa, G. J., Stiernberg, J., Bergmann, J. S., Gordon, E. A., Scott, D., and Fenton, J. W. (1986). Double-signal hypothesis for thrombin initiation of cell proliferation. *Semin. Thromb. Hemost.* **12:**231.

Carson, M. R., Shasby, S. S., and Shasby, D. M. (1989). Histamine and inositol phosphate accumulation in endothelium: cAMP and a G protein. *Am. J. Physiol.* **257:**L259.

Carter, D. T., Hallam, T. J., and Pearson, J. D. (1989a). Protein kinase C activation alters the sensitivity of agonist-stimulated endothelial cell prostacyclin production to intracellular Ca^{2+}. *Biochem. J.* **262:**431.

Carter, A. J., Eisert, W. G., and Muller, T. H. (1989b). Thrombin stimulates inositol phosphate accumulation and prostacyclin synthesis in human endothelial cells from umbilical vein but not from omentum. *Thromb. Haemost.* **61:**122.

Chakraborti, S., Gurtner, G. H., and Michael, J. R. (1989). Oxidant-mediated activation of phospholipase A_2 in pulmonary endothelium. *Am. J. Physiol.* **257:**L430.

Chalifa, V., Mohn, H., and Liscovitch, M. (1990). A neutral phospholiase D activity from rat brain synaptic plasma membranes. *J. Biol. Chem.* **265:**17512.

Chattopadhyay, J., Natarajan, V., and Schmid, H. H. O. (1991). Membrane-associated phospholipase D activity in rat sciatic nerve. *J. Neurochem.* (in press).

Clark, R. B., Salmon, D. M., and Honeyman, T. W. (1980). Phosphatidic acid inhibition of cAMP accumulation in WI-38 fibroblasts: Similarities with carbachol inhibition. *J. Cyclic Nucleotide Res.* **6:**37.

Cockroft, S., and Bar-Saci, D. (1990). Effect of H-ras proteins on the activity of polyphosphoinositide. Phospholipase C in HL60 membranes. *Cell. Signal.* **2:**227.

Cockroft, S., and Gomperts, B. D. (1985). Role of guanine nucleotide regulatory binding proteins in the activation of polyphosphoinositide phosphodiesterase. *Nature* **314:**534.

Cockroft, S., Baldwin, J. M., and Allan, D. (1985). The Ca_{++}-activated polyphosphoinositide phosphodiesterase of human and rabbit neutrophil membranes. *Biochem. J.* **221:**477.

Colden-Stanfield, M., Schilling, W. P., Ritchie, A. K., Esrin, S. G., Navarro, L. T., and Kunze, D. N. (1987). Bradykinin-induced increases in cytosolic calcium and ionic currents in cultured bovine aortic endothelial cells. *Circ. Res.* **61:**632.

Connolly, T. M., Lawing, W. J., Jr., and Majerus, P. W. (1986). Protein kinase C phosphorylates human platelet inositol trisphosphate 5′-phosphomonoesterase, increasing the phosphatase activity. *Cell* **46:**951.

Crapo, S. D., Barry, B. E., Fosue, H. A., and Shelburne, J. (1980). Structural and biochemical changes in rat lungs occurring during exposure to lethal and adaptive doses of oxygen. *Am. Rev. Respir. Dis.* **122:**123.

Crooke, S. T., and Bennett, C. F. (1989). Mammalian phosphoinositide-specific phospholipase C isoenzymes. *Cell. Calcium* **10:**309.

Cross, C. E. (1987). Oxygen radicals and human disease. *Ann. Intern. Med.* **107:**526.

Crouch, M. D., and Lapetina, E. G. (1988a). A role for G_i in control of thrombin receptor–phospholipase C coupling in human platelets. *J. Biol. Chem.* **263:**3363.

Crouch, M. F., and Lapetina, E. G. (1988b). No direct correlation between Ca^{2+} mobilization and dissociation of G_i during platelet phospholipase A_2 activation. *Biochem. Biophys. Res. Commun.* **153:**21.

Davitz, M. A., Hom, J., and Schenkman, S. (1989). Purification of a glycosyl-phosphatidylinositol–specific phospholipase D from human plasma. *J. Biol. Chem.* **264:**13760.

Demolle, D., and Boeynaems, J. M. (1988). Role of protein kinase C in the control of vascular prostacyclin: Study of phorbol esters effect in bovine aortic endothelium and smooth muscle. *Prostaglandins* **35:**243.

Derian, C. K., and Moskowitz, M. A. (1986). Polyphosphoinositide hydrolysis in endothelial cells and carotid artery segments. *J. Biol. Chem.* **261:**3831.

DiCorleto, P. E., and Bowen-Pope, D. F. (1983). Cultured endothelial cells produce a platelet-derived growth factor-like protein. *Proc. Natl. Acad. Sci. USA* **80:**1919.

Dominguez, J. H., Rothrock, J. K., Macias, W. L., and Price, J. (1989). Na^+ electrochemical gradient and Na^+–Ca^{2+} exchange in rat proximal tubule. *Am. J. Physiol.* **257:**F531.

Domino, S. E., Bocckino, S. B., and Garbers, D. L. (1989). Activation of phospholipase D by the fucose-sulfate glycoconjugate that induces an acrosome reaction in spermatozoa. *J. Biol. Chem.* **264:**9412.

Dukes, R. E., Garcia, P. L., and Garcia, J. G. N. (1991). Effect of botulinum toxin C on endothelial cell signal transduction. *FASEB J.* **8:**A2620.

Elliott, S. J., Eskins, S. G., and Schilling, W. P. (1989). Effect of t-butyl-hydroperoxide in bradykinin-stimulated changes in cytosolic calcium in vascular endothelial cells. *J. Biol. Chem.* **264:**3806.

Esmon, C. T., and Owen, W. G. (1981). Identification of an endothelial cell cofactor for thrombin-catalyzed activation of protein kinase C. *Proc. Natl. Acad. Sci USA* **78:**2249.

Exton, J. H. (1990). Signaling through phosphatidylcholine breakdown. *J. Biol. Chem.* **265:**1.

Farrukh, I. S., Michael, J. R., Peters, S. P., Sciuto, M., Adminson, N. F., Freeland, H. S., Paky, A., Spannhake, E. W., Summer, W. R., and Gurtner, G. H. (1988). The role of cyclooxygenase and lipoxygenase mediators in oxidant-induced lung injury. *Am. Rev. Respir. Dis.* **137:**1343.

Fenton, J. W., II. (1988). Regulation of thrombin generation and functions. *Semin. Thromb. Hemost.* **14:**234.

Forsberg, E. J., Feuerstein, G., Shohami, E., and Pollard, H. B. (1987). Adenosine triphosphate stimulates inositol phospholipid metabolism and prostacyclin formation in adrenal medullary endothelial cells by means of P_2-purinergic receptors. *Proc. Natl. Acad. Sci. USA* **84:**5630.

Galdal, K. S., Lybert, T., Evensen, S. A., Nilsen, E., and Prydz, H. (1985). Thrombin induces thromboplastin synthesis in cultured vascular endothelial cells. *Thromb. Haemost.* **54:**373.

Garcia, J. G. N., and Natarajan, V. (1990). Thrombin is a potent activator of human endothelial cell phospholipase D. Regulation by protein kinase C and cytosolic Ca^{2+}. *Clin. Res.* **38:**873A.

Garcia, J. G. N., Birnboim, A. S., Bizios, R., DelVecchio, P. J., Fenton, J. W., II, and Malik, A. B. (1986). Thrombin-induced increases in albumin clearance across cultured endothelial monolayers. *J. Cell. Physiol.* **128:**96.

Garcia, J. G. N., Perlman, M. B., Ferro, T. J., Johnson, A., Jubiz, W., and Malik, A. (1988). Inflammatory events following fibrin microembolization: Alterations in alveolar macrophage and neutrophil function. *Am. Rev. Respir. Dis.* **137:**630.

Garcia, J. G. N., Painter, R. G., Fenton, J. W., English, D., and Callahan, K. S. (1990). Thrombin-induced human endothelial cell PGI_2 biosynthesis. Role of guanine nucleotide-regulatory proteins. *J. Cell. Physiol.* **142:**186.

Garcia, J. G. N., Dominguez, J., and English, D. (1991a). Sodium fluoride induces phosphoinositide hydrolysis, Ca_{++} mobilization and prostacyclin synthesis in cultured human endothelium. Further evidence for regulation by a pertussis toxin-insensitive guanine nucleotide binding protein. *Am. J. Respir. Cell Molec. Biol.* **5:**113–124.

Garcia, J. G. N., Patterson, C. E., Davis, H. W., and Dukes, R. E. (1991b). Role of cholera toxin-sensitive G-proteins in regulation of thrombin-induced barrier dysfunction. *Am. Rev. Respir. Dis.* **143:**A371.

Garcia, J. G. N., Fenton, J. W., and Natarajan, V. (1992a). Thrombin stimulation of human endothelial cell phospholipase D activity. Regulation by protein kinase C and cyclic adenosine 3′5′-monophosphate. *Blood* (in press).

Garcia, J. G. N., Aschner, J., and Malik, A. B. (1992b). Regulation of thrombin-induced endothelial cell prostaglandin synthesis and barrier function. In *Thrombin: Structure and Function.* Edited by L. J. Berliner. Plenum Publishing Co., New York (in press).

Garcia, J. G. N., Stasek, J. E., Natarajan, V., Patterson, C. E., and Dominguez, J. D. (1992c). Role or protein kinase C in the regulation of prostaglandin synthesis in human endothelium. *Am. J. Respir. Cell Molec. Biol.* (in press).

Gelas, P., Ribbes, G., Record, M., Terce, F., and Chap, H. (1989). Differential activation by f Met-Leu-Phe and phorbol ester of a plasma membrane phosphatidylcholine-specific phospholipase D in human neutrophil. *FEBS Lett.* **251:**213.

Gelehrter, T. D., and Sznycer-Laszuk, R. (1986). Thrombin induction of plasminogen activator-inhibitor in cultured endothelial cells. *J. Clin. Invest.* **77:**165.

Gilman, A. G. (1984). G proteins and dual control of adenylate cyclase. *Cell* **36:**577.

Gilman, A. G. (1987). G proteins: Transducers of receptor-generated signals. *Annu. Rev. Biochem.* **56:**615.

Glenn, K. C., and Cunningham, D. D. (1979). Thrombin-stimulated cell division involves proteolysis of its cell surface receptor. *Nature* **278:**711.

Glenn, K. C., Carney, D. H., Fenton, J. W., and Cunningham, D. D. (1980). Thrombin active site regions required for fibroblast receptor binding and initiation of cell division. *J. Biol. Chem.* **255:**6609.

Goldsmith, J. G., and Needleman, S. N. (1982). A comparative study of thromboxane and prostacyclin release from ex-vivo and cultured bovine vascular endothelium. *Prostaglandins* **24:**73.

Goligorsky, M. S., Menton, D. N., Laslo, A., and Lum, H. (1989). Nature of thrombin-induced sustained increase in cytosolic calcium concentration in cultured endothelial cells. *J. Biol. Chem.* **264:**16771.

Gospodarowicz, D., Brown, C. D., Birdwell, C. R., and Zetter, B. R. (1978). Control of proliferation of human vascular endothelial cells. *J. Cell Biol.* **77:**774.

Gurtner, G. H., Knoblanch, A., Smith, P. S., Sies, H., and Adkinson, N. F., Jr. (1983). Oxidant- and lipid-induced pulmonary vasoconstriction mediated by arachidonic acid metabolites. *J. Appl. Physiol.* **59:**953.

Hallam, T. J., and Pearson, J. D. (1986). Exogenous ATP raises cytoplasmic free calcium in Fura-2 loaded piglet aortic endothelial cells. *FASEB Lett.* **207:**95.

Hallam, T. J., Pearson, J. D., and Needham, L. A. (1988). Thrombin-stimulated elevation of human endothelial-cell cytoplasmic free calcium concentration causes prostacyclin production. *Biochem. J.* **251:**243.

Halldorsson, H., Kjeld, M., and Thorgeirsson, G. (1988). Role of phosphoinositides in the regulation of endothelial prostacyclin production. *Arteriosclerosis* **8:**147.

Harlan, J. M., and Callahan, K. S. (1984). Role of hydrogen peroxide in the neutrophil-mediated release of prostacyclin from cultured endothelial cells. *J. Clin. Invest.* **74:**442.

Harlan, J. M., Levine, J. D., Callahan, K. S., Schwartz, B. R., and Harker, L. A. (1984). Glutathione redox cycle protects cultured endothelial cells against lysis by extracellularly generated hydrogen peroxide. *J. Clin. Invest.* **73:**706.

Harlan, J. M., Thompson, P. J., Ross, R. R. and Bowen-Pope, D. F. (1986). α-Thrombin induced release of platelet-derived growth factor-like molecule(s) by cultured human endothelial cells. *J. Cell. Physiol.* **103:**1129.

Heffner, J. E., and Repine, J. E. (1989). Pulmonary strategies of antioxidant-defense. *Am. Rev. Respir. Dis.* **140:**531.

Heller, M. (1978). Phospholipase D. *Adv. Lipid Res.* **16:**267.

Hirata, F., Matsuda, K., Notsu, Y., Hattori, T., and DelCarmine, R. (1981). Phosphoryla tion at a tyrosine residue of lipomodulin in mitogen-stimulated murine thymocytes. *Proc. Natl. Acad. Sci. USA* **81:**9717.

Hokin, M. R., and Hokin, L. E. (1953). Enzyme secretion and the incorporation of P_{32} into phospholipides of pancreas slices. *J. Biol. Chem.* **203:**967.

Hong, S. L. (1980). Effect of bradykinin and thrombin on prostacyclin synthesis in endothelial cells from calf and pig aorta and human umbilical cord veins. *Thromb. Res.* **18:**787.

Hong, S. L., and Deykin, D. (1982). Activation of phospholipases A_2 and C in pig aortic endothelial cells synthesizing prostacyclin. *J. Biol. Chem.* **257:**7151.

Hong, S. L., McLaughlin, N. J., Tzeng, C., and Patton, G. (1985). Prostacyclin synthesis and deacylation of phospholipids in human endothelial cells: Comparison of thrombin, histamine and ionomycin. *Thromb. Res.* **38:**1.

Horie, S., Ishii, H., and Kazama, M. (1990). Heparine-like glycosaminoglycan is a receptor for antithrombin III-dependent but not for thrombin-dependent prostacyclin production in human endothelial cells. *Thromb. Res.* **59:**895.

Huang, C., and Cabot, M. C. (1990). Phorbol diesters stimulate the accumulation of phosphatidate, phosphatidylethanol, and diacylglycerol in three cell types. *J. Biol. Chem.* **265:**14858.

Huang, K-S., Li, S., Fung, W.-J. C., Hulmes, J. D., Reik, L., Pan, Y.-C. C., and Low, M. G. (1990). Purification and characterization of glycosyl-phosphatidylinositol-specific phospholipase D. *J. Biol. Chem.* **265:**17738.

Jacob, R. (1990). Agonist-stimulated divalent cation entry into single cultured human umbilical vein endothelial cells. *J. Physiol.* **421:**55.

Jaffe, E. A., Grulich, J., Weksler, B. B., Hampel, G., and Watanabe, K. (1987). Correlation between thrombin-induced prostacyclin production and inositol trisphosphate and cytosolic free calcium levels in cultured human endothelial cells. *J. Biol. Chem.* **262:**8557.

Jalink, K., Van Corven, E. J., and Moolenaar, W. H. (1990). Lysophosphatidic acid but not phosphatidic acid is a potent Ca^{2+}-mobilizing stimulus for fibroblasts. Evidence for an extracellular site of action. *J. Biol. Chem.* **265:**12232.

Jelsema, C. L., and Axelrod, J. (1987). Stimulation of phospholipase A2 in bovine rod outer segment by the beta-gamma subunits of transducing and its inhibition by the alpha subunit. *Proc. Natl. Acad. Sci.* USA **84:**3623.

Jeremy, J. Y., and Dandona, P. (1988). Fluoride stimulates in vitro vascular prostacyclin synthesis: Interrelationship of G proteins and protein kinase C. *J. Pharm. Pharmacol.* **146:**279.

Johnson, A., and Malik, A. B. (1985). Pulmonary transvascular fluid and protein exchange after thrombin-induced microembolism. *Am. Rev. Respir. Dis.* **132:**70.

Johnson, A. R., Revtyak, G., and Campbell, W. B. (1985). Arachidonic acid metabolites and endothelial injury: Studies with cultures of human endothelial cells. *Fed. Proc.* **44:**19.

Johnson, A., Phillips, P., Hocking, D., Tsan, M.-F., and Ferro, T. (1989). Protein kinase inhibitor promotes pulmonary edema in response to H_2O_2. *Am. J. Physiol.* **256:**H1012.

Jornot, L., Mirault, M. E., and Junod, A. F. (1987). Protein synthesis in hyperoxic endothelial cells: Evidence for translational defect. *J. Appl. Physiol.* **63:**457.

Kajiyama, Y., Murayama, T., and Nomura, Y. (1989). Pertussis toxin-sensitive GTP-binding proteins may regulate phospholipas A_2 in response to thrombin in rabbit platelets. *Arch. Biochem. Biophys.* **274:**200.

Kanzaki, T., Morisake, N., Saito, Y., and Yoshida, S. (1989). Phorbol myristate enhanced specific incorporation of arachidonic acid into phospholipids through lysophospholipid acyltransferase in cultured smooth muscle cells. *Lipids* **24:**1024.

Katada, T., Gilman, A. G., Watanabe, Y., Bauer, S., and Jakobs, K. H. (1985). Protein kinase C phosphorylates the inhibitory guanine-nucleotide-binding regulatory component and apparently suppresses its function in hormonal inhibition of adenylate cylase. *Eur. J. Biochem.* **151:**431.

Kater, L. A., Goetzel, E. J., and Austen, K. F. (1976). Isolation of human eosinophil phospholipase D. *J. Clin. Invest.* **57:**1173.

Kester, M., Simonson, M. S., Mene, P., and Sedov, J. R. (1989). Interleukin-1 generates transmembrane signals from phospholipids through novel pathways in cultured rat mesangial cells. *J. Clin.* Invest. **83:**718.

King, W. G., and Rittenhouse, S. E. (1989). Inhibition of protein kinase C by staurosporine promotes elevated accumulations of inositol trisphosphates and tetrakisphosphate in human platelets exposed to thrombin. *J. Biol. Chem.* **264**(11):6070.

Kiss, Z., and Anderson, W. B. (1989). Phorbol ester stimulates the hydrolysis of phosphatidylethanolamine in leukemia HL-60 NIH 3T3 and baby hamster kidney cells. *J. Biol. Chem.* **264:**1483.

Kitazono, T., Takeshige, K., Cragoe, E. J., and Minakami, S. (1989). Involvement of calcium and protein kinase C in the activation of the Na_+/H_+ exchanger in cultured bovine aortic endothelial cells stimulated by extracellular ATP. *Biochim. Biophys. Acta* **1013:**152.

Knauss, T. C., Jaffer, F. E., and Abboud, H. E. (1990). Phosphatidic acid modulates DNA synthesis, phospholipase C, and platelet-derived growth factor mRNAs in cultured mesangial cells. Role of protein kinase C. *J. Biol. Chem.* **265:**14457.

Kobayashi, M., and Kanfer, J. N. (1987). Phosphatidylethanol formation via transphosphatidylation by rat brain synaptosome phospholipase D. *J. Neurochem.* **48:**1597.

Krishnamurthi, S., Wheeler-Jones, C. P. D., and Kakkar, V. V. (1989). Effect of phorbol ester treatment on receptor-mediated versus G-protein-activator-mediated responses in platelets. Evidence for a two-site action of phorbol ester at the level of G-protein function. *Biochem. J.* **262:**77.

Kroll, M. H., Zovoico, G. B., and Schafer, A. I. (1989). Second messenger function of phosphatidic acid in platelet activation. *J. Cell. Physiol.* **139:**558.

Lambert, T. L., Kent, R. S., and Whorton, A. R. (1986). Bradykinin stimulation of inositol polyphosphate production in porcine aortic endothelial cells. *J. Biol. Chem.* **261:**15288.

Lampugnani, M. G., Pedenovi, M., Dejana, E., Rotilio, D., Donati, M. B., Bussolino, F., Garbarino, G., Ghigo, D., and Bosia, A. (1989). Human α-thrombin induced phos phoinositide turnover and Ca^{2+} movements in cultured human umbilical vein endothelial cells. *Thromb. Res.* **54:**75.

Lapetina, E. G., Billah, M. M., and Cuatrecasas, P. (1981). The initial action of thrombin on platelets. Conversion of phosphatidylinositol to phosphatidic acid preceding the production of arachidonic acid. *J. Biol. Chem.* **256:**5037.

Lapetina, E. G., Lacal, J. C., Reep, B. R., and Vedia, L. M. Y. (1989). A ras-related protein in phosphorylated and translocated by agonists that increase cAMP levels in human platelets. *Proc. Natl. Acad. Sci. USA* **86:**3131.

Levin, E. G., Marzec, U., Anderson, J., and Harker, L. A. (1984). Thrombin stimulates tissue plasminogen activator release from cultured human endothelial cells. *J. Clin. Invest.* **74:**1988.

Levine, J. D., Harlan, J. M., Harker, L. A., Joseph, M. L., and Counts, R. B. (1982). Thrombin-mediated release of factor VIII antigen from human umbilical vein endothelial cells in culture. *Blood* **60:**531.

Lewis, M. S., Whatley, R. E., Cain, P., McIntyre, T. M., Prescott, S. M., and Zimmerman, G. A. (1988). Hydrogen peroxide stimulates the synthesis of platelet-activating factor by endothelium and induces endothelial cell-dependent neutrophil adhesion. *J. Clin. Invest.* **82:**2045.

Lo, W. W. Y., and Fan, T. P. D. (1987). Histamine stimulates inositol phosphate accumulation via the H1-receptor in cultured human endothelial cells. *Biochem. Biophys. Res. Commun.* **148:**47.

Lollar, P., and Owen, W. G. (1980a). Clearance of thrombin from circulation in rabbits by high-affinity binding sites on endothelium. *J. Clin. Invest.* **66:**1222.

Lollar, P., and Owen, W. G. (1980b). Evidence that the effect of thrombin on arachidonate metabolism in cultured human endothelial cells are not mediated by a high affinity receptor. *J. Biol. Chem.* **255:**8031.

Lollar, P., Hoak, J. C., and Owen, W. G. (1980). Binding of thrombin to cultured human endothelial cells. *J. Biol. Chem.* **255:**10279.

Luckoff, A., and Busse, R. (1986). Increased free calcium in endothelial cells under stimulation with adenine nucleotides. *J. Cell. Physiol.* **126:**414.

Lum, H., DelVecchio, P. J., Schneider, A. S., Goligorsky, M. S., and Malik, A. B. (1989) Calcium independence of the thrombin-induced increase in endothelial albumin permeability. *J. Appl. Physiol.* **66:**1471.

Lynch, J. J., Ferro, T. J., Blumenstock, F. A., Brochenauer, A. B., and Malik, A. B. (1990). Increased endothelial albumin permeability mediated by protein kinase C activation. *J. Clin. Invest.* **85:**1991.

Magnusson, M. K., Halldorsson, H., Kjeld, M., and Thorgeirsson, G. (1989). Endothelial inositol phosphate generation and prostacyclin production in response to G-protein activation by AIF_{4-}- *Biochem. J.* **264:**703.

Marcus, A. J. (1978). The role of lipids in platelet function with particular reference to arachidonic acid pathways. *J. Lipid. Res.* **19:**793.

Martin, T. W. (1988). Formation of diacylglycerol by a phospholipase D-phosphatidate phosphatase pathway specific for phosphatidylcholine in endothelial cells. *Biochim. Biophys. Acta* **962:**282.

Martin, T. W., and Michaelis, K. C. (1988). Bradykinin stimulates phosphodiesteric cleavage of phosphatidylcholine in activated endothelial cells. *Biochem. Biophys. Res. Commun.* **157:**1271.

Martin, T. W., and Michaelis, K. (1989). P_2-Purinergic agonists stimulate phosphodiesteratic cleavage of phosphatidylcholine in endothelial cells. Evidence for activation of phospholipase D. *J. Biol. Chem.* **264:**8847.

Martin, T. W., and Wysolmerski, R. B. (1987). Ca^{2+}-dependent and Ca^{2+}-independent pathways for release of arachidonic acid from phosphatidylinositol in endothelial cells. *J. Biol. Chem.* **262:**13086.

Martin, T. W., Feldman, D. R., Goldstein, K. E., and Wagner, J. R. (1989). Long-term phorbol ester treatment dissociates phospholipase D activation from phosphoinositide hydrolysis and prostacyclin synthesis in endothelial cells stimulated with bradykinin. *Biochem. Biophys. Res. Commun.* **165:**319.

Moolenaar, W. H., Aerts, R. J., Tertoolen, L. G. J., and deLaat, S. W. (1986a). The epidermal growth factor-induced calcium signal in A431 cells. *J. Biol. Chem.* **261:**279.

Moolenaar, W. H., Kruijer, W., Tilly, B. C., Verlaan, I., Bierman, A. J., and de Laat, S. W. (1986b). Growth factor-like action of phosphatidic acid. *Nature* **323:**171.

Moriarty, T. M., Padrell, E., Carty, D. J., Omri, G., Landau, E. M., and Iyengar. (1990). G_o Proteins as signal transducer in the pertussis toxin–sensitive phosphoinositol pathway. *Nature* **343:**79.

Moscat, J., Moreno, F., and Garcia-Barreno, P. (1987a). Binding of thrombin to cultured human endothelial cells. *Biochem. Biophys. Res. Commun.* **145:**1302.

Moscat, J., Moreno, F., and Garcia-Barreno, P. (1987b). Mitogenic activity and inositide metabolism in thrombin-stimulated pig aorta endothelial cells. *Biochem. Biophys. Res. Commun.* **145:**1302.

Moscat, J., Moreno, F., Herrero, C., Lopez, Garcia-Barreno, P. (1988). A23187 stimulation of production of inositol phosphates in porcine aorta endothelial cells. *Proc. Natl. Acad. Sci. USA* **85:**659.

Muldoon, L. L., Jamieson, G. A., Jr., and Villereal, M. L. (1987). Calcium mobilization in permeabilized fibroblasts: Effects of inositol trisphosphate, orthovanadate, mitogens, phorbol ester and guanosine trisphosphate. *J. Cell. Physiol.* **130:**29.

Murayama, T., and Ui, M. (1985). Receptor-mediated inhibition of adenylate cyclase and stimulation of arachidonic acid release of 3T3 fibroblasts. Selective susceptibility to islet-activating protein, pertussis toxin. *J. Biol. Chem.* **260:**7226.

Murayama, T., and Ui, M. (1987). Phosphatidic acid may stimulate membrane receptors mediating adenylate cyclase inhibition and phospholipid breakdown in 3T3 fibroblasts. *J. Biol. Chem.* **262:**5522.

Myers, C. L., Lazo, J. S., and Pitt, B. R. (1989). Translocation of protein kinase C is associated with inhibition of 5-HT uptake by cultured endothelial cells. *Am. J. Physiol.* **257:**L253.

Nakashima, S., Hattori, H., Shirato, L., Takenaka, A., and Nozawa, Y. (1988). Differential sensitivity of arachidonic acid release and 1,2-diacylglycerol formation to pertussis toxin, GDP S and NaF in saponin-permeabilized human platelets: Possible evidence for distinct GTP-binding proteins involving phospholipase C and A_2 activation. *Biochem. Biophys. Res. Commun.* **148:**971.

Natarajan, V., and Garcia, J. G. N. (1990a). Involvement of GTP-binding proteins in the activation of bovine endothelial cell phospholipase D. *Clin. Res.* **38:**873A.

Natarajan, V., and Garcia, J. G. N. (1990b). Bradykinin, phorbol esters and aluminum fluoride induce phospholipase D activation of endothelial cells. *FASEB J.* **4:**A1781.

Natarajan, V., and Garcia, J. G. N. (1992). Regulation of phospholipase D in bovine endothelial cells. Evidence for activation by protein kinase C-dependent and -independent mechanisms. *J. Lab. Clin. Med.* (submitted).

Natarajan, V., Schmid, P. C., Reddy, P. V., and Schmid, H. H. O. (1984). Catabolism of *N*-acylethanolamine phospholipids by dog brain preparations. *J. Neurochem.* **42:**1613.

Natarajan, V., Schmid, P. C., and Schmid, H. H. O. (1986). N-acylethanolamine phospholipid metabolism in normal and ischemic rat brain. *Biochim. Biophys. Acta* **878:**32.

Natarajan, V. N., Parinandi, N. L., Schmid, H. H. O., and Garcia, J. G. N. (1991). Exogenous hydroperoxides activate endothelial cell phospholipase D. *Am. Rev. Respir. Dis.* **143:**A573.

Newman, K. B., Michael, J. R., and Feldman, A. M. (1989). Phorbol ester-induced inhibition of the beta-adrenergic system in pulmonary endothelium: Role of a pertussis toxin–sensitive protein. *Am. J. Respir. Cell Molec. Biol.* **1:**517.

Nishizuka, Y. (1986). Studies and perspectives of protein kinase C. *Science* **233:**305.

Ohashi, Y., and Narumiya, S. (1987). ADP-ribosylation of M_r 21,000 membrane protein by type D botulinum toxin. *J. Biol. Chem.* **262:**1430.

Okano, Y., Yamada, K., Yano, K., and Nozawa, Y. (1987). Guanosine 5′-(gamma-thio)triphosphate stimulates arachidonic acid liberation in permeabilized art peritoneal mast cells. *Biochem. Biophys. Res. Commun.* **145:**1267.

Orellana, S., Solski, P. A., and Brown, J. H. (1987). Guanosine 5′-*O*-(thiotriphosphate)-dependent inositol trisphosphate formation in membranes is inhibited by phorbol ester and protein kinase C. *J. Biol. Chem.* **262:**1638.

Parkinson, J. E., Garcia, J. G. N., and Bang, N. U. (1990). Decreased thrombin affinity of cell-surface thrombomodulin following treatment of cultured endothelium with beta-D xyloside. *Biochem. Biophys. Res. Commun.* **169:**177.

Patterson, C. E., Rhoades, R. A., and Garcia, J. G. N. (1992a). Evans Blue–albumin binding as a new marker of transendothelial macromolecule permeability. *J. Appl. Physiol.* (in press).

Patterson, C. E., Dukes, R. E., and Garcia, J. G. N. (1992b). Regulation of thrombin-induced endothelial cell activation by bacterial toxins. *Sem. Thromb. Hemos.* (in press).

Phillips, P. G., Lum, H., Malik, A. B., and Tsan, M. (1989). Phallacidin prevents thrombin-induced increases in endothelial permeability to albumin. *Am. J. Physiol.* **257:**C562.

Pirotton, S., Rasp, E., Demolle, D., Erneux, C., and Boeynaems, J. M. (1987a). Involvement of inositol 1,4,5-trisphosphate and calcium in the action of adenine nucleotides on aortic endothelial cells. *J. Biol. Chem.* **262:**17461.

Pirotton, S., Erneux, B. C., and Bolyraems, J. M. (1987b). Dual role of GTP-binding proteins in the control of endothelial prostacyclin. *Biochem. Biophys. Res. Commun.* **147:**1113.

Pollock, W. K., Rink, T. W., and Irvine, R. (1986). Liberation of [^{3}H]arachidonate acid and changes in cytotoxic free calcium in Fura-2-loaded human platelets stimulated by ionomycin and collagen. *Biochem. J.* **253:**707.

Pollock, W. K., Wreggett, K. A., and Irvine, R. F. (1988). Inositol phosphate production and Ca^{2+} mobilization in human umbilical-vein endothelial cells stimulated by thrombin and histamine. *Biochem. J.* **256:**371.

Prescott, S. M., Zimmerman, G. A., and McIntyre, T. M. (1984). Human endothelial cells in culture produce platelet-activating factor (1-alkyl-2-acetyl-sn-glycero-3-phosphocholine) when stimulated with thrombin. *Proc. Natl. Acad. Sci. USA* **81:**3534.

Putney, J. W., Jr., Weiss, S. J., Van De Walle, C. M., and Haddas, R. A. (1980). Is phosphatidic acid a calcium ionophore under neurohumoral control? *Nature* **284:**345.

Resink, T. J., Grigorian, G. Y., Moldabaeva, A. K., Danilov, S. M., and Buhler, F. R. (1987). Histamine-induced phosphoinositide metabolism in cultured human umbilical vein endothelial cells. Association with thromboxane and prostacyclin release. *Biochem. Biophys. Res. Commun.* **144:**438.

Rizzo, M. T., Tricot, G., Hoffman, R., Jayaram, H. N., Weber, G., Garcia, J. G. N., and English, D. (1990). Inosine monophosphate dehydrogenase inhibitors. Probes for investigations of the functions of guanine nucleotide binding proteins in intact cells. *Cell. Signal.* **2:**509.

Rossi, F., Grzeskowiak, M., Della Bianca, V., Calzetti, F., and Gandini, G. (1990). Phosphatidic acid and not diacylglycerol generated by phospholipase D is functionally linked to the activation of the NADPH oxidase by FMLP in human neutrophils. *Biochem. Biophys. Res. Commun.* **168:**320.

Rotrosen, D., and Gallin, J. I. (1986). Histamine type I receptor occupancy increases endothelial cytosolic calcium, reduces F-actin, and promotes albumin diffusion across cultured endothelial monolayers. *J. Cell Biol.* **103:**2379.

Schmid, P. C., Reddy, P. V., Natarajan, V., and Schmid, H. H. O. (1983). Metabolism of *N*-acylethanolamine phospholipids by a mammalial phosphodiesterase of the phospholipase D type. *J. Biol. Chem.* **258:**9302.

Shasby, D. M., Lind, S. E., Shasby, S. S., Goldsmith, J. C., and Hunninghake, G. W. (1985). Reversible oxidant-induced increases in albumin transfer across cultured endothelium: Alterations in cell shape and calcium homeostatsis. *Blood* **65:**605.

Shasby, D. M., Yorek, M., and Shasby, S. S. (1988). Exogenous oxidants initiate hydrolysis of endothelial cell inositol phospholipids. *Blood* **72:**491.

Shaw, K., and Exton, J. H. (1991). Partial purification from bovine liver plasma membranes of a G-protein activatable β type phosphoinositide-specific phospholipase C. *FASEB J.* **5:**A481.

Shearman, M. S., Sekiguchi, K., and Nishizuka, Y. (1989). Modulation of ion channel activity: A key function of the protein kinase C enzyme family. *Pharmacol. Rev.* **139:**558.

Siess, W., Lapetina, E. G., and Cuatrecasas, P. (1982). Cytochalasins inhibit arachidonic acid metabolism in thrombin stimulated platelets. *Proc. Natl. Acad. Sci. USA* **79:**7709.

Smith, C. D., Cox, C. C., and Snyderman, R. (1986). Receptor-coupled activation of phosphoinositide-specific phospholipase C by an N protein. *Science* **4:**97.

Stasek, J. E., Patterson, C. E., and Garcia, J. G. N. (1990). Cultured bovine pulmonary artery endothelium permeability is modulated by protein kinase C activation and cytoskeletal protein phosphorylation. *Clin. Res.* **38:**849.

Stasek, J. E., Patterson, C. E., and Garcia, J. G. N. (1992a). Protein kinase C phosphorylates caldesmon$_{77}$ and vimentin and enhances albumin permeability across cultured bovine pulmonary artery endothelial cell monolayers. *J. Cell. Physiol.* (in press).

Stasek, J. E., Natarajan, V., and Garcia, J. G. N. (1991). Phosphatidic acid directly activates endothelial cell protein kinase C. *FASEB J.*

Stasek, J. E., and Garcia J. G. N. (1992b). The role of protein kinase C in α-thrombin-mediated endothelial cell activation. *Sem. Thromb. Hemos.* **18:**117.

Stelzner, T. J., Weil, J. V., and O'Brien, R. F. (1989). Role of cyclic adenosine monophosphate in the induction of endothelial barrier properties. *J. Cell. Physiol.* **139:**157.

Takai, T., and Kanfer, J. N. (1979). Partial prufication and properties of rat brain phospholipase D. *J. Biol. Chem.* **254:**9761.

Tate, R. M., Venthuysen, K. M., Shasby, D. M., McMurtry, I. F., and Repine, J. E. (1982). Oxygen radical mediated permeability edema and vasoconstriction in isolated perfused rabbit lungs. *Am. Rev. Respir. Dis.* **126:**802.

Taylor, S. J., Smith, J. A., and Exton, J. H. (1990a). Purification from bovine liver membrane of a guanine nucleotide-dependent activator of phosphoinositide-specific phospholipase C. Immunologic identification as a novel G-protein α subunit. *J. Biol. Chem.* **265:**17150.

Taylor, G. S., Garcia, J. G. N., Dukes, R., and English, D. (1990b). Rapid high performance liquid chromatographic analysis of radiolabeled inositol phosphates. *Anal. Biochem.* **180:**118.

Trotta, R. J., Sullivan, S. G., and Stern, A. (1981). Lipid peroxidation and hemoglobin degradation in red blood cells exposed to *t*-butyl hydroperoxide. Dependence on glucose metabolism and hemoglobin status. *Biochem. Biophys. Acta* **678:**230.

Van Den Bosch, H. (1980). Intracellular phospholipases A. *Biochim. Biophys. Acta* **604:**191.

Vercellotti, G. M., Severson, S. P., Duane, P., and Moldow, C. F. (1990). Hydrogen peroxide alters signal transduction in human endothelial cells. *J. Lab. Clin. Med.* **117:**15.

Voyno-Yasenetskaya, T. A., Tkachuk, V. A., and Checknyova, E. G. (1989a). Genuine nucleotide-dependent, pertussis toxin–sensitive regulation of phosphoinositide turnover by bradykinin in bovine pulmonary artery endothelial cells. *FASEB J.* **3:**44.

Voyno-Yasenetsuaya, T. A., Panchenko, M. P., Nupenko, E. V., Rybin, V. O., and Tkachuk, V. A. (1989b). Histamine and bradykinin stimulate the phosphoinositide turnover in human umbilical vein endothelial cells via different G-proteins. *FEBS Lett.* **259:**67.

Weiss, S. J., Young, J., Lobuglio, A. F., Slivka, A., and Nimeh, N. F. (1981). Role of hydrogen peroxide in neutrophil-mediated destruction of cultured endothelial cells. *J. Clin. Invest.* **68:**714.

Weksler, B. B. (1984). Prostaglandins and vascular function. *Circulation* **70:**63.

Weksler, B. B., Ley, C. W., and Jaffe, E. A. (1978). Stimulation of endothelial cell PGI_2 production by thrombin, trypsin and ionophore A23187. *J. Clin. Invest.* **62:**923.

Werth, D. K., Niedel, J. E., and Pastan, K. (1983). Vinculin, a cytoskeletal substrate of protein kinase C. *J. Biol. Chem.* **258:**11423.

Whorton, A. R., Montgomery, M. E., and Kent, R. S. (1985). Effect of hydrogen peroxide on prostaglandin synthesis and cellular integrity in cultured porcine aortic endothelial cells. *J. Clin. Invest.* **76:**295.

Wysolmerski, R. B., and Lagunoff, D. (1990). Involvement of myosin light-chain kinase in endothelial cell retraction. *Proc. Natl. Acad. Sci. USA* **87:**16.

Yamamoto, K., Tanimoto, T., Kim, S., Kikuchi, A., and Takai, Y. (1989). Small molecular weight GTP-binding proteins and signal transcution. *Clin. Chim. Acta* **185:**347.

Zavoico, G. B., Halenda, S. P., Sha'afi, R., and Feinstein, M. B. (1985). Phorbol myristate acetate inhibits thrombin-stimulated Ca^{2+} mobilization and phosphatidylinositol 4,5-bisphosphate hydrolysis in human platelets. *Proc. Natl. Acad. Sci. USA* **82:**3859.

Zavoico, G. B., Hrbolich, J. K., Gimbrone, M. A., Jr., and Schafer, A. I. (1990). Enhancement of thrombin- and ionomycin-stimulated prostacyclin and platelet-activating factor production in cultured endothelial cells by a tumor-promoting phorbol ester. *J. Cell. Physiol.* **143:**596.

2

Lung Injury and Edema Associated with the Activation of Protein Kinase C

ARNOLD JOHNSON and THOMAS J. FERRO

Stratton Veterans Affairs Medical Center
and Albany Medical College
Albany, New York

I. Introduction

The study of the intracellular mechanisms that couple extracellular stimuli to cellular responses is a new and exciting area of research in the field of pulmonary pathophysiology. In this chapter we focus on the role of the activation of protein kinase C (PKC), a ubiquitous intracellular enzyme with signal transduction activity, in the genesis of noncardiogenic pulmonary edema. The biochemistry and molecular biology of PKC is reviewed in detail elsewhere (Nishizuka, 1986; Shenolikar, 1988; Shearman et al., 1989).

II. Mechanisms of Stimulus–Response Coupling Mediated by PKC Activation

The current understanding of the mechanism of PKC activation is as follows. The process begins when an extracellular molecular stimulus interacts with a receptor in the cell membrane. The ligand–receptor interaction elicits the activation of membrane phospholipase C through the mediation of G proteins (Brown and Birnbaumer, 1988; Fain et al., 1988; Gilman, 1987). The activated phospholipase C catalyzes the hydrolysis of phosphoinositol diphosphate (PIP_2) at the 3-

carbon position of the glycerol backbone of PIP_2. The hydrolysis of PIP_2 results in the release of diacylglycerols and inositol triphosphate (IP_3) (Rando, 1988). IP_3 induces the release of calcium from intracellular stores (Coburn and Baron, 1990), which has a variety of effects. Sources of diacylglycerols other than PIP_2, such as diacylglycerols generated by the action of phospholipase D or the dephosphorylation of phosphatidic acid, may exist (Rando, 1988). The diacylglycerols complex with PKC, calcium, and phosphatidylserine at the cell membrane (Bell, 1986; Wolfson et al., 1985). The PKC is "activated" once associated with diacylglycerols, calcium, and phosphatidylserine, resulting in the phosphorylation of substrate protein by PKC in the cell membrane compartment. PKC-induced phosphorylation results in the activation of the enzyme activity of the substrate protein. Activated PKC phosphorylates many different protein substrates in different cell types, resulting in an array of different biological responses.

Alternative mechanisms for the control of PKC activation and the response mediated by PKC activation may exist. PKC may be directly activated by arachidonic acid metabolites, particularly eicosanoids (Fan et al., 1990; Shearman et al., 1989). PKC activation and activity have been demonstrated in the nuclear membrane (Leach et al., 1989), indicating that the stimulus–response coupling activities of PKC are not limited to the cell outer membrane of the cell. Control of PKC activation exists, mediated by autophosphorylation or by the calpains, which are calcium-activated proteases capable of degrading PKC and releasing the catalytic unit (Shearman et al., 1989). PKC activation causes the activity of phospholipase C to increase (Martin et al., 1989) or decrease (Voyno-Yasenetskaya et al., 1989) in response to bradykinin, indicating that PKC may also alter its own activation by affecting phospholipase C activation. The response induced by PKC activation is also subject to control, because the enzyme activated by PKC may subsequently become dephosphorylated through the actions of phosphatases.

The study of PKC activation and PKC effects is also complicated by the considerable molecular and functional heterogeneity of PKC. At least five different isoforms of PKC exist (Nishizuka, 1986). The molecular weight of PKC is 70 to 80 kD, depending on the isoform (Nishizuka, 1986). Isoforms I, II, and III are the best studied. These three isoforms are derived from the same gene group and contain a phospholipid- and calcium-dependent domain (Fournier et al., 1989; Pelosin et al., 1990). The second group of PKC isoforms, which are derived from more recently cloned genes, differ from the first group in that catalytic activity is calcium independent and is directed toward different substrates (Pelosin et al., 1990). Isoforms of PKC can differ in their ability to respond to arachidonic acid metabolites (Shearman et al., 1989) and in their degree of inhibition of PKC antagonists (Pelosin et al., 1990).

III. Activators and Inhibitors of PKC

PKC activation is defined in most experimental protocols as the translocation of PKC from cytosol to membrane, because the known effects of PKC are limited to the membrane (Bell, 1986; Nishizuka, 1984). Translocation of PKC is detected by studying total PKC activity in the membrane versus cytosol. The total PKC activity of a specimen is defined as maximal (i.e., in the presence of exogenous activators) PKC-specific histone H1 phosphorylation activity (Lynch et al., 1990) or total PKC antigen activity detected using immunoblotting (Stabel et al., 1987).

Differences in conclusions concerning the role of PKC activation in noncardiogenic pulmonary edema or edemagenic cellular effects may be related to the differing nonspecific effects of PKC activators and inhibitors or to differences in the duration of incubation with PKC activators. Two classes of PKC activators, the phorbol esters and the diacylglycerols, are most widely studied. The inhibitors of PKC activation that are most widely used are H7 [1-(5-isoquinolinesulfonyl)-2-methylpiperizine] and staurosporin. H7 is a relatively specific inhibitor of PKC at 25 μM (Lynch et al., 1990), and staurosporin is relatively specific at 100 nM (Johnson et al., 1990). Neither the activators nor the inhibitors have been proved to be fully specific, however, even at low concentrations. The differing nonspecific effects of the various activators and inhibitors may therefore lead to conflicting results, which may be related to non-PKC pathways. The duration of incubation with the PKC activator is also crucial. PKC activation using phorbol myristate acetate (PMA), a phorbol ester purified from croton oil, for 8 to 16 h results in PKC depletion in endothelial cells and the associated lack of PKC-dependent responses. In contrast, briefer exposure of endothelial cells to PMA can lead to the activation of PKC (Lynch et al., 1990). The duration of incubation with the PKC activator must therefore be clarified. Because of the technical difficulties with both PKC activation and inhibition, studies attempting to prove the role of PKC activation in the pathogenesis of pulmonary edema should, whenever possible, use (1) at least two different classes of PKC activators studied at multiple time points and concentrations, with controls; (2) at least two different classes of PKC inhibitors at multiple concentrations, with controls; and (3) direct PKC assay.

IV. Effects of PKC Activation at the Cellular Level

A. Generation of Soluble Mediators

PKC activation may mediate the generation of phlogistic mediators from a variety of cell types found within the normal or inflammatory milieu of the pulmonary vascular compartment. The activities of cell membrane enzymes such as phospholipase A_2, phospholipase D, and phospholipase C, which are involved in the production of phospholipid mediators, are altered by PKC.

The activity of phospholipase A_2 is enhanced by activated PKC in neutrophils and endothelial cells (Zavoico et al., 1990), resulting in increased levels of arachidonic acid (Leyravaud et al., 1989; Zavoico et al., 1990). Levels of arachidonic acid can also increase via the PKC-induced inhibition of acyl-CoA/lysophosphatide acyltransferase, which reincorporates arachidonic acid into lysophosphatides (Pfannkuche et al., 1986). The increased level of arachidonic acid results in enhanced generation of eicosanoids (Parker et al., 1987; Zavoico et al., 1990). The increase in eicosanoid synthesis during acute PKC activation is probably due to increased substrate (arachidonic acid) availability for the cyclooxygenase enzyme complex, and not due to increased cyclooxygenase activity; however, long-term PKC activation can enhance enzyme activity due to de novo synthesis (Zavoico et al., 1990).

The activity of phospholipase D, an enzyme linked to phosphocholine metabolism and ultimately to the generation of platelet activating factor (PAF), may be altered by PKC activation. Phospholipase D activity decreases in endothelial cells in response to bradykinin administered after prolonged incubation with PMA (Martin et al., 1989). Because exposure of cells to PMA results in PKC activation initially, followed by PKC depletion after prolonged exposure (Lynch et al., 1990), the data of Martin et al. may be interpreted as indicating the PKC activation enhances phospholipase D activity in endothelial cells. PMA treatment activates phospholipase D in neutrophils (Reinhold et al., 1990), presumably via PKC activation. In contrast, FMLP increases the phospholipid D activity of neutrophils pretreated with staurosporin, an inhibitor of PKC activity, suggesting possible PKC-mediated inhibition of phospholipase D.

The effects of PKC on phospholipase activity suggest that PKC may have variable or conflicting effects on the release of PAF. On the one hand, PAF generation may be decreased by the removal of choline from phosphocholine via phospholipase D activation. On the other hand, PKC activation could possibly increase PAF generation, because (1) PKC activity enhances acetyltransferase activity in neutrophils (Leyravaud et al., 1989) and endothelial cells (Zavoico et al., 1990), (2) PKC activity enhances phospholipase A_2 activity in neutrophils (Leyravaud et al., 1989) and endothelial cells (Zavoico et al., 1990), and (3) possible PKC-induced inhibition of phospholipase D (Reinhold et al., 1990) could result in decreased removal of choline from phosphocholine, making more substrate for PAF generation available.

A variety of nonlipid mediators of inflammation are altered by PKC activity. Studies indicate decreased binding of PAF (Yamazaki et al., 1989) and LTB_4 (O'Flaherty et al., 1980; Yamzaki et al., 1989) to activated neutrophils and decreased activity of LTD_4 in U-937 cells (Winkler et al., 1988) induced with

PMA. Incubation of smooth muscle cells with PMA decreases the binding of histamine to H_2 receptors (Mitsuhashi and Payan, 1988) and decreases IP_3 formation (Murray et al., 1989). Angiotensin-converting enzyme activity does not change (Myers et al., 1989) as a result of PMA treatment, whereas the uptake of serotonin and resultant PIP_2 synthesis by endothelial cells decreases. Because PIP_2 promotes the action of many inflammatory substances after the initial ligand–receptor interaction [i.e., PAF (Block et al., 1989; Gay and Sitt, 1988a,b), histamine (Murray et al., 1989), muscarinic agonists (Takuwa et al., 1986; Grandordy et al., 1986), and possibly leukotrienes (Grandordy et al., 1986)] prolonged PKC activation using PMA, which may result in feedback inhibition of the transduction pathways of the substance.

The data indicate that PKC activation is associated with alterations of the metabolic pathways potentially involved in the pathogenesis of or protection against pulmonary edema, including those relating to phosphocholine metabolism and PAF generation (Braquet et al., 1989), and arachidonic acid metabolites such as (1) prostaglandins (Brigham et al., 1983; Chopra and Webster, 1988; Downey et al., 1988; Tate et al., 1988), (2) prostacyclin (Czer et al., 1986), (3) thromboxane A_2 (TxA_2) (Farrukh et al., 1985; Munoz et al., 1986), and (4) leukotrienes such as leukotriene B_4 (LTB_4), LTC_4, and LTD_4 (Ford-Hutchinson, 1985; Piper, 1984). The net effect of the altered milieu of soluble mediators resulting from the activation of PKC in the cells of the pulmonary vascular compartment is not immediately obvious. The differences in the conclusions concerning the role of PKC in the control of intracellular lipid metabolism and release of soluble mediators may be related to the use of differing experimental conditions, including (1) differing cell types, (2) differing PKC activators and antagonists, and (3) differing durations of incubation with PKC activators. The consequence of the effects of PKC activation on the metabolism of circulating vasoactive factors and the resultant changes in the control of the pulmonary circulation remain to be determined.

B. Effects on Smooth Muscle Contraction and Pulmonary Vasoreactivity

PKC activation results in alterations in the contractile behavior of smooth muscle in a variety of tissues, based on effects on membrane ionic channels and polarization (Takawa and Park, 1987; Shearman et al., 1989). PKC activators such as phorbol esters and diacylglycerols increase the cellular influx of sodium and calcium ions, which is associated with increases in tension in the tissues of the vasculature (Jiang and Morgan, 1987; Khalil and Van Breemen, 1988), airway (Souhrada and Souhrada, 1989), and trachea (Schramm and Grunstein, 1989). These alterations in ion flux may result in further increases in the activities of the sodium–hydrogen and sodium–potassium pumps, which can eventually result in hyperpolarization and relaxation of the smooth muscle in response to additional PKC activation (Souhrada and Souhrada, 1989; Schramm and Grunstein, 1989). In aortic smooth muscle tissues, PKC activation may in part mediate the tonic contraction induced by phenylephrine in a calcium-free environment as suggested by the use of H7, an inhibitor of PKC activation (Issad et al., 1984). The response to endothelin in aortic strips may also be mediated by the activation of PKC (Sugiura et al., 1989).

PKC activation may alter the pulmonary vasoreactivity induced by the generation of superoxide radical (O_2^-) from endothelial cells (Selvaraj et al., 1987). Reactive oxygen species can influence vasoreactivity (Greenberg et al., 1987; Katusk and Vanhoutte, 1989; Rubanyi and Vanhoutte, 1986; Stewart et al., 1988) by several mechanisms, including (1) the inactivation of endothelium-derived relaxing factor, which is a vasodilator; (2) the independent vasoconstrictor potential of reactive oxygen species; and (3) the generation of plasma-derived chemotactic factors for neutrophils (Petrone et al., 1980).

PKC activation can also sensitize smooth muscle to contraction by other agonists. In arteries from different organs, phorbol esters sensitize the contraction response of smooth muscle to potassium (Nishimura et al., 1990), histamine (Miller et al., 1986), and norepinephrine (Miller et al., 1986), possibly by sensitizing the tissue to calcium. Treatment of abdominal aortic smooth muscle with phorbol esters enhances the serotonin-induced increase in tension. The response to phorbol ester plus serotonin is dependent on an intact endothelium (Consigny, 1989), suggesting the release from PKC-activated endothelial cells of either a vasoconstrictor substance (i.e., reactive oxygen species, endothelin) or an inhibitor (i.e., reactive oxygen species) of a vasodilator substance (i.e., endothelium-derived relaxation factor) (Consigny, 1989). Phorbol esters and diacylglycerols sensitize pulmonary artery tissue to contraction induced by serotonin, KCL, and A23187. Phorbol esters and diacylglycerols also increase the pressor response to KCl and hypoxia in isolated lungs, a response that is blunted using the PKC inhibitor H7 (Orton et al., 1990). The sensitization of airway smooth muscle to ovalbumin (which is manifested as enhanced depolarization and contraction in response to ovalbumin-specific IgG) is inhibited by H7 (Souhrada and Souhrada, 1989), suggesting mediation by PKC activation. The likely mechanism by which PKC activation results in the contraction of smooth muscle is the phosphorylation of components of the "filamin–actin–desmin fibrillar domain," leading to the phase of sustained tonic tension (Rasmussen, 1987). Smooth muscle contraction may also be mediated by the PKC-induced phosphorylation of myosin light chain (Rembold and Murphy, 1988).

C. PKC Activation in Inflammatory Cells

PKC activation (in response to diacylglycerols or PMA) and diacylglycerol generation, in neutrophils, macrophages, and monocytes, is associated with (1) increases in the production of reactive oxygen species (Bass et al., 1988; Badwey et al., 1989; Repine et al., 1974; Wright and Hoffman, 1986), (2) PAF generation (Leyravaud et al., 1989), (3) phagocytosis (Fallman et al., 1989), (4) release of proteases (Naccache et al., 1985; White et al., 1984), and (5) the generation of arachidonic acid metabolites (Pfannkuche et al., 1986). However, the role of PKC activation in the generation of reactive oxygen species from alveolar macrophages (Brieland et al., 1989) and neutrophils (Wright and Hoffman, 1986) has been challenged. PKC activation in platelets is associated with increases in the release of ATP (Watson et al., 1988) and serotonin (Watson et al., 1988). These changes in cell function induced by PKC activation are associated with the phosphorylation of cell proteins of specific molecular weights in the platelet (Block et al., 1989; Watson et al., 1988) and neutrophil (Badwey et al., 1989; Reibman et al., 1988; White et al., 1984).

PKC activation can indirectly cause increases in vascular permeability, vascular pressures, and pulmonary edema, because the phlogistic substances released from PKC-activated inflammatory cells in the circulatory and marginated pool can cause these effects. Reactive oxygen species can injure endothelium, increase permeability, increase leukocyte adherence, and alter endothelial cytoskeleton (Freeman and Crapo, 1982; Johnson et al., 1989; Shasby et al., 1982, 1985; Skoglund et al., 1988). Serotonin (Brigham and Owen, 1975; Demling et al., 1988; Heffner et al., 1987) and many arachidonic acid metabolites (such as LTB_4, LTC_4, LTD_4, 12-hydroxyeicosatetraenoic acid, and TxA_2) have the ability to alter pulmonary hemodynamics and vascular permeability and promote edema. PAF (Braquet et al., 1989) can stimulate neutrophils and monocytes to generate reactive oxygen species and prostaglandins, which in turn affect the pulmonary circulation. PAF is also an important vasoactive substance that causes pulmonary edema (Braquet et al., 1989).

PKC activation can also prime leukocytes for activation by other cellular agonists. For example, PMA treatment primes neutrophils for response to PAF via a PKC- and calcium-dependent mechanism (Gay and Stitt, 1988a,b). Diacylglycerols can prime neutrophils and monocytes to greater stimulation (increase in the respiratory burst) induced by PAF and FMLP. This activity of diacylglycerols, however, may be due to effects other than PKC activation (Bass et al., 1988a,b).

The interaction of endothelium with leukocytes and platelets may be directly modified by PKC activation. Neutrophils (Kamp et al., 1988; Dicorleto and Molte, 1989), macrophages (Issad et al., 1989; Shaw et al., 1990), and platelets (O'Flaherty et al., 1980) may increase adherence to the endothelium in response to PKC activation by PMA or thrombin. In contrast, the adherence of monocytes to the endothelium may be decreased in response to PKC activation (Kamp et al., 1988). PKC activity can increase leukocyte adherence by increasing the expression/affinity of intergrin molecules (CD11/CD18 glycoproteins) in monocytic cells (Skoglund et al., 1988) and neutrophils (Wright and Meyer, 1986). PKC activity can also effect adherence by promoting the phosphorylation of cytoskeletal proteins (Danilov and Juliano, 1989; Pontremoli et al., 1987; Shaw et al., 1990) or by the interaction of intergrins with the cell cytoskeleton, as in the macrophage (Shaw et al., 1990). H_2O_2 may increase the adherence of monocytic cells to plastic via the PKC-induced phosphorylation of proteins of specific molecular weights (Skoglund et al., 1988). PKC activation also results in enhancement of the activity of adhesive ligands (i.e., ELAMS, ICAMS) in human umbilical artery endothelial cells for neutrophils (Lane et al., 1990).

Endogenous factors may induce pro-inflammatory activity by activating PKC in circulating cells. PAF activates PKC in platelets (Block et al., 1989) and neutrophils (Gay and Sitt, 1988a,b). Neutrophil activation induced by "neutrophil activating factor" derived from monocytes is inhibited using staurosporin (Thelen et al., 1988), suggesting mediation by PKC. Thrombin activates PKC in platelets (Watson et al., 1988).

D. Endothelial PKC Activation and the Control of Vascular Permeability

Activated PKC phosphorylates proteins in endothelial cells (Mackie et al., 1986). Basal PKC activity may maintain the normal cytoskeleton, and PKC activation in response to inflammatory factors such as PMA, reactive oxygen species, or thrombin may mediate alterations in the endothelial cytoskeletal morphology (Antonov et al., 1986; Johnson et al., 1989; Phillips et al., 1990; Reinders et al., 1982; Shasby et al., 1982, 1985). Treatment with H7 alters morphology of actin filaments in cultured epithelium and fibroblasts. The H7 effect, however, may be related to signal transduction systems other than PKC, such as other protein kinases dependent on the cofactors cAMP and calcium-calmodulin, which may also be inhibited by H7 (Birrell et al., 1989). Reactive oxygen species mediate the hydrolysis of inositol phospholipids in endothelial (Shasby et al., 1988a) and epithelial (Shasby et al., 1988b) cells, suggesting that reactive oxygen species may indirectly activate PKC via the activation of phospholipase C and the release of diacylglycerols. H_2O_2 causes alterations in cell shape and a redistribution of actin filaments (Shasby et al., 1982, 1985) from the cell periphery to centralized stress fibers. The changes in cell shape and actin filaments are inhibited by H7 (Johnson et al., 1989), suggesting mediation by PKC activation.

Alterations in the endothelial cell cytoskeleton are associated with increases in endothelial permeability (Phillips et al., 1990; Rasio et al., 1989; Shasby et al., 1982, 1985). Reactive oxygen species (Shasby et al., 1985), PMA, and thrombin (Lynch et al., 1990; Phillips et al., 1990) increase permeability to albumin in cultured endothelial cells and cause morphologic evidence of injury (Gartner et al., 1988; Shasby et al., 1985), an effect that is inhibited using H7 (Lynch et al., 1990). PKC activation is associated with the disruption of focal contacts in fibroblasts, suggesting that PKC modulates cytoskeletal proteins such as vinculin, talin, and α-actinin, which are involved in the maintenance of cell adherence and receptor function (Jaken et al., 1989).

E. PKC and the Biological Response to Monokines

Tumor necrosis factor-α (TNF) alters the barrier function of endothelial monolayers via G proteins and increased phospholipase A_2 activity (Brett et al., 1989; Clark et al., 1988). However, specific mechanisms coupling TNF-induced changes in G proteins or phospholipase A_2 activity with permeability have not been identified. PKC activation may mediate the vascular effects of TNF because (1) G proteins may alter PKC activity by inducing phospholipase C activity, (2) TNF and PKC activators such as PMA have similar vascular effects, (3) the response to both TNF and PKC activators is enhanced in the presence of neutrophils (Hocking et al., 1990; Johnson et al., 1990), and (4) TNF and PMA both result in protein phosphorylation (Schutze et al., 1989). Treatment of the endothelium with the PKC inhibitors such as H7 or staurosporin prevents increases in neutrophil adherence induced by endotoxin, TNF, and interleukin-1, possibly due to the decreased expression of ICAM or ELAM on the endothelial surface (Magnuson et al., 1989; Lane et al., 1990).

We investigated the hypothesis that TNF activates pulmonary endothelial PKC. Confluent bovine pulmonary artery endothelial monolayers (Del Vecchio and Smith, 1981) were exposed to TNF (highly purified recombinant human tumor necrosis factor-α from *Escherichia coli*, Cellular Products Inc., Buffalo, NY), heat-inactivated TNF (TNF heated to 90°C for 45 min), or the PKC-activator PMA. Membrane and cytosolic lysate fractions were prepared, and PKC antigenic activity was assessed using Western immunoblot analysis with MC5 monoclonal anti-PKC antibody (Amersham, Arlington Heights, IL). Translocation of PKC antigen activity into the membrane was induced using TNF, 1000 U/mL for 15 min, or PMA, 10^{-6} *M* for 15 min, whereas minimal translocation was noted using TNF, 1000 U/mL for 5 min, or heat-inactivated TNF for 15 min (Fig. 1). Immunofluorescence analysis using the MC5 anti-PKC antibody also showed TNF-induced translocation of PKC (i.e., moderate central fluorescence with moderate peripheral granular and filamentous fluorescence after treatment with TNF, 1000 U/mL for 15 min, or DOG, 4×10^{-5} *M* for 5 min, whereas

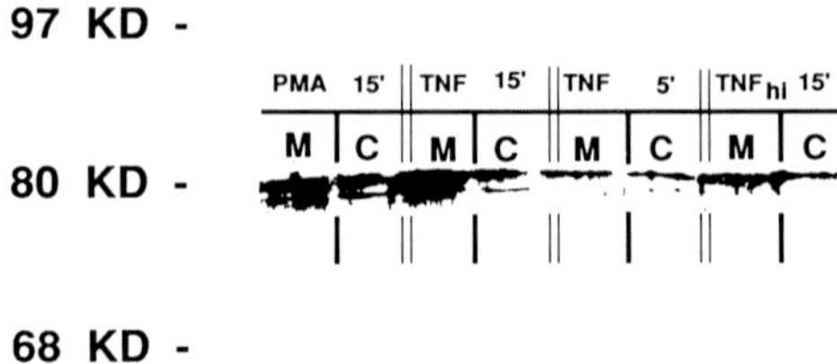

Figure 1 Highly purified recombinant human tumor necrosis factor-α (TNF) induces the translocation of endothelial protein kinase C (PKC), similar to phorbol myristate acetate (PMA). Western immunoblot (100 μg of protein lysate) shows that TNF (1000 U/mL for 15 min) and PMA (10^{-6} *M* for 15 min) induce the translocation of PKC antigen activity from the cytosol into the membrane, whereas TNF (1000 U/mL for 5 min), heat-inactivated TNF (TNF_{hi}), or control do not. Data are representative of four consecutive experiments.

controls showed mostly central fluorescence with minimal peripheral fluorescence); the translocation of PKC-associated immunofluorescence induced by TNF was inhibited using either 10^{-6} *M* calphostin C [a highly specific inhibitor of PKC activation (Kobayashi et al., 1989); Kamiya Biomedical, Thousand Oaks, CA] or IP-300 (rabbit antihuman TNF-α polyclonal antibody for neutralizing; Genzyme, Boston, MA) (Fig. 2). The data indicate that TNF induces the translocation, and thus activation, of pulmonary endothelial PKC via a diacylglycerol-dependent mechanism.

In contrast to the data presented above, Zhang et al. (1988) showed that TNF (at a dose similar to that used in the present study) does not activate PKC in cultured human fibroblasts, and Ritchie et al. (1991) showed that TNF (100 U/mL) caused neither membrane translocation of PKC nor the phosphorylation of the myristoylated alanine-rich C kinase substrate in human umbilical vein endothelium. Thus the biological response to TNF may differ between species, between fibroblasts and endothelial cells, and among endothelial cell types.

V. Effects of Pulmonary PKC Activation

A. Pulmonary PKC Activation in the Isolated Lung

In lungs isolated from various species, including rabbits (Jackson et al., 1986; Shasby et al., 1982), rats (Perry and Taylor, 1988; Perry et al., 1990), guinea pigs (Johnson, 1988), and dogs (Allison et al., 1986, 1988), perfusion with buffer containing PMA without circulating leukocytes increases pulmonary vascular pressures, pulmonary vascular resistance, and causes edema (Figs. 3 and 4; Johnson, 1988). The edema occurs as a result of increases in pulmonary capillary pressures and is not due to increased permeability (Johnson, 1988). PMA in-

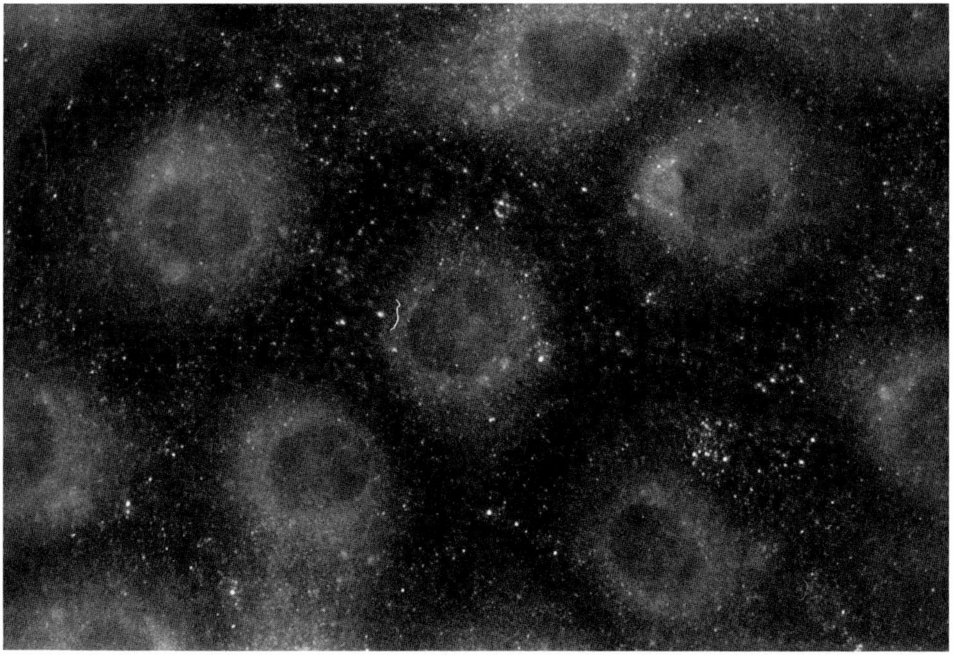

A

Figure 2 Highly purified recombinant human tumor necrosis factor-α (TNF) induces the calphostin C (CAL)-inhibitable translocation of endothelial protein kinase C (PKC)-associated immunofluorescence. Photomicrographs show the following experimental conditions: (A) control; (B) TNF (1000 U/mL for 15 min); (C) TNF+ CAL (10^{-6} *M*). TNF induces the translocation of PKC-associated immunofluorescence from the center to the periphery of the cell, whereas control does not; CAL inhibits the effect of TNF. Data are representative of four consecutive experiments.

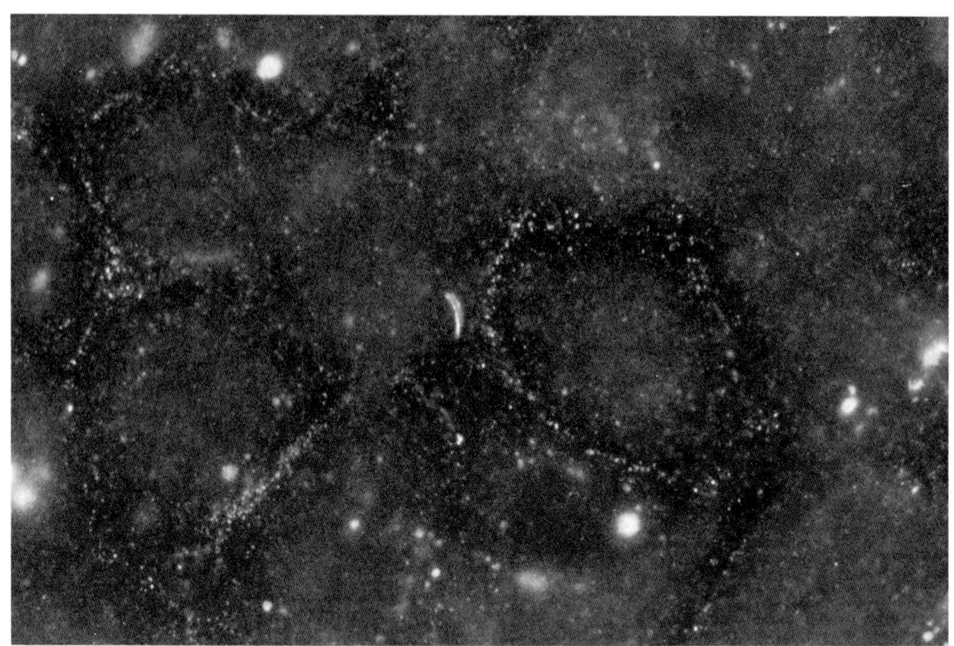

B

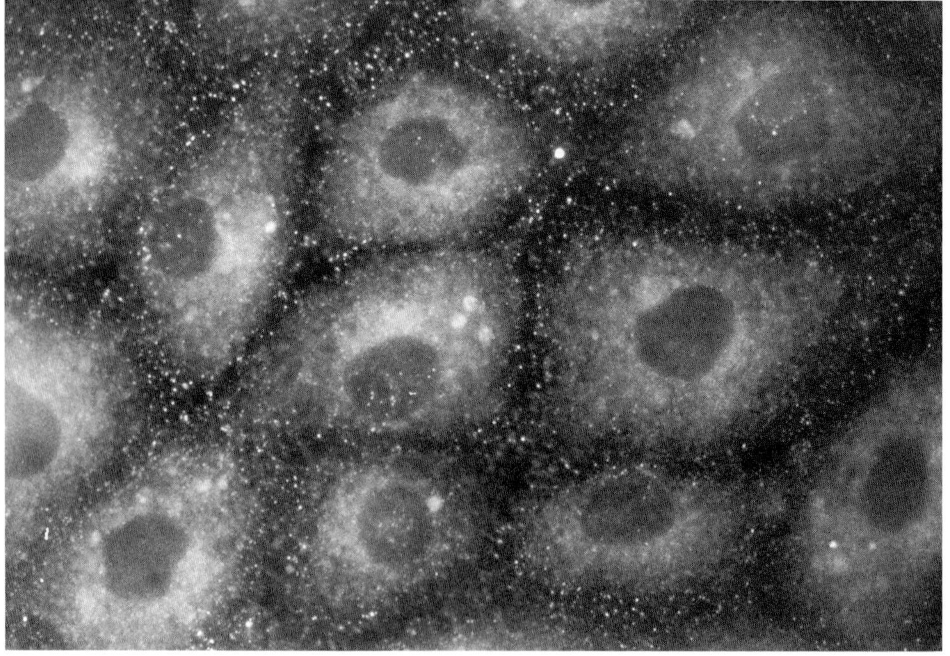

C

Figure 2 *(Continued)*

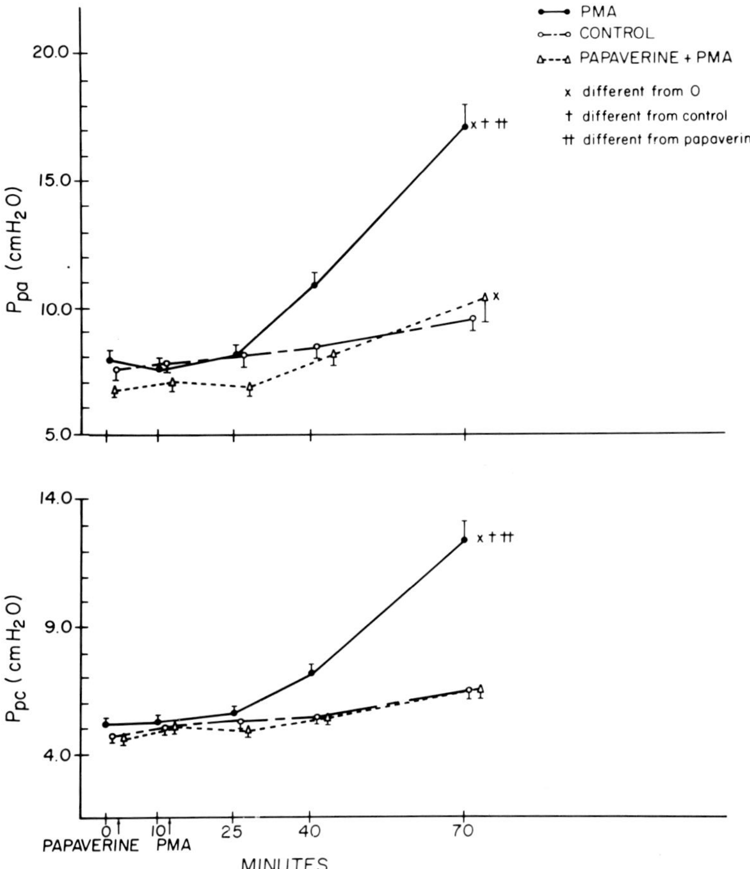

Figure 3 Effect of phorbol myristate acetate (PMA) on pulmonary arterial pressure (P_{pa}) and pulmonary capillary pressure (P_{pc}) in the isolated guinea pig lung perfused with phosphate-buffered Ringer's solution containing 5.5 m*M* dextrose. The PMA (50 n*M*) was added at 0 min, immediately after the 10-min baseline perfusion period. Papaverine (0.03 mg/mL) was added 10 min before the PMA in the papaverine + PMA group. Controls were given PMA vehicle only. PMA causes increases in P_{pa} and P_{pc}, which are inhibited by papaverine. (From Johnson, 1988.)

creases vascular permeability in the isolated lung only in the presence of circulating neutrophils, as shown using dogs (Allison et al., 1986, 1988), rats (Perry and Taylor, 1988; Perry et al., 1990), and rabbits (Jackson et al., 1986; Shasby et al., 1983). Monocytes can also contribute to PMA-induced injury in the rat lung (Perry et al., 1990). In the rabbit (Pitt et al., 1987), intratracheal instillation of PMA increases epithelial permeability, whereas in the rat, endothelial per-

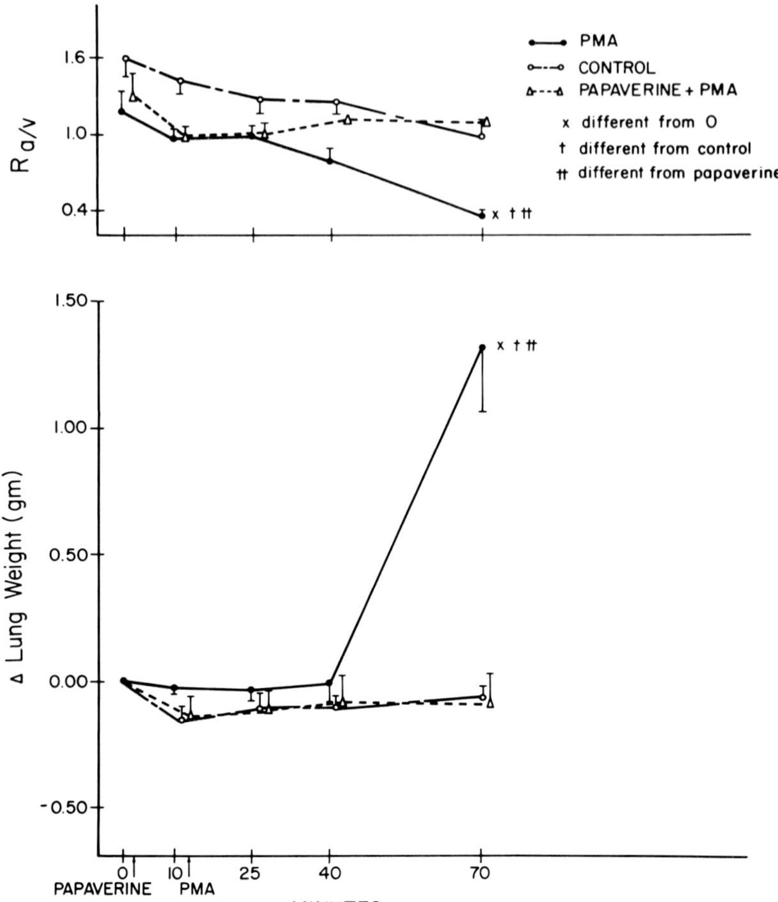

Figure 4 Effect of phorbol myristate acetate (PMA) on the pulmonary arterial/venous resistance ratio ($R_{a/v}$) and change in (Δ) lung weight in the isolated guinea pig lung perfused with phosphate-buffered Ringer's solution containing 5.5 m*M* dextrose. The PMA (50 n*M*) was added at 0 min, immediately after the 10-min baseline perfusion period. Papaverine (0.03 mg/mL) was added 10 min before the PMA in the papaverine + PMA group. Controls were given PMA vehicle only. PMA causes increases in $R_{a/v}$ and lung weight, which are inhibited by papaverine. (From Johnson, 1988.)

meability is increased (Perry and Taylor, 1989). The permeability changes are independent of neutrophils and inhibited using catalase (Pitt et al., 1989).

The study of pulmonary PKC activation has been extended by perfusing the isolated lung with dioctanoylglycerol, a diacylglycerol capable of PKC activation. Dioctanoylglycerol perfusion results in increases in pulmonary vascular resistance, pulmonary capillary pressure, and edema (Fig. 5; Johnson et al., 1990). The diacylglycerol challenge is associated with an increase in the capillary filtration coefficient, indicating an increase in vascular permeability. The capillary filtration coefficient increase occurs independent of circulating leukocytes and thus may be a direct effect of dioctanoylglycerol on the pulmonary microvascular endothelium. In contrast, PMA increases vascular permeability in the isolated lung only in the presence of circulating leukocytes, as noted above (Allison et al., 1986, 1988; Perry and Taylor, 1988; Perry et al., 1990; Jackson et al., 1986; Shasby et al., 1983). The ability of one PKC activator (i.e., dioctanoylglycerol) to alter pulmonary vascular permeability directly, whereas the other PKC activator (i.e., PMA) does not, may be related to the differing effects of the two compounds on non-PKC pathways. This difference does not rule out a role for PKC activation in vascular permeability increases, however, because the neutrophil dependence of the effect of PMA may be ex-

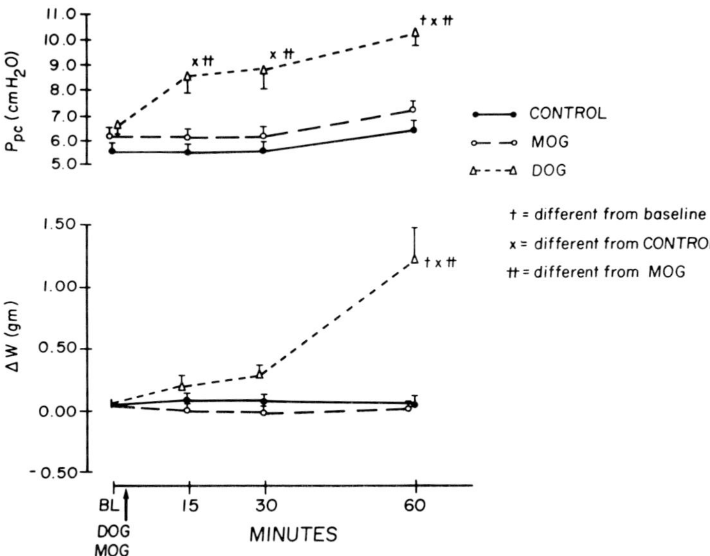

Figure 5 Effect of dioctanoylglycerol (DOG) on pulmonary capillary pressure (P_{pc}) and lung weight gain (ΔW) in the isolated guinea pig lung perfused with phosphate-buffered Ringer's solution containing 5.5 m*M* dextrose. The DOG (20 μ*M*) was added at 0 min, immediately after the 10-min baseline perfusion period. The control was monooctanoylglycerol (20 μ*M*), a diacylglycerol that does not activate PKC. DOG increases in P_{pc} and lung weight, whereas MOG does not. (From Johnson et al. 1990.)

plained by the activation of "protective" non-PKC pathways, which may only be overcome by the addition of neutrophils.

PMA treatment probably increases vascular pressures indirectly via the release of soluble mediators, as opposed to a direct effect on the smooth muscle of the vasculature leading to vasoconstriction. Metabolites of arachidonic acid are important mediators of the pulmonary vascular effects of PMA. In the in situ dog lung, pretreatment with the TxA_2 synthetase inhibitor OKY-046 attenuates the increases in pulmonary vascular resistance and prevents the increase in permeability after PMA treatment (Allison et al., 1986). This observation has been verified in the guinea pig because pretreatment with the TxA_2 synthetase inhibitor prevents the increases in vascular pressures, edema, and TxA_2 levels in response to PMA (Johnson, 1988). Leukotrienes may also be important mediators of the pulmonary vascular effects of PMA. PMA treatment of dog lung tissue releases leukotrienes (Sprague et al., 1988), and the effect of PMA in isolated guinea pig lungs is attenuated with the 5-lipoxygenase inhibitor U60,257 and the peptidoleukotriene receptor blocker FPL-55712 (Johnson, 1988). Despite the variety of extracellular effectors mediating the pulmonary vascular response to PMA, a common intracellular pathway might exist. The response to PMA appears to be mediated by intracellular calcium, because verapamil attenuates the pressure response and prevents the permeability increase after PMA challenge (Allison et al., 1986).

Reactive oxygen species also have a role in lung injury induced by PMA and neutrophils. Pretreatment with catalase or deferroxamine reduces the hemodynamic and permeability responses to perfusion of dog lungs with PMA-containing blood (Allison et al., 1988). Catalase has a similar effect on guinea pig lungs perfused with dioctanoylglycerol plus neutrophils (Johnson et al., 1990). In addition, dimethylthiourea prevents the hemodynamic responses to PMA plus neutrophils in rabbit lungs (Jackson et al., 1986). The protective effect of the antioxidants is related to neutrophil-derived reactive oxygen species, because antioxidants do not prevent the PMA response in the absence of neutrophils (Allison et al., 1988; Johnson, 1988). In addition, H_2O_2-induced edema in the isolated guinea pig lung is inhibited using the PKC inhibitor H7 (Fig. 6; Johnson et al., 1989), suggesting that PKC activation may result from as well as lead up to the release of reactive oxygen species. Thus PKC-activating inflammatory mediators may promote the release of reactive oxygen species, which may promote tissue injury directly, or via further PKC activation.

PMA can also effect the metabolic state of the isolated lung. In the airway, the clearance of mannitol and inulin is increased after the tracheal instillation of PMA in isolated lungs, suggesting increases in epithelial permeability (Pitt et al., 1987). The increased clearance (permeability) is prevented using catalase and is

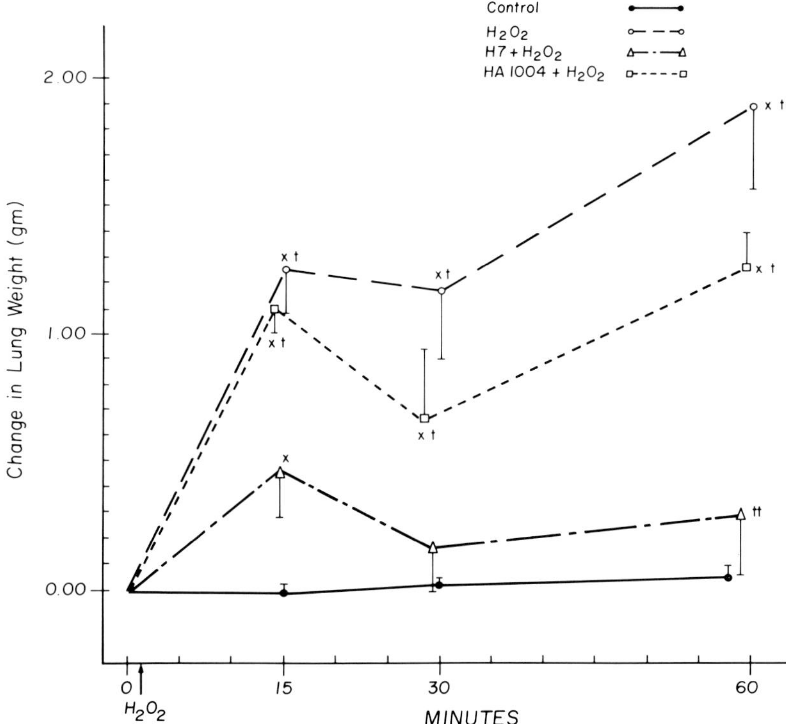

Figure 6 Effect of inhibition of protein kinase (PKC) activation on H_2O_2-induced increase in lung weight in the isolated guinea pig lung perfused with phosphate-buffered Ringer's solution containing 5.5 m*M* dextrose. The H_2O_2 (0.1 m*M*) was added at 0 min, immediately after the 10-min baseline perfusion period. The PKC inhibitor H7 (30 μ*M*) or the control HA1004 (30 μ*M*) was added 10 min before the H_2O_2 in the H_2O_2 + H7 and H_2O_2 = HA1004 groups. The inhibition of PKC activation prevents H_2O_2-induced lung weight gain. (From Johnson et al., 1989.)

independent of circulating neutrophils, implicating pulmonary macrophages as mediators (Pitt et al., 1987). The removal of serotonin (Merker and Gillis, 1988; Weng and Pitt, 1990) and propranolol (Merker and Gillis, 1988) is reduced with PMA treatment of isolated rat or rabbit lungs. PMA may induce this response either by decreasing surface area or by promoting endothelial injury. The effect of PMA on serotonin extraction is prevented using the PKC inhibitor staurosporin (Weng and Pitt, 1990).

B. Pulmonary PKC Activation In Vivo

There is conclusive evidence that intravenous, intraperitoneal, and/or airway challenge with PMA increases vascular permeability, manifested as increases in (1) radiolabeled albumin in the interstitium, (2) bronchoalveolar lavage protein content, (3) flow of protein rich lymph, and (4) extravascular lung water. These data have been obtained using rabbits (O'Flaherty et al., 1980; Taylor et al., 1985; Kuroda et al., 1987; Pitt et al., 1987), mice (Struhar and Harbeck, 1987) rats (Johnson and Ward, 1982; Perry and Taylor, 1988), monkeys (Revak et al., 1985), dogs (Dorinsky et al., 1988; Mizer et al., 1989; Stephenson et al., 1990), and sheep (Loyd et al., 1983; Dyer and Snapper, 1986). There is also morphologic evidence of lung injury (O'Flaherty et al., 1980; Kuroda et al., 1987), characterized by (1) interstitial and alveolar edema, (2) hemorrhage, (3) increases in interstitial and alveolar neutrophils and platelets, and (4) ruffling, vacuolization, and disruption of endothelial and epithelial cells. PMA causes leukopenia and hypoxemia in the sheep (Loyd et al., 1983; Dyer and Snapper, 1986) and dog (Stephenson et al., 1990). In the sheep, increases in (1) pulmonary lymph flow with elevated protein content that suggest increased permeability, (2) pulmonary vascular resistance, (3) pulmonary arterial pressure, and (4) TxA_2 are noted.

The changes noted after intravenous challenge with PMA are mediated by neutrophils in rabbits and rats, because neutrophil-derived H_2O_2 reaction products are increased (Kuroda et al., 1987) with PMA treatment, and neutrophil depletion prevents the PMA response (Taylor et al., 1985; Kuroda et al., 1987; Perry and Taylor, 1988). The dependence on neutrophils for the response to PMA in vivo, however, varies with the species and with the route of PMA challenge. In sheep, the response to intravenous PMA is independent of circulating neutrophils, suggesting that other cell types, such as the intravascular macrophage, are important (Dyer and Snapper, 1986; Warner and Brain, 1990). The airway instillation of PMA in rabbits causes neutrophil-independent lung injury (Johnson and Ward, 1982), which suggests participation of the alveolar macrophage in the PMA effect. In the rat, the increased pulmonary vascular permeability following airway instillation of PMA may depend, however, on the presence of neutrophils (Perry and Taylor, 1988).

There are many soluble mediators of the response to PMA in vivo. Reactive oxygen species are released by neutrophils activated with either PMA or diacylglycerols (Bass et al., 1988; Badwey et al., 1989; Repine et al., 1974; Wright and Hoffman, 1986). Treatment with intravenous superoxide dismutase + catalase or dimethylthiourea prevents the PMA response in rabbits, but not the neutrophil-induced pneumonitis (Kuroda et al., 1987). Superoxide dismutase or catalase alone offer little protection, implicating $OH^{\cdot}$ as the mediator of the PMA response in vivo (Kuroda et al., 1987). In the airway instillation model, catalase prevents the PMA response, but superoxide dismutase has no effect (Johnson and Ward, 1982), which suggests H_2O_2 generated from alveolar macrophages cause lung injury. In the monkey, PMA instillation causes the generation of reactive oxygen species and proteases, which can contribute to lung injury (Revak et al., 1985). In the sheep cyclooxygenase inhibition blunts the initial increase in pulmonary arterial pressure and hypoxia after intravenous PMA; however, the later alterations in pulmonary hemodynamics are not affected (Newman et al., 1984). The use of cyclooxygenase inhibitors is inconclusive since the synthesis of both constrictor and dilator prostaglandins are inhibited, and shunting to leukotriene synthesis may occur. In the dog, TxA_2 receptor and synthetase antagonists prevented the hypoxemia and blunted the edema but had no effect on the increase in pulmonary arterial pressures after PMA (Stephenson et al., 1990). In contrast, anti-TxA_2 agents prevent the increase in pulmonary vascular resistance after PMA treatment in the isolated lung, as noted above. This apparent discrepancy in the role of TxA_2 during PMA-induced lung injury can be attributed to the generation of different mediators with blood perfusion (Allison et al., 1986; Stephenson et al., 1990) compared to perfusion with acellular buffer used in the isolated lung studies (Johnson, 1988).

Pulmonary PKC activation in vivo is also characterized by alterations of the metabolic function of the lung. In rabbits, PMA increases the K_M value for [^{3}H]BPAP and [^{14}C]AMP but not for serotonin (McCormick et al., 1987; Havill et al., 1989). The increases in K_m value are independent of vascular surface area and injury (McCormick et al., 1987; Havill et al., 1989). These data suggest alterations in angiotensin converting enzyme and 5′-nucleotidase activity induced by PKC activation.

VI. Summary

The studies reviewed above support the hypothesis that pulmonary PKC activation serves as a pro-inflammatory intracellular signal transduction system mediating noncardiogenic pulmonary edema (Fig. 7). Substances with potentially anti-edemagenic properties, such as PGE_1 and PGE_2 (Brigham et al., 1983; Chopra and Webster, 1988; Downey et al., 1988; Tate et al., 1988), and PGI_2 (Czer et al., 1986), may also be generated during PKC activation, but the balance seems to favor a pro-inflammatory state.

The PKC activation of both resident cells of the normal lung (i.e., endothelial, fibroblast, smooth muscle, alveolar macrophage, and marginated macrophages and neutrophils) and of the circulating pool of cells (i.e., platelets, monocytes, and neutrophils) may result in pro-inflammatory responses. In the lung, PKC activation mediates, at least in part, the production of phlogistic signals, which include PAF, TxA_2, leukotrienes, and reactive oxygen species. PKC

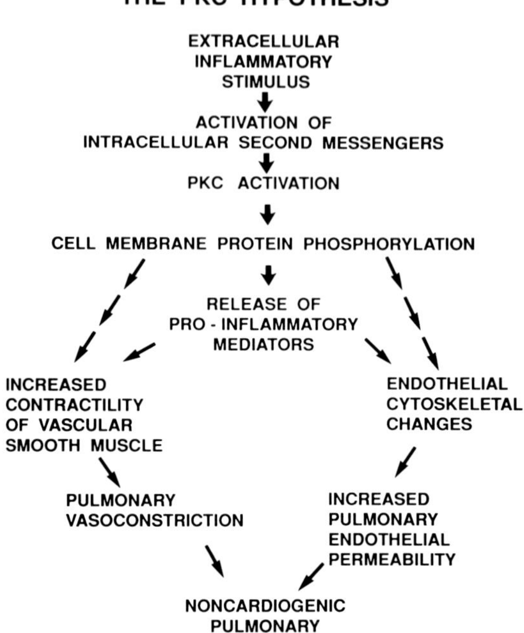

Figure 7 Summary of the proposed schema for the mediation of noncardiogenic pulmonary edema by the activation of pulmonary PKC.

activation can also mediate the response (vasoconstriction, bronchoconstriction, increased permeability, cell adherence) to these inflammatory substances. These substances are known to cause increases in vascular permeability and pressures, hypoxemia, altered lung mechanics, and morphologic signs of vascular injury in different models of pulmonary edema.

Prolonged PKC activation probably decreases the potency of inflammatory signals, due to feedback inhibition of the initial ligand–receptor interaction, G protein, and phospholipase alterations. The implications of this phenomenon in the response to inflammatory signals at the organ level remains to be determined.

The role of PKC in mediating alterations in pulmonary function during different states of pulmonary pathology must be explored. The hypothesis that PKC activation mediates the changes in pulmonary vascular resistance and pressure, airway function, and vascular and airway permeability during the noncardiogenic pulmonary edema associated with sepsis, hyperoxia, intravascular coagulation, smoke and chemical inhalation, and other challenges require further study. If there is a component of PKC activation mediating the inflammatory injury of noncardiogenic pulmonary edema, the inhibition of pulmonary PKC activation at the bedside may prove to be efficacious for management of adult respiratory distress syndrome (ARDS).

Acknowledgments

Supported by the Research Service, Department of Veterans Affairs (A.J), National Institute of Health (NHLBI) (A.J.), the American Heart Association of New York State (A.J.), the American Lung Association of New York State (T.J.F.), and the Potts Memorial Foundation, Catskill, NY (T.J.F., A.J.).

References

Allison, R. C., Marble, K. T., Hernandez, E. M., Townsley, M. I., and Taylor, A. E. (1986). Attenuation of permeability lung injury after phorbol myristate acetate by verapamil and OKY-046. *Am. Rev. Respir. Dis.* **134:**93–100.

Allison, R. C., Hernandez, E. M., Prasad, V. R., Grisham, M. B., and Taylor, A. E. (1988). Protective effects of O_2 radical scavengers and adenosine in PMA-induced lung injury. *J. Appl. Physiol.* **64:**2175–2182.

Antonov, A. S., Lukashev, M. E., Romanov, Y. A., Tkachuk, V. A., Repin, V. S., and Smirnov, V. N. (1986). Morphological alterations in endothelial cells from aorta and umbilical vein induced by forskolin and phorbol 12-myristate 13-acetate: A synergistic action of adenylate cyclase and protein kinase C activators. *Proc. Natl. Acad. Sci. USA* **83:**9704–9708.

Bach, M. K. (1983). *The Leukotrienes: Their Structure, Actions and Role in Disease.* Scope Publications, Kalamazoo, Mich.

Bacon, K. B., and Camp, R. D. R. (1990). Interleukin (IL)-8 induced in vitro human lymphocyte migration is inhibited by cholera and pertussis toxin and inhibitors of protein kinase C. *Biochem. Biophys. Res. Commun.* **169:**1999–1104.

Badwey, J. A., Heyworth, P. G., and Karnovsky, M. L. (1989). Phosphorylation of both 47 and 49 kDa proteins accompanies superoxide release by neutrophils. *Biochem. Biophys. Res. Commun.* **158:**1029–1035.

Bass, D. A., McPhail, L. C., Schmitt, J. D., Morris-Natsclke, S., McCall, C. E., and Wykle, R. L. (1988a). Selective priming of rate and duration of the respiratory burst of neutrophils by 1,2-diacyl and 1-*O*-alkyl-2-acyl diglycerides. *J. Biol. Chem.* **264:**19610–19617.

Bass, D. A., Gerad, C., Olbrantz, P., Wilson, J., McCall, C. E., and McPhail, L. C. (1988b). Priming of the respiratory burst of neutrophils by diacylglycerol. *J. Biol. Chem.* **262:**6643–6649.

Bell, R. M. (1986). Protein kinase C activation by diacylglycerol second messengers. *Cell* **45:**631–632.

Birrel, G. B., Hedberg, K. K., Habliston, D. L., and Griffith, O. H. (1989). Protein kinase C inhibitor H7 alters the actin cytoskeleton of cultured cells. *J. Cell. Physiol.* **141:**74–84.

Block, L. H., Abraham, W. M., Groscurth, P., Qiao, B. Y., and Perruchoud, A. P. (1989). Platelet-activating factor (PAF) dependent biochemical, morphologic and physiologic responses to human platelets. Demonstration of translocation of protein kinase C associated with protein phosphorylation. *Am. J. Respir. Cell Mol. Biol.* **1:**277–288.

Braquet, P., Touqui, L., Shen, T. Y., and Vargaftig, B. B. (1989). Perspectives in platelet activating factor research. *Pharmacol. Rev.* **39:**97–145.

Brett, J., Gerlach, H., Nawroth, P., Steinberg, S., Godman, G., and Stern, D. (1989). Tumor necrosis factor cachectin increases permeability of endothelial cell monolayers by a mechanism involving regulatory G proteins. *J. Exp. Med.* **169:**1977–1991.

Brieland, J. K., Balazovich, K., and Fantone, J. C. (1989). The effect of acute inflammatory lung injury on the respiratory burst and protein kinase C activity of rat pulmonary alveolar macrophages. *Am. Rev. Respir. Dis.* **139:**378–381.

Brigham, K. L., and Owen, P. J. (1975). Mechanism of the serotonin effect on lung transvascular fluid flux and protein movement in awake sheep. Circ. Res. 36: 761–770.

Brigham, K. L., Ogletree, M., Snapper, J. S., Hinson, I., and Parker, R. (1983). Prostaglandins and lung injury. *Chest* **83:**705–725.

Brown, A. M., and Birnbaumer, L. (1988). Direct G protein gating of ion channels. *Am. J. Physiol.* **23:**H401–H410.

Choppa, J., and Webster, R. O. (1988). PGE_1 inhibits neutrophil adherence and neutrophil mediated injury to cultured endothelial cells. *Am. Rev. Respir. Dis.* **138:**915–920.

Clark, M. A., Chen, M. J., Crooke, S. T., and Bomalaski, J. S. (1988). Tumor necrosis factor (cachectin) induces phospholipase A_2 activity and synthesis of a phospholipase A_2-activating protein in endothelial cells. *Biochem. J.* **250:**125–132.

Coburn, R. F., and Barron, C. B. (1990). Coupling mechanisms in airway smooth muscle. *Am. J. Physiol.* **2:**L119–L133.

Consigny, P. M. (1989). Phorbol amplification of serotonin induced arterial contractions is endothelium-dependent. *Am. J. Physiol.* **26:**H1174–H1180.

Czar, G. T., Marsh, J., Konopka, R., and Moser, K. M. (1986). Low dose PGI_2 prevents monocrotaline-induced thromboxane production and lung injury. *J. Appl. Physiol.* **60:**464–471.

Danilov, Y. N., and Juliano, R. L. (1989). Phorbol ester modulation of integrin-mediated cell adhesion: A post-receptor event. *J. Cell Biol.* **108:**1925–1933.

Del Maestro, R. F., Thaw, H. H., Bjork, J., Planker, M., and Arfos, K. E. (1980). Free radicals as mediators of tissue injury. *Acta Physiol. Scand.* **492:**43–57.

Del Vecchio, P. J., and Smith, J. R. (1981). Expression of angiotensin converting enzyme activity in cultured pulmonary artery endothelial cells. *J. Cell. Physiol.* **108:**337–345.

Demling, R. H., Wong, C., Fox, R., Hechtman, H., and Huval, W. (1989). Relationship of increased lung serotonin levels to endotoxin induced pulmonary hypertension in sheep: Effects of a serotonin antagonist. *Am. Rev. Respir. Dis.* **132:**1257–1261.

DiCorleto, P. E., and Motte, C. A. (1989). Thrombin causes increased monocyte cell adhesion to endothelial cells through a protein kinase C–dependent pathway. *Biochem. J.* **264:**71–77.

Dorinsky, P. M., Costello, J. L., and Gadek, J. E. (1988). Oxygen distribution and utilization after phorbol myristate acetate induced lung injury. *Am. Rev. Respir. Dis.* **138:**1454–1463.

Downey, G. P., Gumbay, R. S., Doherty, D. E., LaBrecque, J. F., Henson, J. E., Henson, P. M., and Worthen, G. S. (1988). Enhancement of pulmonary inflammation by PGE_2: Evidence for a vasodilator effect. *J. Appl. Physiol.* **64:**728–741.

Dyer, E. L., and Snapper, J. R. (1986). Role of circulating granulocytes in sheep lung injury produced by phorbol myristate acetate. *J. Appl. Physiol.* **60:**576–589.

Fain, J. N., Wallace, M. A., and Wojcikiewicz, R. J. H. (1988). Evidence for involvement of guanine nucleotide binding regulatory proteins in the activation of phosphoapaces by hormones. *FASEB J.* **2:**2569–2574.

Fallman, M., Lew, D. P., Stendahl, O., and Anderson, T. (1989). Receptor-mediated phagocytosis in human neutrophils is associated with increased formation of inositol phosphates and diaglycerol. *J. Clin. Invest.* **84:**886–891.

Fan, X., Huang, X., DaSilva, C., and Castagna, M. (1990). Arachidonic acid and related methyl ester mediate protein kinase C activation in intact platelets through the arachidonate metabolism pathways. Biochem. Biophys. Res. Commun. 169:933–940.

Farrukh, I. S., Michael, J. R., Summer, W. R., Adkinson, N. F., and Gurtner, G. H. (1985). Thromboxane induced pulmonary vasoconstriction: Involvement of calcium. *J. Appl. Physiol.* **58:**34–44.

Ford-Hutchinson, A. W. (1985). Leukotrienes: Their formation and role as inflammatory mediators. *Fed. Proc.* **44:**19–24.

Fournier, A., Hardy, S. J., Clark, K. J., and Murray, A. W. (1989). Phorbol ester induces differential membrane association of protein kinase C subspecies in human platelets. *Biochem. Physiol. Res. Commun.* **161:**556–561.

Freeman, B. A., and Crapo, J. D. (1982). Free radicals and tissue injury. *Lab. Invest.* **47:**412–426.

Furchgott, R. F. (1983). Role of endothelium in responses of vascular smooth muscle. *Circ. Res.* **53:**558–573.

Gartner, S. L., Sieckmann, D. G., Kang, Y. H., Watson, L. P., and Homer, L. D. (1988). Effects of lipopolysaccharide lipid A, lipid A, lipid X and phorbol ester on cultured bovine endothelial cells. *Lab. Invest.* **59:**181–191.

Gay, J. C., and Sitt, E. S. (1988a). Platelet-activating factor induces protein kinase activity in the particulate fraction of human neutrophils. *Blood* **71:**159–165.

Gay, J. C., and Stitt, E. S. (1988b). Enhancement of phorbol ester-induced protein kinase activity in human neutrophils by platelet activating factor. *J. Cell. Physiol.* **137:**439–447.

George, J. N., Pickett, E. B., Soiecerman, S., McEver, R. P., Kunicki, T. J., Kieffer, N., and Newman, R. J. (1986). Platelet surface glycoproteins. J. Clin. Invest. **78**: 340–348.

Gilman, A. G. (1987). G proteins: Transducers of receptor-operated signal. *Annu. Rev. Biochem.* **56:**615–619.

Grandordy, B. M., Cuss, F. M., Sampson, A. S., Palmer, J. B., and Barnes, P. J. (1986a). Phosphatidylinositol response to cholinergic agonists in airway smooth muscle: Relationship to contraction and muscarinic receptor occupancy. *J. Pharmacol. Exp. Ther.* **238:**273–279.

Grandordy, B. M., Meldrum, L., Sturton, R. G., and Barnes, P. J. (1986b). Leukotriene C_4 and D_4 induce contractions and formation of inositol phosphates in airway lung parenchyma. *Am. Rev. Respir. Dis.* **113:**A-113.

Greenberg, B., Rloden, K., and Barnes, P. J. (1987). Endothelium-dependent relaxation of human pulmonary arteries. *Am. J. Physiol.* **252:**H434–H438.

Havill, A. M., Riggs, D., Pitt, B. R., and Gillis, N. C. (1989). Resolution of impaired pulmonary function and pulmonary hypertension after phorbol ester administration in rabbits. *Am. Rev. Respir. Dis.* **140:**782–788.

Hefner, J. E., Sahn, S. A., and Repine, J. E. (1989). The role of platelets in the adult respiratory distress syndrome: Culprits or bystanders? *Am. Rev. Respir. Dis.* **135:**482–492.

Hidaka, H., Inagaki, M., Kawwomoto, S., and Sasaki, Y. (1984). Isoquinolinesulfonamides novel and potent inhibitors of cyclic nucleotide protein kinase and protein kinase C. *Biochemistry* **23:**5036–5041.

Issaad, C., Ventura, M. A., and Thomopoulos, P. (1989). Biphasic regulation of macrophage attachment by activators of cyclic adenosine monophosphate dependent kinase and protein kinase C. *J. Cell. Physiol.* **140:**317–322.

Jackson, J. H., White, C. W., McMurty, I. F., Berger, E. M., and Repine, J. E. (1986). Dimethylthiourea decreases acute lung edema on phorbol myristate acetate treated rabbits. *J. Appl. Physiol.* **61:**353–360.

Jaken, S., Leach, K., and Kiauck, T. (1989). Association of type 3 protein kinase C with focal contacts in rat embryo fibroblasts. *J. Cell. Biol.* **109:**697–704.

Jiang, M. J., and Morgan, K. G. (1987). Intracellular calcium levels in phorbol ester induced contraction of vascular smooth muscle. *Am. J. Physiol.* **253:**1365–1371.

Johnson, A. (1988). PMA induced pulmonary edema: Mechanism of the vasoactive effect. *J. Appl. Physiol.* **65:**2302–2312.

Johnson, K. J., and Ward, P. A. (1982). Acute and progressive lung injury after contact with phorbol myristate acetate. *Am. J. Pathol.* **107:**29–35.

Johnson, A., Phillips, P., Hocking, D., Tsan, M. F., and Ferro, T. J. (1989). A protein kinase inhibitor prevents pulmonary edema in response to H_2O_2. *Am. J. Physiol.* **25:**H1012–H1022.

Johnson, A., Hocking, D. L., and Ferro, T. J. (1990). Mechanisms of pulmonary edema induced by a diacylglycerol second messenger. *Am. J. Physiol.* H85–H91.

Kamp, D. W., Bauer, K. D., Rubin, D. B., and Dunn, M. M. (1988). Tumor promoting phorbol esters inhibit monocyte adherence to endothelial cells. *J Appl. Physiol.* **66:**437–442.

Kamp, D. W., Bauer, K. D., Knap, A., and Dunn, M. M. (1989). Contrasting effects of inflammatory stimuli on neutrophil and monocyte adherence to endothelial cells. *J. Appl. Physiol.* **67:**556–562.

Katusic, Z. S., and Vanhoutte, P. M. (1989). Superoxide anion is an endothelium derived contracting factor. *Am. J. Physiol.* **26:**H28–H33.

Khalil, R. A., and Van Breeman, C. (1988). Sustained contraction of vascular smooth muscle-calcium influx on C kinase activation. *J. Pharmacol. Exp. Ther.* **244:** 557–542.

Kobayashi, E., Nakamo, H., Morimoto, M., and Tamaoki, T. (1989). Calphostin C (UCN-1028C), a novel microbial compound, is a highly potent and specific inhibitor of protein kinase C. *Biochem. Biophys. Res. Commun.* **159:**548–553.

Kuroda, M., Murakami, K., and Ishikawa, Y. (1987). Role of hydroxyl radical derived from granulocytes in lung injury induced by phorbol myristate acetate. *Am. Rev. Respir. Dis.* **136:**1435–1444.

Lane, T. A., Lamkin, G. E., and Wancewicz, E. V. (1990). Protein kinase C inhibitors block the enhanced expression of intercellular adhesion molecule-1 on endothelial cells activated by interleukin-1, lipopolysaccride and tumor necrosis factor. *Biochem. Biophys. Res. Commun.* **172:**1273–1281.

Leach, K. L., Powers, E. A., McGuire, J. C., Dong, L., Kiley, S. C., and Jaken, S. (1988). Monoclonal antibodies specific for type 3 protein kinase C recognize district domains of protein kinase C and inhibit functional activity. *J. Biol. Chem.* **263:**13223–13230.

Leach, K. L., Powers, E. A., Ruff, V. A., Jaken, S., and Kaufmann, S. (1989). Type 3 protein kinase C localization to the nuclear envelop of phorbol ester treated NTH 3T3 cells. *J. Cell Biol.* **109:**685–695.

Leyravaud, S., Bossant, M. J., Joly, F., Bessou, G., Benveniste, J., and Ninio, E. (1989). Biosynthesis of PAF-acether: Phorbol myristate acetate induced PAF-acether biosynthesis and acetlyltransferase activation in human neutrophils. *J. Immunol.* **143:**245–249.

Liles, W. C., Meir, K. E., and Henderson, W. R. (1988). Phorbol myristate acetate and the calcium ionophore A23187 synergistically induce release of LTB_4 by human neutrophils: Involvement of protein kinase C activation in regulation of the 5-lipooxygenase pathway. *J. Immunol.* **138:**3396–3402.

Loyd, J. E., Newman, J. H., English, D., Ogletree, M. L., Meyrick, B. O., and Brigham, K. L. (1983). Lung vascular effects of phorbol myristate acetate in awake sheep. *J. Appl. Physiol.* **54:**267–276.

Lynch, J. J., Ferro, T. J., Blumenstock, F. A., Brockenauer, A. M., and Malik, A. B. (1990). Increased endothelial permeability mediated by protein kinase C. *J. Clin. Invest.* **85:**1991–1998.

Mackie, K., Lai, Y., Nairn, A. C., Greengard, P., Pitt, B. R., and Slaso, J. (1986). Protein phosphorylation in cultured endothelial cells. *J. Cell. Physiol.* **128:**367–374.

Magnuson, D. K., Maier, R. V., and Pohlman, T. H. (1989). Protein kinase C: A potential pathway of endothelial cell activation by endotoxin, tumor necrosis factor and interleukin-1. *Surgery* **106:**216–223.

Martin, T. W., Feldman, D. R., Goldstein, K. E., and Wagner, J. R. (1989). Long term phorbol ester treatment dissociates phospholipase D activation from phosphoinositide hydrolysis and prostacyclin synthesis in endothelial cells stimulated with bradykinin. *Biochem. Biophys. Res. Commun.* **165:**319–326.

McCormick, J. R., Chrzanowski, R., Andreani, J., and Catravas, J. D. (1987). Early pulmonary endothelial enzyme dysfunction after phorbol ester in conscious rabbits. *J. Appl. Physiol.* **63:**1972–1978.

McDonald, J. A. (1989). Receptors for extracellular matrix components. *Am. J. Physiol.* **257:**L331–L332.

Merker, M. P., and Gillis, C. N. (1988). Propanolol and serotonin removal in lung injury. *J. Appl. Physiol.* **65:**2579–2584.

Miller, J. R., Hawkins, D. J., and Wells, J. N. (1986). Phorbol esters alter the contractile responses of porcine coronary artery. *J. Pharmacol. Exp. Ther.* **239:**38–42.

Mitsuhashi, M., and Payan, D. G. (1988). Phorbol ester mediated desensitization of histamine H_2 receptors on a cultured smooth muscle cell line. *Life Sci.* **43:**1433–1440.

Mizer, L. A., Weisbrode, S. E., and Dorinsky, P. M. (1989). Neutrophil accumulation and structural changes in nonpulmonary organs after acute lung injury induced by phorbol myristate acetate. *Am. Rev. Respir. Dis.* **139:**1017–1029.

Mukaida, N., Yagisawa, H., Kawai, T., and Kasahara, T. (1988). The role of protein kinase C activation in signal transmission by interleukin-2. *Biochem. Biophys. Res. Commun.* **154:**187–193.

Munoz, N. M., Shioya, T., Murphy, T. M., Primack, S., Dame, C., Sands, M. F., and Leff, A. R. (1986). Potentiation of vagal contractile response by thromboxane mimetic U-46619. *J. Appl. Physiol.* **61:**1173–1179.

Murray, R. K., Bennett, C. F., Fluharty, S. J., and Kotikoff, M. I. (1989). Mechanism of phorbol ester inhibition of histamine induced IP_3 formation in cultured airway smooth muscle. *Am. J. Physiol.* **1:**L209–L216.

Myers, C. L., Lazo, J. S., and Pitt, B. R. (1989). Translocation of protein kinase C is associated with inhibitors of 5-HT uptake by cultured endothelial cells. *Am. J. Physiol.* **1:**L253–L258.

Naccache, P. H., Molski, T. F. P., Borgeat, P., and Shaafi, R. I. (1985). Intracellular calcium redistribution and its relationship to f-Met-Leu-Phe, leukotriene B_4 and phorbol ester induced rabbit neutrophil degranulation. *J. Cell. Physiol.* **122:** 273–280.

Nairn, A. C., Hemmings, H. C., and Greengard, P. (1985). Protein kinase C in the brain. *Annu. Rev. Biochem.* **54:**931–976.

Newman, J. H., Loyd, J. E., Ogletree, M. L., Meyrick, B. O., and Brigham, K. L. (1984). Cyclooxygenase inhibition during phorbol-induced granulocyte stimulation in awake sheep. *J. Appl. Physiol.* **56:**999–1007.

Nishimura, J., Klalid, R. A., Dreuth, J. P., and Breeman, C. V. (1990). Evidence for increased myofilament Ca^{2+} sensitivity in norepinephrine activated vascular smooth muscle. *Am. J. Physiol.* **259:**H2–H8.

Nishizuka, Y. (1984). The role of protein kinase C in cell surface signal transduction and tumor-promotion. *Nature* **308:**693–698.

Nishizuka, Y. (1986). Studies and perspectives of protein kinase C. *Science* **233:**305–312.

O'Flaherty, J. T., Cousant, S., Lineberger, A. S., Bond, E., Bass, A., Dechatelet L. R., Leake, E. S., and McCall, C. E. (1980). Phorbol myristate acetate: In vivo effects upon neutrophils, platelets and the lung. *Am. J. Pathol.* **101:**79–90.

O'Flaherty, J. T., Redman, J. F., and Jacobson, D. P. (1990). Mechanisms invoked in the bidirectional effects of protein kinase C activators on neutrophil responses to leukotriene B_4. *J. Immunol.* **144:**1909–1913.

Orton, E. C., Raffestin, B., and McMurtry, I. F. (1990). Protein kinase C influences rat pulmonary vascular reactivity. *Am. Rev. Respir. Dis.* **141:**654–658.

Parker, J., Daniel, L. W., and Waite, M. (1987). Evidence of protein kinase C involvement in phorbol ester-stimulated arachidonic and acid release and prostaglandin synthesis. *J. Biol. Chem.* **262:**5385–5393.

Pelosin, J. M., Keramidas, M., Souvignet, C., and Chambaz, E. M. (1990). Differential inhibition of protein kinase C subtypes. *Biochem. Biophys. Res. Commun.* **169:**1040–1048.

Perry, M., and Taylor, A. E. (1988). Phorbol myristate acetate-induced injury of isolated perfused rat lungs: Neutrophil dependence. *J. Appl. Physiol.* **65:**2164–2169.

Perry, M. L., Kayes, S. G., Barnard, J. W., and Taylor, A. E. (1990). Effects of phorbol myristate acetate stimulated human leukocytes rat lung. *J. Appl. Physiol.* **68:**235–240.

Petrone, W. F., English, D. K., Wong, K., and McCord, J. M. (1980). Free radicals and inflammation: Superoxide dependent activation of a neutrophil chemotactic factor in plasma. *Proc. Natl. Acad. Sci. USA* **77:**1159–1163.

Pfannkuche, H. J., Kaever, V., and Resch, K. (1986). A possible role of protein kinase C in regulating prostaglandin synthesis of mouse peritoneal macrophages. *Biochem. Biophys. Res. Commun.* **139:**604–611.

Phillips, G., Lum, H., Malik, A. B., and Tsan, M. F. (1990). Phallacidin prevents thrombin induced increases in endothelial permeability to albumin. *Am. J. Physiol.* **257:** 562–567.

Piper, P. J. (1984). Formation and actions of leukotrienes. *Physiol. Rev.* **64:**744–761.

Pitt, B. R., Cole, J. S., Davies, P., and Gillis, C. N. (1987). Rapid increases in respiratory epithelial permeability occur after intratracheal instillation of PMA. *J. Appl. Physiol.* **63:**242–301.

Pontremoli, S., Melloni, E., Michetti, M., Sparatore, B., Salamino, F., Sacco, O., and Horecker, B. L. (1987). Phosphorylation and proteolytic modification of specific cytoskeletal proteins in human neutrophils stimulated by phorbol 12-myristate 13-acetate. *Proc. Natl. Acad. Sci. USA* **84:**3604–3608.

Rando, R. R. (1988). Regulation of protein C activity by lipids. *FASEB J.* **2:**2348–2355.

Rasio, E. A., Bendayaiv, M., Goresky, C. A., Alexander, J., Steven, and Shepro, D. (1989). Effect of phallodin on structure and permeability of rete capillaries in the normal and hypoxic state. *Circ. Res.* **65:**591–599.

Rasmussen, H., Takuwa, Y., and Park, S. (1987). Protein kinase C in the regulation of smooth muscle contraction. *FASEB J.* **1:**177–185.

Reibman, J., Korchak, H. M., Vosshall, L. B., Haines, K. A., Rich, A. B., and Weissmann,

G. (1988). Changes in diacylglycerol labeling, cell shape and protein phosphoriylation distinguish ''triggering'' from ''activation'' of human neutrophils. *J. Biol. Chem.* **263:**6322–6328.

Reinders, J. M., Vervoorn, R. C., Verwe, C. L., Van Mourik, J. A., and De Groot, P. G. (1982). Perturbation of cultured human vascular endothelial cells by phorbol ester or thrombin alters the cellular von Willebrand factor distribution. *J. Cell. Physiol.* **153:**79–87.

Reinhold, S. L., Prescott, S. M., Zimmerman, G. A., and McIntyre, T. M. (1990). Activation of human neutrophil phospholipase D by three separable mechanisms. *FASEB J.* **4:**208–214.

Rembold, C. M., and Murphy, R. A. (1988). [Ca^{2+}]-dependent myosin phosphorylation in phorbol ester stimulated smooth muscle contraction. *Am. J. Physiol.* **255:**C719–C723.

Repine, J. E., White, J. G., Clawson, C. C., and Holmes, B. M. (1974). Effects of phorbol myristate acetate on the metabolism and ultrastructure of neutrophils in chronic granulomatous disease. *J. Clin. Invest.* **54:**83–90.

Reyak, S. D., Rice, C. L., Schraufshatter, A., Halsey, W. A., Bohl, B. P., Clancy, R. M., and Cockrane, C. G. (1985). Experimental pulmonary inflammatory injury in the monkey. *J. Clin. Invest.* **76:**1182–1192.

Ritchie, A. J., Johnson, D. R., Ewenstein, B. M., and Pober, J. S. (1991). Tumor necrosis factor induction of endothelial cell surface antigens is independent of protein kinase C activation or inactivation. *J. Immunol.* **146:**3056–3062.

Royall, J. A., Berkow, R. L., Beckman, J. S., Cunningham, M. K. Matalon, S., and Freeman, B. A. (1989). Tumor necrosis factor and interleukin 1α increase vascular endothelial permeability. *Am. J. Physiol.* **257:**L399–L410.

Rubanyi, G. M., and Vanhoutte, P. M. (1986). Oxygen derived free radicals endothelium and responsiveness of vascular smooth muscle. *Am. J. Physiol.* **250:**H813–H821.

Schramm, C. M., and Grunstein, M. M. (1989). Mechanisms of protein kinase C regulation of airway contractility. *J. Appl. Physiol.* **66:**1935–1941.

Schutze, S., Scheurich, P., Pfizenmaier, K., and Kronke, M. (1989). Tumor necrosis factor signal transduction: Tissue specific serine phosphorylation of a 26 kDa cytostolic protein. *J. Biol. Chem.* **264:**3562–3567.

Selvaraj, P. M., Goodwin, J. D., and Ryan, V. S. (1987). Superoxide anion release by pulmonary endothelium: Response to phorbol ester and calcium ionophore. *Fed. Proc.* **46:**1401.

Shasby, D. M., Shasby, S. S., Sullivan, J. M., and Peach, M. J. (1982a). Role of endothelial cell cytoskeleton in control of endothelial permeability. *Circ. Res.* **51:**657–661.

Shasby, D. M., Vanbenthuysen, K. M., Tate, R. M., Shasby, S. S., McMurtry, I., and Repine, J. E. (1982b). Granulocytes mediate acute edematous lung injury in rabbits and in isolated rabbit lungs perfused with phorbol myristate acetate role of oxygen radicals. *Am. Rev. Respir. Dis.* **125:**443–447.

Shasby, D. M., Shasby, S. S., and Peach, M. J. (1983). Granulocytes and phorbol myristate acetate increase permeability to albumin of cultured endothelial monolayers and isolated lungs. *Am. Rev. Respir. Dis.* **127:**72–76.

Shasby, D. M., Lind, S. E., Shasby, S. S., Goldsmith, J. C., and Hunninghake, G. W. (1985). Reversible oxidant induced increases in albumin transfer across cultured endothelium: Alterations in cell shape and calcium homeostasis. *Blood* **65:** 605–614.

Shasby, D. M., Yorek, M., and Shasby, S. S. (1988a). Exogenous oxidants initiate hydrolysis of endothelial cell in inositol phospholipids. *Blood* **72:**491–499.

Shasby, D. M., Winter, M., and Shasby, S. S. (1988b). Oxidants and conductance of cultured epithelial cell monolayer inositol phospholipid hydrolysis. *Am. J. Physiol.* **255:**781–788.

Shaw, L. M., Messier, J. M., and Mercurio, A. M. (1990). The activation dependent adhesion of macrophages to laminin involves cytoskeletal anchoring and phosphorylation of the $\alpha_6\beta_1$ integrin. *J. Cell Biol.* **110:**2167–2174.

Shearman, M. S., Sekiguchi, K., and Nishizuka, Y. (1989). Modulation of ion channel activity: A key function of the protein kinase C enzyme family. *Pharmacol. Rev.* **41:**212–239.

Shenolikar, S. (1988). Protein phosphorylation: Hormones, drugs and bioregulation. *FASEB J.* **2:**2753–2764.

Skoglund, G., Cotgreave, I., Rincon, J., Patarroyo, M., and Ingelman-Sunberg, M. (1988). H_2O_2 activates CD11/CD18 dependent cell adhesion. *Biochem. Biophys. Res. Commun.* **157:**443–449.

Souhrada, M., and Souhrada, J. F. (1989a). The role of protein kinase C in sensitization and antigen response of airway smooth muscle. *Am. Rev. Respir. Dis.* **140:**1567–1572.

Souhrada, M., and Souhrada, J. F. (1989b). Sodium and calcium influx induced by phorbol ester airway smooth muscle cells. *Am. Rev. Respir. Dis.* **139:**927–932.

Sprague, R. S., Stephenson, A. H., Dahms, T. E., and Lonigro, A. J. (1988). Synthesis of leukotrienes by dog lung tissue fragments in response to phorbol myristate acetate. *FASEB J.* **2:**A1185.

Stabel, S., Rodriguez-Pena, A., Young, S., Rosengurt, E., and Parker, P. J. (1987). Quantitation of protein kinase C by immunoblot: Expression in different cell lines and response to phorbol esters. *J. Cell. Physiol.* **130:**111–117.

Stephens, K. E., Ishizaka, A., Larrk, J. W., and Raffin, T. A. (1988). Tumor necrosis factor causes increased pulmonary permeability and edema. *Am. Rev. Respir. Dis.* **137:**1364–1370.

Stephenson, A. H., Sprague, R. S., Dahms, T. E., and Lonigro, A. J. (1990). Thromboxane does not mediate pulmonary hypertension in phorbol ester induced acute lung injury in dogs. *J. Appl. Physiol.* **69:**345–352.

Stewart, D. J., Pohl, U., and Bassenoce, E. (1988). Free radicals inhibit endothelium dependent dilation in the coronary resistance bed. *Am. J. Physiol.* **24:**H765–H769.

Struhar, D., and Harbeck, R. J. (1987). Inhibition of induced acute lung edema by a novel protein kinase C inhibitor. *FASEB J.* **1:**116–118.

Sugiura, M., Inagami, T., Hare, G. M. T., and Johns, J. A. (1990). Endothelium action: Inhibition by a protein kinase C inhibitor and involvement of phosphoinositols. *Biochem. Biophys. Res. Commun.* **158:**170–176.

Takuwa, Y., and Park, S. (1987). Protein kinase C in the regulation of smooth muscle contraction. *FASEB J.* **1:**177–185.

Takuwa, Y., Takuwa, N., and Rasmussen, H. (1986). Carbachol induces a rapid and sustained hydrolysis in bovine tracheal smooth muscle. Measurements of the mass of polyphosoinositides, 1,2-diacylglycerol and phosphatidic acid. *J. Biol. Chem.* **261:**14670–14675.

Tamaoki, T., Nomoto, H., Takahashi, I., Kato, Y., Morimoto, M., and Tomita, F. (1986). Staurosporine a potent inhibitor of phospholipid/Ca^{+2} dependent protein kinase. *Biochem. Biophys. Res. Commun.* **135:**397–402.

Tate, G. A., Mandell, B. F., Schumacher, H. R., and Zurier, R. B. (1988). Suppression of acute inflammation of 16-methyl prostaglandin E_1. *Lab. Invest.* **59:**192–199.

Taylor, R. G., McCall, C. E., Thrall, R. S., Woodruff, R. D., and O'Flaherty, J. T. (1985). Histopathologic features of phorbol myristate acetate–induced lung injury. *Lab. Invest.* **52:**61–70.

Thelen, M., Peveri, P., Kernen, P., Tscharner, V. V., Wals, A., and Baggiolini, M. (1988). Mechanisms of neutrophil activation by NAF, a novel monocyte derived peptide agonist. *FASEB J.* **2:**2702–2706.

Tracey, K. J., Beutler, B., Lowry, S. F., Merryweather, J., Wolpe, S., Milsark, I., Hariri, R., Fahey, T., Zentella, A., Albert, J., Shires, G. T., and Cerami, A. (1986). Shock and tissue injury induced by recombinant human cachectin. *Science* **234:**470–474.

Voyno-Yasenetskaya, T. A., Tkachuk, V. A., Cheknyova, E. G., Panchenko, M. P., Grigorian, G. Y., Vavrek, R. J., Stewart, J. M., and Ryan, U. S. (1989). Guanine nucleotide-dependent pertussis toxin–insensitive regulation of phosphoinositide turnover by bradykinin in bovine pulmonary artery endothelial cells. *FASEB J.* **3:**44–51.

Warner, A. E., and Brain, J. D. (1990). The cell biology and pathogenic role of pulmonary intravascular macrophage. *Am. J. Physiol.* **2:**L1–L12.

Watson, P., McNally, J., Shipman, L. J., and Godfrey, P. P. (1988). The action of the protein kinase C inhibitor staurosporine on human platelets. *Biochem. J.* **249:** 345–350.

Weng, W., and Pitt, B. R. (1990). Activation of protein kinase C inhibits extraction of serotonin by perfused rat lung in situ. *Am. J. Physiol.* **2:**L289–L293.

White, J. R., Huang, C. K., Hill, J. M., Naccache, P. H., Becker, E. L., and Shaafi, R. I. (1984). Effect of phorbol 12-myristate 13-acetate and its analogue 4-phorbol 12,13 didecanoate on protein phosphorylation and lysozomal enzyme release in rabbit neutrophils. *J. Biol. Chem.* **259:**8605–8611.

Winkler, J. D., Sarau, H. M., Foley, J. J., and Crooke, S. T. (1982). Phorbol 12-myristate 13-acetate inhibition of leukotriene D_4-induced signal transduction was rapidly reversed by staurosporine. *Biochem. Biophys. Res. Commun.* **157:**571–529.

Wolfson, M., McPhail, L. C., Nasrallah, V. N., and Snyderman, R. (1985). Phorbol myristate acetate mediates redistribution of protein kinase C in human neutrophils: Potential role in the activation of the respiratory burst enzyme. *J. Immunol.* **135:**2057–2062.

Wright, C. D., and Hoffman, M. D. (1986). The protein kinase C inhibitors H-7 and H-9 fail to inhibit human neutrophil activation. *Biochem. Biophys. Res. Commun.* **135:**749–755.

Wright, S. D., and Meyer, B. C. (1986). Phorbol esters cause sequential activation and deactivation of complement receptors on polymorphonuclear leukocytes. *J. Immunol.* **136:**1759–1764.

Yamazaki, M., Gomez-Cambronero, J., Durstin, M., Molski, T. F. P., Becker, E. L., and Shaafi, R. I. (1989). Phorbol 12–myristate 13–acetate inhibits binding of leukotriene B_4 and platelet activating factor and the responses they produced in neutrophils: Site of action. *Proc. Natl. Acad. Sci. USA* **86:**5791–5794.

Zavoico, G. B., Hrbolich, J. K., Gimbrone, M. A., Jr., and Schafer, A. I. (1990). Enhancement of thrombosis and ionomycin stimulated prostaglandin and platelet activating factor production in cultured endothelial cells by a tumor promoting phorbol ester. *J. Cell. Physiol.* **143:**596–605.

Zhang, Y., Lin, J. X., Yip, Y. K., and Vilcek, J. (1988). Enhancement of cAMP levels of protein kinase activity by tumor necrosis factor and interleukin-1 in human fibroblasts: Role in the induction of interleukin-6. *Proc. Natl. Acad. Sci. USA* **85:**6802–6805.

3

The Role of cAMP in the Regulation of Pulmonary Vascular Permeability

G. H. GURTNER

New York Medical College
Valhalla, New York

A. KNOBLAUCH

Kantonsspital St. Gallen
St. Gallen, Switzerland

A. M. SCIUTO

U.S. Army Medical Research Institute
of Chemical Defense
Aberdeen Proving Grounds, Maryland

I. Introduction

Drugs that increase cAMP are useful therapeutic and investigative tools. It is well accepted that these drugs are potent bronchodilators and vasodilators because of their action on smooth muscle. The mechanisms of action, however, appear to be complex and multifactorial; this is reviewed below. The smooth muscle elements action and myosin are present in the cytoskeleton of pulmonary endothelial cells, and contraction of these elements could open tight junctions between cells and increase vascular permeability (Becker and Machman, 1973; DeClerck et al., 1981; Wong et al., 1983). Cyclic AMP–induced inhibition of this process may prevent increase permeability in lung injury, and relaxation of contracted cells may reverse the pathophysiological events in lung injury. There is evidence that in systemic and bronchial vessels, development of gaps between endothelial cells increases vascular permeability (Majno and Palade, 1961; Majno et al., 1967; Svensjo et al., 1979; Pietra et al., 1971). More recently, it has become increasingly clear that the same phenomenon occurs in the pulmonary circulation in several models of acute lung injury and has also been demonstrated using pulmonary endothelial cell monolayers. Although cAMP has direct antipermeability effects, other actions of this second messenger, such as inhibition of mediator production, can also affect pulmonary vascular permeability.

II. Effects of cAMP in Acute Lung Injury

The effects of drugs that increase cAMP have been investigated in several lung injury models using isolated lungs or intact animals. When used as a pretreatment or treatment, isoproterenol or aminophylline can protect against acid aspiration lung injury in rabbits (Mizus et al., 1985), or peroxide-induced lung injury in rabbits (Farrukh et al., 1988). Pretreatment with PGE_1 or dibutyryl cAMP also protected against peroxide-induced injury. Pretreatment with isoproterenol protected against thrombin-induced injury in intact sheep (Minnear et al, 1986). Pretreatment with β adrenergic drugs, aminophylline, or dibtyryl cAMP prevented edema formation in phosgene-exposed rabbit lungs (Kennedy et al., 1989). Pretreatment or treatment with isoproterenol or aminophylline protected against endotoxin injury in the pig lung (Walman et al., 1984; Parker et al., 1984). In these experiments, blood-perfused lungs from 20-kg pigs were studied. When we studied the effect of endotoxin alone, it was administered in a continuous infusion until pulmonary artery pressure reached twice the basal level. The same endotoxin dosages were administered to isolated lungs pretreated with a continuous infusion of isoproterenol. Several doses of isoproterenol were investigated; however, we found complete inhibition of endotoxin-induced vasoconstriction and lung weight gain at infusions as small as 0.5. μg/min. Since isoproterenol presented both endotoxin-induced pulmonary hypertension and lung weight gain, we attempted to differentiate experimentally between vascular pressure effects from those caused by changes in vascular permeability by changing left atrial pressure before and after endotoxin administration. These observations are shown in Fig. 1.

The results show that pretreatment with isoproterenol completely protected against endotoxin-induced injury. In addition, weight gain in the isoproterenol-treated lungs prior to administration of endotoxin was significantly lower than in the untreated lungs at positive (but not at negative) left atrial pressure. This observation suggests that cAMP may have a physiological role in the regulation of pulmonary vascular permeability.

The drugs used in these studies increase tissue cAMP by different mechanisms: Dibutyryl cAMP is a form of cAMP; isoproterenol activates adenyl cyclase associated with the β adrenergic receptor; PGE1 activates an adenylate cyclase, which is not associated with the β adrenergic receptor and aminophylline inhibits cAMP phosphodiesterase (Farrukh et al., 1987). The common mechanism of protective action appears to be the increase in cAMP.

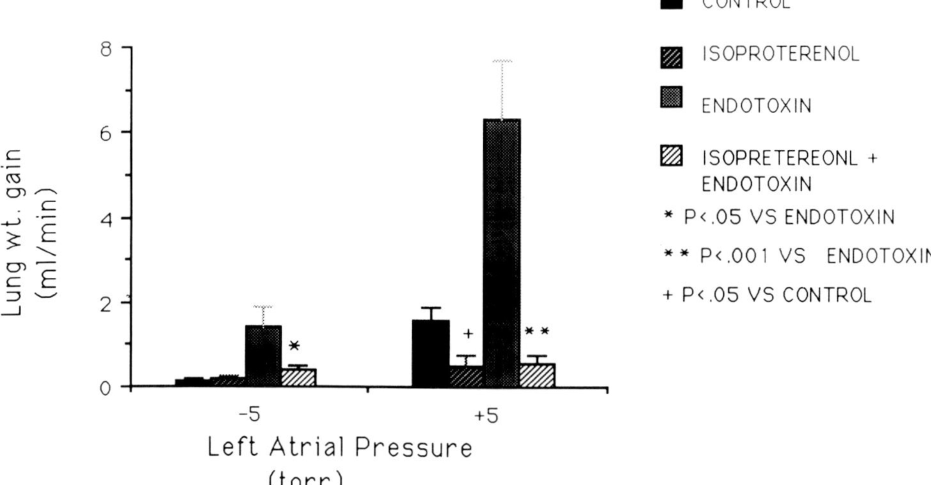

Figure 1 Lung weight gain in the experimental groups at two left atrial pressures. In the endotoxin group, weight gain was significantly greater than control at both left atrial pressures. Pretreatment with isoproterenol presented endotoxin-induced weight gain. Administration of 20 mg of the β adrenergic blocker propranolol reversed the protective effect of isoproterenol. Propranolol also blocks the protective effects of isoproterenol in acid aspiration lung injury. (From Mizus et al., 1985.)

III. Effects of Drugs That Increase cGMP in Acute Lung Injury

We investigated the effect of sodium nitroprusside (SNP), a drug that increases cGMP using the peroxide injury model (Jafri and Gurtner 1990) and found that SNP did not protect against oxidant challenge. We subsequently investigated the effects of dibutyryl cGMP and 8-bromo cGMP and found that these forms of cGMP did not have antipermeability effects. Since all of these compounds are potent vasodilators, we conclude that the antipermeability effects of drugs that increase cAMP could not be due to their vasodilator action alone.

IV. Temporal Nature of cAMP-Related Protection

Posttreatment with drugs that increase cAMP can also protect if the agents are administered early in the course of the pathophysiological events. Aminophylline administered 30 min after acid aspiration challenge completely arrests edema formation (Mizus et al., 1985). Aminophylline administered soon after peroxide challenge blocks edema formation (Farrukh et al., 1987). Beta adrenergic drugs, dibutyryl cAMP, or aminophylline administered approximately 30 min after phosgene exposure are effective in blocking edema formation (Kennedy et al., 1989).

In contrast, if treatment is delayed, the salutary effects of these drugs are less clear. Aminophylline or β adrenergic drugs administered approximately 6 h after *Pseudomonas* challenge to sheep lowered pulmonary vascular pressure and lymph protein clearance; however, the authors believed that these effects could be explained by the reduction in vascular pressure alone (Foy et al., 1979). Since these drugs have acute antipermeability effects in sheep (Minnear et al., 1986) and since they protect acutely in endotoxin injury (Walman et al., 1984), the diminished effectiveness observed after delayed administration may reflect irreversible changes. This phenomenon may explain why some of the agents have not been effective in treatment of full-blown adult respiratory distress syndrome (ARDS) (Silverman et al., 1990) and suggest the importance of early treatment. This is discussed below in greater detail.

V. Effects of cAMP on the Permeability of Endothelial Cell Monolayers

Several groups have investigated the effects of increased cAMP on the permeability of pulmonary artery endothelial cells grown on porous filters (Shasby et al., 1982; Stelzner et al., 1990). The baseline permeability of these monolayers can be reduced approximately 10-fold by cholera toxin or forskolin, both of which cause substantial elevation of cAMP (Stelzner et al., 1989). Although these agonists have not been tested in isolated lungs, drugs that increase cAMP do not decrease lung weight gain in uninjured isolated lungs perfused in zone 2 conditions (i.e., left atrial pressure < alveolar pressure) (Fig 1). The observations taken together suggest that normal vascular endothelium in vivo affords tighter barrier under normal conditions than do endothelial cell monolayers. Under conditions in which left atrial pressure exceeds alveolar pressure by 10 to 15 torr, isoproterenol significantly reduces lung weight gain (Fig. 1). A similar effect of aminophylline was observed in buffer-perfused rabbit lungs (Kennedy et al., 1989). These findings suggest that even modest elevation of pulmonary microvascular pressure can increase vascular permeability and that this is prevented by increased cAMP.

VI. Effects of cAMP on Mediator Production

A. Animal Experiments

We and other investigators find that mediators derived from arachidonic acid are of primary importance in peroxide- or phosgene-induced lung injury (Farrukh et al., 1988; Guo et al., 1990; Gurtner, 1987). Phosgene-induced lung injury is oxidant in nature and appears to be caused by inactivation of antioxidant sulfhydryls by direct chemical reaction. Drugs that increase cAMP can protect against both types of lung injury (Farrukh et al., 1987; Kennedy, et al., 1989). Since these drugs have been shown to prevent or reverse endothelial contraction and act as vasodilators, we thought this to be the most likely mechanism of protection. Therefore, the observation that aminophylline or isoproterenol could inhibit thromboxane and peptide leukotriene production in the phosgene model was not anticipated. The data are shown in Fig. 2; aminophylline or isoproterenol significantly inhibited phosgene-induced edema formation and the production of peptide leukotrienes (C_4/D_4/E_4) and thromboxane. The mechanism of protection in this injury model is not clear since drugs that increase cAMP have direct antipermeability effects as well. A similar protective effects occurs with administration of 4,8,11,14-eicosapentanyoic (ETYA), which blocks all pathways of arachidonic acid metabolism or by peptide leukotriene receptor antagonists (Farrukh et al., 1988; Guo et al., 1990).

The direct antipermeability effects of drugs that increase cAMP can be clearly seen in the acid aspiration injury model, in which inhibition of AA mediator production by ETYA or ibuprofen significantly increases lung weight gain, probably by inhibition of thromboxane-induced vasoconstriction in the injured area (Mizus et al., 1984). In these experiments we measured the effect of inhibitors of arachidonic acid metabolism on the rate of lung weight gain, pulmonary artery pressure, and mediator production in an acid lung injury model. Experiments were carried out using isolated lungs of 2 to 3 kg male NZW rabbits perfused at 60 mL/min with autologous blood diluted 1:1 with Krebs–Henseleit buffer. The lungs were challenged with 2mL/kg of 0.1 *n*HC1 administered intratracheally. The inhibitors used were ibuprofen 12.5 mg/kg or 100 10μM ETYA. The results are shown in Fig. 3. In an uninjured control group, lung weight and PPa did not increase. In the acid control group PPa increased significantly and thromboxane B_2 was produced. Ibuprofen or ETYA prevented the generation of thromboxane and the increase in PPa after acid. Despite eliminating the pulmonary hypertension, lung weight gain was significantly increased by either ibuprofen or ETYA. The mechanism may involve inhibition of a protective AA metabolite or an increase in microvascular pressure by reducing vas-

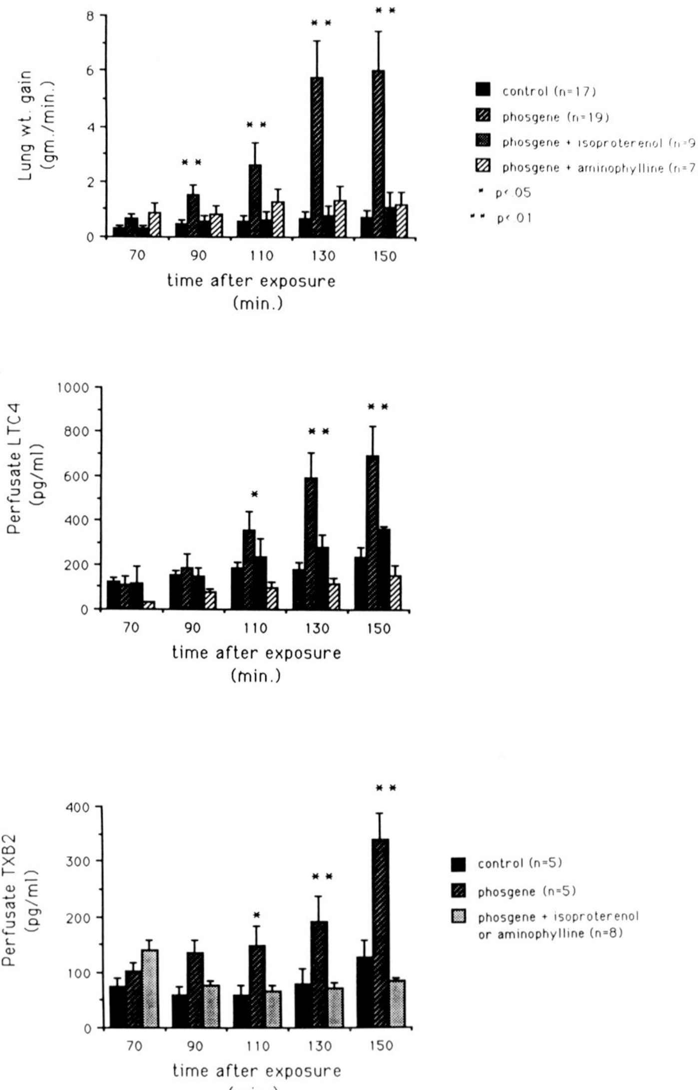

Figure 2 Lung weight gain and perfusate concentrations of LTC_4 and TxB_2 in isolated perfused rabbit lung experiments. The animals were exposed to a cumulative dose of 1500 ppm/min (i.e., 300 ppm for 5 min), anesthetized, and killed by rapid exsanguination. A detailed description of the preparation and assays is included in the Farrukh et al. (1988) and Kennedy et al. (1989) references. The lungs were studied from 70 to 150 min after exposure. Phosgene caused pulmonary edema and significant increases in LTC_4 and TxB_2 in the phosgene group. These changes were inhibited by aminophylline and isoproterenol.

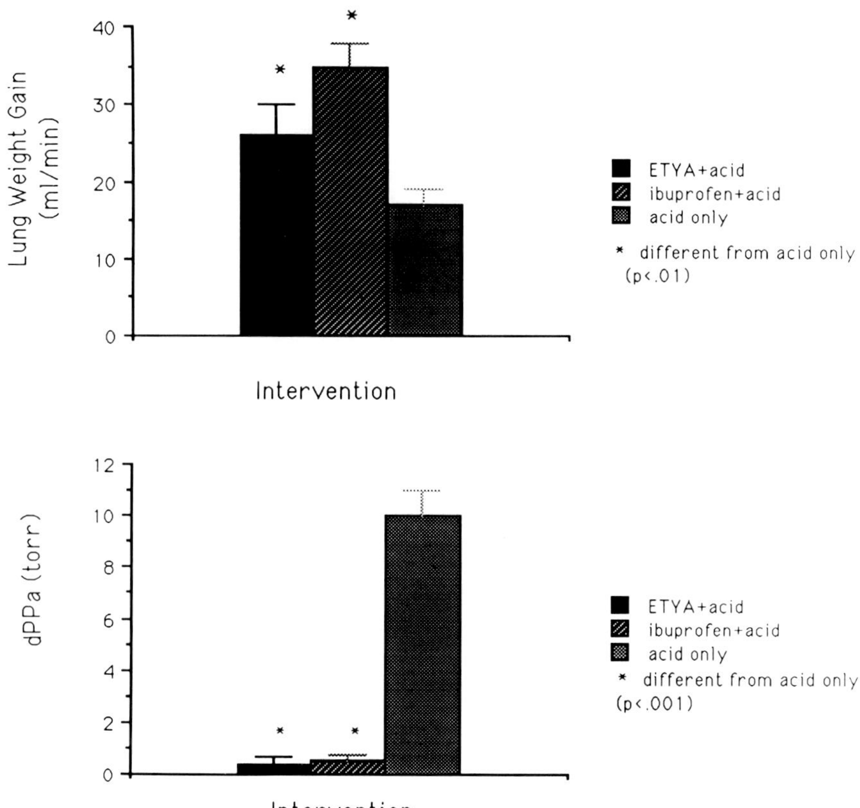

Figure 3 Cumulative weight gain and increase in pulmonary artery pressure (dPPa) 30 min after acid challenge. All groups show severe injury in comparison with uninjured lungs, which do not gain weight over this time period. Pretreatment with ETYA or ibuprofen augments edema formation and blocks the increase in pulmonary artery pressure in the acid-only group. Perfusate thromboxane concentration was 577 ± -54 pg/mL in the acid-only group and was undetectable in the ETYA or ibuprofen groups. The mechanism may involve inhibition of a protective vasoconstrictor metabolite or an increase in microvascular pressure by reducing vascular resistance upstream from the exchanging vessels. These observations taken together with our published work on the effects of drugs that increase cAMP in the acid aspiration injury model (Mizus et al., 1985) lead us to conclude that AA mediators do not play a significant role in acid aspiration injury and provide strong evidence for direct antipermeability effects of cAMP.

cular resistance upstream of the exchanging vessels. These results, taken together with the previous results showing protection by drugs that increase cAMP (Mizus et al., 1985), confirm the direct antipermeability effects of cAMP in the aspiration model.

B. Experiments Using Cultured Cells

Drugs that increase cAMP can inhibit production of cyclooxygenase and lipoxygenase mediators in several different cells and human lung tissue (Kuehl et al., 1987; Mandl et al., 1988; Peachell et al., 1988). The mechanism of this inhibition is not clear but may be mediated by cAMP-dependent protein kinase since the inhibitory effect can be caused by the dissociated catalytic subunit of the enzyme (Mandl et al., 1988). Since cyclooxygenase and lipoxygenase mediators are reduced similarly, and since cAMP causes a decrease in the level of free arachidonic acid, the site of inhibition could be on phospholipase A_2 or C (Kuehl et al., 1987).

In addition to its inhibitory action on production of AA mediators, increased cAMP has been shown to inhibit release of histamine from human lung mast cells and basophils (Peachell et al., 1988) and to inhibit superoxide production by neutrophils (Kuehl et al., 1987). The mechanism of inhibition is unknown but may be related to cellular calcium levels. In aortic endothelial cells, dibutyryl-cAMP attenuates the increase in intracellular calcium caused by ATP (Luckhoff et al., 1990). Cyclic AMP can also stimulate calcium uptake by sarcoplasmic reticulum in aortic endothelial cells (Watras, 1988). It also seems possible that the inhibition of AA mediator production could have a similar mechanism.

VII. Cyclic AMP and the Immune System

Drugs that increase cAMP have been shown to suppress immunological responses. This may be caused partially by inhibition of mediator and superoxide production; however, there appear to be direct effects as well. These drugs can suppress lymphocyte natural killer activity by inhibiting target cell bindings (Ullberg et al., 1983); interleukin-2-induced proliferation of lymphocytes can be blocked at an early differentiation step by these compounds (Johnson et al., 1988). Both of these actions could be related to the effects of cAMP on the cytoskeleton. Treatment with corticosteroids or cyclosporine markedly increases the adenylate cyclase activity in lymphoid membranes from kidney transplant patients (Michael and Brodde, 1989); the authors speculate that activation of adenylate cyclase might be involved in the immunosuppressive effects of these drugs.

Aminophylline can also inhibit pulmonary host defense in mice (Nelson et al., 1985). Killing of aerosolized gram-positive or gram-negative bacteria was inhibited in a dose-related manner. Susceptibility of host-defense immunosuppression was greater to the gram-negative bacterium (P. *mirabilis*) than to the gram-positive organism (*Staphylococcus aureus*). At doses of aminophylline of 40 or 80 mg/kg there was proliferation rather than killing of *Proteus mirabilis* in the lungs of challenged mice. These observations suggest caution in the use of drugs that increase cAMP in patients with pulmonary infections; however, the immunosuppressive effects of aminophylline were found only at doses that are substantially greater than those used clinically. Since there is no clear relationship between pulmonary infection and chronic aminophylline therapy in asthmatics, the use of these drugs in generally accepted doses appears to be safe.

VIII. Mechanisms of Action of cAMP and cGMP on Vascular Permeability and Vasomotor Tone

Although cAMP has clear antipermeability effects in lungs and endothelial cell monolayers, its mechanisms of action appear to be complex and multifactorial. Cyclic AMP appears to have several mechanisms of action, which at present cannot be related to a unique biochemical event. In smooth muscle, cAMP protein kinase–mediated phosphorylation of myosin light-chain kinase reduces the enzyme's affinity for the calcium calmodulin complex (Nishikawa et al., 1984). This phenomenon could explain a vasodilator effect of the cAMP; however, increases in cGMP that do not alter the affinity of calcium for the calcium calmodulin complex also cause vasodilation (Adelstein, et al., 1982). Although these observations do not explain the similar vasodilation caused by cAMP and cGMP, they could explain the difference in antipermeability effects of drugs that increase cAMP from those that increase cGMP (Jafri and Gurtner, 1990). Other observations which suggest that cAMP may inhibit protein kinase C in platelets also support the hypothesis that cAMP effects are mediated through the action of its protein kinase; cGMP has similar activity (Waldman and Walter, 1989). This effect might explain the similar vasodilator properties of cAMP and cGMP but not the different effects on vascular permeability. Cyclic AMP does not seem to inhibit phospholipase C mediate signal transduction since it did not prevent accumulation of IP2 or IP3 in the experiments of Waldman and Walter or in human umbilical endothelial cells stimulated with histamine (Carson et al., 1989). Cyclic AMP also decreases cellular calcium in some tissues—for example, in aortic endothelial cells stimulated with ATP (Luckoff et al., 1990). The mechanism may be related to the decrease in calcium influx caused by isoproterenol in rabbit aortic rings during potassium-induced depolarization (Meisheri and van Breeman, 1982). Cyclic AMP also increases calcium efflux from smooth muscle cells (Scheid and Fay, 1984). The calcium-lowering properties of cAMP are not seen in all tissues; for example, cAMP does not reduce calcium in human umbilical endothelial cells stimulated with histamine (Carson et al., 1989).

An important event in smooth muscle contraction is the phosphorylation of myosin (de Lanerolle et al., 1982). Myosin dephosphorylation has also been shown to be essential for cAMP-dependent and cAMP-independent relaxation of tracheal smooth muscle (de Lanerolle, 1988). The role of cAMP protein kinase is not known in cAMP-mediated phenomena other than the phosphorylation of myosin light-chain kinase. The report of a relatively specific inhibitor of cAMP protein kinase suggests future experiments to define its role further (Smith et al., 1990).

IX. Possible Therapeutic Strategy for the Use of Drugs That Increase cAMP in Acute Lung Injury

The compelling experimental evidence for a direct antipermeability effect of these drugs in several lung injury models, as well as the observations that these drugs can inhibit production of AA mediators, strongly suggest that these agents may be useful in the prevention and perhaps treatment of acute lung injury. Clinical studies on the use of drugs in treatment of the adult respiratory distress syndrome have been hampered by the difficulties inherent in definition of the clinical syndrome. In addition, delayed treatment may be less effective than treatment of patients at risk. Since drugs that increase cAMP are widely used and have relatively low toxicity, their use is clearly feasible. However, there has not been an adequate clinical trial of the drugs in human lung injury. The negative results of trials of PGE1 therapy in ARDS patients may not represent a convincing negative test of the hypothesis, because treatment was begun after full-blown development of the syndrome (Silverman et al., 1990). In addition, administration of PGE_1 may not be the optimal test of the cAMP-mediated antipermeability hypothesis because PGE_1-induced increase in cAMP increases can be down regulated by pro-inflammatory mediators (Garcia-Sainz, 1991). A better test of the hypothesis might involve use of the drugs in patients at risk for ARDS or the use of drugs such as aminophylline, which have direct effects. The immunosuppresive potential of these drugs might pose a relative contraindication for their use in septic lung injury.

References

Adelstein, R. S., Sellers, J. R., Conti, M. A., Pato, M. D., and deLanerolle, P. (1982). Regulation of smooth muscle contractile proteins by calmodulin and cAMP. *Fed. Proc.* **41:**2873–2878.

Becker, C. G., and Machman, R. L. (1973). Contractile proteins of endothelial cells, platelets, and smooth muscle. *Am. J. Pathol.* **71:**1–22.

Carson, M. R., Shasby, S. S., and Shasby, D. M. (1989). Histamine and inositol phosphate accumulation in endothelium: cAMP and a G protein. *Am. J. Pathol.* **257:**L259–L264.

DeClerck, F., DeBrabender, M., Meels, H., and Vande, V. (1981). Direct evidence for the contractile capacity of endothelial cells. *Thromb. Res.* **23:**505–520.

de Lanerolle, P. (1988). cAMP, myosin dephoshorylation, and isometric relaxation of airway smooth muscle. *J. Appl. Physiol.* **64(2):**705–709.

de Lanerolle, P., Condit, J. R., Tanenbaum, M., and Adelstein, R. S. (1982). Myosin phosphorylation, agonist concentration and contraction of tracheal smooth muscle. *Nature* **298:**871–872.

Farrukh, I. S., Gurtner, G. H., and Michael, J. R. (1987). Pharmacological modification of acute lung injury: Role of cyclic AMP. *J. Appl. Physiol.* **62:**47–54.

Farrukh, I. S., Michael, J. R., and Gurtner, G. H. (1988). Role of cyclooxygenase and lipoxygenase mediators in edema formation in oxidant lung injury. *Am. Rev. Respir. Dis.* **137:**1343–1349.

Foy, T., Marrion, J., Brigham, K. L., and Harris T. R. (1979). Isoproterenol and aminophylline reduce lung capillary filtration during high permeability. *J. Appl. Physiol.* **46:**146–151.

Garcia-Sainz, J. A. (1991). Cell responsiveness and protein kinase C: Receptors, G proteins and membrane effectors. *News Physiol. Sci.* **6:**169–173.

Guo, Y. L., Kennedy, T. P., Michael, J. R., Sciuto, A. M., Ghio, A. J., Adkinson, N. F., Jr., and Gurtner, G. H. (1990). Mechanisms of phosgene-induced lung toxicity: Role of arachidonate mediators. *J. Appl. Physiol.* **69:**1615–1622.

Jafri, M. H. Jr., and Gurtner, G. H. (1990). A drug that increased cGMP blocks thromboxane induced pulmonary hypertension and reduces edema formation in oxidant lung injury. *Am. Rev. Resp. Dis. 141 (4)*: A293.

Johnson, K. W., Davis, B. H., and Smith, K. A. (1988). cAMP antagonizes interleukin 2-promoted T-cell cycle progression at a discrete point in early G1. *Proc. Natl. Acad. Sci. USA* **85:**6072–6076.

Kennedy, T. P., Michael, J. R., Hoidal, J. R., Hasty, D., Sciuto, A. M., Hopkins, C., Lazar, R., Tolley, E., and Gurtner, G. H. (1989). Dibutyryl cAMP, aminophylline and beta adrenergic agonists protect against pulmonary edema caused by phosgene. *J. Appl. Physiol.* **67:**2542–2552.

Kuehl, F. A., Zanetti, M. E., Soderman, D. D., Miller, D. K., and Ham, E. A. (1987). Cyclic AMP-dependent regulation of lipid mediators in white cells. *Am. Rev. Resp. Dis.* **136:**210–213.

Luckhoff, A., Mulsch, A., and Busse, R. (1990). cAMP attenuates autacoid release from endothelial cells: Relation to internal calcium. *Am. J. Physiol.* **258:** H960–H966.

Majno, G., and Palade, G. E. (1961). Studies on inflammation. The effect of histamine and serotonin on vascular permeability: An electron microscopic study. *J. Biophys. Biochem. Cytol.* **21:**833–847.

Majno, G., Gilmore, V., and Lenethal, M. (1967). On the mechanism of vascular leakage caused by histamine-type mediators. *Circ. Res.* **21:**833–847.

Mandl, J, Mucha, I., Banhegyi, G., Meszaros, G., Farago, A., Spolarics, Z., Machovich,

R., Antoni, F., and Garzo, T. (1988). cAMP dependent inhibition of thromboxane A2 prostacyclin and PGF2 synthesis in mouse hepatocytes. *Prostaglandins* **36:**(6).

Meisheri, K. D., and van Breemen, C. (1982). Effects of β-adrenergic stimulation on calcium movements in rabbit aortic smooth muscle: relationship with cyclic AMP. *Am. J. Physiol.* **331:**429–441.

Michel, M. C. and Brodde, O. E. (1989). Lymphocyte adenylate cyclase activity in immunosuppressed patients. *Eur. J. Clin. Pharmacol.* **37:**41–43.

Minnear, F. L., Johnson, A., and Malik, A. B. (1986). β-Adrenergic modulation of pulmonary transvascular fluid and protein exchange. *J. Appl. Physiol.* **60:**266–274.

Mizus, I., Michael, J. R., and Gurtner, G. H. (1984). Inhibitors of arachidonic acid metabolism increase edema in acid lung injury. *Fed. Proc.* **43:**884.

Mizus, I., Summer, W., and Gurtner, G. (1985). Isoproterenol and aminophylline attenuate pulmonary edema after acid lung injury. *Am. Rev. Respir. Dis.* **131:**256–259.

Nelson, S., Summer, W. R. and Jakab, G. J. (1985). Aminophylline-induced suppression of pulmonary antibacterial defenses. *Am. Rev. Respir. Dis.* **131:**923-927.

Nishikawa, M., DeLanerolle, P., Lincoln, T. M., and Adelstein, R. S. (1984). Phosphorylation of mammalian myosin light chain kinases by the catalytic subunit of cyclic AMP–dependent protein kinase and by cyclic GMP-dependent protein kinase. *J. Biol. Chem.* **259:**8429–8436.

Parker, S. D., Walman, A. T., Traystman, R. J., and Gurtner, G. H. (1984). Effects of endotoxin in the isolated perfused pig lung. *Anesthesiology* **61(3A):**A139.

Peachell, P. T., MacGlashan, D. W., Lichtenstein, L. M., Jr., and Schleimer, R. P. (1988). Regulation of human basophil and lung mast cell function by cyclic adenosine monophosphate. *J. Immunol.* **140:**571–579.

Pietra, G. G., Szidon, J. P., Leventhal, M. M. and Fishman, A. P. (1971). Histamine and interstitial pulmonary edema in the dog. *Cir. Res.* **29:**323–337.

Scheid, C. R. and Fay, F. S. (1984). β-Adrenergic effects on transmembrane ^{45}Ca fluxes in isolated smooth muscle cells. *Am. J. Physiol.* **246:**431–438.

Shasby, D. M. Shasby, S. S., Sullivan, J. M., and Peach, M. J. (1982). Role of endothelial cell cytoskeleton in control of endothelial permeability. *Cir. Res.* **51:**657–661.

Silverman, H. J., Slotman, G., Bone, R. C., Maunder, R., Hyers, T. M., Kerstein, M. D., and Ursprung, J. J. (1990). Effects of prostraglandin E1 on oxygen delivery and consumption in patients with the adult respiratory distress syndrome. *Chest* **98:**405–410.

Smith, M. K., and Colbran,, R. J. and Soderling, T. R. (1990). Specificities of autoinhibitory domain peptides for four protein kinases. *J. Biol. Chem.* **265:**1837–1840.

Stelzner, T. J., Weil, J. V. and OBrien, R. F. (1989). Role of cyclic adenosine monophosphate in the induction of endothelial barrier properties. *J. Cell. Physiol.* **139:** 157–166.

Svensjo, E., Arfors, K. E., Raymond, R. M., and Giegh, G. T. (1979). Morphological and physiological correlation of brandykinin induced macromolecular efflux. *Am. J. Physiol.* **236:**H600–H606.

Ullberg, M., Jondal, M., Lanefelt, F., and Fredholm, B. B. (1983). Inhibition of human

NK cell cytotoxicity by induction of cyclic AMP depends on impaired target cell recognition. *Scand. J. Immunol.* **17:**365–373.

Waldmann, R., and Walter, U. (1989). Cyclic nucleotide elevating vasodilators inhibit platelet aggregation at an early step of the activation cascade. *Eur. J. Pharmacol.* **159:**317–320.

Walman, A. T., Parker, S. D., Traystman, R. J., and Gurtner, G. H. (1984). Isoproterenol protects against pulmonary edema in endotoxin lung injury. *Anesthesiology* **61(3A):**A113.

Watras, J. (1988). Regulation of calcium uptake in bovine aortic sacroplasmic reticulum by cyclic AMP-dependent protein kinase. *J. Mol. Cell. Cardiol.* **20:**711–723.

Wong, A. J., Pollard, T. D., and Herman, I. M. (1983). Actin filament stress fibers in vascular endothelial cells in vivo. *Science* **219:**867–869.

4

Cytoarchitectural Aspects of Endothelial Barrier Function in Response to Oxidants and Inflammatory Mediators

PATRICIA G. PHILLIPS and MIN-FU TSAN

Stratton Veterans Affairs Medical Center
and Albany Medical College
Albany, New York

I. Introduction

The venular endothelial cell plays a pivotal role in the active regulation of microvascular membrane permeability to macromolecules. The first morphological evidence that endothelial cells were active functional units of the vasculature came from the work of Magno et al., who demonstrated that inflammatory mediators histamine and bradykinin produced widened endothelial junctions or gaps in postcapillary venules subsequent to active contraction (Magno, et al., 1969). Others observed that immune complexes and leukocytes, as well as inflammatory mediators, could produce cell separations, and that some vasoactive agents could inhibit mediator-stimulated gap formation (Grega, et al., 1981; Hurley, 1983). These findings suggested that there is dynamic regulation of membrane permeability. The discovery that endothelial cells contain actomyosin, antigenically related to smooth-muscle actomyosin (Becker and Nachman, 1973), as well as other cytoskeletal elements associated with cell mobility and contractility (Drenckhahn and Groschel-Stewart, 1980; Drenckhahn, 1983), lent further support to Magno's hypothesis concerning endothelial contractility and the regulation of permeability.

Traditionally, vascular permeability has been studied in intact animals or in isolated-perfused organ preparations. These studies have provided essential information characterizing the sites of leakage of macromolecules from the vasculature. However, in recent years, there has been increasing emphasis on the study of molecular mechanisms involved in the regulation of permeability. The advent of the ability to grow endothelial cells in culture has provided the opportunity to investigate biochemical aspects of barrier function in a setting where structure, function, and molecular mechanisms can be studied in parallel.

In this chapter we address the cytoarchitectural aspects of barrier function. The term *cytoarchitectural* refers to the putative role of the actin microfilament system in the regulation of permeability. Actin comprises 10% of cellular protein. It is responsible for many of the mechanical functions of cells (reviewed by Rungger-Brandle and Gabbiani, 1983), is an important building block in the scaffold support structure of cells (Stossel, 1984) is thought to participate in cell-to-substrate anchoring (reviewed by Geiger, 1983; Burridge et al., 1987), and perhaps most importantly in the context of this review, is thought to participate in the formation and maintenance of cell-to-cell tight junctions (Wong and Gotlieb, 1986).

II. Structure of Endothelial Tight Junctions

Early ultrastructural studies of vascular permeability involved the use of electron-dense tracers to map the dimensions of pores between endothelial cells, thought to be likely sites of a paracellular pathway for solute passage (Bruns and Palade, 1968; Karnovsky, 1969; Simionescu et al., 1975; Simionescu, 1983). Tight junctions, as viewed by electron microscopy, appeared to be sites of fusion of adjacent cell membrane leaflets. However, Karnovsky noted that horseradish peroxidase (molecular diameter 5nm) gained access to space between plasma membranes in junctional regions of capillaries, implying that the junctions were permeable. These junctions offered some restriction to passage of molecules such as microperoxidase, but were not absolute barriers. Additional structural information was provided by using freeze-fracture technique (Simionescu et al., 1975; Schneeberger, 1981). These techniques though useful, provided only indirect information about the lines of contact between cells, since the networks of ridges and grooves in the freeze-fracture replicas are located in a plane next to the paracellular pathway and may not represent a direct correlation between the networks and the lines of contact (Simionescu et al., 1975). Essential information about the three-dimensional structure of the endothelial junction was obtained by Bundgaard (1984) using serial-section electron microscopy. He derived three-dimensional reconstructions which suggested that endothelial cell junctions were organized as irregular networks of lines of contact between neighboring cells. Pathways circumventing the lines of contact were followed through the entire junctional region, providing a tortuous pathway connecting luminal and abluminal aspects of the cell. Individual lines of contact exhibited discrete discontinuties, approximately 4 nm wide. The reconstruction demonstrated patent gaps of various sizes through the junctional region and supported the notion that the paracellular pathway in capillary endothelium was permeable not only to small solutes, but also to certain macromolecules. Figure 1 is a schematic drawing of the organization of a tight junction in capillary endothelium.

Ultrastructural studies had demonstrated that actin and other cytoskeletal

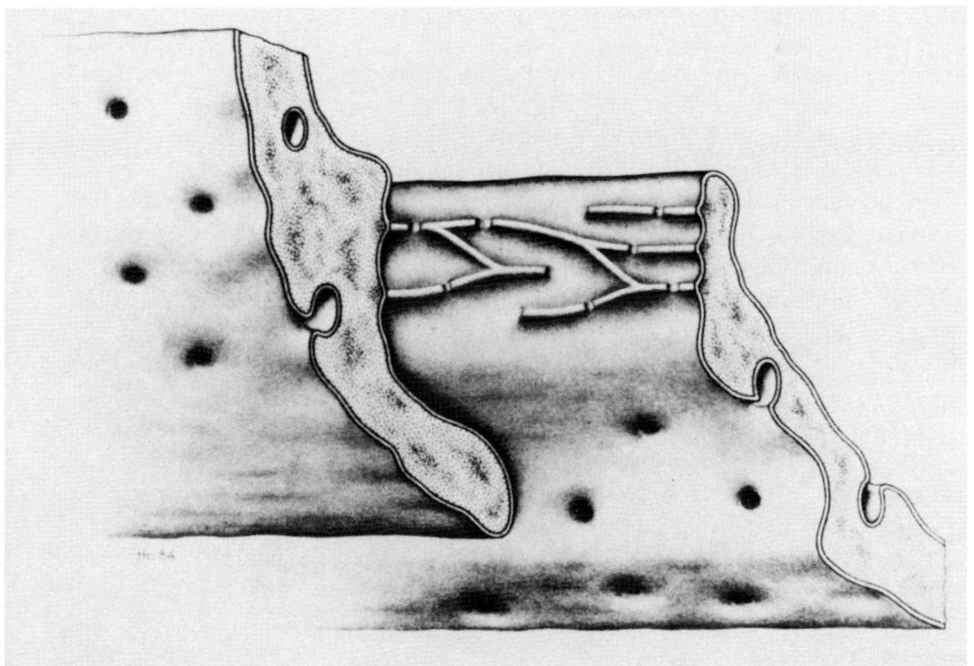

Figure 1 Schematic drawing of the organization of tight junctions of capillary endothelium. A small segment of a capillary wall is viewed from the pericapillary space. The junctional region on the lateral surface of an endothelial cell is exposed. Three-dimensional reconstructions based on consecutive thin sections have shown that the punctuate junctions in random individual thin sections represent an irregular network of lines of contact. Passage of hydrophilic solutes through the junctional region can occur by circumvention of lines of contact and via discrete interruptions in the lines. The pathways are accessible to hydrophilic solutes of dimensions at least up to the size of small proteins (From Bundgaard, 1984.)

proteins known to be involved in contractility were closely associated with endothelial cell junctions (Becker and Nachman, 1973; Drenckhahn, 1983). Further, in 1980, Hammersen, reviewing the literature concerning endothelial contractility, noted 82 publications on this topic. He questioned the ability of endothelial cells to contract and proposed instead that actin filaments functioned to anchor cells to substrate and in providing tensile force to stabilize endothelial shape within the monolayer (Hammersen, 1980). There is evidence that actin filaments may function in all of these roles, each of them contributing to endothelial monolayer homeostasis.

III. Actin Microfilament System in Endothelial Cells: General Considerations

Actin filaments are distributed in two main locations in endothelial cells. This is true both in situ and in cells growing in culture, although there are some anatomically related differences in the distribution of filaments in situ (White, et al., 1983; Gotlieb, et al., 1984; Gabbiani, et al., 1983; Kim et al., 1989). The predominant structure in confluent endothelial cells is the circumferential band (peripheral band), which delineates the margins of cells. Figure 2 shows a comparison of rhodamine phalloidin–stained actin filaments in calf pulmonary en-

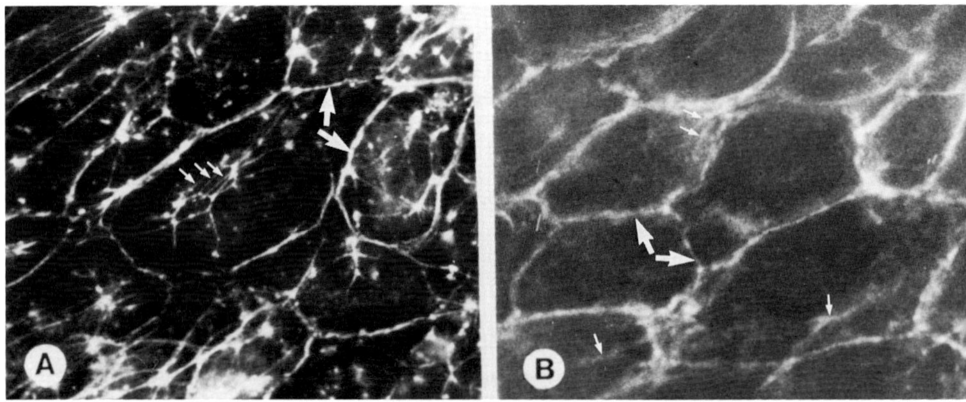

Figure 2 Rhodamine phalloidin staining of endothelial cells to demonstrate actin filament distribution. Cells or vessel segments were fixed, permeabilized, stained with rhodamine phalloidin and examined by fluorescence microscopy. (A) Confluent bovine pulmonary artery endothelial cells growing on polycarbonate filters; (B) endothelial cells viewed in situ in guinea pig pulmonary artery. Large arrows point to peripheral actin bands in individual endothelial cells; small arrows point to individual stress fibers.

dothelial cells cultured on a polycarbonate filter with in situ staining in guinea pig pulmonary artery. Peripheral bands of actin are clearly visible in both monolayers and appear structurally similar.

Microfilaments are also distributed as stress fibers in the cytoplasm of cells. Stress fibers are usually abundant in cells cultured on plastic or glass, while the occurrence of these structures varies in situ, with increases in fiber number and thickness observed in areas of vessels exposed to rapid flow or mechanical stress (White et al., 1983; Franke et al., 1984; Kim et al., 1989).

These two types of actin filaments exhibit different sensitivities to disruptive agents (Wong and Gotlieb, 1986) and are thought to serve different functions. Stress fibers are generally associated with conditions where the need for increased adherence to substrate is essential: that is, with increased mechanical stress, as well as in wound healing, liver regeneration, and in certain metastastic states (reviewed by Rungger-Brandle, and Gabbiani, 1983). A number of actin stress fibers terminate in specialized structures called focal contacts, which are involved in the formation of adhesion plaques between cells and extracellular matrix (Wehland et al., 1979; Lazarides and Burridge, 1975). These foci also function as sites of communication between the cell and its external environment (Burridge et al., 1987), so that the potential exists for signals to be transferred from the matrix to the cell body where functional changes might be mediated via the cytoskeleton.

Actin filaments localized in the cell periphery are currently believed to function as a scaffold support system, stabilizing cells side to side in the monolayer (Stossel, 1984). As endothelial cells become confluent, they shift their mode of anchoring from one that emphasizes cell-to-substrate attachment, characterized by numerous stress fibers and focal contacts, to one that favors cell-to-cell stabilization, characterized by prominent peripheral bands. These peripheral bands are thought to link with other cytoskeletal proteins, such as vinculin and α-actinin to form a type of adherens junction (Wong and Gotlieb, 1986). This junction appears to be similar to the zonula adherens of epithelial cells, which is closely associated with a perijunctional ring of actomyosin filaments (PAMR) (reviewed by Gumbiner, 1987a and Madara, 1989).

Actin filaments have been shown to insert directly into the plasma membrane, where they serve to partition certain intramembrane proteins into discrete areas, preventing lateral diffusion of these proteins within the plasma membrane (Gabbiani et al., 1978; Koch and Smith, 1978; Moore et al., 1978; Wu et al., 1982; reviewed by Geiger, 1983). It has been suggested that actin might serve to position and stabilize intramembrane proteins, such as those that compose the junctional strands. The number and complexity of these strands are thought to regulate the permeability of cell monlayers (Meza et al., 1980).

IV. Functional Links Between the Cytoskeleton and Tight Junctions

A. Epithelium

Epithelial cell systems have provided useful models for studying the putative relationship between tight junctions and the cytoskeleton, since the cytoskeletal networks in these cells have been extensively characterized (reviewed by Gumbiner, 1987). The tight junctions of epithelial and endothelial cells both possess a peripheral ring of actin and myosin filaments lying adjacent to the lateral membrane at the site of the junctional complex, an anatomical location ideally suited for regulation of paracellular permeability. The tight junction of epithelial cells is termed the zonula occludens (ZO) (Farquhar and Palade, 1963; reviewed by Gumbiner, 1987). The ZO consists of a narrow belt that wraps around the epithelial cells at the apical pole. A perijunctional ring of actin and myosin (PAMR) appears to associate with the lateral plasma membrane just below the ZO. Recently, Madara (1987), using detergent extraction procedures to prepare cytoskeletons of whole intestinal absorptive cells, determined that individual elements of the perijunctional cytoskeleton, including actin microfilaments, were associated with tight junctions by means of plaquelike densities in areas of the lateral membrane at the site of the tight junction. Insertion of actin filaments appears to be not only below the ZO, as reported earlier, but also directly into the area of the tight junction. These associations are not diffuse but occur only in areas in the lateral membranes that are thought to represent specific intrajunctional sites of the barrier to transepithelial permeability. Figure 3 is a schematic illustration depicting the structural relationship between the tight junction and the cytoskeleton in intestinal epithelial cells.

Functional links between the cytoskeleton and the ZO were first described in cultured renal epithelium (Meza et al., 1980) and in gallbladder epithelium (Bentzel et al., 1980) using pharmacological agents known to target the cytoskeleton. Meza et al. studied the effect of cytochalasin B (CB), an agent that disrupts actin microfilaments, on occluding epithelial junctions. CB abolished electrical resistance of these monolayers, a change that was preceded by pronounced disorganization in the microfilament network, particularly the loss of cortical actin filaments. This agent also markedly inhibited resealing of junctions that had been opened by removal of extracellular calcium. These investigators suggested that the microfilaments might be involved in the redistribution of the surface components that constituted occluding junctions (junctional strands).

Bentzel studied the effect of plant cytokinins on *Necturus* gallbladder, a representative leaky epithelium. Concomitant with morphological changes in actin filaments, cytokinins induced rapid increases in transepithelial resistance and potential difference (Bentzel et al., 1980). When the intramembranous struc-

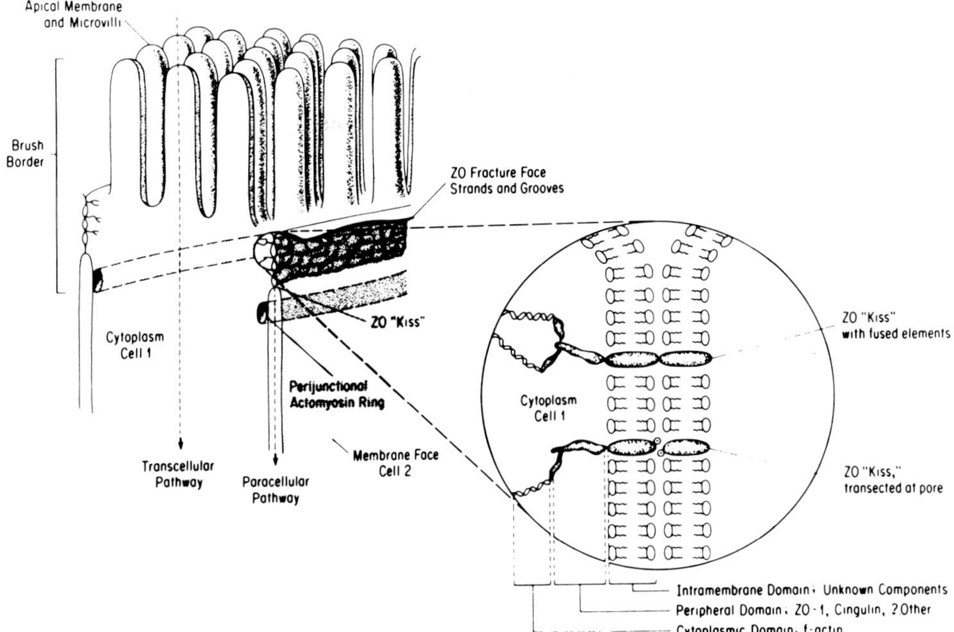

Figure 3 Schematic illustrations depicting tight junction (ZO) location and structure in intestinal epithelial cells. On the left is shown the brush border region of a transected cell. Fragments of the lateral membranes of flanking, neighbor cells are shown. The membrane face of the neighboring cell in the foreground is shown to highlight the freeze-fracture appearance of the ZO. The inset displays a speculative model of the molecular substructure of the ZO. Note that not only might the cytoskeleton modulate the ZO indirectly by tensile forces within a perijunctional actomyosin ring which circumferentially wraps the cell and inserts on the lateral membrane just below the ZO (left), but direct cytoskeletal–ZO interactions also appear to occur (inset). (From Madara, 1989).

ture of the tight junction was studied by freeze-fracture, peak cytokinin-induced increments in transepithelial resistance were associated with a more complex rearrangement of the tight junctional meshwork of strands rather than an increased number of strands. They invoked recruitment or rearrangement of existing strands as a possible mechanism for stabilization of the junction. Others have observed the importance of cytoskeletal elements in the induction and assembly of tight junctions (Montesano et al., 1975; 1976; Saxon et al., 1978).

The perijunctional ring of actin and myosin (PAMR) is thought to be a contractile ring, based on studies of isolated brush borders of epithelial cells, which have an extensive microfilament network bounded by the PAMR. These structures showed morphologic changes suggestive of ring contraction in the presence of divalent cations and ATP (Rodewald et al., 1976; Burgess, 1982; Keller and Mooseker, 1982), as well as phosphorylation of myosin in parallel (Keller and Mooseker, 1982).

It remained to be determined whether epithelial cells in intact monolayers were also capable of contraction. Pitelka demonstrated that mechanical tension generated within epithelial cells by removal of calcium or seeding them at low densities affected the position of strands in tight junctions (Pitelka and Taggart, 1983). Withdrawal of calcium caused a strong centripetal contraction of the cell body, destabilizing the tight junctional strands and increasing their lateral mobility.

Madara expanded the studies of Meza with cytochalasin D (CD) to examine the nature of the permeability lesion induced by this agent (Madara et al., 1986). Using ultrastructure and Ussing chamber techniques, he demonstrated maximal decreases in transepithelial resistance and junctional charge selectivity with CD. Analysis of simultaneous flux studies with sodium and nonabsorbable extracellular tracer mannitol suggested that CD opened a transjunctional shunt, which could fully account for increased sodium permeability and thus decreased resistance. Ultrastructural studies revealed that CD produced condensation of actin filaments in the PAMR. Quantitative freeze-fracture demonstrated marked alterations in occluding junction structure, including diminished strand number and reduced strand–strand cross-linking. In subsequent studies with CD, Madara demonstrated that despite enhanced junctional permeability to ions and mannitol, there was no gross disruption of epithelial integrity, since permeation to larger molecules such as inulin was unaffected. Further, the alteration in tight junction structure and permeability elicited by CD could be prevented by prior treatment of cells with uncoupler 2,4-dinitrophenol, suggesting the involvements of a contractile event, probably contraction of the PAMR (Madara et al., 1987). The contractile event did not lead to loss of monolayer confluency, despite disruption of barrier function measured by electrical resistance, suggesting the possibility of subtle changes in tight junction structure mediated by the cytoskeleton. This finding was reaffirmed in studies with *Clostridium difficile* toxin A, which abolished transepithelial electrical resistance while monolayers were still confluent, as assessed by electron microscopy and Normarski optics. Most notable was the loss of cortical actin staining over the same time course (Hecht et al., 1988).

Although actin filaments have been shown to have sites of insertion directly in the membrane at the level of both the ZO and the zonula adherens, other cytoskeletal proteins may also play a role in the control of permeability barriers. Recently, two other proteins, ZO-1 and cingulin, have been isolated in preparations enriched for tight junctions (Stevenson et al., 1989). ZO-1 is a phosphoprotein found in endothelial and epithelial cells, which is thought to be a likely candidate for linking actin filaments to the ZO.

B. Endothelium

Although the anatomical links between the tight junction and the cytoskeleton, particularly the PAMR, in endothelial cells have not been characterized as extensively as they have been for the epithelium, it has been suggested that the peripheral band of endothelial cells may show similar structure–function relationships (Wong and Gotlieb, 1986).

The current concept that actin peripheral filaments participate in regulation of endothelial permeability has been derived from a series of studies similar to those utilized to study the epithelium. Cell culture models for studying permeability involve the use of cells from a variety of vascular sites grown on suitably treated porous supports (reviewed by Albelda et al., 1988). The transendothelial movement of a number of macromolecules has been studied, usually with radiolabeled macromolecules, and appears to increase when the cells are perturbed by a number of agents. Electrical resistance across monolayers is generally low, although the values are similar to the measurement across frog mesenteric capillaries (Crone and Christensen, 1981). Whereas the epithium maintains high resistance to both small and large molecules, nonbrain endothelium is characterized by relatively low resistance to small ion flux (i.e., low electrical resistance) and relatively high resistance to macromolecules. The endothelial barrier was six times as permeable to small molecules (1.4 nm molecular radius) as the epithelial barrier, yet only twice as permeable to larger molecules, such as albumin (Albelda et al., 1988). It has been suggested that the measurement of electrical resistance may not accurately reflect endothelial macromolecular permeability and may not be as useful as it has been in the study of epithelial barriers (Albelda et al., 1988; Navab et al., 1986; Milton and Knutson, 1990).

The first studies to investigate the putative link between cytoskeleton and permeability involved correlation of in situ injury with culture studies of morphology using comparable concentrations of the injurious agent. Utilizing an isolated-perfused lung preparation, Shasby demonstrated that pretreatment with cytochalasin B (CB) led to increased vascular permeability, as evidenced by increased lung wet weight and increased lavage albumin to perfusate albumin concentration. He observed changes in cell shape and actin filament distribution in cultured cells exposed to CB and suggested that a similar mechanism might be responsible for the in situ increases in lung vascular permeability (Shasby et al., 1982).

Ultrastructural studies were performed on rats exposed to the sedative ethchlorvynol, which causes the development of reversible pulmonary edema. The injury was associated morphologically with the formation of endothelial blebs and gap formation (Wysolmerski and Lagunoff, 1984). In subsequent studies with cultured endothelial cells exposed to comparable concentrations of this agent, cells lost their peripheral actin bands and formed gaps, attaching to each other by filamentous processes (Wysolmerski and Lagunoff, 1985). Both of these studies linked changes in actin filament distribution to in situ loss of barrier function by extrapolation of cellular findings to the intact vasculature.

Studies on the effects of hyperoxia on endothelial barrier function were performed in a cultured endothelium monolayer system in which function (Garcia et al., 1986; Cooper et al., 1987) and structure could be examined in parallel (Phillips and Tsan, 1988). When endothelial cells were exposed to 95% oxygen for 3 days, they demonstrated significant increases in permeability to albumin (Table 1). This impairment of barrier function occurred in the absence of cytotoxicity or loss of cells from the monolayer. However, the permeability increase at day 3 coincided with dramatic changes in actin filament distribution (Fig. 4). Two features were observed: first, an increase in number and thickness of actin stress fibers, which was evident by 48 h and more obvious at 72 h, and second, disruption or absence of the actin peripheral band at 72 h. The time course for loss of barrier function at 3 days in this endothelial cell permeability/morphology model correlated well with the onset of interstitial edema observed in animal models of hyperoxia (Kistler et al., 1967; Kapanci et al., 1969; Bowden and Adamson, 1974; Crapo et al., 1980).

Although the loss of cortical actin filament probably contributes to the loss of barrier function at 3 days, the increase in actin stress fibers may play a dif-

Table 1 Effect of Hyperoxia on Permeability of Cultured Endothelial Monolayers to [^{125}I]Albumin[a]

	[^{125}I]Albumin clearance rate (μL/min)		
	1 day	2 days	3 days
Normoxia	0.30 ± 0.10 (5)	0.26 ± 0.06 (4)	0.26 ± 0.03 (13)
Hyperoxia	0.34 ± 0.08 (5)	0.26 ± 0.05 (4)	0.63 ± 0.08* (13)

[a]Values are means ± SE for number of experiments given in parentheses. Each experiment was done in triplicate or quadruplicate, and results were averaged. Confluent endothelial monolayers on synthetic polycarbonate membranes were exposed to normoxia (95% air, 5% CO_2) or hyperoxia (95% O_2, 5% CO_2) for up to 3 days. At various intervals, clearance of [^{125}I]Albumin across endothelial monolayers was determined.

*$p < 0.001$ (vs. normoxia).

Source: Phillips and Tsan, 1988.

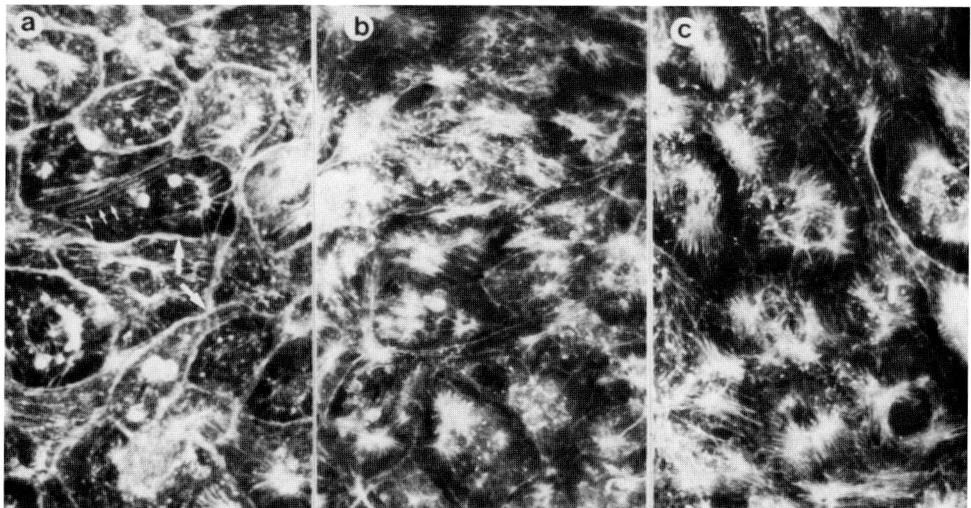

Figure 4 Rhodamine phalloidin staining of confluent bovine pulmonary artery endothelial cells growing on polycarbonate filters (filters form the base of chambers used for measuring permeability to [^{125}I]-albumin). After exposure to normoxia or hyperoxia, monolayers were fixed, permeabilized, stained with rhodamine phalloidin, and examined by fluorescence microscopy. Large arrows, peripheral bands; small arrows, individual stress fibers. (a) control (normoxia); (b) hyperoxia for 2 days; (c) hyperoxia for 3 days. Magnification × 412. (From Phillips, and Tsan, 1988.)

ferent role in this model. Phillips et al. subsequently demonstrated that the increase in stress fibers correlated with increased cell-substrate anchoring, since oxygen-exposed cells demonstrated substantially increased adherence to substrate (Phillips et al., 1988). An additional observation that hyperoxia lead to degradation of endothelial cell subcellular matrix suggested that hyperoxia-exposed cells may respond to loss of anchoring substratum by shifting actin filament distribution from peripheral side-to-side stabilization (peripheral bands) to increased stress fiber and focal contract formation in order to maintain monolayer integrity, despite increased permeability (Phillips et al., 1990). These observations are consistent with those of Madara (Madara et al., 1987; Hecht et al., 1988), in which impaired barrier function and disruption of peripheral actin were seen in apparently confluent monolayers.

Hyperoxic injury is thought to result from the intracellular generation of elevated levels of oxygen radical species which overwhelm the natural antioxidant capacity of the body (Freeman and Crapo, 1982; reviewed by White and Repine, 1985). Infiltration of activated neutrophils also contributes substantially to the pathology (Fox et al., 1981). To simulate the oxidant generation by neutrophils, cultured endothelial cells were exposed to a xanthine/xanthine oxidase oxygen radical generating system (Shasby et al., 1985). Oxidant injury resulted in reversible increases in monolayer permeability to albumin as well as cell shape changes. Since some oxidized lipids can act as calcium ionophores (Serhan et al., 1981), Shasby tested the effect of calcium ionophore A23187 on permeability and shape changes in this system. Since the ionophore-induced changes mimicked those observed with oxidative injury, they suggested that cell shape changes were related to oxidant-induced changes in calcium homeostasis, possibly mediated by the cytoskeleton (Shasby et al., 1985). The work of Rotrosen and Gallin with the effect of histamine on cultured endothelial cell permeability and actin content also supported a role of cytosolic calcium in the regulation of endothelial shape change and endothelial monolayer permeability (Rotrosen and Gallin, 1986).

Exposure of cultured endothelial cells to hydrogen peroxide resulted in loss of peripheral actin filaments and increased stress fiber formation (Johnson et al., 1989), features very similar to those observed after 3 days of hyperoxia (Phillips and Tsan, 1988). The time course of this loss in cortical actin closely paralleled increased permeability in isolated-perfused guinea pig lung in response to hydrogen peroxide. Of particular interest was the observation that both the permeability changes (in situ) and the loss of the actin peripheral bands (in culture) could be blocked by an inhibitor of protein kinase C (PKC). Although the actin structural changes were similar to those observed with long-term oxygen exposure, the mechanisms of these changes are likely to be different, since hyperoxia is accompanied by changes in other support systems, such as extracellular matrix, which may serve to modify the actin distribution (Phillips et al., 1990).

Hydrogen peroxide was shown to initiate hydrolysis of endothelial cell membrane phospholipids via phoslipase A- and C-dependent pathways. Shasby et al. (1988a) suggested that this process might contribute to oxidant-mediated changes in barrier function, possibly through activation of PKC. Implications of these findings in the potential regulation of actin filament polymerization and distribution are discussed in Section V.

In order to study the effect of an agent known to cause changes in actin distribution and permeability in culture (Stolpen et al., 1986; Brett et al., 1989; Royall et al., 1989), these parameters were studied in situ in an isolated-perfused lung preparation from guinea pigs pretreated for 16 h with tumor necrosis factor (TNF) (Hocking et al., 1990). These preparations showed lung weight gain as well as an increase in lung wet/dry weight ratios, indicating the formation of pulmonary edema. In situ staining of pulmonary arteries to visualize actin filaments revealed a characteristic ruffling of cortical actin, occurring with the same time dependence as the loss of barrier function. The ruffling of the actin peripheral filament border suggested instability of this structure and, consequently, of the tight junctions which it helps to maintain.

Cortical actin filament disruption occurs in parallel with loss of barrier function in a number of injury models. If this structure is essential in the maintenance of permeability barrier, stabilization of actin with phallacidin, which prevents actin depolymerization (Weiland, 1977; Gabbiani et al., 1975), should prevent loss of barrier functions. This hypothesis was tested in a thrombin-induced increase in permeability model (Phillips et al., 1989). Pretreatment with phallacidin resulted in time-dependent binding of the compound to existing filament networks. Stabilization of actin filaments prevented the loss of peripheral actin filaments and completely ablated thrombin-induced permeability (Fig. 5 and Table 2). Further, Alexander et al., demonstrated that phalloidin pretreatment of cells on microcarrier bead significantly reduced permeability increases by histamine, bradykinin, thromboxane A_2 mimetic, and cytochalasin B while increasing the number of stress fibers (Alexander et al., 1988). Serotonin (5-HT) has been shown to promote junctional tone between adjacent endothelial cells both in vivo (Shepro et al., 1984; Grega et al., 1986) and in vitro (Bottaro et al., 1986). The mechanism of this stabilization was investigated using electron immunocytochemistry, which demonstrated that 5-HT was internalized by endothelial cells and bound to actin filaments and in dense areas of filament interactions (Mineau-Hanschke et al., 1989). The authors suggested that 5-HT helped to regulate endothelial junctional stability by promoting actin filament formation and stability, as had been demonstrated by Montesano for the phalloidin-mediated induction of tight junctions from preexisting tight junctional elements (Montesano et al., 1976). Rasio demonstrated that phalloidin pretreatment provided protection against structural and functional damage induced by hyperoxia-reperfusion in rete capillaries (Rasio et al., 1989).

Saponin-permeabilized endothelial cells have been shown to contract upon exposure to calcium and ATP, resulting in thiophosphorylation of myosin via a calmodulin/myosin light-chain kinase-dependent reaction (Wysolmerski and Lagunoff, 1990). This contraction resulted in retraction of cells from each other and the formation of gaps which would increase permeability, as suggested by Magno. However, formation of gaps large enough to be visible at the light microscopic level, as described in this study, may not be necessary for impairment of barrier function. There is evidence that disruption of cortical actin filaments can result in more subtle injury, even in apparently confluent monolayers (Wong and Gottlieb, 1986; Phillips and Tsan, 1988; Phillips et al., 1989; Hecht et al., 1988).

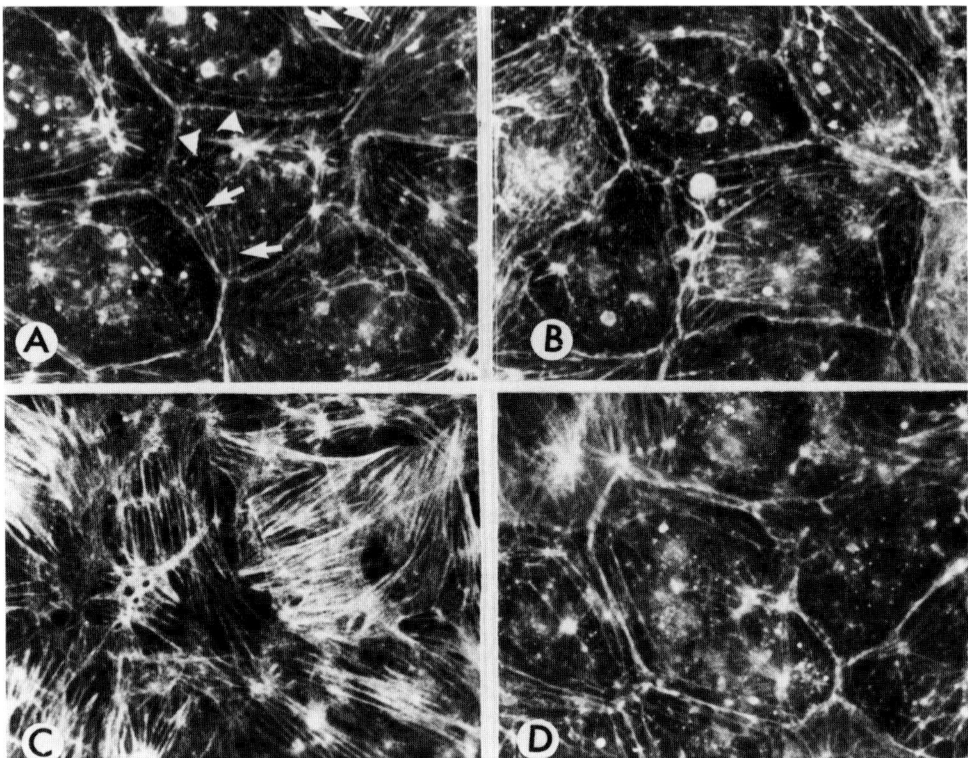

Figure 5 Rhodamine–phalloidin staining of endothelial monolayers growing on polycarbonate filters. (A) control. (B) 7-Nitrobenz-2-oxa-1,3-diazole (NBD) -conjugated-phallacidin (O.3 μM) pretreated for 3 hr. (C) α thrombin (10^{-7}M) treatment for 30 min. (D) Pretreatment with 0.3 μ*M* NBD-phallacidin for 3 h and then α-thrombin for 30 min. Arrowheads, actin peripheral bands; arrows, each arrow points to an individual stress fiber. Magnification × 1240. (From Phillips et al., 1989.)

V. Unifying Concepts

The temporal association of cortical actin disruption with impaired barrier function has been demonstrated in epithelial and endothelial cell systems, in both acute and chronic injury models. In most cases the permeability changes observed were reversible, consistent with the concept that the tight junction is a dynamic structure. Tight junctions assemble and disassemble either partially or

Table 2 Effect of Phallacidin on Thrombin-Induced Permeability of Endothelial Monolayers to [^{125}I]Albumin[a]

Pretreatment	[^{125}I]Albumin clearance rate (μL/min) Control	Thrombin	Thrombin/control ratio
Media	0.266 ± 0.03 (18)	0.425 ± 0.04* (18)	1.59
NBD-P	0.272 ± 0.08 (4)	0.282 ± 0.06 (4)	1.04
P	0.286 ± 0.05 (5)	0.334 ± 0.06 (5)	1.16
NBD	0.236 ± 0.07 (2)	0.356 ± 0.01* (2)	1.51

[a]Confluent endothelial monolayers on membrane filters were pretreated for 3 h with one of the agents above prior to exposure to either control media or α-thrombin (1×10^{-7} *M*), and clearance of [^{125}I]albumin was determined. The thrombin/control ratio was obtained by dividing the [^{125}I]albumin clearance rate with thrombin challenge by this rate for each respective control group. Values are means ± SE of the results.

NBD-P, NBD-conjugated phallacidin; P, phallacidin; NBD, NBD chloride.

*$p < 0.005$ vs. its respective control.

Source: Phillips et al., 1989.

completely during many developmental and physiological processes. Electrophysiological experiments have demonstrated the rapid recovery of tight junctions after injury (Hudspeth, 1982; Kachar and Pinto Da Silva, 1981). Tight junction recovery did not require protein synthesis (Martinez-Palomo et al., 1980), implying that tight junction precursor molecules are available in the cell membrane and can be recruited. Taken collectively, the evidence presented in this review suggests that actin filaments may participate in the organization and maintenance of these junctional proteins. Chronic models for barrier function impairment (such as hyperoxia) may be more complex with respect to actin rearrangements, occurring with a different time course and involving other support systems in remodeling the endothelium. Nevertheless, the loss of peripheral actin may still signal loss of important junction stabilizing structures.

The integrity of tight junctions has long been known to depend on extracellular calcium (Sedar and Forte, 1964; Gumbiner and Simons, 1987; Martinez-Palomo et al., 1980; Pitelka et al., 1983b). The calcium dependence probably results indirectly from calcium effects on other junctional elements rather than from direct effects on the tight junction itself (Gumbiner, 1987). Such junctional elements might include actin, myosin, or the cadherins, which are species-specific calcium-binding proteins such as uvomorulin, which has been shown to participate in the formation of various types of cell adherence junctions (Gumbiner and Simons, 1987; Hirano et al., 1987).

A number of agonists, such as histamine, epinephrine, and acetyl choline, exert some of their effects by raising calcium concentration in the cytosol of target cells. A rise in cytosolic calcium leads to an increase in Ca^{2+} bound to calmodulin and subsequent interaction of this complex with specific or multifunctional calmodulin-dependent protein kinases. Involvement of this complex in the activation of myosin light-chain kinase would favor the process of contraction (reviewed by Exton, 1985). Actin associated with tight junctions might also be subject to regulation by calcium-dependent actin-binding proteins gelsolin, villin, and fragmin, which nucleate actin filament assembly, sever actin filaments along their length, and block actin monomer exchange at their fast-growing ends (Stossel, 1984). These proteins may be important in mediating rapid cell shape changes which involve actin.

It has been suggested that stimuli such as oxidants or inflammatory mediators might function by redistributing actin or cytoskeletal regulatory proteins between the cytosol and the membrane, as has been described in studies of the neutophil response to chemotactic factors (reviewed by Omann et al., 1987). Oxidants have been shown to increase phospholipase A- and C-mediated hydrolysis of cell membrane lipids, leading to the production of diglycerides, phophatidic acid, and inositol polyphosphates in endothelial and epithelial cells (Shasby et al., 1988a,b).

Polyphosphoinsositides, phosphatidyl inositol monophosphate, and phosphatidylinositol 4,5-bisphosphate (PIP_2) modulate the actin-binding, filament-severing and end-binding functions of gelsolin (Lind et al., 1987; Janmey and Stossel, 1987). Regulation of gelsolin by intracellular messengers calcium and polyphosphoinositides allows for formation of several different gelsolin–actin intermediates with distinct functional properties that may be involved in changes in the state of cytoplasmic actin following cell stimulation (Janmey et al., 1987). It has been demonstrated that gelsolin binds to actin filament ends within cells, and that it functions in both cytoplasmic and membrane domains (Hartwig, et al., 1989). In recent reports, PIP_2 has also been shown to interact directly with actin-binding protein profilin. The rapid interaction of PIP_2 with profilin and profilin–actin complexes caused rapid dissociation of the complex with concomitant polymerization of actin (Lassing and Lindberg, 1985).

Further, in vitro studies have demonstrated the formation of supramolecular complexes composed of actin, α-actinin, palmitic acid, and diacylglycerol (DAG), suggesting that modification of membrane lipids could affect the interactions of actin and α-actinin within the membrane as well as the state of actin polymerization. Oxidative activation of phopholipase C-type activity would probably result in the activation of protein kinase C (PKC). Recently, Hocking et al. have demonstrated inhibition of oxidant-mediated cytoskeletal and permeability changes by PKC inhibitor 1-(5-isoquinolinesulfonyl)-2-methylpiperazine dihydrochloride (H7) (Hocking et al., 1990). Type 3 PKC has been found localized in the focal contents of cells (Jaken et al., 1989) at sites of attachment and communication between the cell and extracellular matrix.

VI. Future Directions

As outlined in previous sections, there is considerable evidence to suggest that the actin filament network participates in the maintenance of endothelial barrier function. It is also clear that the actin filaments themselves are subject to modulation by a number of agents. Future research to address the regulation of permeability that occurs rapidly and/or reversibly should include studies with newly isolated junctional proteins such as ZO-1 and cingulin, to determine their involvement in formation and maintenance of tight junctions. Of considerable interest, too, will be investigations of the roles of actin-regulating proteins such as gelsolin and profilin in these settings, particularly with regard to their interactions with inositol phospholipids in transmembrane signaling. In terms of injury models in which the permeability lesion develops with time and appears to involve remodeling of the endothelium, it will be important to study the interactions of cells with their supporting substratum. These interactions are mediated via focal contacts, which serve as sites of attachment between the matrix and cytoskeleton. A number of enzymes with regulatory potential have been localized at the cytoplasmic face of focal contacts (i.e., PKC, plasminogen activators) (reviewed by Burridge et al., 1987).

VII. Summary

Endothelial and epithelial cells both possess tight junctions which selectively limit the passage of macromolecules through the paracellular pathway between cells. Anatomically associated with this tight junction is a perijunctional ring of actin and myosin filaments, which in epithelial cells has been shown to insert directly into plaques intimately associated with the tight junction. Experiments with pharmacologic agents known to target the cytoskeleton have demonstrated close correlations between the actin filament status and maintenance of barrier function. In addition, the disruption of peripheral actin filaments is a consistent feature of a number of injury models associated with the development of pulmonary edema, suggesting functional relevance for this structure in the control of permeability. Since actin filaments insert directly into cell membranes, oxidative (or other) changes that perturb the lipid composition of the membranes may alter the polymerization state of actin filaments as well as the distribution of actin/α-actinin bound to junctional complexes.

References

Albeida, S. M., Sampson, P. M., Haselton, F. R., McNiff, J. M., Mueller, S. N., Williams, S. K., Fishman, A. P., and Levine, E. M. (1988). Permeability characteristics of cultured endothelial cell monolayers, *J. Appl. Physiol.* **64:**308.

Alexander, J. S., Hechtman, H. B., and Shepro, D. (1988). Phalloidin enhances endothelial barrier function and reduces inflammatory permeability in vitro. *Microvasc. Res.* **35:**308.

Becker, C. G., and Nachman, R. L. (1973). Contractile proteins of endothelial cells, platelets, and smooth muscle. *Am. J. Pathol.* **71:**1.

Bentzel, C. J., Hainau, B., Ho, S., Hui, S. W., Edelman, A., Anagnostopoulos, T., and Benedetti, E. L. (1980). Cytoplasmic regulation of tight-junction permeability. Effect of plant cytokinins, *Am. J. Physiol.* **239:**C89.

Bottaro, D., Shepro, D., and Hechtman, H. B. (1986). Heterogeneity of intimal and microvessel endothelial cell barriers, *Microvasc. Res.* **32:**389.

Bowden, D. H., and Adamson, I. Y. R. (1974). Endothelial regeneration as a marker of the differential vascular responses in oxygen-induced pulmonary edema. *Lab. Invest.* **30:**350.

Brett, J., Gerlach, H., Nawroth, P., Steinberg, S., Godman, G., and Stern, D. (1989). Tumor necrosis factor/cachectin increases permeability of endothelial cell monolayers by a mechanism involving regulatory G proteins. *J. Exp. Med.* **169:**1977.

Bruns, R. R., and Palade, G. E. (1968). Studies on blood capillaries. I. General organization of blood capillaries in muscle. *J. Cell Biol.* **37:**244.

Bundgaard, M. (1984). The three-dimensional organization of tight junctions in capillary endothelium revealed by serial-section electron microscopy. *J. Ultrastruct. Res.* **88:**1.

Burgess, D. R. (1982). Reactivation of intestinal epithelial brush border motility: ATP-dependent contraction via a terminal web contractile ring. *J. Cell Biol.* **95:**853.

Burridge, K., Molony, L., and Kelley, T. (1987). Adhesion plaques: Sites of transmembrance interaction between the extracellular matrix and actin cytoskeleton, *J. Cell Sci. Suppl.* **8:**211.

Cooper, J. A., Del Vecchio, P. J., Minnear, F. L., Burhop, K. E., Selig, W. M., Garcia, J. G. N., and Malik, A. B. (1987). Measurement of albumin permeability across endothelial monolayers in vitro. *J. Appl. Physiol.* **62:**1076.

Crapo, J. D., Barry, B. E., Foscue, H. A., and Shelburne, J. (1980). Structural and biochemical changes in rat lungs occurring during exposures to lethal and adaptive doses of O_2. *Am. Rev. Respir. Dis.* **122:**123.

Crone, C., and Christensen, O. (1981). Electrical resistance of a capillary endothelium. *J. Gen. Physiol.* **77:**349.

Drenckhahn, D. (1983). Cell motility and cytoplasmic filaments in vascular endothelium. *Prog. Appl. Microcirc.* **1:**53.

Drenckhahn, D., and Groschel-Stewart, U. (1980). Localization of myosin actin, and tropomysin in rat intestinal epithelium: Immunohistochemical studies at the light and electron microscope levels. *J. Cell Biol.* **86:**475.

Exton, J. H. (1985). Role of calcium and phosphoinositides in the actions of certain hormones and neurotransmitters. *J. Clin. Invest.* **75:**1753.

Farquhar, M. G., and Palade, G. E. (1963). Junctional complexes in various epithelia. *J. Cell Biol.* **17:**375.

Franke, R. P., Grafe, M., Schnittler, H ., Seiffge, D., Mittermayer, C., and Drenckhahn, D. (1984). Induction of human vascular endothelial stress fibers by fluid shear stress. *Nature (Lond).)* **307:**648.

Freeman, B. A., and Crapo, J. D. (1982). Biology of disease: Free radicals and tissue injury, *Lab. Invest.* **47:**412.

Fox, R. B., Hoidal, J. R., Brown, D. M., and Repine, J. E. (1981). Pulmonary inflammation due to oxygen toxicity: Involvement of chemotactic factors and polymorphonuclear leukocytes. *Am. Rev. Respir. Dis.* **123:**521.

Gabbiani, G., Montesano, R., Tuchweber, B., Milagros, S., and Orci, L. (1975). Phalloidin-induced hyperplasia of actin filaments in rat hepatocytes. *Lab. Invest.* **33:**562.

Gabbiani, G., Chaponnier, C., Zumbe, A., and Vassalli, P. (1977). Actin and tubulin cocap surface immunoglobulins in murine B lymphocytes. *Nature (Lond.)* **269:**695.

Gabbiani, G., Gabbiani, F., Lombardi, D., and Schwartz, S. M. (1983). Organization of actin cytoskeleton in normal and regenerating arterial endothelial cells. *Proc. Natl. Acad. Sci. USA* **80:**2361.

Garcia, J. G. N., Siflinger-Birnboim, A., Bizios, R., DelVecchio, P. J., Fenton, J. W., II, and Malik, A. B. (1986). Thrombin-induced increases in albumin permeability across cultured endothelial monolayers. *J. Cell. Physiol.* **128**:96.

Geiger, B. (1983). Membrane–cytoskeleton interactions. *Biochim. Biophys. Acta* **737:**305.

Gotlieb, A. I., Spector, W., Wong, M. K. K., and Lacey, C. (1984). In vitro reendothelialization: Microfilament bundle re-organization in migration of porcine endothelial cells. *Arteriosclerosis* **4:**91.

Grega, G. J., Svensjo, E., and Haddy, F. J. (1981). Macromolecular permeability of the microvascular membrane: Physiological and pharmacological regulation, *Microcirculation* **1:**325.

Grega, G. J., Adamski, S. W., and Dobbins, D. E. (1986). Physiological and pharmacological evidence for the regulation of permeability. *Fed. Proc.* **45:**96.

Gumbiner, B. (1987a). Structure, biochemistry, and assembly of epithelial tight junctions. *Am. J. Physiol.* **253** (*Cell. Physiol.* **22**):C749.

Gumbiner, B., and Simons, K. (1987). The role of uvomorulin in the formation of epithelial occluding junctions. In *Junctional complexes of Epithelial Cells* Edited by M. Stoker, Wiley, Chichester, West Sussex, England, p. 168.

Hammersen, F. (1980). Endothelial contractility: Does it exist? *Adv. Microcirc.* **9:**95.

Hartwig, J. H., Chambers, K. A., and Stossel, T. P. (1989). Association of gelsolin with actin filaments and cell membranes of macrophages and platelets. *J. Cell Biol.* **108:**467.

Hecht, G., Pothoulakis, C., LaMont, J. T., and Madara, J. L. (1988). Clostridium difficile toxin A perturbs cytoskeletal structure and tight junction permeability of cultured human intestinal epithelial monolayers. *J. Clin. Invest.* **82:**1516.

Hirano, S., Nose, A., Hatta, K., Kawakami, A., and Takeichi, M. (1987). Calcium-dependent cell–cell adhesion molecules (cadherins): Subclass specifications and possible involvement of actin bundles. *J. Cell Biol.* **105:**2501.

Hocking, D. C., Phillips, P. G., Ferro, T. J., and Johnson, A. (1990). Mechanisms of pulmonary edema induced by tumor necrosis factor-alpha. *Circ. Res.* **76:**68.

Hudspeth, A. J. (1982). The recovery of local transepithelial resistance following single-cell lesion. *Exp. Cell Res.*, **138:**331.

Hurley, J. V. (1983). *Acute inflammation*, 2nd ed. Churchill Livingstone, Melbourne, Australia.

Jaken, S., Leach, K., and Klauck, T. (1989). Association of type 3 PKC with focal contacts in rat embryo fibroblasts. *J. Cell Biol.* **109:**697.

Janmey, P. A., and Stossel, T. P. (1987a). Modulation of gelsolin function by phosphatidylinositol 4,5-biphosphate, *Nature (Lond.)* **325:**362.

Janmey, P. A., Iida, K., Lin, H. L., and Stossel, T. P. (1987). Polyphosphoinositide micelles and polyphosphoinoside-containing vescicles dissociate endogenous gelsolin–actin complexes and promote actin assembly from the fast growing end of actin filaments blocked by gelsolin. *J. Biol. Chem.* **262:**12228.

Johnson, A., Phillips, P. G., Hocking, D., Tsan, M.-F., and Ferro, T. J. (1989). Protein kinase inhibition prevents pulmonary edema in response to H_2O_2. *Am. J. Physiol.* **256:**H1012.

Kachar, B., and Pinto Da Silva, P. (1981). Rapid massive assembly of tight junction strands. *Science Wash. D.C.* **213:**541.

Kapanci, Y., Weibel, E. R., Kaplan, H. P., and Robinson, F. R. (1969). Pathogenesis and reversibility of the pulmonary lesions of oxygen toxicity in monkeys. *Lab. Invest.* **20:**101.

Karnovsky, M. J. (1969). The ultrastructural basis of capillary permeability studied with peroxidase as a tracer. *J. Cell Biol.* **35:**213.

Keller, T. C. S., and Mooseker, M. S. (1982). Ca^{+2}-calmodulin dependent phosphorylation of myosin, and its role in brush border contraction in vitro. *J. Cell Biol.* **95:**943.

Kim, D. W., Langille, B. L., Wong, M. K. K., and Gotlieb, A. I. (1989). Patterns of endothelial microfilament distribution in the rabbit aorta in situ. *Circ. Res.* **64:**21.

Kistler, G. S., Caldwell, P. R. B., and Weibel, E. R. (1967). Development of fine structural damage to alveolar and capillary lining cells in oxygen-poisoned rat lungs. *J. Cell Biol.* **33:**605.

Koch, L. E., and Smith, M. E. (1978). An association between actin and the major histocompatibility antigen H-2. *Nature (Lond)* **273:**:274.

Lassing, I., and Lindberg, U. (1985). Specific interaction between phosphatidylinositol 4,5-bisphosphate and profilactin, *Nature (Lond)* **314:**472.

Lazarides, E., and Burridge, K. (1975). Alpha-actinin: Immunoflourescent localization of a muscle structural protein in non-muscle cells. *Cell* **6:**289.

Lind, S. E., Janmey, P. A., Chaponnier, C., Herbert, T. J., and Stossel, T. P. (1987).

Reversible binding of actin to gelsolin and profilin in human platelet extracts. *J. Cell Biol.* **105:**833.

Madara, J. L. (1987). Intestinal absorptive cell tight junctions are linked to cytoskeleton. *Am. J. Physiol.* **253** (*Cell Physiol.* **22**):C854.

Madara, J. L., Barenberg, D., and Carlson, S. (1986). Effects of cytochalasin D on occluding junctions of intestinal absorptive cells: Further evidence that the cytoskeleton may influence paracellular permeability and junctional charge selectivity. *J. Cell Biol.* **102:**2125.

Madara, J. L., Moore, R., and Carlson, S. (1987). Alteration of intestinal tight junction structure and permeability by cytoskeletal contraction. *Am. J Physiol.* **253** (*Cell Physiol.* **22**)**:**C854.

Madara, J. L. (1989). Loosening tight junctions. Lessons from the intestine. *J. Clin. Invest.* **83:**1089.

Magno, G., Shea, S. M., and Leventhal, M. (1969). Endothelial contraction induced by histamine-type mediators: An electron microscopic study. *J. Cell Biol.* **42:**647.

Martinez-Palomo, A., Meza, I., Beaty, G., and Cerijido, M. (1980). Experimental modulation of occluding junctions in a cultured transporting epithelium. *J. Cell Biol.* **87:**736.

Meza, I., Ibarra, G., Sabanero, M., Martinez-Palomo, A., and Cerijido, M. (1980). Occluding junctions and cytoskeletal components in a cultured transporting epithelium. *J. Cell Biol.* **87:**746.

Milton, S. G. and Knutson, V. P. (1990). Comparison of the function of the tight junctions of endothelial cells and epithelial cells in regulating the movement of electrolytes and macromolecules across the cell monolayer. *J. Cell. Physiol.* **144:**498.

Mineau-Hanschke, R., Hechtman, H. B., and Shepro, D. (1989). Endothelial cell junctional integrity modulation by serotonin: An ultra structural analysis, *Tissue Cell* **21:**161.

Montesano, R., Friend, D. S., Perrelet, A., and Orci, L. (1975). In vivo assembly of tight junctions in fetal rat liver. *J. Cell Biol.* **67:**310.

Montesano, R., Gabbiani, G., Perrelet, A., and Orci, L. (1976). In vivo induction of tight junction proliferation in rat liver. *J. Cell Biol.* **68:**793.

Moore, P. B., Ownby, C. L., and Carraway, K. L. (1978). Interaction of cytoskeletal elements with the plasma membrane sarcoma 180 acites tumor cell. *Exp. Cell Res.* **115:**331.

Navab, M., Hough, G. P., Berliner, J. A., Frank, J. A., Fogelman, A. M., Haberland, M. E., and Edwards, P. A. (1986). Rabbit beta-migrating very low density lipoproteins increases endothelial macromolecular transport without altering electrical resistance. *J. Clin. Invest.* **78:**389.

Omann, G. M., Allen, R. A., Bokoch, G. M., Painter, R. G., Traynor, A. E., and Sklar, L. A. (1987). Signal transduction and cytoskeletal activation in the neutrophil. *Physiol. Rev.* **67:**285.

Phillips, P. G. and Tsan, M.-F. (1988). Hyperoxia causes increased albumin permeability of cultured endothelia monolayers. *J. Appl. Physiol.* **64:**1196.

Phillips, P. G., Higgins, P. J., Malik, A. B., and Tsan, M.-F. (1988). Effect of hyperoxia on the cytoarchitecture of cultured endothelial cells. *Am. J. Pathol.* **132:**59.

Phillips, P. G., Lum, H., Malik, A. B., and Tsan, M.-F. (1989). Phallacidin prevents thrombin-induced increases in endothelial permeability to albumin. *Am. J. Physiol.* **257:** (*Cell. Physiol.* **26**):C562.

Phillips, P. G., Birnby, L., DiBernardo, L. A., Ryan, T. J., and Tsan, M.-F. (1992) Hyperoxia increases plasminogen activator activity of cultured endothelial cells. *Am. J. Physiol.* **262** (*Lung Cell Mol. Physiol.* **6**):L21.

Pitelka, D. R., and Taggart, B. N. (1983). Mechanical tension induces lateral movement of intramembrane components of the tight junction. Studies on mouse mammary cells in culture. *J. Cell Biol.* **96:**606.

Pitelka, D. R., Taggart, B. N., and Hamamoto, S. T. (1983). Effect of extracellular calcium depletion on membrane topography and occluding junctions of mammary epithelial cells in culture. *J. Cell Biol.* **96:**613.

Rasio, E. A., Bendayan, M., Goretsky, C. A., Alexander, J. S., and Shepro, D. (1989). Effect of phalloidin on structure and permeability of rete capillaries in normal and hypoxic state. *Circ. Res.* **65:**591.

Rodewald, R., Newman, S. B., and Karnovsky, M. J. (1976). Contraction of isolated brush borders from intestinal epithelium. *J. Cell Biol.* **70:**541.

Rotrosen, D., and Gallin, J. I. (1986). Histamine type I receptor occupancy increases endothelial cytosolic calcium, reduces F-actin, and promotes albumin diffusion across cultured monolayers. *J. Cell Biol.* **103:**2379.

Royall, J. A., Berkow, R. L., Beckman, J. S., Cunningham, M. K., Matalon, S., and Freeman, B. A. (1989). Tumor necrosis factor and interleukin 1-alpha increase vascular endothelial permeability. *Am. J. Physiol.* **257** (*Lung Cell Mol. Physiol.* **1**):L399.

Rungger-Brandle, E., and Gabbiani, G. (1983). The role of cytoskeletal and cytocontractile elements in pathologic processes. *Am. J. Pathol.* **110:**361.

Saxon, M. E., Popov, V. I., Kirkin, A. H., and Allakhverdov, B. L. (1978). De novo formation of tight-like junctions induced with phalloidin between mouse lymphocytes. *Naturwissenschaften* **65:**S62.

Schneeberger, E. E. (1981). Segmental differentiation of endothelial intercellular junctions in intra-ascinar arteries and veins of the rat lung. *Circ. Res.* **49:**1102.

Sedar, A. W., and Forte, J. G. (1964). Effect of calcium depletion on the junctional complexes between oxyntic cells of gastric glands. *J. Cell Biol.* **22:**173.

Serhan, C., Anderson, P., Goodman, E., Dunham, P., and Weissman, G. (1981). Phosphatidic and oxidized fatty acids are calcium ionophores. *J. Biol. Chem.* **256:**2736.

Shasby, D. M., Shasby, S. S., Sullivan, J. M., and Peach, M. J. (1982). Role of endothelial cytoskeleton in control of endothelial permeability. *Circ. Res.* **51:**657.

Shasby, D. M., Lind, S. E., Shasby, S. S., Goldsmith, J. C., and Hunninghake, G. W. (1985). Reversible oxidant-induced increases in albumin transfer across cultured endothelium: Alterations in cell shape and calcium homeostasis. *Blood* **65:**605.

Shasby, D. M., Yorek, M., and Shasby, S. S. (1988a). Endogenous oxidants initiate hydrolysis of endothelial cell inositol phopholipids. *Blood* **72:**491.

Shasby, D. M., Winter, M., and Shasby, S. S. (1988b). Oxidants and conductance of cultured epithelial cell monolayer inositol phospholipid hydrolysis. *Am. J. Physiol.* **255** (*Cell. Physiol.* **24**):C781.

Shepro, D., Welles, S. L., and Hechtman, H. B. (1984). Vasoactive agonists prevent erythrocyte extravasation in thrombocytopenic hamsters. *Thromb. Res.* **35:**421.

Simionescu, N. (1983). Cellular aspects of transcapillary exchange. *Physiol. Rev.* **63:**1536.

Simionescu, N., Simionescu, M., and Palade, G. E. (1975). Permeability of muscle capillaries to small heme peptides. Evidence for the existence of patent transendothelial channels. *J. Cell Biol.* **64:**586.

Stevenson, B. R., Heintzelman, M. B., Anderson, J. M., Citi, S., and Mooseker, M. S. (1989). ZO-1 and cingulin: Tight junction proteins with distinct identities and localizations. *Am. J. Physiol.* **257** (*Cell. Physiol.* **26**):C621.

Stolpen, A. H., Guinan, E. C., Fiers, W., and Pober, J. S. (1986). Recombinant tumor necrosis factor and immune interferon act singly and in combination to reorganize human vascular endothelial cell monolayers. *Am. J. Pathol.* **123:**16.

Stossel, T. P. (1984). Contribution of actin to the structure of the cytoplasmic matrix. *J. Cell Biol.* **99:**15s.

Wehland, J., Osborn, M., and Weber, K. (1979). Cell-to-substratum contacts in living cells: A direct correlation between interference-reflection and indirect-immunoflouresence microscopy using antibodies against actin and alpha-actinin. *J. Cell Sci*: **37:**257.

Weiland, T. (1977). Modifications of actin by phallatoxins. *Naturewissenschaften* **64:**303.

White, C. W., and Repine, J. E. (1985). Pulmonary antioxidant defense mechanisms. *Exp. Lung Res.* **8:**81.

White, G. E., Gimbrone, M. A., and Fujiwara, K. (1983). Factors influencing the expression of stress fibers in vascular endothelial cells in situ. *J. Cell Biol.* **97:**416.

Wong, M. K. K., and Gotlieb, A. I. (1986). Endothelial cell monolayer integrity I. Characterization of dense peripheral band of microfilaments. *Arteriosclerosis* **6:**212.

Wu, E.-S., Tank, D. W., and Webb, W. W. (1982). Unconstrained lateral diffusion of concanavalin A receptors on bulbous lymphocytes. *Proc. Natl. Acad. Sci.* USA **79:**4962.

Wysolmerski, R., and Lagunoff, D. (1984). Ethchlorvynol-induced pulmonary edema in rats. An ultrastructural study. *Am. J. Pathol.* **115:**447.

Wysolmerski, R., and Lagunoff, D. (1985). The effect of ethchlorvynol on cultured endothelial cells. A model for the study of the mechanism of increased vascular permeability. *Am. J. Pathol.* **119:**505.

Wysolmerski, R. B., and Lagunoff, D. (1990). Involvement of myosin light-chain kinase in endothelial cell retraction. *Proc. Natl. Acad. Sci. USA* **87:**16.

5

Modification of Lipid Composition to Reduce Susceptibility of Vascular Endothelial Cells to Oxidant Injury: A Novel Defense Strategy

C. MICHAEL HART

Indiana University Medical Center
Indianapolis, Indiana

EDWARD R. BLOCK

University of Florida College of Medicine
Veterans Affairs Medical Center
Gainesville, Florida

I. Introduction

Partially reduced oxygen species (PROS), including hydrogen peroxide (H_2O_2), superoxide ion ($O_2^{\overline{\bullet}}$), and hydroxy radical ($OH\bullet$), have been implicated in the pathogenesis of many forms of tissue injury (Cross, 1987). These species are intermediates in the tetravalent reduction of oxygen and normally are found in cells in small amounts (Freeman and Crapo, 1982). Nonenzymatic (e.g., vitamin E and glutathione) and enzymatic (e.g., superoxide dismutase, catalase, and glutathione peroxidase) factors protect the cell from the damaging effects of PROS by converting them into less reactive chemical species. This balance of oxidants and antioxidants maintains the proper redox environment essential for normal cellular function. When the burden of oxidants on the cell increases, the antioxidant defenses may be overwhelmed. PROS can then chemically react with cellular lipids, proteins, carbohydrates, and nucleic acids, leading to structural and chemical modifications that result in cell dysfunction or death.

Within the lung, the pulmonary vascular endothelium constitutes a cellular compartment that is sensitive to the deleterious effects of PROS (Bishop et al., 1985; Suttorp and Simon, 1982; Weiss et al., 1981). Structural (Crapo et al., 1978; Kistler et al., 1967; Lee et al., 1983) and biochemical (Block and Stalcup, 1981; Crapo et al., 1980; Rubin et al., 1983) studies confirmed that the vascular endothelium is injured early in the course of oxidant injury. The endothelial cell is subject to attack by PROS when the lung is exposed to hyperoxia (Fridovich, 1978; Turrens, et al., 1982) or redox cycling agents (Cross, 1987). In addition, PROS originating predominantly from activated inflammatory cells, consisting mainly of H_2O_2 (Weiss et al., 1981), can interact with the endothelial cell surface (Shasby et al., 1983; Babior, 1978; Sacks et al., 1978) in disorders involving lung inflammation. Consequently, an increased burden of PROS can disturb the oxidant–antioxidant balance in the pulmonary vascular endothelium and result in abnormal endothelial function. Both in vivo and in vitro models have demonstrated that oxidants cause perturbations in endothelial permeability (Shasby et al., 1982; Harlan et al., 1981; Newman et al., 1983), thrombogenicity (Crapo et al., 1983), and metabolic function (Block and Stalcup, 1981). In the human, the ultimate clinical manifestation of oxidant-induced pulmonary endothelial cell derangement is noncardiogenic pulmonary edema (Baldwin et al., 1986; Brigham and Meyrick, 1984; Cochrane et al., 1983).

Strategies to protect cells from oxidant injury have traditionally focused on methods of augmenting the antioxidant defense mechanisms within the cell (Heffner and Repine, 1989). Increasing the intracellular levels of antioxidant enzymes such as catalase (Buckley et al., 1987), glutathione peroxidase (Ody and Junod, 1985), or superoxide dismutase (Freeman et al., 1983) has successfully prevented oxidant injury in several experimental models. Unfortunately, the short half-lives of these antioxidant enzymes in the circulation detracts from their efficacy in preventing oxidant injury when administered intravenously. In addition, antioxidant enzyme molecules are inefficiently transported into the cell interior. Endothelial cells are susceptible not only to PROS generated outside the cell (e.g., those released by leukocytes), but also to PROS generated within the cell. Thus intracellular targeting of antioxidants constitutes an additional challenge in the delivery of antioxidant enzymes.

Alternative methods for augmenting antioxidant potential include increasing intracellular levels of vitamin E (Suttcorp et al., 1986), glutathione (Tsan et al., 1985), and other nonenzymatic antioxidants. Recruitment of platelets (Heffner et al., 1988) or red blood cells (Toth et al., 1984) also decreases oxidant injury in tissues. Like the antioxidant enzymes, these nonenzymatic antioxidants are difficult to deliver to intracellular compartments. Thus, although a variety of compounds enhance the antioxidant capabilities of cells and tissues, the inability to deliver these molecules to precise intracellular targets presents theoretical as well as practical limitations for their clinical efficacy.

Several different areas of investigation now suggest that modification of cellular lipids may alter tissue oxidant susceptibility (Sosenko et al., 1988; Ruch et al., 1989; Diplock et al., 1988). The nature and extent of lipid modifications that must occur to modulate tissue oxidant injury have not been fully characterized. Although previous studies (reviewed below) evaluating the effects of lipid alterations on oxidant injury have produced conflicting results, most investigators have implicated alterations in the extent of unsaturation of constituent fatty acids. PROS tend to react with the loosely bound electrons of carbon double bonds found in abundance in the fatty acyl chains of cell membrane lipid bilayers (Horton and Fairhurst, 1987). Electron abstraction from carbon double bonds within membrane fatty acyl chains generates lipid radicals that can promote and amplify lipid peroxidation and structural derangements (Horton and Fairhurst, 1987). Thus alteration of the number and location of fatty acyl carbon double bonds present in cell lipids constitutes an alternative approach to modifying the susceptibility of tissues to injury from PROS.

II. Background

Several different lines of investigation using a variety of experimental models have examined the relationship between fatty acid modifications and the susceptibility to oxidant injury. For instance, based on observations that poikilotherms (Clements, 1971) and younger animals (Clark and Lambertsen, 1971) display a greater resistance to the deleterious effects of hyperoxia and have greater degrees of unsaturation in their lung fatty acids, Kehrer and Autor (1978) demonstrated that saturated fatty acid–enriched diets increased mortality in rats subsequently exposed to hyperoxia. This dietary manipulation produced an increase in the saturated fatty acid content of lung triglycerides but had minimal effects on the fatty acid composition of lung phospholipids. Similarly, Sosenko and co-workers (1988, 1989) found that newborn rats were more resistant to the lethal effects of hyperoxia when their lung lipids were enriched with polyunsaturated fatty acids. In the same study, enriching newborn rat lung lipids with saturated fatty acids increased the mortality rate in animals exposed to hyperoxia compared to control animals. The alterations in the fatty acid composition of rat lung lipids that enhanced resistance to hyperoxia were not associated with changes in antioxidant enzyme activities (Sosenko, et al., 1988) or prostaglandin metabolites (Sosenko et al., 1989). Similarly, Kennedy and co-workers (1989) found that adult rats fed diets enriched with polyunsaturated fatty acids and then treated with intratracheal bleomycin manifested less morphometric evidence of lung injury. Most recently, Dennery and colleagues (1990) evaluated the susceptibility to hyperoxic injury of rabbit tracheal epithelial cells in monolayer culture. Cells cultured in lipid-supplemented media, producing fatty acid profiles with greater amounts of polyunsaturated fatty acids (PUFA), were compared to cells cultured in media without lipid supplementation. The lipid-supplemented cells, compared to unsupplemented cells, were more resistant to hyperoxic injury and produced fewer lipid peroxidation products. These studies support the concept originally proposed by Dormandy (1969) that cellular polyunsaturated fatty acids in cytoplasmic or neutral lipid pools (e.g., in triglycerides) could scavenge PROS, thereby protecting membrane-unsaturated bonds from oxidant injury and could preserve the integrity of critical membrane functions.

In contrast, traditional biochemical theory predicts that enrichment of membranes with PUFA should heighten susceptibility to oxidant injury by increasing the number of sites prone to oxidant attack (Horton and Fairhurst, 1987). Several investigations in different systems support this concept. Freeman and associates (1983) demonstrated enhancement of hyperoxic injury in cultured porcine endothelial cells enriched with PUFA and protection from hyperoxic injury when these cells were incubated with liposomes composed of saturated fatty acids. Ruch and co-workers (1989) found that cultured hepatocytes became more resistant to H_2O_2 toxicity with increasing culture duration. Resistance was associated with reductions in the PUFA content of hepatocyte triglyceride and phospholipid pools and with increases in the oleic acid (18:1ω9) content of esterified and free fatty acid pools. Rietjens and colleagues (1987) noted that enriching the phospholipids of rat alveolar macrophages with PUFA enhanced their susceptibility to oxidant gases. Changes in macrophage fatty acid composition rather than alterations in membrane fluidity were responsible for the observed changes in oxidant susceptibility. Similarly, in a series of investigations, Balasubramanian et al. (1988, 1989) and Diplock and co-workers (1988) noted that compared to other tissues, rat intestinal mucosae contained increased amounts of an inhibitor of lipid peroxidation. Upon further characterization, this inhibitor was found to consist of a combination of fatty acids. Palmitoleic (16:1) and oleic (18:1) acids were determined to be the functional components of the inhibitory mixture and successfully reduced lipid peroxidation in two separate in vitro systems. Malis et al. (1990) noted that enrichment of mitochondrial membranes with ω3 fatty acids enhanced mitochondrial damage caused by exposure to oxidant stress (xanthine/xanthine oxidase). These investigators found that ω3 fatty acid enrichment also enhanced oxidant-induced phospholipase A_2 activity and postulated that the enhanced degrees of fatty acid unsaturation stimulated lipid peroxidation, leading to the observed enhancement of phopholipase activity. Finally, Schatte and Mathias (1982) found that mortality in rats exposed to hyperoxia was proportional to the dietary content of polyunsaturated fatty acids. Taken together, these studies provide both in vivo and in vitro evidence that reduction in cellular polyunsaturated fatty acids and augmentation of monounsaturated fatty acids reduced cell or tissue susceptibility to oxidant injury.

In summary, this collection of studies demonstrates that the relationship between the degree of fatty acid unsaturation and susceptibility to oxidant injury remains controversial. Clearly, however, modification of lipid composition appears to alter the process of oxidant-induced injury. The lack of consensus among these studies evaluating the relationship between lipid composition and oxidant injury may relate to the wide variety of experimental models studied. For instance, dietary manipulations in intact animals can be expected to modify not only the fatty acid composition of specific tissues, but may also modify other factors important in the generation of oxidant-induced injury. For example, fatty acid modifications can alter neutrophil function and the generation of arachidonic acid metabolites. These alterations could in turn modify the interactions of the vascular endothelium with circulating blood cells. Therefore, a potential disadvantage of models using whole animals and dietary manipulations rests in the difficulty inherent in attributing alterations in oxidant susceptibility solely to the induced alterations in tissue lipid composition. Although problems also exist with in vitro models using cultured cells isolated from the intact lung, our current technical inability to sort the wide variety of lung cells prevents the characterization of in vivo lipid modifications in specific cell types.

Within the lung, the vascular endothelium is felt to be particularly susceptible to the deleterious effects of hyperoxia. Dietary modifications have been shown to alter the fatty acid composition of whole lung lipid extracts. However, the precise effects on endothelial cell lipid composition remain to be discerned. As an alternative to studying pulmonary vascular injury in vivo, we have developed a model of oxidant-induced lung injury using cultured monolayers of porcine pulmonary artery endothelial cells (PAEC). We selected this model because Kaduce and colleagues (1982) have previously demonstrated that the fatty acid composition of cultured PAEC can be altered rapidly and extensively by modifying the lipid composition of the cell culture medium. The obvious limitation of this approach is that to be clinically useful the impact of lipid manipulations on the animal as a whole must be considered. However, this model has enabled us better to define the relationship between fatty acyl composition and susceptibility to oxidant injury by supplementing the culture medium of PAEC monolayers with a variety of exogenous fatty acids. Both supplemented and nonsupplemented cells are then subjected to oxidant (hyperoxia, H_2O_2, or enzymatically generated H_2O_2) or nonoxidant conditions, after which the extent of cell injury is determined. Our results indicate that transient manipulations of PAEC culture media produce persistent alterations in the fatty acid composition and the susceptibility of these cells to oxidant injury. These results suggest that lipid modifications may represent a new modality for augmenting the resistance of cells and tissues to oxidant injury. These findings, as well as several potential mechanisms by which fatty acids alter oxidant injury, are reviewed below.

III. Experimental Protocol

The general experimental protocol that we have used to evaluate the effects of supplemental fatty acids on oxidant- induced PAEC cytotoxicity involves selecting matched dishes of PAEC 3 to 4 days postconfluency. The maintenance medium is thoroughly decanted from each dish and replaced with 4 mL of maintenance medium supplemented with either fatty acid dissolved in absolute ethanol or an equal volume of absolute ethanol vehicle (ETOH) alone, giving a final ETOH concentration of 0.1%. Preliminary experiments demonstrated no differences in cell morphology, oxidant susceptibility, or membrane fluidity in ETOH-supplemented versus unsupplemented cells. Both ETOH- and fatty acid–supplemented dishes are incubated for 3 h at 37°C in humidified 5% CO_2–air. After 3 h, dishes of cells are examined with a phase-contrast microscope, morphologic differences are noted, and supplemented media are discarded. Each dish is then washed with three 2-mL aliquot of sterile Hanks' balanced salt solution (HBSS) before being replenished with maintenance medium and returned to the incubator for subsequent studies. In selected experiments, dishes were studied immediately after the removal of supplemented medium before replacing the maintenance medium.

PAEC were subjected to oxidant stress by exposure to hyperoxia (95% O_2–5% CO_2 for 66 h), H_2O_2 (100 μ*M* in HBSS for 30 min), glucose–glucose oxidase, (30 m*M* glucose plus 50 to 100 mU glucose oxidase for 30 min), or to nonoxidant control conditions consisting of air–5% CO_2 for 66 h, HBSS alone for 30 min, or glucose alone for 30 min, respectively. In all experiments, cell injury was assessed by measuring the release of intracellular lactate dehydrogenase (LDH). In preliminary experiments, LDH release was found to be at least as sensitive as other commonly measured parameters of cell cytotoxicity, including release of radiolabeled compounds (e.g., [^{3}H]adenine) and exclusion of trypan blue. LDH release also correlated with morphologic evidence of injury as seen with phase-contrast microscopy.

IV. Experimental Results

A. Effects of Supplemental Fatty Acids on Oxidant-Induced PAEC Injury

Our initial studies evaluated the effects of *cis*-vaccenic acid (18:1ω7, CVA), a monounsaturated fatty acid, on PAEC oxidant susceptibility. Previous work from our laboratory demonstrated that incubation with 0.1 m*M* CVA for 3 h altered the fatty acid composition of PAEC phospholipids, produced a peak of sufficient magnitude to allow for adequate resolution during gas chromatographic analysis of fatty acid composition, and induced changes in the biophysical state of PAEC membranes (Block and Edwards, 1987). These studies also demonstrated that supplementation with CVA had no effect on the protein content or cell number compared to ETOH-supplemented cells either immediately or 72 h after supplementation (Table 1). Similarly, supplementation with CVA had little effect on endothelial cell morphology as assessed by phase-contrast microscopy. Finally, LDH release was similar in ETOH- and CVA-supplemented cells exposed to control conditions. In contrast, incubation with CVA had a profound effect on subsequent hyperoxic injury in PAEC (Fig. 1). As expected, hyperoxia injured cells, causing a five-fold increase in the LDH release compared to that of ETOH-treated control cells (ETOH-C = 7 ± 1% vs. ETOH-O_2 = 35 ± 6%; $p < 0.05$). However, LDH release in hyperoxic cells pretreated with CVA was significantly less than that in hyperoxic cells pretreated with the ethanol vehicle alone (ETOH-O_2 = 35 ± 6% vs. CVA-0_2 = 20 ± 4%; $p < 0.05$).

CVA also had a profound effect on subsequent injury seen in PAEC exposed to H_2O_2 (Fig. 2). These effects were seen when cells were supplemented with CVA and immediately exposed to H_2O_2 as well as when cells were supplemented with CVA and were then incubated with maintenance medium for 24 to 72 h before exposure to H_2O_2. LDH release in control cells pretreated with CVA was similar to that of control cells pretreated with vehicle at all time points. As expected, H_2O_2 exposure injured cells, causing at least a three-fold increase in LDH release compared to that of ETOH-treated control cells. However, LDH release in cells supplemented with CVA and treated with H_2O_2 was significantly

Table 1 Effect of CVA Supplementation on PAEC Protein Content and Cell Density[a]

	Time after supplementation	
	0 h	72 h
Protein (μg/dish)		
ETOH	567 ± 8	570 ± 3
CVA	573 ± 5	587 ± 7
Cell density (× 10^6/dish)		
ETOH	3.1 ± 0.7	3.1 ± 0.1
CVA	3.1 ± 0.7	3.1 ± 0.1

[a]Cells were incubated for 3 h in maintenance medium supplemented with 0.1 m*M cis*-vaccenic acid (CVA) or 0.1% ethanol (ETOH) vehicle. Cell protein content and density were determined as reported previously (Hart et al., 1990) both immediately after supplementation (0 h) and after a 3-day (72-h) incubation in maintenance medium. Protein values are expressed in micrograms per 60-mm dish of cells, and cell density measurements represent millions of cells per 60-mm culture dish. The data represent the average values ± SEM from four to six experiments.

Source: Hart et al., 1990.

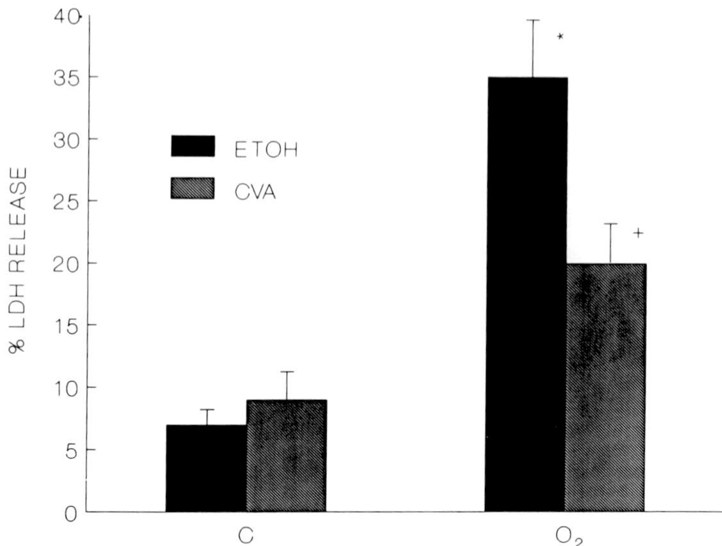

Figure 1 Lactate dehydrogenase (LDH) release from PAEC exposed to control (C: 20% O_2, 5% CO_2, 75% N_2) or hyperoxic (O_2: 95% O_2, 5% CO_2) conditions for 66 h. Cells from each condition were supplemented for 3 h with 0.1 m*M* CVA or 01.% ETOH vehicle. Each bar represents the mean LDH release ± SEM for five experiments. * $p < 0.05$ vs. ETOH–C; $^{+}$ $p < 0.05$ vs. ETOH–O_2. (From Hart et al., 1990.)

less than that in cells supplemented with ETOH and exposed to H_2O_2. Morphologic alterations revealed by phase-contrast microscopy correlate well with LDH release and indicate that vehicle-supplemented cells exposed to H_2O_2 were more extensively injured than CVA-supplemented cells exposed to H_2O_2 (Fig. 3).

To confirm that supplemental CVA was incorporated into PAEC lipids, endothelial cell lipids were extracted into chloroform–methanol, separated into subclasses using thin-layer chromatography, and the fatty acid composition of the individual lipid subclasses analyzed using gas chromatography as reported previously (Hart et al., 1990). The results shown in Table 2 illustrate that supplementation with CVA caused dramatic increases in the amount of 18:1ω7 in the phospholipid, free fatty acid, and triglyceride fractions of supplemented PAECs. The increases in this monounsaturated fatty acid were associated with reductions in the mole percentage of saturated fatty acids and/or PUFA. These alterations in fatty acid composition were seen 24 h following CVA supplementation (Table 2) as well as 48 h following CVA supplementation (data not shown). Taken together, these results confirm (1) that the CVA-induced alterations in lipid composition persisted for at least 48 h after supplementation, and (2) that a single supplemental fatty acid when added to the culture medium of

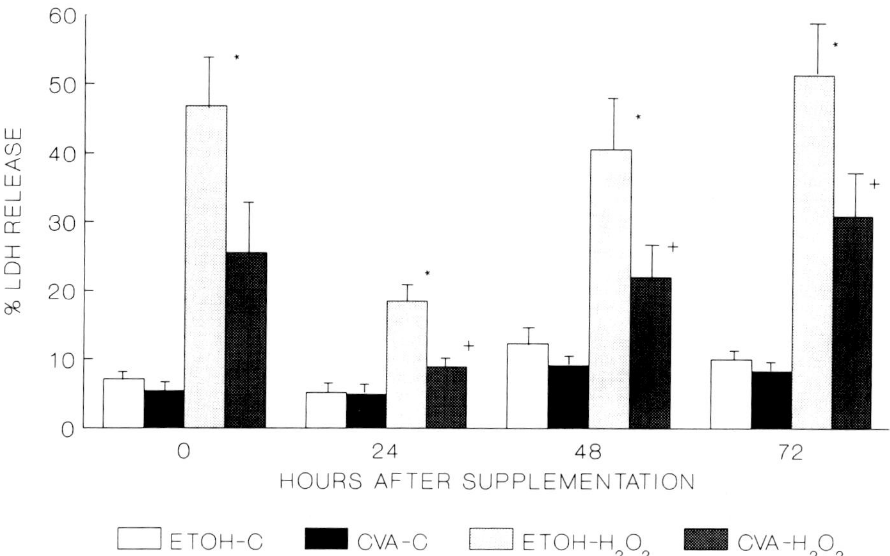

Figure 2 Lactate dehydrogenase (LDH) release from PAEC exposed to nonoxidant control (C) or oxidant (H_2O_2) conditions. Cells were supplemented for 3 h with 0.1 m*M* CVA or 0.1% ETOH vehicle. After supplementation, cells were immediately exposed (0 h) to C or 0.1 m*M* H_2O_2 or allowed to incubate in maintenance medium for 24 to 72 h before exposure to C or H_2O_2. Each bar represents the mean LDH release ± SEM for four to six experiments. $^*p < 0.05$ vs. ETOH–C; $^+p < 0.05$ vs. ETOH–H_2O_2. (From Hart et al., 1990.)

PAECs alters not only fatty acid composition but the subsequent susceptibility of the cells to oxidant injury. This oxidant protective effect could be attributed to the fatty acid because similarly treated cells receiving the ethanol vehicle alone were not protected.

We next evaluated the effects of supplementation with a variety of exogenous fatty acids on oxidant injury in PAECs. Figure 4 demonstrates that supplementation with oleic acid (18:ω9) protected PAECs from oxidant injury in a fashion similar to supplementation with CVA. Oleic acid, an isomer of CVA, is the most abundant octadecanoic acid in human serum. Figure 4 shows that supplementation with 0.1 m*M* 18:1ω9 for 3 h caused no significant increase in LDH release compared to cells supplemented with ETOH alone. As expected, H_2O_2 caused significant cell injury at all time points, manifested by a two- to 10-fold increase in LDH release compared to ETOH control cells. As reported previously (Harlan et al., 1984), the oxidant susceptibility of PAEC varies between lines and passages of cells, accounting for the range of LDH release observed in ETOH–H_2O_2 cells. Despite variations in the absolute magnitude of cell injury,

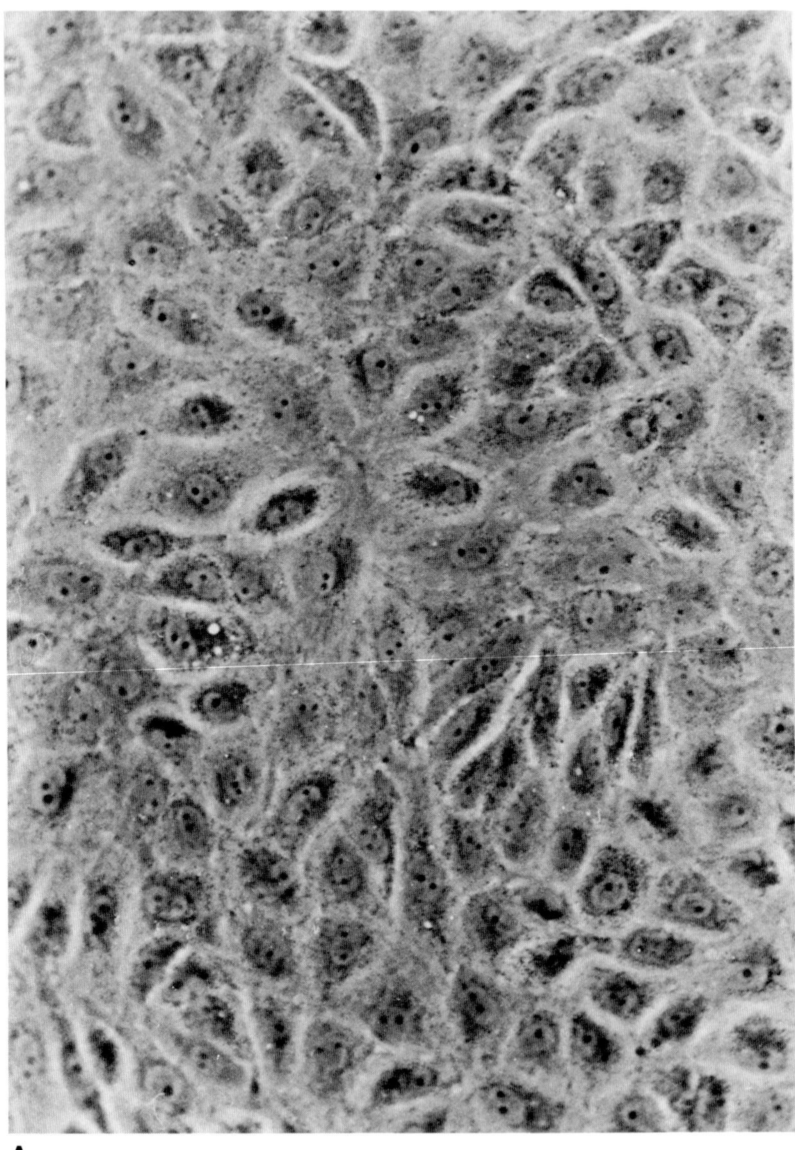

Figure 3 Phase-contrast micrographs (x200) of PAEC monolayers from various treatment groups. Cells were supplemented with 0.1 m*M* *cis*-vaccenic acid (CVA) or 0.1% ethanol (ETOH) vehicle for 3 h, then incubated in maintenance medium for 24 h before exposure to 100 μ*M* H_2O_2 in HBSS or to HBSS alone for 30 min. Photomicrographs were taken 2 h after HBSS or H_2O_2 incubation. (A) ETOH/HBSS; (B) CVA/HBSS; (C) ETOH/H_2O_2; (D) CVA/H_2O_2. (From Hart et al., 1990.)

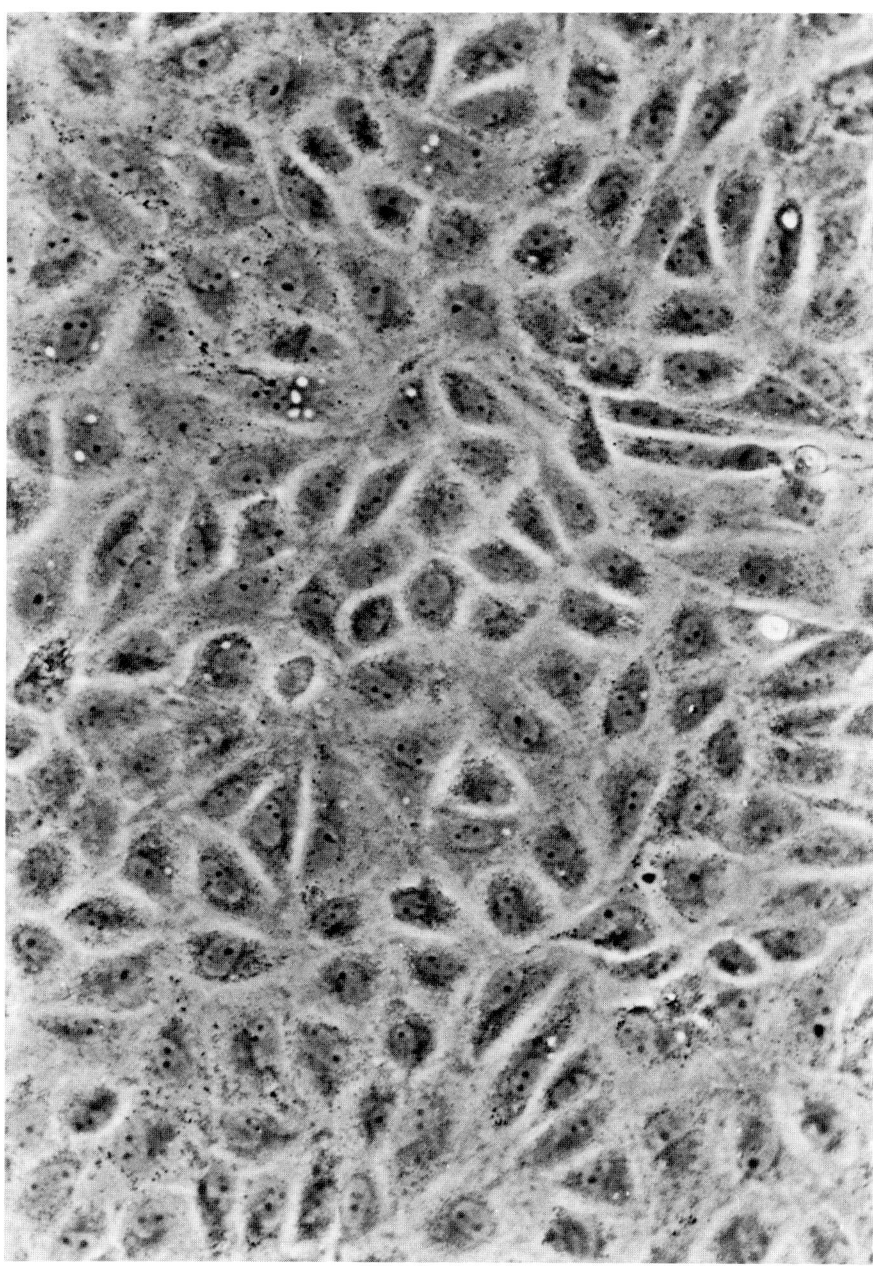

B

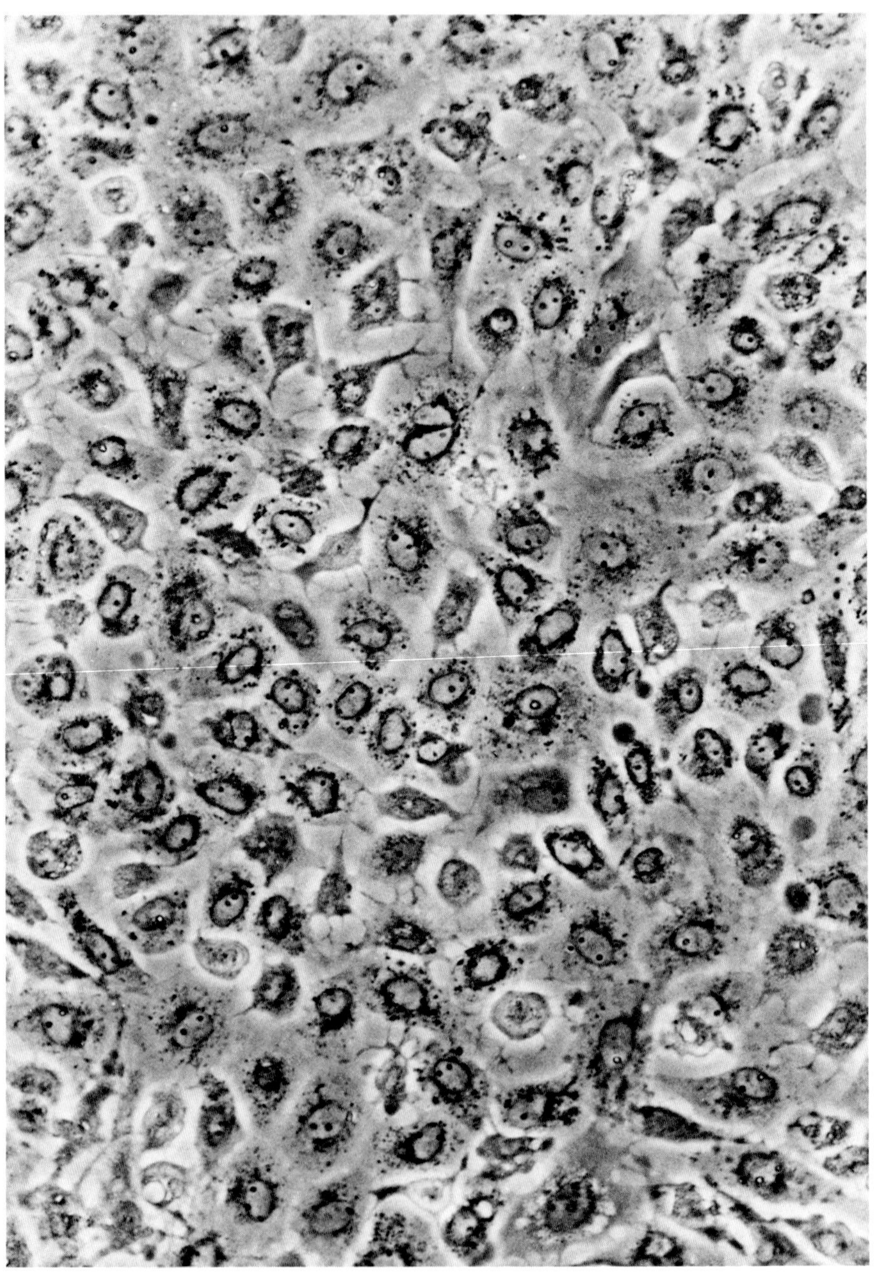

C

Figure 3 (*continued*)

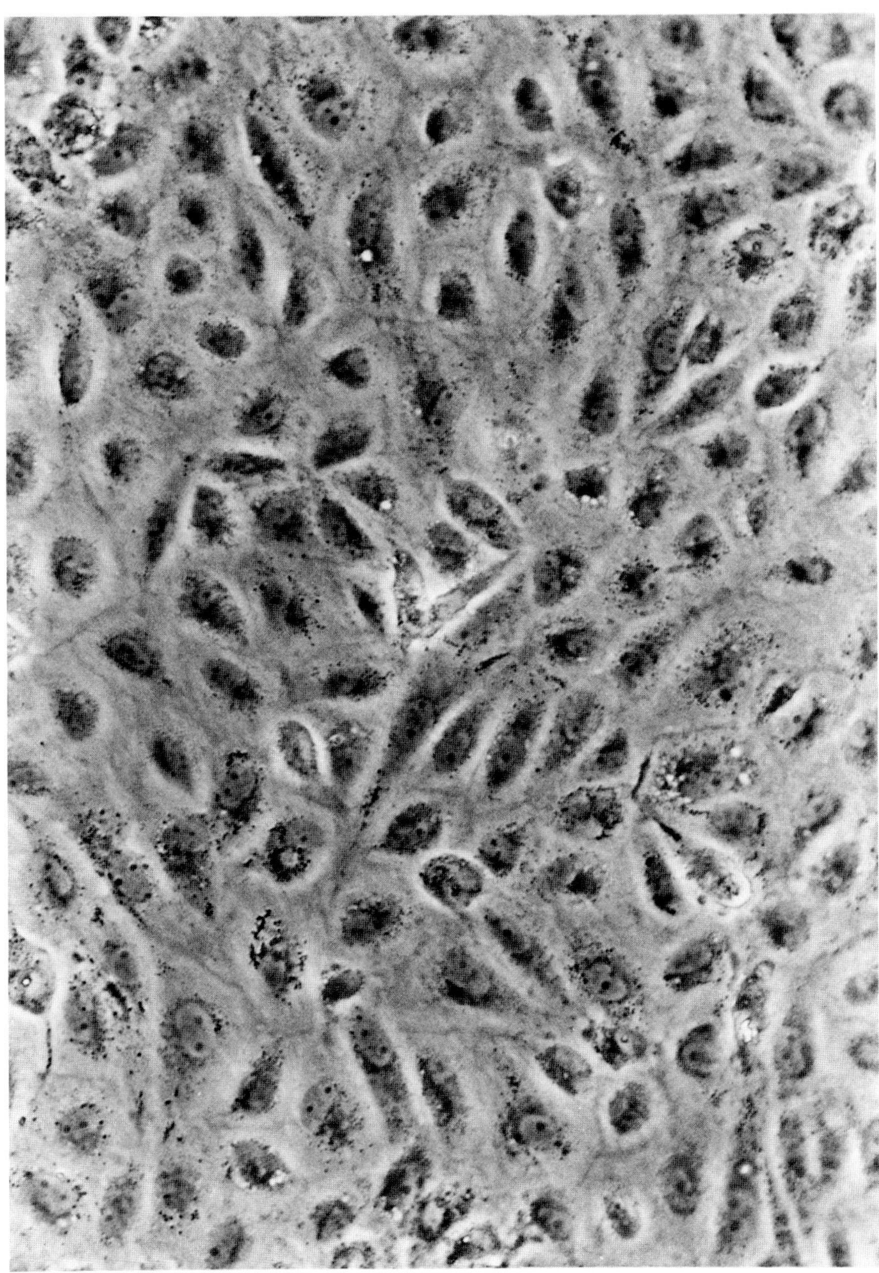

D

Table 2 Effects of CVA Incubation on the Fatty Acid Composition of PAEC Lipids[a]

Fatty acid[b]	Phospholipids				Free fatty acids				Triglycerides			
	Ethanol		CVA		Ethanol		CVA		Ethanol		CVA	
	AVG	SEM	AVG	SEM	AVG	SEM	AVG	SEM	AVG	SEM	AVG	SEM
14:0	1.4	0.3	0.7	0.1	1.3	0.6	1.1	0.4	7.1	2.5	1.8	0.2
14:1	0.4	0.0	0.3	0.0	0.9	0.1	0.7	0.2	2.1	0.6	1.0	0.1
16:0	26.5	2.6	19.5	1.2	24.2	2.3	16.8	0.7	36.2	4.5	11.8	0.4
16:1	4.3	0.4	3.4	0.2	3.8	1.2	3.1	0.7	2.3	0.3	3.6	0.1
18:0	17.8	1.4	14.1	0.5	19.4	1.2	15.0	2.4	18.1	0.9	6.1	0.4
18:1	20.2	0.6	14.8	0.5	20.2	1.3	13.7	0.2	12.6	0.6	7.9	0.1
18:1ω7	10.0	0.5	28.2	2.2	12.0	1.0	38.0	3.6	9.4	0.7	56.3	0.5
18:2	1.2	0.2	1.0	0.1	1.4	0.1	0.9	0.3	ND		0.9	0.0
18:3	0.8	0.1	0.5	0.0	0.4	0.4	ND		ND		1.1	0.2
20:1	0.6	0.0	0.7	0.1	0.3	0.3	0.6	0.3	ND		2.9	0.4
20:4	6.8	2.4	7.5	2.1	5.9	0.7	5.0	0.9	3.4	3.0	1.3	0.4
22:4	3.1	0.4	2.9	0.4	1.5	0.3	1.2	0.1	0.1	0.1	1.2	0.1
22:5	1.7	0.7	1.7	0.6	2.2	0.5	2.1	0.4	7.4	3.7	1.4	0.7
22:6	1.7	0.7	1.7	0.6	0.9	0.7	0.9	0.4	ND		0.9	0.4
Sat[c]	47.1	4.0	35.4	1.4	45.9	1.8	33.6	2.8	61.9	3.3	20.1	0.6
Mono[c]	35.9	1.3	48.2	3.0	37.4	3.7	55.9	4.5	27.1	0.6	72.4	0.9
Poly[c]	17.3	5.2	16.7	4.3	17.0	5.4	10.5	1.8	11.0	3.2	7.5	1.3

[a]Endothelial cell lipid classes were extracted, separated, and analyzed using thin-layer and gas chromatography as reported previously (Hart et al., 1990). Values are in mol % and represent the average of four determinations ± SEM from PAEC supplemented with 0.1 m*M* *cis*-vaccenic acid (CVA) or 0.1% ethanol vehicle for 3 h and then incubated in maintenance medium for 24 h before cell collection and lipid extraction. ND, not detected.

[b]Only major fatty acid components are listed. Abbreviations represent number of carbon atoms:number of double bonds. 18:1ω7 is CVA.

[c]Values are the sum of saturated (SAT), monounsaturated (MONO), and polyunsaturated fatty acids (POLY) in mol % within each treatment group.

Source: Hart et al., 1990.

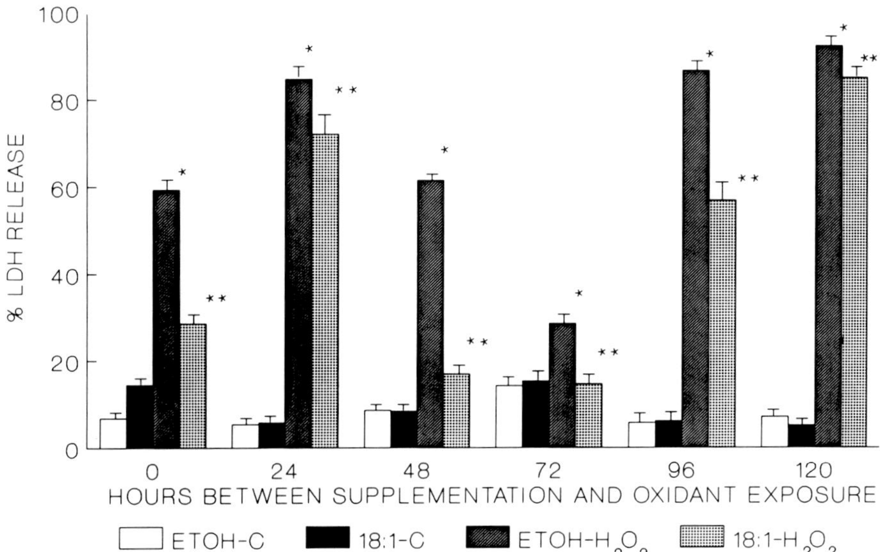

Figure 4 Lactate dehydrogenase (LDH) release from PAEC supplemented with oleic acid (18:1) or ethanol vehicle (ETOH) for 3 h. After supplementation, cells were immediately exposed (0 h) to C or 100 μ*M* H_2O_2 or allowed to incubate in maintenance media 24 to 120 h before exposure to C or H_2O_2. Each bar represents mean LDH release ± SE for six experiments. **p* < 0.01 vs. ETOH–C; ***p* < 0.05 vs. ETOH–H_2O_2. (Modified from Hart et al., 1991.)

supplementation with 18:1ω9 resulted in significant and consistent reductions in subsequent H_2O_2–induced injury, whether the oxidant exposure occurred immediately (0 h), 24, 48, 72, 96, or 120 h after 18:1ω9 supplementation. In addition, 18:1 supplementation protected PAECs from oxidants generated enzymatically with glucose plus glucose oxidase (Fig. 5). In summary, two monounsaturated fatty acid isomers, CVA (18:1ω7) and oleic acid (18:1ω9), protect PAECs from sources of oxidant stress as varied as hyperoxia, reagent H_2O_2, and enzymatically generated H_2O_2.

Supplementation with stearic acid (18:0), a saturated fatty acid, produced similar results (Fig. 6). Rather than supplementing PAECs with an ethanolic solution of stearate, the sodium salt of stearate was used in aqueous solution. LDH release from control cells supplemented with 18:0 was similar to that of control cells supplemented with vehicle. LDH release from oxidant-exposed vehicle-supplemented cells was three times greater than that in vehicle-supplemented control cells. However, like supplementation with 18:1 fatty acids, supplementation with 18:0 protected cells against subsequent H_2O_2 exposure.

In contrast to the effects of saturated and monounsaturated 18-carbon fatty

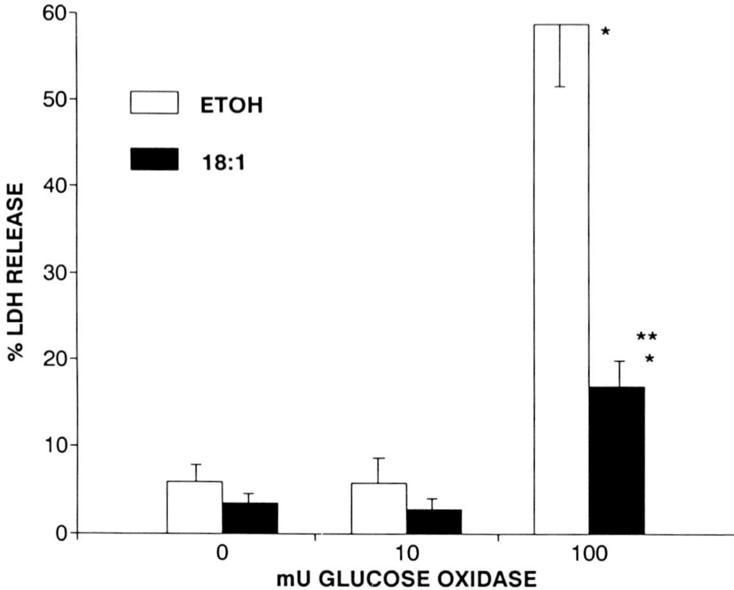

Figure 5 Lactate dehydrogenase (LDH) release from PAEC supplemented with oleic acid (18:1) or ethanol vehicle (ETOH) for 3 h. After supplementation, cells were incubated in maintenance medium for 24 h prior to exposure to 30 m*M* glucose in HBSS or to glucose/HBSS plus 0, 10, or 100 mU glucose oxidase for 30 min. Each bar represents the mean LDH release ± SE for three dishes of PAEC. $*p < 0.01$ vs. similarly supplemented dishes treated with 0 mU glucose oxidase; $**p < 0.01$ vs. ETOH–100 mU glucose oxidase.

acids on oxidant-exposed PAECs, supplementation with PUFA produced very different results. When PAECs were supplemented with linolenic acid (18:3ω6), there was no significant increase in LDH release compared to that of vehicle-treated control cells (Fig. 7). However, prior supplementation with 18:3ω6 resulted in a significant increase in LDH release in oxidant-exposed cells. Similarly, supplementing PAECs with eicosatrienoic acid, 20:3ω3, caused no significant increases in LDH release in control cells, whereas it greatly enhanced the LDH release from oxidant-exposed cells (Fig. 8). Taken together, these results indicate that supplemental saturated and monounsaturated fatty acids can reduce the oxidant susceptibility of PAECs, whereas comparable supplementation with polyunsaturated fatty acids enhances subsequent oxidant injury in PAECs.

To determine if the addition of supplemental fatty acids could modify PAEC injury once the oxidative process was initiated, we modified our experimental protocol as follows. After first exposing PAEC to control (HBSS) or oxidant (100 μ*M* H_2O_2 in HBSS) conditions for 30 min, each dish was

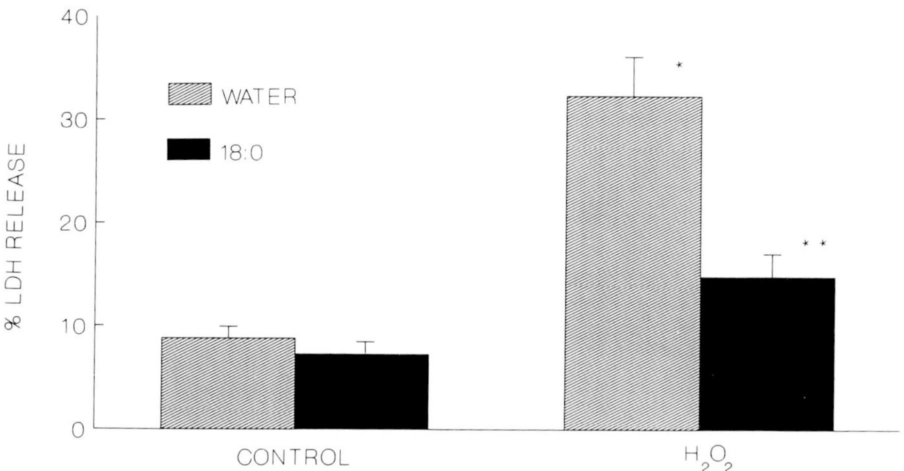

Figure 6 Lactate dehydrogenase (LDH) release from PAEC supplemented with stearic acid (18:0) and then exposed to oxidant (H_2O_2) or control conditions. Cells were supplemented with 0.1 m*M* 18:0 or 0.1% aqueous vehicle (water) for 3 h. After supplementation, cells were immediately exposed to control or H_2O_2. Each bar represents mean LDH release ± SE for 12 determinations $*p < 0.01$ vs. water–control; $**p < 0.01$ vs. water–H_2O_2. (From Hart et al., 1991.)

replenished with maintenance medium supplemented with 0.1 m*M* CVA (18:1ω7), linolenic acid (18:3ω6), or ethanol vehicle alone (0.1%) and allowed to incubate for 3 h before determining the extent of PAEC injury. Figure 9 demonstrates that incubation in CVA-supplemented medium reduced cytotoxicity in PAEC previously exposed to H_2O_2. In contrast, Fig. 10 illustrates that incubation in linolenic acid–supplemented medium enhanced the development of injury in PAEC previously exposed to H_2O_2. These findings demonstrate that supplemental fatty acids modulate oxidant-induced PAEC cytotoxicity whether exposure to the supplemental fatty acid occurs before or 30 min after the initiation of oxidant stress.

B. Potential Mechanisms of Fatty Acid–Induced Modulation of Oxidant Injury

Alterations in Antioxidant Enzyme Activity

Although fatty acids can have numerous effects on cells (Stubbs and Smith, 1984; Spector and Yorek, 1985), the mechanism by which they alter oxidant injury in tissues remains unclear. We have explored several potential

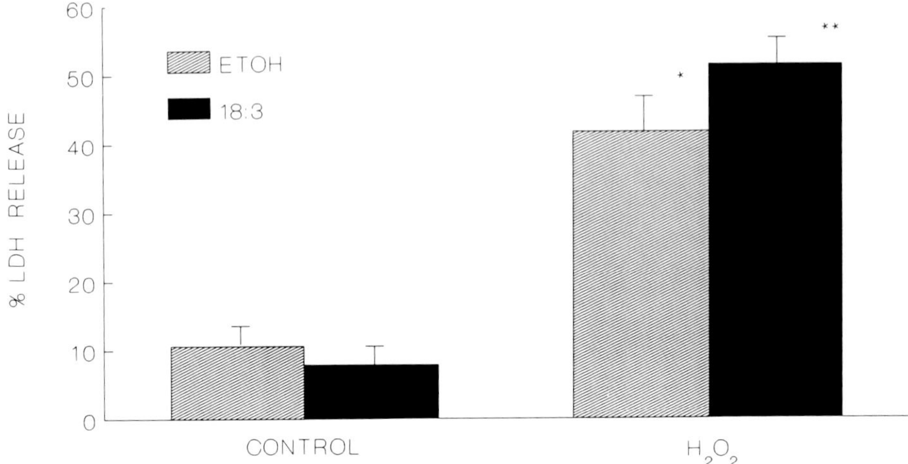

Figure 7 Lactate dehydrogenase (LDH) release from linolenic acid–supplemented (18:3) PAEC exposed to oxidant (H_2O_2) or control conditions. Cells were supplemented with either 0.1 m*M* 18:3(ω6) or 0.1% ethanol vehicle (ETOH) for 3 h. After supplementation, cells were incubated in maintenance medium for 24 h before exposure to control or H_2O_2. Each bar represents the mean LDH release from six experiments ± SE. $^*p < 0.005$ vs. ETOH–control; $^{**}p < 0.01$ vs. ETOH-H_2O_2. (From Hart et al., 1991.)

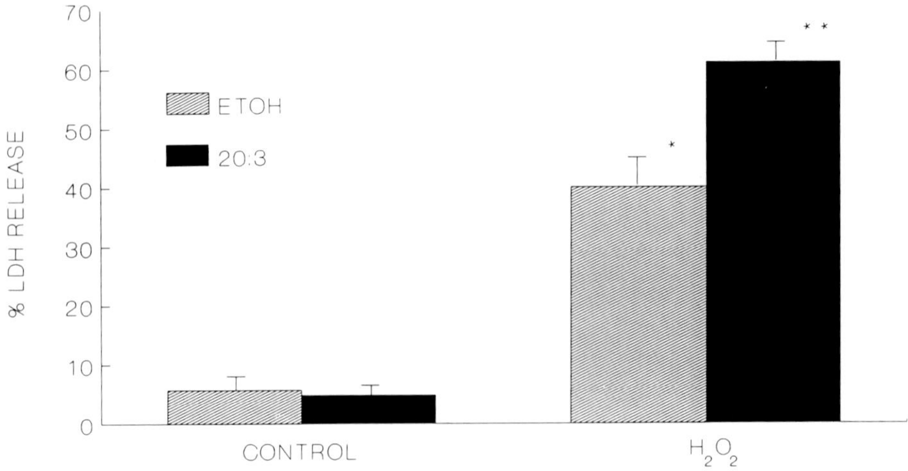

Figure 8 Lactate dehydrogenase (LDH) release from eicosatrienoic acid-supplemented (20:3) exposed to oxidant (H_2O_2) or control conditions. Cells were supplemented with either 0.1 m*M* 20:3(ω3) or 0.1% ethanol vehicle (ETOH) for 3 h. After supplementation, cells were immediately exposed to control or H_2O_2. Each bar represents the mean LDH release ± SE from four experiments. $^*p < 0.01$ vs. ETOH–control; $^{**}p < 0.01$ vs. ETOH–H_2O_2. (From Hart et al., 1991.)

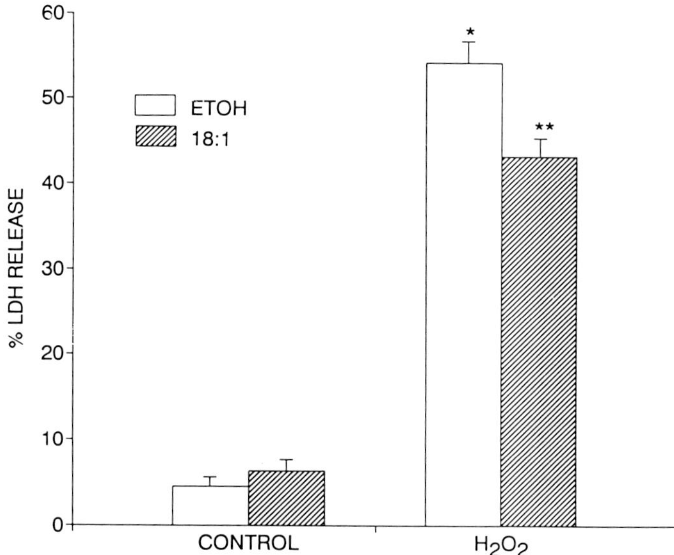

Figure 9 Lactate dehydrogenase (LDH) release from PAEC exposed to control or oxidant (H_2O_2) conditions prior to incubation in CVA-supplemented medium. Cells were first exposed to a control solution (HBSS alone) or to 100 μ*M* H_2O_2 in HBSS for 30 min. After washing, each monolayer was replenished with maintenance medium containing either ethanol vehicle (ETOH) alone (0.1%) or 0.1 m*M* CVA (18:1) in ethanol and incubated for 3 h. Each bar represents the mean LDH release ± SE from nine dishes of PAEC. *$p < 0.05$ vs. control–ETOH; **$p < 0.05$ vs. H_2O_2–ETOH.

mechanisms by which fatty acid alterations might modulate oxidant injury. Because modifications in cell culture medium can influence oxidant susceptibility (Bishop et al., 1985), we investigated whether fatty acid supplementation might enhance PAEC antioxidant enzyme activities. As shown in Table 3, CVA had no significant effect on antioxidant enzyme activities at a time when protection was afforded and thus is unlikely to explain its ability to protect cells from oxidant exposure.

Alterations in DNA Repair or Synthesis

Alternatively, CVA might enhance the ability of PAEC to repair oxidant-induced injury, allowing greater resistance to oxidant stress. Both hyperoxia and H_2O_2 have been shown to depress the ability of endothelial cells to incorporate thymidine into DNA (Clement et al., 1985; Junod et al., 1985), and H_2O_2 has been shown to produce DNA damage in cultured cells (Mello Filho et al., 1984; Schraufstatter et al., 1986; Junod et al., 1989). We therefore evaluated the effects

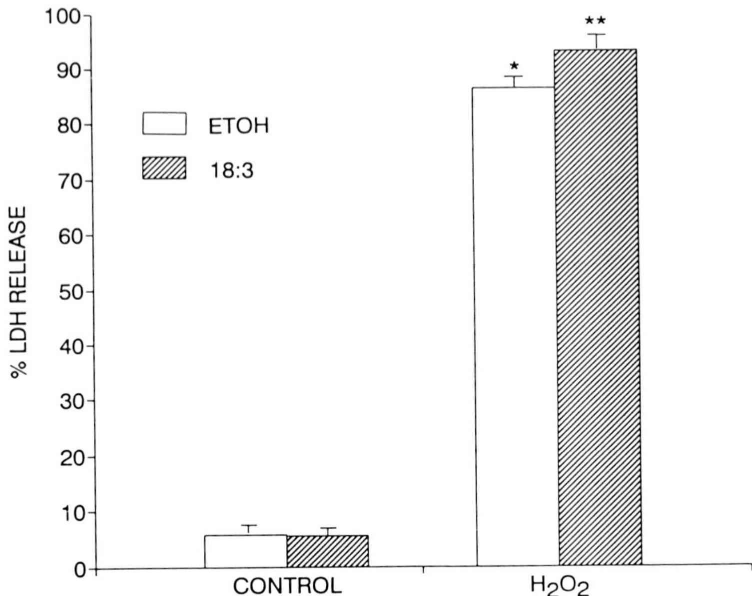

Figure 10 Lactate dehydrogenase (LDH) release from PAEC exposed to control or oxidant (H_2O_2) conditions prior to incubation in linolenic acid–supplemented medium. Cells were first exposed to a control solution (HBSS alone) or to 100 μ*M* H_2O_2 in HBSS for 30 min. After washing, each monolayer was replenished with maintenance medium containing either ethanol vehicle (ETOH) alone (0.1%) or 0.1 m*M* linolenic acid (18:3) in ethanol and incubated for 3 h. Each bar represents the mean LDH release ± SE for six dishes of PAEC. *$p < 0.01$ vs. control–ETOH, **$p < 0.05$ vs. H_2O_2–ETOH.

Table 3 Effect of CVA Incubation on Antioxidant Enzyme Activities in PAEC[a]

Incubation	GSH-Per	G-6-PD	GSH-Red	CAT	SOD
ETOH	28.5 ± 3.8	64.3 ± 6.5	34.9 ± 4.6	17.1 ± 1.2	0.56 ± 0.06
CVA	25.5 ± 2.9	61.8 ± 8.0	38.2 ± 2.7	15.8 ± 1.5	0.50 ± 0.06

[a]PAEC were incubated for 3 h in maintenance medium supplemented with either 0.1 m*M cis*-vaccenic acid (CVA) or 0.1% ethanol vehicle (ETOH) before collecting the cells and determining the activities of the following antioxidant enzymes: glutathione peroxidase (GSH-Per), glucose-6-phosphate dehydrogenase (G-6-PD), glutathione reductase (GSH-Red), catalase (CAT), and superoxide dismutase (SOD). Antioxidant enzyme activities were determined as reported previously (Hart et al., 1990). Values are the mean enzyme activity in units ± SEM from five experiments.
Source: Hart et al., 1990.

Table 4 Effect of CVA Supplementation on Thymidine Uptake and Incorporation into PAEC Exposed to Hydrogen Peroxide[a]

Supplementation-treatment	24 h	72 h
Uptake		
Ethanol–HBSS	52.5 ± 8.9	9.7 ± 0.8
Ethanol–H_2O_2	22.3 ± 2.1*	5.5 ± 0.7*
CVA–HBSS	66.0 ± 10.6†	18.4 ± 0.9‡
CVA–H_2O_2	25.8 ± 3.7*	6.9 ± 0.5*,†
Incorporation		
Ethanol–HBSS	28.7 ± 4.9	25.0 ± 4.8
Ethanol–H_2O_2	8.2 ± 1.2*	4.3 ± 0.5*
CVA-HBSS	30.4 ± 4.7	40.9 ± 4.4‡
CVA–H_2O_2	8.7 ± 1.2*	6.8 ± 0.7*,‡

[a]PAEC were supplemented with either *cis*-vaccenic acid (CVA) or ethanol and incubated in maintenance medium for 24 or 72 h before exposure to control (HBSS) or oxidant (H_2O_2) conditions. Thymidine uptake and incorporation were determined as previously described (Hart et al., 1990). Values are the mean ± SEM of 14 dishes and are expressed as pmol thymidine/mg cell protein.
*$p < 0.01$ vs. similarly supplemented control dishes.
†$p < 0.05$ vs. similarly exposed ETOH-supplemented cells.
‡$p < 0.01$ vs. similarly exposed ETOH-supplemented cells.
Source: Hart et al., 1990.

of CVA supplementation and oxidant exposure on the uptake and incorporation of thymidine into PAECs. These results (Table 4) confirm previous reports that oxidant injury depresses the ability of cultured endothelial cells to take up and incorporate thymidine into DNA. The CVA-induced enhancement of thymidine uptake and incorporation remains unexplained. It is unlikely, however, that this effect of CVA explains its protective effects on cells subsequently exposed to H_2O_2 because thymidine uptake and incorporation were reduced more (as percentage of control cells) in CVA-supplemented cells treated with H_2O_2 than in cells supplemented with the ethanol vehicle alone and subsequently exposed to H_2O_2. Thus thymidine uptake and incorporation studies suggest that supplemental CVA protects PAECs from oxidant injury via mechanisms that are unrelated to DNA repair or synthesis.

Modifications in the Biophysical Properties of PAEC Membranes

Because supplementation with CVA has a fluidizing effect on PAEC membranes, CVA could protect against oxidant injury by compensating for oxidant-induced reduction in PAEC membrane fluidity (Patel and Block, 1988). To determine the effects of supplemental fatty acids on the physical state of PAEC

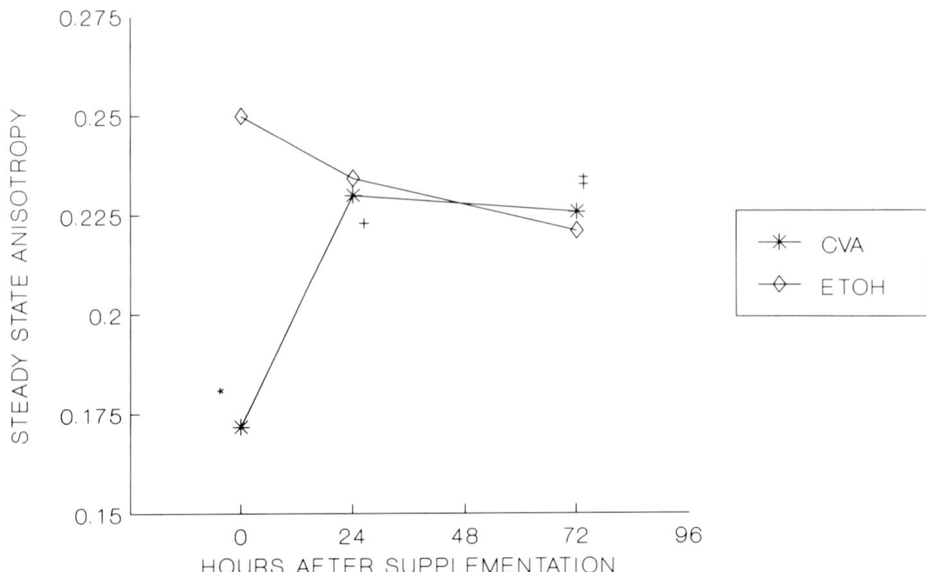

Figure 11 Effect of CVA or ETOH vehicle on steady-state anisotropies for DPH incorporated into PAEC. Confluent monolayers were incubated for 3 h in maintenance medium supplemented with 0.1 m*M* CVA or ETOH vehicle. Cells were studied immediately after supplementation (0 h) or incubated for an additional 24 or 72 h in maintenance medium before collection and incubation with DPH. The data are steady-state anisotropy values in arbitrary units and represent the means from four to five dishes of PAEC. Standard deviations for all groups were less than 2% and are not shown. $^*p < 0.001$; $^+p < 0.01$; ‡ $p < 0.05$ versus ETOH-supplemented cells at similar time after supplementation. (From Hart et al., 1990.)

membranes, the fluorescence polarization of 1,6-diphenyl-1,3,5- hexatriene (DPH) was measured as reported previously (Block and Edwards, 1987; Hart et al., 1990). DPH is a fluorescent aromatic hydrocarbon that partitions into the central and mid-acyl side-chain regions of PAEC plasma membranes. As the order of the membrane is increased, the motion of the probe is hindered, resulting in a change in its fluorescence polarization. Steady-state fluorescence anisotrophies were measured as described previously (Block and Edwards, 1987). Decreases in anisotropy reflect decreases in order, which are associated with increases in membrane fluidity. Figure 11 demonstrates that CVA fluidizes the membranes of PAEC for at least 24 h after supplementation. By 72 h after supplementation this fluidizing effect has resolved. However, as shown earlier in Figs. 2 and 3, PAEC are protected from H_2O_2-induced injury from 0 to 72 h after supplementation. These results indicate that the fatty acid–induced oxidant protection and the alterations in PAEC membrane fluidity are unrelated. Furthermore, supplementation with CVA failed to protect PAEC against a nonoxidant

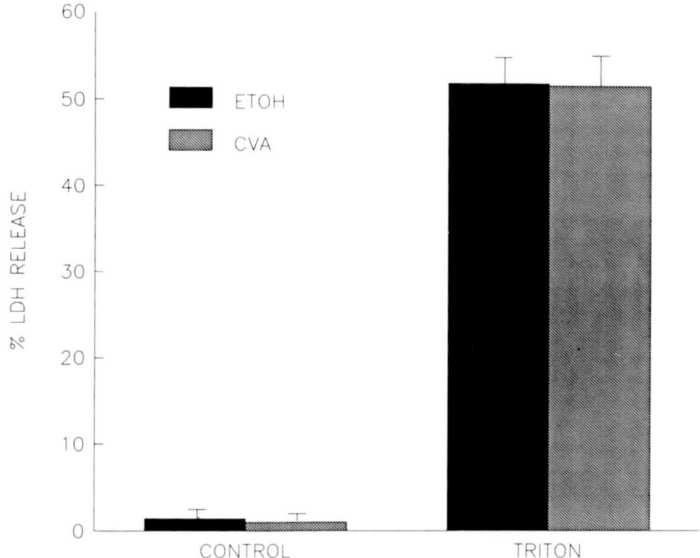

Figure 12 Lactate dehydrogenase (LDH) release from PAEC exposed to 0.005% Triton X-100 in HBSS or to HBSS alone for 60 min. Cells were supplemented with 0.1 m*M* CVA or 0.1% ETOH vehicle for 3 h, then incubated for 24 h in maintenance medium before exposure to Triton. Each bar represents the mean LDH release ± SEM from eight dishes. (From Hart et al., 1990.)

form of cytotoxicity. Figure 12 demonstrates that supplementation with CVA failed to protect the PAEC membrane from detergent-induced cell lysis. This lack of protection in supplemented cells provides additional evidence that the effects of supplemental fatty acids are specific to oxidant injury, are not seen with nonoxidant, surface-active perturbants, and are not related to alterations in the physical state of the membrane.

Modification of Extracellular H_2O_2 Concentration

Because supplemental fatty acids may be released from cultured cells (Hennig et al., 1984), we questioned whether supplemental fatty acids might protect PAEC from oxidant stress by scavenging extracellular oxidants. We therefore conducted experiments to determine if fatty acid supplementation altered the concentration of H_2O_2 in the medium bathing PAEC monolayers. The H_2O_2 concentrations of both oxidant-containing media (100 μ*M* H_2O_2 in HBSS) and of control media (HBSS alone) were determined both before and after incubation with cells that had been supplemented with ethanol or 18:1 24 h previously.

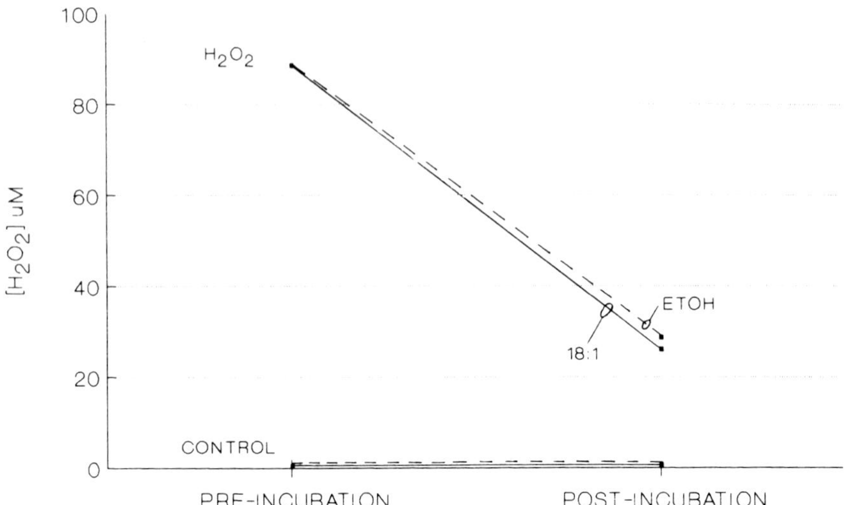

Figure 13 H_2O_2 concentrations in oxidant (H_2O_2) and control media before and after incubation with PAEC previously supplemented with ethanol vehicle or oleic acid. Dishes of PAEC were incubated for 3 h in media supplemented with 0.1 m*M* oleic acid (18:1) or ethanol vehicle (ETOH). Oxidant medium was prepared by dissolving reagent H_2O_2 in HBSS and control medium consisted of HBSS alone. Aliquots of H_2O_2 and control media were assayed for H_2O_2 as described by Hyslop and Sklar (1984). Next, each medium was added to dishes of PAEC supplemented with ETOH or 18:1 and allowed to incubate for 30 min. At the end of this incubation aliquots of media were again assayed for H_2O_2 concentration. Each point is the mean H_2O_2 concentration of four determinations (SEM < 1%).

H_2O_2 concentrations were determined according to the methods of Hyslop and Sklar (1984). Figure 13 illustrates that H_2O_2 concentrations were undetectable in the control media. By contrast, the initial H_2O_2 concentrations in the medium bathing oxidant-exposed cells were approximately 90 μ*M* and decreased to approximately 30 μ*M* in both ethanol and 18:1 supplemented cells after a 30-min incubation. These results demonstrate that supplementation with a monounsaturated fatty acid failed to affect the uptake of H_2O_2 into PAEC or to alter the scavenging of extracellular H_2O_2.

Changes in Oxidant-Induced Lipid Peroxidation

To better define the relationship between the susceptibility of PAEC to oxidant injury and the degree of saturation of supplemental fatty acids, we measured products of lipid peroxidation in oxidant-stressed PAEC. Lipid peroxidation was induced by incubating supplemented cells with either a free radical–generating system or with H_2O_2, as described previously (Hart et al., 1990). Table 5 il-

Table 5 Production of Lipid Peroxidation Products in Pulmonary Artery Endothelial Cells Supplemented with *cis*-Vaccenic Acid, Oleic Acid, Linolenic Acid, or Ethanol Vehicle[a]

Supplementation	nmol TBARS/mg protein
ETOH	0.62 ± 0.04
18:1ω7	0.46 ± 0.02*
ETOH	1.78 ± 0.04
18:1ω9	1.38 ± 0.07†
ETOH	0.41 ± 0.03
18:3ω6	1.19 ± 0.21‡

[a]PAEC were incubated for 3 h in media supplemented with either a 0.1 m*M* ethanolic solution of *cis*-vaccenic acid (18:1ω7), oleic acid (18:1ω9), or linolenic acid (18:3ω6), or with 0.1% ethanol vehicle (ETOH). Cells were then collected and incubated with a free radical–generating system as described previously (Hart et al., 1991). Results are the mean ± SEM of TBARS generated/mg cell protein from four to six assays. Treatments had no significant effect on protein values.
*$p < 0.02$ vs. ETOH.
†$p < 0.01$ vs. ETOH.
‡$p < 0.05$ vs. ETOH.
Source: Hart et al., 1991.

lustrates that supplementation with 18:1ω7 or 18:1ω9 caused a significant reduction in the amount of thiobarbituric acid–reactive substances (TBARS) generated when cells were exposed for 30 min to a free radical–generating system consisting of dihydroxyfumarate and $FeCl_3$ chelated with adenosine diphosphate. By contrast, supplementation with 18:3ω6 followed by incubation with a free radical–generating system resulted in significant increases in TBARS production compared to vehicle-supplemented cells. Similar results were obtained when supplemented PAEC were exposed to H_2O_2 for 30 min. Cells supplemented with 18:1 fatty acids and exposed to H_2O_2 produced fewer products of lipid peroxidation than did vehicle-supplemented companion cells (Fig. 14). On the other hand, supplementation with 18:3ω6 produced increases in H_2O_2-induced products of lipid peroxidation (Fig. 15). The amount of TBARS measured in control and oxidant-exposed cells differed between experiments (Table 5 and Figs. 14 and 15). These differences may be explained by interexperimental variations in the amount of endogenous and exogenous iron present when cells were exposed to the free radical–generating system as well as by variables inherent in the TBARS assay(Beuge and Aust, 1978). These studies lend further support to the hypothesis that supplemental fatty acids alter the course of oxidant injury in PAEC by modifying the propensity of cell lipids to undergo oxidant-induced peroxidative reactions.

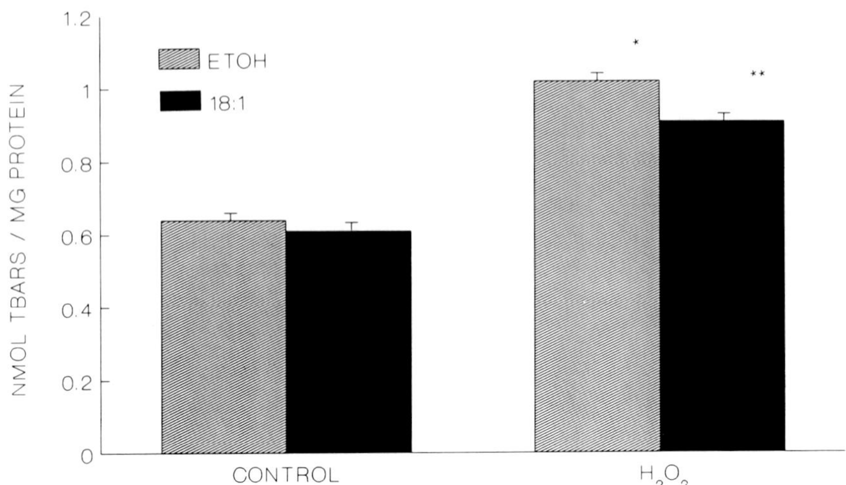

Figure 14 Products of lipid peroxidation generated by exposing supplemented PAEC to oxidant (H_2O_2) or control conditions. Cells were supplemented with (a) 0.1 m*M* CVA or 0.1 m*M* oleic acid (18:1) or (b) 0.1% ethanol vehicle (ETOH) for 3 h. After supplementation, cells were incubated in maintenance medium for 24 h before exposure to control or H_2O_2. The extent of lipid peroxidation in each group was estimated by measuring thiobarbituric acid– reactive substances (TBARS) and protein remaining in cells and released into the culture medium as reported previously (Hart et al., 1991). There were no significant differences between the mean protein values from the various treatment groups. Each bar represents the mean TBARS (cells + medium) ± SEM from 12 flasks. Results are expressed as nmol TBARS//mg protein. $*p < 0.01$ vs. ETOH–control; $**p < 0.01$ vs. ETOH–H_2O_2. (From Hart et al., 1991.)

Alterations in PAEC Lipid Composition and Reactivity

To evaluate and characterize the alterations in lipid composition induced by supplementing PAEC with exogenous fatty acids, we performed a variety of qualitative and quantitative lipid analyses on PAEC. As reviewed earlier, previous hypotheses regarding the ability of supplemental fatty acids to modulate oxidant injury emphasized changes in the lipid composition of either membrane or nonmembrane lipid pools., Therefore, to better characterize the distribution of oleic acid in our model, we performed studies that included radiolabeled oleic acid. In these experiments, trace amounts of radiolabeled oleic acid were added to the supplemented medium (Hart et al., 1991), and PAECs were collected and analyzed 0 to 72 h after supplementation. Table 6 shows that immediately (0 h) after supplementation with 18:1ω9, 72% of the incorporated supplemental fatty

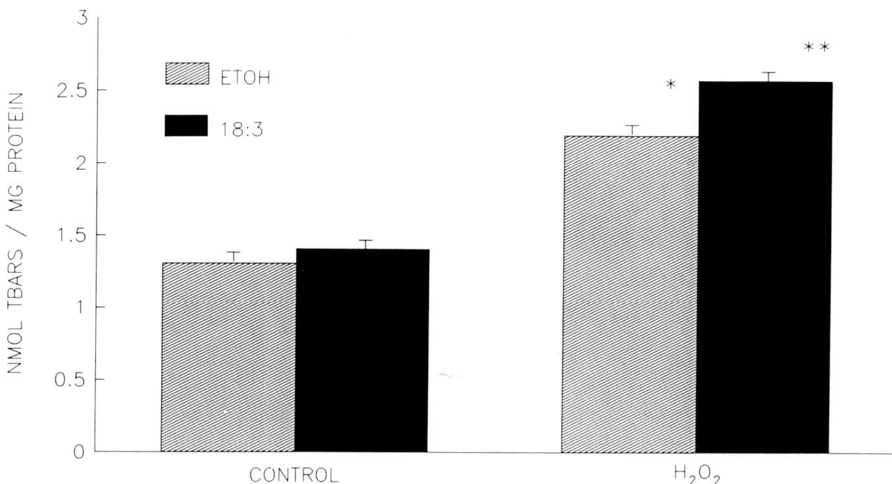

Figure 15 Products of lipid peroxidation generated by exposing linolenic acid–supplemented (18:3) PAEC to oxidant (H_2O_2) or control conditions. Cells were supplemented with 0.1 m*M* 18:3ω6 or 0.1% ethanol vehicle (ETOH) for 3 h. After supplementation cells were incubated in maintenance medium for 24 h before exposure to control or H_2O_2. The amount of lipid peroxidation was estimated by measuring thiobarbituric acid–reactive substances (TBARS) and protein remaining in cells and released into the culture medium. There were no significant differences between the mean protein values from the various treatment groups. Each bar represents the mean TBARS (cells + medium) ± SEM from six flasks. Results are expressed as nmol TBARS/mg protein. $^*p < 0.01$ vs. ETOH–control; $^{**}\,p < 0.01$ vs. ETOH–H_2O_2. (From Hart et al., 1991.)

acid was found in the trigylceride fraction. However, in those cells that were incubated in maintenance medium for 24 to 72 h after supplementation, greater amounts of the supplemental fatty acid were incorporated into the phospholipid fraction, and progressively smaller amounts of 18:1ω9 were found in triglyceride and free fatty acid fractions. Although cells initially took up approximately the same amount of the supplemental radiolabel (18.9 to 22.1%), the cell-associated activity seen immediately after supplementation decreased at later time points, due to release of the radiolabel into the maintenance medium. Thus although the supplemental monounsaturated fatty acid initially incorporated predominantly into the triglyceride (nonmembrane) fraction, over the ensuing 24 to 48 h the vast majority of the 18:1ω9 was found in the phospholipid (membrane) fraction. Despite redistribution of the supplemental fatty acid between intracellular lipid compartments, 18:1ω9-supplemented cells were protected from oxidant injury for 0 to 72 h after fatty acid supplementation, as shown in Fig. 4. These studies suggest that neither the specific lipid compartment into which supplemental monounsaturated fatty acid incorporates nor its subsequent intracellular redistribution over time influences the effects of supplemental fatty acids on susceptibility of PAECs to oxidant injury.

To define further the relationship between lipid modifications induced by oleic acid supplementation and oxidant susceptibility, we performed quantitative fatty acid analyses on PAECs after supplementation and also after supplementation and oxidant exposure (submitted for publication). Flasks of PAEC were incubated with ETOH- or 18:1-supplemented medium for 3 h, washed, and then incubated in maintenance medium for 0 to 72 h. Selected flasks were exposed to oxidant or control conditions for 30 min, followed by a 2-h incubation in maintenance medium prior to cell collection. Cell lipids were extracted (Folch et al., 1957) and separated into phospholipid, cholesterol, free fatty acid, and triglyceride fractions using thin-layer chromatography plates (Hart et al., 1990; Rastogi and Nordoy, 1980). After collection, methyl heptadecanoate was added to each fraction as an internal standard. Fractions were then derivatized (Morrison and Smith, 1964) and analyzed with gas chromatography (Hart et al., 1990). These analyses demonstrated that the phospholipid fraction contained the majority of PAEC fatty acids. Supplementation with oleic acid increased the 18:1 content of all fractions at all intervals after supplementation. The increases in 18:1 content were accompanied by decreases in the content of other constituent fatty acids, including both saturated and polyunsaturated fatty acids. The most dramatic effect of oleic acid was seen in the triglyceride fraction immediately after supplementation when oleic acid increased the 18:1 content to levels 100-fold greater than vehicle-supplemented cells. This large increase in the triglyceride fatty acids of supplemented PAEC resolved by 24 h after supplementation. These findings are consistent with previous reports (Denning et al., 1983) and with the data in Table 6 demonstrating that supplemental fatty acids are initially incorporated into the triglyceride fraction and are either released into the culture medium or transferred to the phospholipid fraction during subsequent maintenance culture. This apparent increase in PAEC triglyceride content immediately after oleic acid supplementation was confirmed with a biochemical assay that measures triglyceride content by detecting its glycerol backbone. In contrast to its effects on the amount of PAEC triglyceride, oleic acid supplementation had no effect on the phospholipid content of PAEC.

We also evaluated the combined effects of oleic acid supplementation and oxidant exposure on the fatty acid profiles of PAEC lipid fractions. Oleic acid supplementation increased the 18:1 content of all fractions at all time points, similar to the findings in PAECs that were supplemented but never exposed to control or oxidant conditions. Compared to control cells, H_2O_2-exposed PAECs had less phospholipid PUFA, consistent with oxidant-induced peroxidation of

Table 6 Distribution of Supplemental Oleic Acid in Pulmonary Artery Endothelial Cells[a]

Lipid class	Hours after supplementation			
	0	24	48	72
Phospholipid	50.3 (13.2)[b]	128.5 (78.9)	185.1 (90.4)	180.1 (91.4)
Triglyeride	276.0 (72.4)	108.3 (6.7)	4.1 (2.0)	3.9 (2.0)
Free fatty acid	18.0 (4.7)	12.4 (7.6)	8.0 (3.9)	6.3 (3.2)
CPM released (media)	—	195.3	120.7	174.4
Cell-associated CPM	381.0	162.9	204.7	197.1
Total CPM[c]	381.0 (22.1)	358.2 (20.8)	325.4 (18.9)	371.5 (21.6)

[a]PAEC were incubated in media supplemented with 0.1 m*M* oleic acid containing 1.7×10^6 CPM of [^{3}H]oleic acid for 3 h at 37°C. After supplementation, PAECs were washed thoroughly and collected immediately (0 h) or after a 24 to 72 h of incubation in maintenance media.
[b]Each value represents the mean CPM $\times 10^3$ (% total) from three separate dishes at each time point. Only the major lipid classes are reported, so the sum of the values in parentheses (CPM in lipid class ÷ total cell-associated CPM × 100) does not equal 100%.
[c]Total CPM was calculated as the sum of the cell-associated radioactivity for each time point plus the activity released into the maintenance media for the 24- to 72-h cultures. The values in parentheses (total CPM ÷ amount of radiolabel initially added to cells × 100) represent the fraction of the supplemental fatty acid that was initially taken up by the cells.
Source: Hart et al. 1991.

PAEC phospholipid fatty acids. Oxidant-induced loss of PUFA from the triglyceride fraction was not observed, a finding that would have suggested that the PAEC neutral lipid fraction was serving as an oxidant sink. Because oxidant susceptibility has been postulated to relate to the degree of fatty acid unsaturation in tissue lipids (Freeman et al., 1983; Ruch et al., 1989; Hart et al., 1990, 1991; Kehrer and Autor, 1978; Sosenko et al., 1989; Dormandy, 1969), we calculated the total number of fatty acid double bonds within each lipid fraction. Oleic acid supplementation failed to consistently reduce the number of fatty acid double bonds in PAEC phospholipid fractions. Due to oxidant-induced loss of PUFA from phospholipids, H_2O_2 exposure decreased the number of phospholipid double bonds compared to similarly supplemented control cells. In the triglyceride fraction, oleic acid supplementation increased the number of double bonds above vehicle-supplemented cells at 0 h only, and oxidant exposure failed to reduce the number of double bonds. Therefore, quantitative fatty acid analyses in fatty acid supplemented and oxidant-exposed cells failed to support our previous hypothesis that oleic acid protected PAECs by reducing the number of double bonds in phospholipid fatty acids. Similarly, these analyses failed to support the notion that supplemental fatty acids alter oxidant injury by changing the number of nonmembrane fatty acid double bonds.

V. Summary and Conclusions

Fatty acid supplementation produces persistent alterations in the composition of PAEC lipids. Saturated and monosaturated fatty acids are associated with increased resistance to oxidant injury, whereas supplementation with PUFA can result in enhanced susceptibility to oxidant injury in PAEC. The mechanism responsible for this modulation of oxidant injury remains undefined. Previous hypotheses have provided potential explanations for the ability of fatty acids to modulate oxidant injury. The first, based on the chemical reactivity of fatty acid double-bond systems, postulates that reducing the unsaturation of cell lipids by replacing PUFA with exogenous saturated or monounsaturated fatty acids should reduce oxidant reactivity and confer increased resistance to oxidant injury. An alternative theory suggests that supplemental lipids are incorporated into non-membrane intracytoplasmic pools of neutral lipids and that by increasing the number of fatty acid double bonds in this lipid fraction, intracellular free radicals would be directed away from the structural lipids of cell membranes. As a result, enrichment with PUFA is predicted to enhance resistance to oxidant injury by providing an intracellular oxidant ''sink.'' The current results, however, do not support either of these theories. Triglyceride fatty acids and double-bond numbers are increased immediately after supplementation only. Therefore, the ''sink'' theory cannot adequately explain the observed oxidant protection 24 to 72 h after oleic acid supplementation. The ''biochemical'' theory fails to explain adequately the observed protection because the number of phospholipid double bonds is not consistently reduced by oleic acid supplementation.

Although our results suggest that alterations of double-bond numbers do not fully explain the effects of lipid modifications on oxidant susceptibility, it is apparent that alterations in membrane fatty acid composition do modulate oxidant susceptibility. The lipid analyses reported above examine the effects of fatty acid supplementation and oxidant exposure on whole cell lipid classes. Quantitatively small but functionally important alterations in the fatty acid composition of subcellular organelle membranes (e.g., mitochondrial or microsomal membranes) could account for the alterations observed in oxidant susceptibility. Because the plasma membrane accounts for approximately 50% of PAEC phospholipids (Sekharam et al., 1990), subtle changes in the fatty acid composition of subcellular organelles could be masked by analyses at the whole cell level. Similarly, the fatty acid analyses of total phospholipids may overshadow important alterations in the composition of phospholipid subclasses. For instance, altering the fatty acid composition of phosphoinositol species could potentially influence transmembrane signaling events, modifying the substrate for phospholipases and the subsequent generation of arachidonic acid metabolites and diacylglycerol. However, because phosphatidylinositol comprises a relatively small percentage of plasma membrane phospholipids, such alterations could be missed in the analysis of total phospholipid.

Finally, supplemental fatty acids may alter oxidant injury in cells by mechanisms that are not directly related to effects on lipid composition. Fatty acids have been shown to modify the intracellular distribution and concentration of divalent cations [e.g., Ca^{2+} (Serhan et al., 1981; Croset et al., 1989) and Fe^{2+} (Simpson and Peters, 1987)], to influence the intracellular generation of reactive oxygen species (Chan et al., 1988, Bawdey et al., 1981; Peterson et al., 1988), and to alter eicosanoid metabolism (Spector and Yorek, 1985; Higgs et al., 1986; Lee, 1989). Fatty acid–induced alteration of such events could then modify the generation of injury to oxidant-exposed cells and tissues.

VI. Future Directions

The studies discussed in this chapter serve to illustrate the dynamics of lipid composition in cultured cells when challenged with exogenous fatty acids. Supplemental fatty acids are taken up by cells from the culture medium and are redistributed within the cell over time. These fatty acids produce persistent alterations in PAEC lipid composition and oxidant susceptibility as well as in the generation of lipid peroxidation products. In addition, supplemental fatty acids alter the development of PAEC cytotoxicity even if oxidant exposure has already occurred (Figs. 9 and 10). These data emphasize that in combination with oxidant stress, the administration of exogenous PUFA to humans could have deleterious effects not seen in healthy human subjects. Furthermore, a major limitation of antioxidant defense strategies has been that in most models, successful oxidant protection requires initiation of treatment prior to or in the early stages of oxidant stress, a limitation that lipid modification may potentially overcome (Fig. 9). However, the precise relationships between fatty acyl structure and susceptibility to injury must be defined before the full potential of lipid alterations in antioxidant defense strategies can be appreciated.

The complexities of cellular lipid metabolism coupled with the constantly evolving and interactive nature of the many events postulated to be important in the generation of oxidant injury present a seemingly insurmountable challenge for the elucidation of the precise mechanism whereby lipid modifications alter oxidant injury. The experimental results presented herein strive to characterize a model of oxidant injury to lung endothelial cells. Although several potential mechanisms that might explain fatty acid–induced modulation of oxidant injury have been explored in this model, many more remain. Our results, along with those of others, demonstrate the potential utility of lipid alterations in protecting tissues from oxidant stress. In light of recent advances in the understanding of dietary lipids and their impact on the pathogenesis of cardiovascular disease, continued investigation into lipid composition and its effects on oxidant injury will probably provide new insights into the pathogenesis of oxidant injury and present avenues for the development of novel antioxidant defense strategies.

Acknowledgments

The authors thank Mrs. Dana Dunn and Mrs. Anne Crawford in their secretarial assistance, and Ms. Janet Wooten for her help in editing the manuscript. This work was supported by the Medical Research Service of the Department of Veterans Affairs (ERB) and by Grants HL-35908 and HL-27791 from the NIH Heart, Lung, and Blood Institute (ERB).

References

Babior, B. M. (1978). Oxygen-dependent microbial killing by phagocytes. *N. Engl. J. Med.* **298:**659.

Balasubramanian, K. A., Manohar, M., and Mathan, V. I. (1988). An unidentified inhibitor of lipid peroxidation in intestinal mucosa. *Biochim. Biophys. Acta* **962:**51.

Balasubramanian, K. A., Nalini, S., Cheeseman, K. H., and Slater, T. F. (1989). Nonesterified fatty acids inhibit iron-dependent lipid peroxidation. *Biochim. Biophys. Acta* **1003:**232.

Baldwin, S. R., Grum, C. M., Boxer, L. A., Simon, R. H., Ketai, L. H., and Devall, L. J. (1986). Oxidant activity in expired breath of patients with adult respiratory distress syndrome. *Lancet* **1:**11.

Bawdey, J. A., Curnutte, J. T., and Karnovsky, M. L. (1981). *cis*-Polyunsaturated fatty acids induce high levels of superoxide production by human neutrophils, *J. Biol. Chem.* **256:**12640.

Beuge, J. A., and Aust, S. D. (1978). Microsomal lipid peroxidation. In *Methods in Enzymology*. Edited by S. Fleischer and L. Packer. Academic Press, New York, p. 302.

Bishop, C. T., Mirza, Z., Crapo, J. D., and Freeman, B. A. (1985). Free radical damage to cultured procine aortic endothelial cells and lung fibroblasts: Modulation by culture conditions. *In Vitro Cell. Dev. Biol.* **21**(4):229.

Block, E. R., and Edwards, D. A. (1987). Effect of plasma membrane fluidity on serotonin transport by endothelial cells. *Am. J. Physiol.* **253:**C672.

Block, E. R., and Stalcup, S. A. (1981). Depression of serotonin uptake by cultured endothelial cells exposed to high O_2 tension. *J. Appl. Physiol.* **50**(6):1212.

Brigham, K. L., and Meyrick, B. (1984). Interactions of granulocytes with the lungs. *Circ. Res.* **54:**623.

Buckley, B. J., Tanswell, A. K., and Freeman, B. A. (1987). Liposome-mediated augmentation of catalase in alveolar type II cells protects against H_2O_2 injury. *J. Appl. Physiol.* **63**(1):359.

Chan, P. H., Chen, S. F., and Yu, A. C. H. (1988). Induction of intracellular superoxide radical formation by arachadonic acid and by polyunsaturated fatty acids in primary astrocytic cultures. *J. Neurochem.* **50:**1185.

Clark, J. M., and Lambertsen, C. J. (1971). Pulmonary oxygen toxicity: A Review. *Pharmacol. Rev.* **23:**37.

Clement, A., Hubscher, U., and Junod, A. F. (1985). Effects of hyperoxia on DNA synthesis in cultured porcine aortic endothelial cells. *J. Appl. Physiol.* **59:**1110.

Clements, J. A. (1971). Comparative lipid chemistry of lungs. *Arch. Intern. Med.* **127:**387.

Cochrane, C., Spragg, G. R., and Revak, S. D. (1983). Pathogenesis of the adult respiratory distress syndrome: evidence of oxidant activity in bronchoalveolar lavage fluid. *J. Clin. Invest.* **71:**754.

Crapo, J. D., Peters-Golden, M., Marsh-Salin, J., and Shelburne, J. S. (1978). Pathologic changes in the lungs of oxygen-adapted rats: A morphometric analysis. *Lab. Invest.* **39:**640.

Crapo, J. D., Barry, B. E., Foscue, H. A., and Shelburne, J. (1980). Structural and biochemical changes in rat lungs occurring during exposures to lethal and adaptive doses of oxygen. *Am. Rev. Respir. Dis.* **122:**123.

Crapo, J. D., Freeman, B. A., Barry, B. E., Turrens, J. F., and Young, S. L. (1983). Mechanisms of hyperoxic injury to the pulmonary microcirculation. *Physiologist* **26:**170.

Croset, M., Black, J. M., Swanson, J. E., and Kinsella, J. E. (1989). Effects of dietary n-3 polyunsaturated fatty acids on phospholipid composition and calcium transport in mouse cardiac sarcoplasmic reticulum. *Lipids* **24:**278.

Cross, C. E. (1987). Oxygen radicals and human disease. *Ann. Intern. Med.* **107:**526.

Dennery, P. A., Kramer, C. M., and Alpert, S. E. (1990). Effect of fatty acid profiles on the susceptibility of cultured rabbit tracheal epithelial cells to hyperoxic injury. *Am. J. Respir. Cell Mol. Biol.* **3:**137.

Denning, G. M., Figard, P. H., Kaduce, T. L., and Spector, A. A. (1983). Role of triglycerides in endothelial cell arachidonic acid metabolism. *J. Lipid Res.* **24:**993.

Diplock, A., Balasubramanian, K. A., Manohar, M., Mathan, V. I., and Ashton, D. (1988). Purification and characterization of the inhibitor of lipid peroxidation from intestinal mucosae. *Biochim. Biophys. Acta* **962:**42.

Dormandy, T. L. (1969). Biological rancidification. *Lancet* **2:**684.

Folch, J., Lees, M., and Sloane-Stanley, G. H. (1957). A simple method for the isolation and purification of total lipids from animal tissues. *J. Biol. Chem.* **226:**497.

Freeman, B. A., and Crapo, J. D. (1982). Biology of disease-free radicals and tissue injury. *Lab. Invest.* **47:**412.

Freeman, B. A., Young, S. L., and Crapo, J. D. (1983). Liposome-mediated augmentation of superoxide dismutase in endothelial cells prevents oxygen injury. *J. Biol. Chem.* **258**(20):12534.

Fridovich, I. (1978). The biology of oxygen radicals. *Science* **201:**875.

Harlan, J. M., Killen, P. D., Harker, L. A., Striker, G. E., and Wright, D. G. (1981). Neutrophil-mediated endothelial injury in vitro. Mechanisms of cell detachment. *J. Clin. Invest.* **68:**1394.

Harlan, J. M., Levine, J. D., Callahan, K. S., Schwartz, B. R., and Harker, L. A. (1984). Glutathione redox cycle protects cultured endothelial cells against lysis by extracellularly generated hydrogen peroxide. *J. Clin. Invest.* **73:**706.

Hart, C. M., Tolson, J. K., and Block, E. R. (1990). Fatty acid supplementation protects pulmonary artery endothelial cells from oxidant injury. *Am. J. Respir. Cell Mol. Biol.* **3:**479.

Hart, C. M., Tolson, J. K., and Block, E. R. (1991). Supplemental fatty acids alter lipid peroxidation and oxidant injury in endothelial cells. *Am. J. Physiol.* **260:**L481.

Heffner, J. E., and Repine, J. E. (1989). Pulmonary strategies of antioxidant defense. *Am. Rev. Respir. Dis.* **140:**531.

Heffner, J. E., Katz, S. A., Halushka, P. V., and Cook, J. A. (1988). Human platelets attenuate oxidant injury in isolated rabbit lungs. *J. Appl. Physiol.* **65:**1258.

Hennig, B., Shasby, D. M., Fulton, A. B., and Spector, A. A. (1984). Exposure to free fatty acid increases the transfer of albumin across cultured endothelial monolayers. *Arteriosclerosis* **4:**489.

Higgs, E. A., Moncada, A., and Vane, J. R. (1986). Prostaglandins and thromboxanes from fatty acids. *Prog. Lipid Res.* **25:**5.

Horton, A. A., and Fairhurst, S. (1987). Lipid peroxidation and mechanisms of toxicity. *CRC Crit. Rev. Toxicol.* **18**(1):27.

Hyslop, P. A., and Sklar, L. A. (1984). A quantitative fluorimetric assay for the determination of oxidant production by polymorphonuclear leukocytes: Its use in the simultaneous flourimetric assay of cellular activation processes. *Anal. Biochem.* **141:**280.

Junod, A. F., Clement, A., Jornot, L., and Petersen, H. (1985). Differential effects of hyperoxia and hydrogen peroxide on thymidine kinase and adenosine kinase activities of cultured endothelial cells. *Biochim. Biophys. Acta* **847:**20.

Junod, A. F., Jornot, L., and Peterson, H. (1989). Differential effects of hyperoxia and hydrogen peroxide on DNA damage, polyadenosine disphosphate-ribose polymerase activity, and nicotinamide adenine dinucleotide and adenosine triphosphate contents in cultured endothelial cells and fibroblasts. *J. Cell. Physiol.* **140:**177.

Kaduce, T. L., Spector, A. A., and Bar, R. S. (1982). Linolenic acid metabolism and prostaglandin production by bovine pulmonary artery endothelial cells. *Arteriosclerosis* **2:**380.

Kehrer, J. P., and Autor, A. P. (1978). The effect of dietary fatty acids on the composition of adult rat lung lipids: Relationship to oxygen toxicity. *Toxicol. Appl. Pharmacol.* **44:**423.

Kennedy, J. I., Chandler, D. B., Fulmer, J. D., Wert, M. D., and Grizzle, W. E. (1989). Dietary fish oil inhibits bleomycin-induced pulmonary fibrosis in the rat. *Exp. Lung Res.* **15:**315.

Kistler, G. S., Caldwell, P. R. B., and Weibel, E. R. (1967). Development of fine structural damage to alveolar and capillary lining cells in oxygen poisoned rat lungs. *J. Cell Biol.* **32:**605.

Lee, T. H. (1989). Pharmacological modulation of leukotriene and platelet activating factor biosynthesis and activities by alternative dietary fatty acids. *Clin. Exp. Allergy* **19:**15.

Lee, S. L., Douglas, H. J., Deneke, S. M ., and Fanburg, B. L. (1983). Ultrastructural changes in bovine pulmonary artery endothelial cells exposed to 80% O_2 in vitro. *In Vitro Cell. Dev. Biol.* **19:**714.

Malis, C. D., Weber, P. C., Leaf, A., and Bonventre, J. V. (1990). Incorporation of marine lipids into mitochondrial membranes increases susceptibility to damage by calcium and reactive oxygen species: Evidence for enhanced activation of phospholipase A2 in mitochondria enriched with n-3 fatty acids. *Proc. Natl. Acad. Sci. USA* **87:**8845.

Mello Filho, A. C., Hoffman, M. E., and Meneghini, R. (1984). Cell killing and DNA damage by hydrogen peroxide are mediated by intracellular iron. *Biochem. J.* **218:**273.

Morrison, W. R., and Smith, L. M. (1964). Preparation of fatty acid methyl esters and dimethylacetals from lipids with boron fluoride–methanol. *J. Lipid Res.* **5:**600.

Newman, J. H., Loyd, J. E., English, D. K., Ogletree, M. L., Fulkerson, W. J., and Brigham, K. L. (1983). Effects of 100% oxygen on lung vascular function in awake sleep. *J. Appl. Physiol.* **54:**1379.

Ody, C., and Junod, A. F. (1985). Effect of variable glutathione peroxidase activity on H_2O_2-related cytotoxicity in cultured aortic endothelial cells. *Proc. Soc. Exp. Biol. Med.* **180:**103.

Patel, J. M., and Block, E. R. (1988). The effect of oxidant gases on membrane fluidity and function in pulmonary endothelial cells. *Free Radic. Biol. Med.* **4:**121.

Peterson, D. A., Mehta, N., Butterield, J., Husak, M., Christopher, M. M., Jagarlaupaudi, S., and Eaton, J. W. (1988). Polyunsaturated fatty acids stimulate superoxide formation in tumor cells: A mechanism for specific cytotoxicity and a model for tumor necrosis factor. *Biochem. Biophys. Res. Commun.* **155:**1033.

Rastogi, B. K., and Nordoy, A. (1980). Lipid composition of cultured human endothelial cells. *Thromb. Res.* **18:**629.

Rietjens, I. M. C. M., van Tilburg, C. A. M., Coener, T. M. M., Alink, G. M., and Konings, A. W. T. (1987). Influence of polyunsaturated fatty acid composition and membrane fluidity on ozone and nitrogen dioxide sensitivity of rat alveolar macrophages. *J. Toxicol. Environ. Health.* **21:**45.

Rubin, D. B., Housset, B., Jean-Mairet, Y., and Junod, A. F. (1983). Effects of hyperoxia on biochemical indexes of pig aortic endothelial cell function. *In Vitro Cell. Dev. Biol.* **19:**625.

Ruch, R. J., Crist, K. A., and Klaunig, J. E. (1989). Effects of culture duration on hydrogen peroxide-induced hepatocyte toxicity. *Toxicol. Appl. Pharmacol.* **100:**451.

Sacks, T., Moldow, C. F., Craddock, P. R., Bowers, T. K., and Jacob, H. S. (1978). Oxygen radicals mediate endothelial cell damage by complement stimulated granulocytes. An in vitro model of immune damage. *J. Clin. Invest.* **61:**1161.

Schatte, C. L., and Mathias, M. M. (1982). Effect of dietary fat on pulmonary enzymes and toxicity during normobaric hyperoxia. *Aviat. Space Environ. Med.* **53**(7):629.

Schraufstatter, I. U., Hyslop, P. A., Hinshaw, D. B., Spragg, R. G., Sklar, L. A., and Cochrane, C. G. (1986). Hydrogen peroxide–induced injury of cells and its prevention by inhibitors of poly (ADP-ribose) polymerase. *Proc. Natl. Acad. Sci. USA* **83:**4908.

Sekharam, K. M., Patel, J. M., and Block, E. R. (1990). Effect of polyunsaturated fatty acids and phospholipids on [^{3}H]-vitamin E incorporation into pulmonary artery endothelial cell membrane. *J. Cell. Physiol.* **145:**555.

Serhan, C., Anderson, P., Goodman, E., Dunham, P., and Weismann, G. (1981). Phosphatidate and oxidized fatty acids are calcium ionophores. *J. Biol. Chem.* **256:**2736.

Shasby, D. M., Vanbenthuysen, K. M., Tate, R. M., Shasby, S. S., McMurty, I., and Repine, J. E. (1982). Granulocytes mediate acute edematous lung injury in rabbits and in isolated rabbit lungs perfused with phorbol myristate acetate: Role of oxygen radicals. *Am. Rev. Respir. Dis.* **125:**443.

Shasby, D. M., Shasby, S. S., and Peach, M. J. (1983). Granulocytes and phorbol myristate acetate increase permeability to albumin of cultured endothelial monolayers and isolated perfused lungs. Role of oxygen radicals and granulocyte adherence. *Am. Rev. Respir. Dis.* **:127**:72.

Simpson, R. J., and Peters, T. J. (1987). Transport of Fe^{2+} across lipid bilayers: Possible role of free fatty acids. *Biochim. Biophys. Acta* **898:**187.

Sosenko, I. R. S., Innis, S. M., and Frank L. (1988). Polyunsaturated fatty acids and protection of newborn rats from oxygen toxicity. *J. Pediatr.* **112:**630.

Sosenko, I. R. S., Innis, S. M., and Frank L. (1989). Menhaden fish oil, n-3 polyunsaturated fatty acids, and protection of newborn rats from oxygen toxicity. *Pediatr. Res.* **25**(4):399.

Spector, A. A., and Yorek, M. A. (1985). Membrane lipid composition and cellular function. *J. Lipid Res.* **26:**1015.

Stubbs, C. D., and Smith, A. D. (1984). The modification of mammalian membrane polyunsaturated fatty acid composition in relation to membrane fluidity and function. *Biochim. Biophys. Acta* **779:**89.

Suttorp, N., and Simon, M. L. (1982). Lung cell oxidant injury: Enhancement of polymorphonuclear leukocyte-mediated cytotoxicity in lung cells exposed to sustained in vitro hyperoxia. *J. Clin. Invest.* **70:**342.

Suttorp, N., Toepfer, W., and Roka, L. (1986). Antioxidant defense mechanisms of endothelial cells: Glutathione redox cycle versus catalase. *Am. J. Physiol.* **251:**C671.

Toth, K. M., Clifford, D. P., Berger, E. M., White, C. W., and Repine, J. E. (1984). Intact human erythrocytes prevent hydrogen peroxide–mediated damage to isolated perfused rat lungs and cultured bovine pulmonary artery endothelial cells. *J. Clin. Invest.* **74:**292.

Tsan, M. F., Danis, E. H., Del Vecchio, P. J., and Rosano, C. L. (1985). Enhancement of intracellular glutathione protects endothelial cells against oxidant damage. *Biochem. Biophys. Res. Commun.* **127:**270.

Turrens, J. F., Freeman, B. A., and Crapo, J. D. (1982). The effect of hyperoxia on superoxide production by lung submitochondrial particles. *Arch. Biochem. Biophys.* **217:**401.

Weiss, S. J., Young, J., LoBuglio, A. F., Slivka, A., and Nimeh, N. F. (1981). Role of hydrogen peroxide in neutrophil-mediated destruction of cultured endothelial cells. *J. Clin. Invest.* **68:**714.

6

Induced Expression of p52(PAI-1) in the Cellular Response to Hyperoxia: Common Changes in Gene Expression Elicited by Growth Factors and Hyperoxic Stress

PAUL J. HIGGINS

Albany Medical College
Albany, New York

I. Pulmonary Tissue Response to Hyperoxia

A number of excellent studies have detailed pulmonary structural and biochemical changes as a consequence of exposure to supraphysiologic concentrations of oxygen (e.g., Crapo et al., 1980; Chvapil and Peng, 1975; Thet et al., 1986; Durr et al., 1987). At the cellular level, the first visible indications of hyperoxic lung injury include swelling of alveolar epithelial cells and alterations in the morphology of specific subcellular organelles (i.e., mitochondria and microsomes) (Freeman et al., 1982). Both acute and chronic regimens of hyperoxic stress produce alterations in alveolar membrane permeability, swelling of the vascular endothelium, breakdown of endothelial barrier function with (resulting edema), and subsequent decreases in respiratory function. Ultrastructural and morphometric studies have clearly demonstrated that one of the earliest morphologic events associated with hyperoxic lung injury involves focal swelling of capillary endothelial cells and concomitant development of interstitial edema (Bowden and Adamson, 1974; Crapo et al., 1980). The reparative phase, which follows acute or chronic hyperoxic injury, involves generalized proliferation of various lung cell populations, including fibroblasts, smooth muscle, type II epithelial, and endothelial cells (Crapo et al., 1980; Jones et al., 1984; Coflesky et al., 1988; Bowden and Adamson, 1974; Adamson and Bowden, 1974; Thet et al., 1986).

The cell types involved in this proliferative response are generally similar in both types of injury models. Increases in the number of fibroblasts and myofibroblasts and deposition of extracellular matrix (ECM) (i.e., collagen, fibronectin), however, appear to be significantly greater and more persistent following chronic hyperoxic lung injury as compared to acute hyperoxic stress (Durr et al., 1987). These specific cell populations probably contribute significantly to the development of fibrosis and subsequent pulmonary hypertension (Jones et al., 1984; Chvapil and Peng, 1975; Coflesky, et al., 1987).

II. Analysis of Hyperoxia-Associated Changes in Cellular Gene Expression

Changes in gene expression play an important role in tissue remodeling following hyperoxic lung injury (Horowitz et al., 1989, 1990). Among the important candidate proteins that might contribute to posthyperoxic trauma include autocrine/paracrine growth factors, proteases and protease inhibitors, chemotactic factors, and various structural proteins, in particular those involved in construction of the ECM (e.g., White et al., 1990).

Cell proliferation in the hyperoxic-stressed lung appears to be a consistent response to this type of injury (e.g., Crapo et al., 1980). A major fraction of the responding population involves cells of connective tissue origin, such as fibroblasts and smooth muscle cells. Platelet-derived growth factor (PDGF) is an important mitogen for cells of mesenchymal cell origin; both smooth muscle cells and fibroblasts possess receptors for PDGF and are readily stimulated by this growth factor in vitro (Bowen-Pope and Ross, 1982). PDGF-B chain mRNA abundance in lung tissue was, in fact, found to increase significantly (2.5-fold) by day 3 of hyperoxic stress and remained elevated up to at least day 7 (Fabisiak et al., 1989). This relatively early increase in lung PDGF-B mRNA content during the time course of hyperoxic lung injury preceded onset of DNA synthesis and induced increases in actin mRNA cytoplasmic abundance (the latter reflecting hyperplasia of smooth muscle cells, myofibroblasts, and interstitial fibroblasts) associated with subsequent tissue remodeling. Production of PDGF (and perhaps other stimulatory cytokines or growth factors) within the oxygen-damaged lung may represent early autocrine or paracine stress–response mechanisms. In the chronic hyperoxia model, however, such inductions may be important in the subsequent reparative response but, if inappropriately regulated, may lead to aberrant ECM accumulation and eventual fibrosis (Fabisiak et al., 1989). Growth factor–induced deposition of ECM is a complex event involving orchestrated changes in the expression of structural genes (i.e., fibronectin, collagen), matrix-degrading proteases, and specific protease inhibitors. Indeed, mRNA for tissue inhibitor of metalloproteinases (TIMP), a 28-kD secreted glycoprotein which inhibits collagenase and stromelysin (Matrisian, 1990), is increased sixfold in the lung tissue of hyperoxia-treated rabbits (Horowitz et al., 1989). Expression of the TIMP gene is positively influenced by the tumor promotor 12-O-tetradecanoylphorbol-13-acetate and PGDF, as are the proto-oncogenes c-*myc*, c-*fos*, and c-*sis* (Horowitz, 1989, for a discussion). Should TIMP induction in the oxygen-damaged lung occur via a signaling pathway similar to that utilized by phorbol esters, hyperoxia may activate a specific set of growth regulatory and tissue pattern–forming genes (see also below for induction by hyperoxia of the expression of the c-*fos* and p52 genes in rat cells). It is tempting to speculate that TIMP and other induced regulators of the pericellular proteolytic environment may function to alter deposition or stability of ECM proteins, contributing, thereby, to development of the fibrotic phase of hyperoxic lung injury.

TIMP is not the only potential regulator of cell shape and substrate adhesion/ECM to be induced as a consequence of hyperoxic stress. Pig endothelial (PE) and rat kidney (NRK) cells exhibited similar cytoarchitectural responses to hyperoxic stress as did calf pulmonary artery endothelial (CPAE) cells (White et al., 1990). Exposure of these cells to hyperoxic environments resulted in a marked increase in substrate adherence, increased cytoskeletal-associated actin content, development of dense ventral microfilament (MF) stress fibers, and thickened vinculin-containing MF termini [i.e., focal contacts (FCs)] (Phillips et al., 1988; White et al., 1990). Mechanisms underlying such morphologic adaptations are largely unknown, but induction of specific adhesion-associated cytoskeletal elements (FCs) (Burridge, 1986) probably relates to the marked substrate adherence of hyperoxia-stressed cells (Phillips et al., 1988). Specific aspects of this adaptive response to hyperoxia, however, resemble cytoarchitectural events initiated by the growth regulatory agents sodium butyrate (NaB) (Ryan and Higgins, 1988) and transforming growth factor-B (TGF-B) (Wood et al., 1991). NaB- and TGF-B-directed MF network remodeling in NRK cells, for example, involves increased deposition of newly synthesized actin into the cytoskeletal framework, stimulated α-actinin and vinculin synthesis, formation of vinculin-containing FCs, and enhanced substratum adhesiveness (Altenburg et al., 1976; Ryan et al., 1987; Ryan and Higgins, 1988; Higgins and Ryan, 1989a). The increased spreading/substratum adhesion typical of hyperoxia-stressed PE and NRK cells (White et al., 1990) is consistently associated with hyperinduction and substrate deposition of a glycoprotein of 45 kD (p45; in PE cells) and 52 kD (p52; in NRK cells) (Fig. 1). Subsequent biochemical comparisons of the endothelial and nonendothelial p45-p52 proteins have revealed them to be homologous (Higgins and Ryan, 1992). These same proteins were also inducible in endothelial cells and fibroblasts upon exposure to NaB, TGF-B, and PDGF (Higgins et al., 1991; Wood et al., 1991).

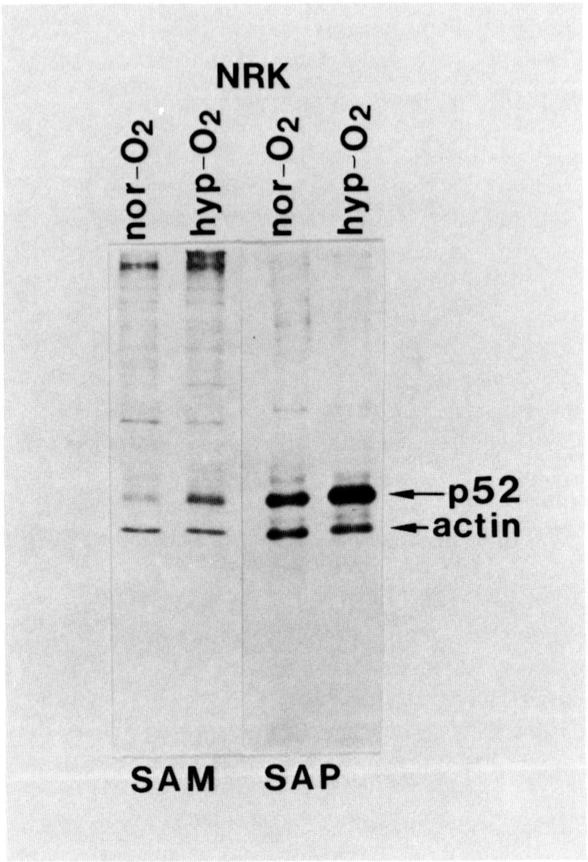

Figure 1 Hyperoxia-associated increased deposition of p52 into two cellular subcompartments enriched in ECM and cell-to-substrate adhesive elements. NRK cells were cultured in normoxic (nor-O_2; 20% O_2) of hyperoxic (hyp- O_2; 95% O_2) environments for 2 days, then labeled with [^{35}S]methionine under nor-O_2 conditions. EDTA-resistant substrate-attached material (SAM) (containing ECM and contact structures) and saponin-resistant proteins (SAP) (consisting of the ventral undersurface residue and associated focal contact structures) remaining after removal of cells with a stream of buffer (see Higgins and Ryan, 1989a for details as to extract preparation) were solubilized in sample buffer and the constituent proteins fractionation on sodium dodecyl sulfate (SDS)–10% acrylamide slab gels. Exposure to hyp-O_2 environments consistently resulted in an approximately fivefold increase in SAM or SAP fraction-associated p52 deposition.

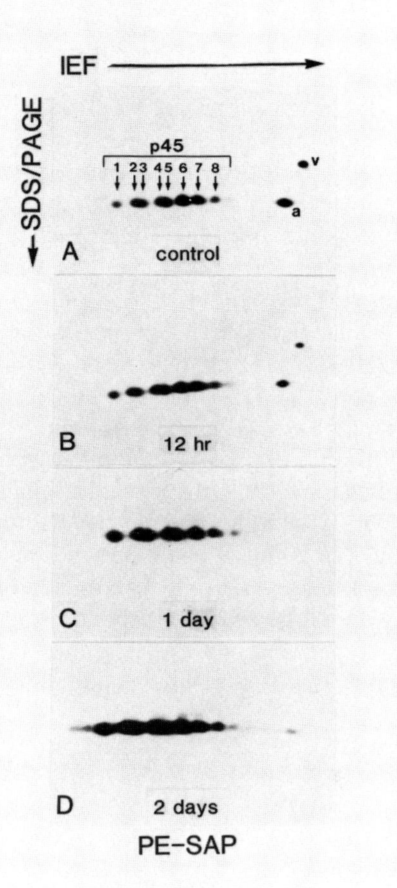

Figure 2 Two-dimensional electrophoretic profiles of SAP fraction protein from PE cells cultured in normoxic (control; 20% O_2) (A) or hyperoxic (95% O_2; 12 h–2 days) (B–D) environments. First dimension IEF gels were loaded with equivalent cpm, trichloroacetic acid–insoluble. [^{35}S]methionine-labeled SAP fraction protein; second dimension fractionation utilized SDS–10% acrylamide slab gels (Higgins and Ryan, 1989a). Scanning densitometry of fluorographs indicated that the relative content of p45 in the SAP fraction of PE cells increased as early as 12 h after exposure to hyperoxic stress (White et al., 1990). The positions of the SAP fraction cytoskeletal proteins actin (a) and vimentin (v) are indicated as are the eight distinct isoforms of p45. (From White et al., 1990.)

In TGF-B- or NaB-treated NRK cells, as is true for hyperoxia-stressed PE cells, increased p52/p45 is an early aspect of the inductive response, occurring within 12 h of initial inducer exposure and prior to obvious changes in cell shape (Ryan and Higgins, 1989a; White et al., 1990) (Figs. 1 and 2). Retrospective analysis of the time course of NaB- and hyperoxia-stimulated p52/p45 substrate deposition by their respective cell types revealed that such ECM accumulation occurred prior to FC formation and MF reorganization (Ryan and Higgins, 1988; Phillips et al., 1988; White et al., 1990; Higgins et al., 1992). p52-like proteins distribute to the ventral undersurface "carpet" of various cell types, including avian and rodent fibroblasts (Neyfakh and Svitkina, 1983; Higgins and Ryan, 1989), human mesothelial, endothelial, and fibrosarcoma cells (Rheinwald et al., 1987; Pollanen et al., 1988), and porcine endothelial cells (White et al., 1990; Higgins et al., 1991 for a review). While such proteins display intermediate filament like solubility properties (Ryan and Higgins, 1987; Higgins and Ryan, 1989b; Santaren and Bravo, 1987), p52 did not reassociate into pelletable structures under standard intermediate filament disassembly/reassembly conditions capable of discriminating intermediate filaments from nuclear lamin proteins (Ryan and Higgins, 1987). Comparison of the available two-dimensional profiles of PE and NRK substrate-attached proteins (White et al., 1990; Higgins et al., 1989, 1990, 1991) with the REF52 global protein database (Garrels, 1989) led to the identification of p52 and p45 as the rat and pig counterparts of murine "p45" (Santaren and Bravo, 1987; Garrels and Franza, 1989).

III. p52 Is Plasminogen Activator Inhibitor Type 1

Processing of the mature 52-kD p52 glycoprotein occurs via at least two posttranslational additions of complex oligosaccharide units to a core peptide of 43 kD (p43), resulting in the generation of an intermediate 50-kD (p50) and mature 52-kD glycoprotein, both of which serve as substrates for subsequent addition of sialic acid residues (Higgins et al., 1989, 1990). Two-dimensional electrophoretic mapping of the p52 isoforms expressed by rat cells (Fig. 3) revealed a marked similarity in electrophoretic microheterogeneity of p50/p52 to gp50 (Baumann and Held, 1981). gp50 appears identical to a specific serine protease inhibitor (SERPIN) family member, plasminogen activator inhibitor type 1 (PAI-1) (Sprengers and Kluft, 1987), and to known PAI-1 proteins of other species (e.g., IIP48 and mesosecrin) (Thalacker and Nilsen-Hamilton, 1987; Rheinwald et al., 1987; Zeheb et al., 1987). These comparative data suggested that p52 may, indeed, be rat PAI-1 (rPAI-1). Antibodies to NRK p52 (anti-p52), in fact, specifically immunoprecipitated both p50 and p52 from the secreted protein fraction of NRK cells (Higgins et al., 1991). These identical proteins were immunoprecipitated from the same preparation with antisera to

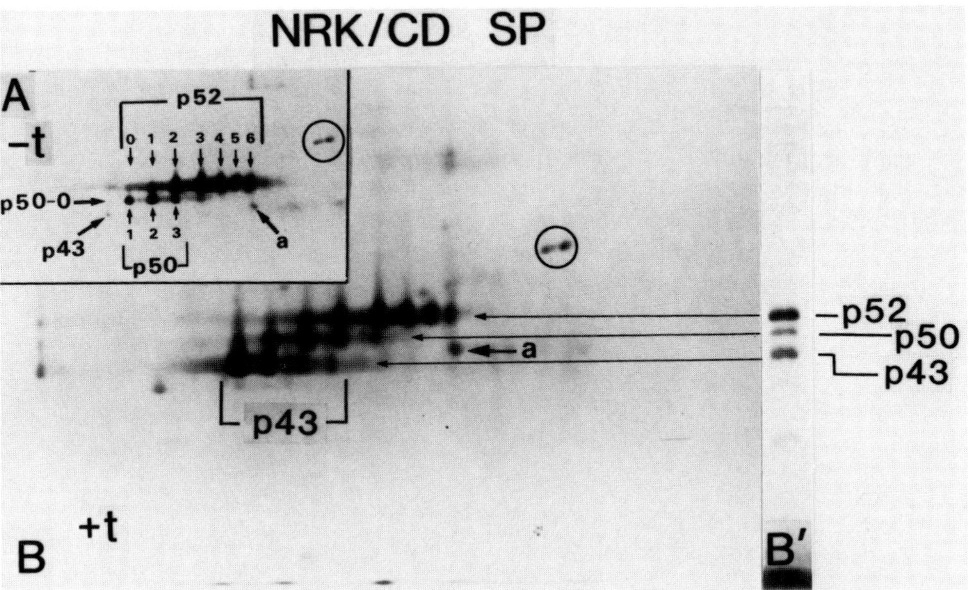

Figure 3 Demonstration of the complexity of the mature p52 protein, its intermediate isoform p50, and the core p43 protein in the secreted protein fraction of NRK cells. [^{35}S]methionine secreted proteins (SP) from cytochalasin D–stimulated NRK cells were used for two-dimensional mapping since exposure to CD results in a 10-fold increase in p52 mRNA gene transcription and is a convenient hyperinducer of p52 expression in NRK cells (Higgins et al., 1989, 1990). Cells were labeled in the presence (+) or absence (–) of the N-glycosylation inhibitor tunicamycin (t); treatment with tunicamycin results in an accumulation of p43 species, thus allowing for assessment of microheterogeneity within this molecular mass category. In the absence of tunicamycin, only a single minor 43-kD species is resolved as compared to four distinct p50 variants (p50-0 to p50-3) and at least seven isoforms of the mature 52-kD protein (p52-0 to p52-6) (A). Cells labeled in the presence of a suboptimal concentration of tunicamycin exhibit a significant increase in the microheterogeneity of p43, which probably represents non-N-linked post-translational modifications to the core protein backbone (B). Because of this diversity in p52 composition, the nomenclature p52(PAI-1) is retained until it is ascertained that each species actually functions as a PAI. The small amount of actin (a) evident in the secreted protein fraction serves as an internal marker, as does osteopontin (circled). Two-dimensional maps (A,B) served to positively identify p52, p50, and p43 in one-dimensional separations (B′) of the products of immunoprecipitation (refer to Figs. 4 and 5).

human and bovine PAI-1 as well as with antibodies to rPAI-1 (Fig. 4). That the proteins so immunoprecipitated by antibodies to bovine PAI-1 were, in fact, p50 and p52 was confirmed by two-dimensional electrophoretic analysis (Fig. 5) and proteolytic digestion/peptide fragment sizing, in each case, of the products of

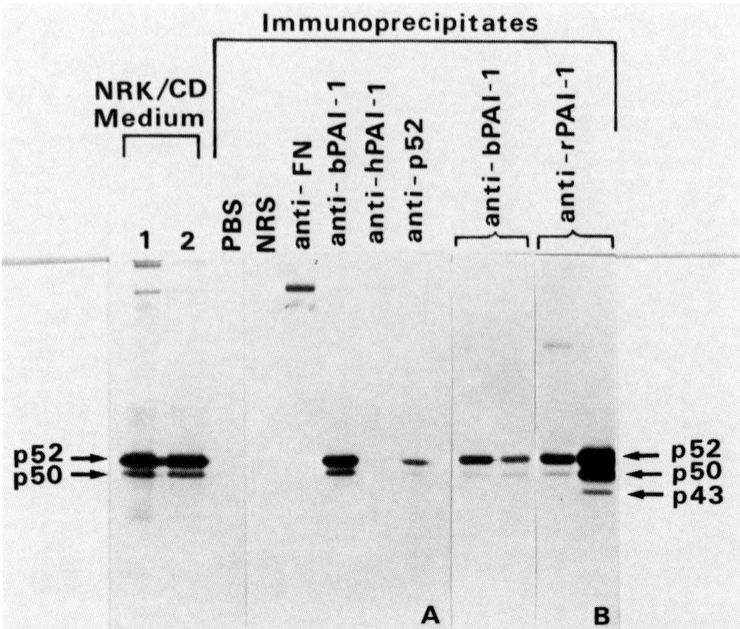

Figure 4 Electrophoretic analysis of immunoprecipitation products generated using antibodies to p52 and PAI-1. [^{35}S]methionine-labeled secreted proteins from NRK/CD cells (Higgins et al., 1990), undiluted or diluted with an equal volume of 2X immunoprecipitation buffer (lanes 1 and 2), provided internal p50/p52 standards (A). Phosphate-buffered saline (PBS), normal rabbit serum (NRS), and antifibronectin (FN) serum were substituted for the primary antisera to p52 or PAI-1 in control immunoprecipitation reactions. Antisera to bovine (b) and human (h) PAI-1 both precipitated proteins with the identical mobilities of p50/p52. The relatively faint bands developed with the anti-hPAI-1 serum was expected due to the low affinity of this antibody preparation for rat PAI-1. Antisera to bPAI-1, p52, and rPAI-1 each recognized the unglycosylated 43-kD core protein (p43) as well as the intermediate (p50) and mature (p52) isoforms (B). p43 is evident only for the immune precipitates obtained with anti-r-PAI-1 serum (in B) due to the exposure selected. (From Higgins et al., 1990.)

immunoprecipitation (Fig. 6). The two-dimensional electrophoretic microheterogeneity of p52, moreover, was identical in apparent pI distribution to the seven distinct isoforms of bovine PAI-1 resolved in two-dimensional gels by reverse fibrin autoradiography (van Mourik et al., 1984). Western blotting additionally indicated that the 50- and 52-kD matrix-associated proteins were the only proteins recognized by antibodies to rPAI-1 (Higgins, et al., 1991).

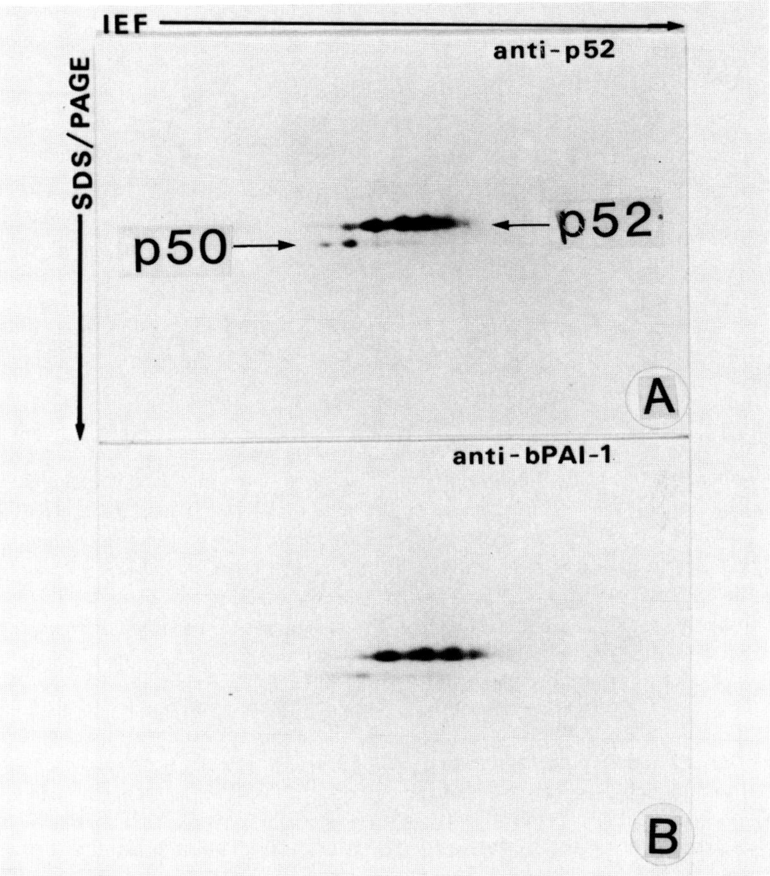

Figure 5 Two-dimensional electrophoretic analysis of NRK/CD-secreted proteins immunoprecipitated with antisera to gel-purified p52 (A) or bPAI-1 (B). (Modified from Higgins et al., 1990.)

IV. Potential Molecular Mechanisms Underlying Control of ECM-Regulating Gene Expression by Growth Factors and Hyperoxic Stress

TGF-B plays a critical role in control of the composition of the ECM by stimulating synthesis of fibronectin, collagen, and chondroitin-dermatan sulfate proteoglycans (Westerhausen et al., 1991 for references). Importantly, TGF-B also inhibits ECM degradation by repressing growth factor induction of serine-, thiol-, and metalloproteases as well as by increasing the synthesis/secretion of

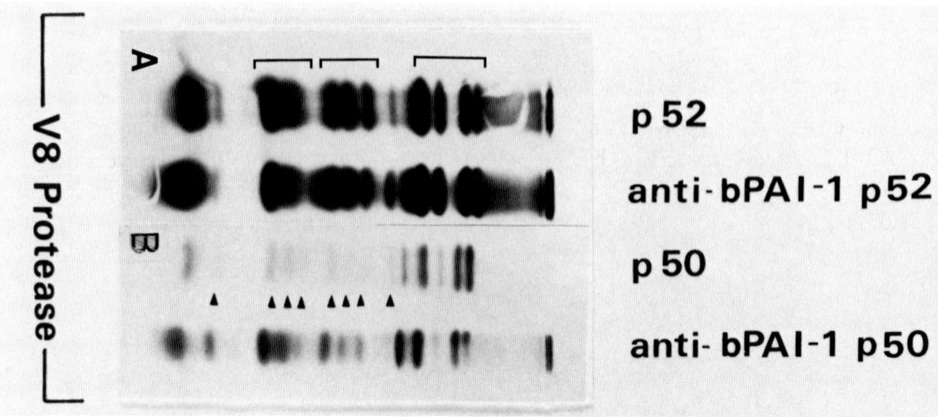

Figure 6 Identification of the anti-PAI-1 reactive 50- and 52- kD proteins as p50 and p52 using proteolytic cleavage. Bands containing [^{35}S]methionine-labeled p50 and p52 were cut out of one-dimensional electrophoretic separations of NRK/CD-secreted proteins and digested with V8 protease, as were bands containing anti-bPAI-1 immunoprecipitated 50- and 52-kD proteins (as in Fig. 4). Electrophoresis of digestion products in SDS–15% acrylamide gels indicated that p50/p52 and the anti-bPAI-1-immunoprecipitated 50- and 52-kD proteins were probably the same, due to the identity of the fragmentation profiles. Arrowheads point to faint bands. Brackets indicate characteristic V8 protease band groups. (Modified from Higgins et al., 1990.)

PAI-1 and TIMP (Sporn et al., 1987). The net result of TGF-B action in the majority of cell systems examined is, therefore, decreased proteolytic activity in the immediate pericellular environment. Of particular interest are the recent findings that two pulmonary fibrosis-inducing agents, bleomycin and hyperoxic stress, also stimulate expression of TGF-B mRNA in rat endothelial cells and fibroblasts and that hyperoxia further induces expression of the c-*fos* proto-oncogene (Phan et al., 1991; Higgins et al., in preparation). TGF-B autocrine or paracrine stimulation may, if inappropriately regulated, lead to chronic excessive ECM accumulation as a consequence of the differential action of this growth factor on expression of specific proteases (metalloproteinases, PA) and their inhibitors (TIMP, PAI-1).

How might TGF-B effect changes in gene expression related to the control of synthesis of ECM constitutents and their organization? TGF-B inhibits the expression of at least one metalloproteinase, stromelysin, via a 5′ flanking sequence in the stromelysin promotor region referred to as a TGF-B-inhibitory element (TIE) (Matrisian, 1990). The transcriptional effector c-FOS (the protein product of the c-*fos* gene) (Curran and Franza, 1988) has been implicated in stromelysin suppression by TGF-B since c-FOS appears to be required for TGF-

B action (Westerhausen et al., 1991 for references) and FOS is present in the protein complex which recognizes the stromelysin promoter (Matrisian, 1990). c-FOS interacts with the c-JUN proto-oncogene protein to form heterodimeric transcriptional units which recognize a specific DNA sequence referred to as an AP-1 (activator protein-1) binding site (Curran and Franza, 1988). Interestingly, the NaB-mediated induction of PAI-1 expression in cultured rat cells (e.g., Ryan and Higgins, 1989; Higgins and Ryan, 1989) also appears to involve c-FOS (Higgins and Tanaka, 1991 for a review). Although there are some differences in the FOS protein induced in cultured cells by NaB as compared to FOS induced by growth factors, gel shift experiments indicated that the stimulated FOS protein has an unimpaired capacity to participate in the formation of transcriptional complexes with the JUN/AP-1 protein (Narranjo et al., 1990). FOS and JUN may play significant roles in diverse signalling events related to control of ECM constituents. Indeed, sequence analysis of the 5′ flanking region of the rat p52(PAI-1) gene revealed various potential regulatory elements, most notably a closely grouped array of AP-1-like sites spanning the region from –592 to –2112 nucleotides upstream from the coding start sequence (Bruzdzinski, et al., 1990). Since the collagenase promoter also possesses AP-1 sites (Matrisian, 1990), control of expression of ECM-degrading (i.e., collagenase) and protective (i.e., PAI-1) proteins at the molecular level is likely to be quite complex and probably cell-type specific with regard to growth factor requirements. A hint of the complexity inherent in molecular controls is evidenced by the recent finding of two distinct TGF-B-inducible elements in the 5′ region of the human PAI-1 gene at sites –791 to –546 and –328 to –187 nucleotides upstream from the cap site (Westerhausen et al., 1991). Although these segments do not possess an AP-1 consensus sequence, the region –672 to –666 resembles an AP-1-like sequence (GGAGTCA) and position –244 to –238 encodes an NF-1 (nuclear factor-1)-like site. Therefore, at least two distinct trans-acting factors, would appear to mediate TGF-B initiated signal transduction events at the level of the human PAI-1 gene promoter.

V. Conclusions

The relevance of TGF-B and c-*fos* mRNA induction by fibrotic stimulators (e.g., bleomycin, hypoxia) (Phan et al., 1991; Higgins et al., in preparation) to the associated changes in expression of ECM constituents evident in various endothelial and fibroblastoid cell types (e.g., White et al., 1990) remains to be determined. The spectrum of trans-acting transcriptional control factors (such as AP-1, NF-1, and related effectors) and cis elements involved in ECM gene expression, the recognition of both positive and negative transcriptional regulation, and the identification of multiple controlling sequences in genes encoding not only ECM structural proteins but matrix-active proteases and their specific inhibitors are just beginning to be defined. It is apparent, however, that certain common pathways of intracellular signal transduction are involved in the cellular response to environmental stimuli (e.g., hyperoxic stress) and at least some polypeptide growth factors. Definition of the specific molecular targets involved, and the extent to which signaling events converge, are critical to our further understanding of fibrotic syndromes of pulmonary and nonpulmonary tissues.

Acknowledgments

Supported by grants from NIH, the American Cancer Society, Angio-Medical Corporation, Boehringer Mannheim Italia, and the Veterans Administration. The author thanks D. Higgins for manuscript preparation and my colleagues (M. Ryan, J. E. White, P. G. Phillips, and L. Staiano-Coico) for helpful discussions.

References

Adamson, I. Y. R., and Bowden, D. H. (1974). Type 2 cell as a progenitor of alveolar epithelial regeneration. A cytodynamic study in mice after exposure to oxygen. *Lab. Invest.* **30:**35–42.

Altenburg, B. C., Via, D. P., and Steiner, S. H. (1976). Modification of the phenotype of murine sarcoma and virus–transformed cells by sodium butyrate. *Exp. Cell Res.* **102:**223–231.

Baumann, H., and Held, W. A. (1981). Biosynthesis and hormone-regulated expression of secretory glycoproteins in rat liver and hepatoma cells. Effect of glucocorticoids and inflammation. *J. Biol. Chem.* **256:**10145–10155.

Bowden, D. H., and Adamson, I. Y. R. (1974). Endothelial regeneration as a marker of the differential vascular responses in oxygen-induced pulmonary edema. *Lab. Invest.* **30:**350–374.

Bowen-Pope, D. F., and Ross, R. (1982). Platelet-derived growth factor. II. Specific binding to cultured cells. *J. Biol. Chem.* **257:**5161–5171.

Bruzdzinski, C. J., Riordan-Johnson, M., Nordby, E. C., Suter, S. M., and Gelehrter, T. D. (1990). Isolation and characterization of the rat plasminogen activator inhibitor-1 gene. *J. Biol. Chem.* **265:**2078–2088.

Burridge, K. (1986). Cell substratum adhesive structures. *Cancer Rev.* **4:**18–78.

Chvapil, M., and Peng, Y.-M. (1975). Oxygen and lung fibrosis. *Arch. Environ. Health* **30:**528–532.

Coflesky, J. T., Jones, R. C., Reid, L. M., and Evans, J. N. (1987). Mechanical properties and structure of isolated pulmonary arteries remodelled by chronic hyperoxia. *Am. Rev. Respir. Dis.* **136:**388–394.

Coflesky, J. T., Adler, K. B., Woodcock-Mitchell, J., Mitchell, J., and Evans, J. (1988)

Proliferative changes in the pulmonary arterial wall during short-term hyperoxic injury to the lung. *Am. J. Pathol.* **117:**273–285.

Crapo, J. D., Barry, B. E., Foscue, H. A., and Shelburne, J. (1980). Structural and biochemical changes in rat lungs occurring during exposure to lethal and adaptive doses of oxygen. *Am. Rev. Respir. Dis.* **112:**123–143.

Curran, T., and Franza, B. R. (1988). FOS and JUN: The AP-1 connection. *Cell* **55:** 395–397.

Durr, R. A., Bubaybo, B. A., and Thet, L. A. (1987). Repair of chronic hyperoxic lung injury: Changes in lung ultrastructure and matrix. *Exp. Mol. Pathol.* **47:**219–240.

Fabisiak, J. P., Evans, J. N., and Kelley, J. (1989). Increased expression of PDGF-B (c-*sis*) mRNA in rat lung precedes DNA synthesis and tissue repair during chronic hyperoxia. *Am. J. Respir. Cell Mol. Biol.* **1:**181–189.

Freeman, B. A., Topolosky, M. K., and Crapo, J. D. (1982). Hyperoxia increases oxygen radical production in rat lung homogenates. *Arch. Biochem. Biophys.* **216:**477–484.

Garrels, J. I. (1989). The QUEST system for quantitative analysis of two-dimensional gels. *J. Biol. Chem.* **264:**5269–5268.

Garrels, J. I., and Franza, B. R. (1989). The REF52 protein database. Methods of database construction and analysis using the QUEST system and characterizations of protein patterns from proliferating and quiescent REF52 cells. *J. Biol. Chem.* **264:** 5283–5298.

Higgins, P. J., and Ryan, M. P. (1989a). Biochemical localization of the transformation-sensitive 52 kDa (p52) protein to the substratum contact regions of cultured rat fibroblasts. Butyrate induction, characterization, and quantification of p52 in v-*ras* transformed cells. *Biochem. J.* **257:**173–182.

Higgins, P. J., and Ryan, M. P. (1989b). Cytoarchitectural of *ras* oncogene-expressing tumor cells: Butyrate modulation of substate adhesion, cytoskeletal actin content and subcellular microfilament distribution. *Int. J. Biochem.* **21:**1143–1151.

Higgins, P. J., and Ryan, M. P. (1992). Regulation of p52(PAI-1), actin, and p21*ras* in butyrate-induced flat revertants of v-*ras*-transformed rat kidney cell. *Biochem. J.* (in press).

Higgins, P. J., and Tanaka, Y. (1991). Cytoarchitectural response and expression of c-*fos*/-52 genes during enhancement of butyrate-initiated differentiation of human colon carcinoma cells by 1,25-dihydroxyvitamin D_3 and its analogs. In *Calcium, Vitamin D, and Prevention of Colon Cancer.* Edited by M. Lipkin. Boca Raton, Fla., CRC Press, pp. 305–326.

Higgins, P. J., Ryan, M. P., and Chaudhari, P. (1989). Cytochalasin D-mediated hyperinduction of the substrate-associated 52-kilodalton protein p52 in rat kidney fibroblasts. *J. Cell. Physiol.* **139:**407–417.

Higgins, P. J., Ryan, M. P., Zeheb, R., Gelehrter, T. D., and Chaudhari, P. (1990). p52 induction of cytochalasin D in rat kidney fibroblasts: Homologies between p52 and plasminogen activator inhibitor type-1. *J. Cell. Physiol.* **143:**321–329.

Higgins, P. J., Chaudhari, P., and Ryan, M. P. (1991). Cell-shape regulation and matrix protein p52 content in phenotypic variants of *ras*-transformed rat kidney fibroblasts. Functional analysis and biochemical comparison of p52 with proteins implicated in cell-shape determination. *Biochem. J.* **273:**651–658.

Horowitz, S., Dafai, N., Shapiro, D. L., Holm, B. A., Notter, R. H., and Quible, D. J. (1989). Hyperoxic exposure alters gene expression in the lung. Induction of the tissue inhibitor of metalloproteinases mRNA and other mRNAs. *J. Biol. Chem.* **264:**7092–7095.

Horowitz, S., Shapiro, D. L., Finkelstein, J. N., Notter, R. H., Johnston, C. J., and Quible, D. J. (1990). Changes in gene expression in hyperoxia-induced neonatal lung injury. *Am. J. Physiol.* **258:**L107–L111.

Jones, R., Zapol, W. M., and Reid, L. (1984). Pulmonary artery remodelling and pulmonary hypertension after exposure to hyperoxia for 7 days: A morphometric and hemodynamic study. *Am. J. Pathol.* **132:**563–573.

Matrisian, L. (1990). Metalloproteinases and their inhibitors in matrix remodelling. *Trends Genet.* **6:**121–215.

Narranjo, J. R., Mellstrom, B., Auwerx, J., Mollinedo, F., and Sassone-Corsi, P. (1990). Unusual c-*fos* induction upon chromaffin PC12 differentiation by sodium butyrate: Loss of *fos* autoregulatory function. *Nucl. Acids Res.* **18:**3605–3615.

Neyfakh, A. A., and Svitkina, T. M. (1983). Isolation of focal contact membrane using saponin. *Exp. Cell Res.* **149:**582–586.

Phan, S. H., Gharaee-Kermani, M., Wolber, F., and Ryan, U. S. (1991). Stimulation of rat endothelial cell transforming growth factor-B production by bleomycin. *J. Clin. Invest.* **87:**148–154.

Phillips, P. G., Higgins, P. J., Malik, A. B., and Tsan, M. -F. (1988). Effect of hyperoxia on the cytoarchitecture of cultured endothelial cells. *Am. J. Pathol.* **132:**59–72.

Pollanen, J., Hedman, K., Nielsen, L. S., Dano, K., and Vaheri, A. (1988). Ultrastructural localization of plasma membrane-associated urokinase-type plasminogen activator at focal contacts. *J. Cell Biol.* **106:**87–95.

Rheinwald, J. G., Jorgensen, J. L. Hahn, W. C., Terpstra, A. J., O'Connell, T. M., and Plummer, K. K. (1987). Mesosecrin: A secreted glycoprotein produced in abundance by human mesothelial, endothelial and kidney epithelial cells in culture. *J. Cell Biol.* **104:**263–275.

Ryan, M. P., and Higgins, P. J. (1987). Discrimination between the nuclear lamin and intermediate filament (cytokeratin/vimentin) proteins of rat hepatic tumor cells by differential solubility and electrophoretic criteria. *Int. J. Biochem.* **19:**1187–1192.

Ryan, M. P., and Higgins, P. J. (1988). Cytoarchitecture of Kirsten sarcoma virus-transformed rat kidney fibroblasts: butyrate-induced reorganization within the actin microfilament network. *J. Cell. Physiol.* **137:**25–34.

Ryan, M. P., Borenfreund, E., and Higgins, P. J. (1987). Butyrate-induced cytoarchitectural reorganization of Mallory body-containing rat hepatic tumor cells. *J. Natl. Cancer Inst.* **79:**555–567.

Santaren, J. F., and Bravo, R. (1987). Immediate induction of a 45 K secreted glycoprotein by serum and growth factors in quiescent mouse 3T3 cells. Two-dimensional gel analysis. *Exp. Cell Res.* **168:**494–506.

Sporn, M. B., Roberts, A. B., Wakefield, L. M., and de Crombrugghe, B. (1987). Some recent advances in the chemistry and biology of transforming growth factor-beta. *J. Cell Biol.* **105:**1039–1045.

Sprengers, E. D., and Kluft, C. (1987). Plasminogen activator inhibitors. *Blood* **69:** 381–387.

Thalacker, F. W., and Nilsen-Hamilton, M. (1987). Specific induction of secreted proteins by transforming growth factor-B and 12-*O*-tetradecanoylphorbol-13-acetate. Relationship with an inhibitor of plasminogen activator. *J. Biol. Chem.* **262:** 2283–2290.

Thet, L. A., Parra, S. C., Shelburne, J. D. (1986). Sequential changes in lung morphology during the repair of acute oxygen-induced lung injury in adult rats. *Exp. Lung Res.* **11:**209–228.

van Mourik, J. A., Lawrence, D. A., and Loskutoff, D. J. (1984). Purification of an inhibitor of plasminogen activator (antiactivator) synthesized by endothelial cells. *J. Biol. Chem.* **259:**14914–14921.

Westerhausen, D. R., Hopkins, W. E., and Billadello, J. J. (1991). Multiple transforming growth factor-B-inducible elements regulate expression of the plasminogen activator inhibitor type-1 gene in Hep G2 cells. *J. Biol. Chem.* **266:**1092–1100.

White, J. E., Tsan, M. -F., Phillips, P. G. and Higgins, P. J. (1990). The substrate-associated protein p45 of porcine endothelial cells: Multiple isoforms, cytoskeletal-like properties and induction by hyperoxic stress. *Int. J. Biochem.* **22:**1159–1164.

Wood, P. A., Ryan, M. P., and Higgins, P. J. (1991). Transforming growth factor-B partially restores cytoskeletal structure and matrix p52 protein expression in *ras* oncogene-transformed KNRK fibroblasts and in sodium butyrate-treated KNRK cells. *Proc. Am. Assoc. Cancer Res.* (in press).

Zeheb, R., Rafferty, U. M., Rodriguez, M. A., Andreasen, P., and Gelehrter, T. D. (1987). Immunoaffinity purification of HTC rat hepatoma cell plasminogen activator-inhibitor-1. *Thromb. Haemost.* **58:**1017–1023.

7

Molecular Mechanisms of Cytokine-Induced Tolerance to Acute Oxidant Lung Injury

CARL W. WHITE

National Jewish Center for Immunology and Respiratory Medicine
University of Colorado Health Sciences Center
Denver, Colorado

I. Introduction

Endotoxin (Frank, et al., 1978, 1980) and interleukin-1 plus tumor necrosis factor (White et al., 1987, 1989; White and Ghezzi, 1989) induce an impressive protection of rats against lethal pulmonary oxygen toxicity. An explanation of the molecular mechanisms responsible for this adaptive response is evolving as multiple groups are actively pursuing the question of how cytokine-mediated protection against oxidant injury occurs.

Although the findings of several groups working in multiple systems, both in vivo and in cell culture, are initially disparate, there are a few generalizations which are suggested by this body of work. First, endotoxin and endotoxin-induced cytokines appear to induce a state of increased oxidative stress in vivo (Chang, et al., 1988) and in vitro (Matsubara and Ziff, 1986; Matthews et al., 1987; Yamauchi et al., 1989; Zimmerman et al., 1989; Brigham et al., 1987). Second, both endotoxin and the cytokines tumor necrosis factor (TNF) and interleukin-1 (IL-1) amplify this oxidative stress, at least in part through the additional recruitment [Pohlman et al., 1986; Bevilacqua, et al., 1985; Goldblum et al., 1987a, b; Movat et al., 1987; Smith et al., 1989) and activation (Guthrie et al., 1984; Urban et al., 1986; Klebanoff et al., 1986; Tsujimoto et al., 1986; Berkow et al., 1987; Larrick et al., 1987) of neutrophils and other inflammatory cells. Injurious proteases as well as oxidants may be produced and be active through these mechanisms (Smedley, et al., 1986). Nonetheless, both tumor necrosis factor and endotoxin can directly damage endothelial and other cell types (Sato et al., 1986; Stolpen et al., 1986; Horvath et al., 1988; Royall et al., 1989). Third, induction of protective antioxidants by endotoxin and by both tumor necrosis factor and interleukin-1 can occur both in vivo and in cultured cells (Frank et al., 1980; Hass et al., 1989; Wong and Goeddel, 1988; Asayama et al., 1985; Shiki et al., 1987; Visner et al., 1990; Masuda et al., 1988; White et al., 1989). Depending on the system, there are differences in which superoxide dismutase, copper,zinc (cytoplasmic) or manganese (mitochondrial), is induced and over what time course. Enzymes of the glutathione redox cycle and hexose monophosphate shunt may be less impressively and consistently induced initially (White et al., 1989). A link between an initial burst of oxidants and the rise in antioxidants resulting from endotoxin or cytokine exposure, although suspected, has not yet been demonstrated directly. Effects of endotoxin in inducing antioxidants may not always require the production of cytokines. It is not clear which responses require products of the arachidonate cascade, although much work suggests their involvement, possibly secondarily (Chang et al., 1987, 1989; Brigham et al., 1987). The possibility that cytokines actually could decrease production of toxic O_2 metabolites, as suggested in other models of tolerance (Ischiropoulos et al., 1989) by certain critical cell types or organelles, largely has been unexplored. Finally, it is tempting to speculate that induction of antioxidants may contribute as a common mechanism to multiple forms of tolerance. These include the tolerance to (1) pulmonary oxygen toxicity or other forms of acute lung injury (Frank et al., 1980; White et al., 1987; Gordon et al., 1987), (2) radiation toxicity (Smith et al., 1958; Neta et al., 1986, 1987), (3) bone marrow toxicity following cytotoxic drugs (Stork et al., 1989), and (4) lethal bacterial challenge or to endotoxin, TNF, and/or IL-1-induced shock and multiple organ damage induced by interleukin-1 and/or tumor necrosis factor and often by endotoxin itself (Madonna et al., 1986; Patton et al., 1987; Vogel et al., 1988; Ozaki et al., 1987; Van der Meer et al., 1988; Alexander et al., 1991). Certainly, each of these systems is quite complex, and other factors, such as induction of growth factors and resulting changes in cell populations, could also be critical in many of these forms of protection. However, it remains possible that early changes in antioxidants are either required or permissive for these additional forms of adaptation.

II. Endotoxin-Induced Tolerance To Hyperoxia and Copper,Zinc Superoxide Dismutase

Frank and co-workers initially demonstrated the protective effect of endotoxin against pulmonary O_2 toxicity and related mortality in rats (Frank et al., 1978, 1980; Hass et al., 1989). An association between the development of endotoxin-mediated tolerance and increases in total lung superoxide dismutase (SOD) activity has been demonstrated repeatedly. Species such as mice, which did not develop endotoxin-related tolerance, also did not show increases in SOD activity. That such an increase in lung copper,zinc superoxide dismutase activity could effectively decrease lethal pulmonary oxygen toxicity in mice, once this had occurred, is suggested by our recent studies in transgenic mice, which overexpress the human gene for this protein (White et al., 1991). The copper chelator diethyldithiocarbamate (DDC) also prevents the tolerance in endotoxin-treated rats, presumably by decreasing Cu,Zn SOD activity (Frank et al., 1980). Block demonstrated that metabolic functions of the lung, namely clearance of serotonin and norepinephrine, which normally are impaired by brief or prolonged hyperoxic exposures, are preserved by endotoxin pretreatment (Block, 1983).

In adult rats given endotoxin, the increase in lung Cu,Zn SOD activity is due to an increased rate of synthesis of Cu,Zn SOD which occurs in endotoxin-injected rats *only* if they are also exposed to hyperoxia (0.95×1 atm) (Hass et al., 1989). Detailed analyses have shown an actual *decrease* in Cu,Zn SOD protein synthesis both in air- and O_2-exposed rats following endotoxin treatment at a time when Cu,Zn SOD mRNA is increased almost 50% in both groups (Iqbal et al., 1989). Similarly, lung slices exposed to oxygen synthesize increased amounts of Cu,Zn SOD protein following endotoxin compared to saline pretreatment (Hass et al., 1982). Thus although endotoxin alone increases Cu,Zn SOD mRNA concentration, concomitant O_2 exposure is needed to produce increased Cu,Zn SOD protein (Iqbal et al., 1989). This differs from exposure to hyperoxia alone in adult rats, where a translationally mediated increase in Cu,Zn SOD synthesis (126% of air control after 12 h) occurs. This increase is transient and does not result in increased lung SOD activity after 72 h in these animals (most do not survive). Although these adult rats do not increase Cu,Zn SOD mRNA or become tolerant during such lethal O_2 exposure, they will do so if given a ''rest period'' (24 h) after 48 h of exposure and then are reexposed to hyperoxia. This same Cu,Zn SOD mRNA increase occurs in neonatal rats during prolonged, continuous exposure to hyperoxia. Thus concomitant exposure to endotoxin and hyperoxia in adult rats is able to effect an adaptive response which occurs spontaneously in newborns (Frank, 1985; Hass et al., 1989).

III. Cytokine-Induced Tolerance to Hyperoxia

The extent to which locally or systemically produced cytokines such as interleukin-1 or tumor necrosis factor contribute to these effects of endotoxin in inducing O_2 tolerance is not clear. However, it is known that monocytes and alveolar macrophages can produce both of these cytokines in response to endotoxin (Matthews, 1981; Dinarello, 1984, 1988; Beutler and Cerami, 1987). In addition, both of these cytokines can circulate following production by fixed phagocytes of the reticuloendothelial system. This is especially true for tumor necrosis factor, but much less so for IL-1 (Michie et al., 1988) which is heavily cell-bound compared to TNF (Ghezzi et al., 1991). Furthermore, other cell types, such as endothelial cells, also can produce IL-1 locally in response to such stimuli as endotoxin, tumor necrosis factor, and IL-1 itself (Dinarello et al., 1986a; Libby et al., 1986). However, it appears probable that in inducing antioxidants in cultured endothelium and in lung slices, endotoxin may be acting, at least in part, through direct actions not requiring cytokine production. However, it seems likely that cytokines would act to potentiate the induction of antioxidants produced due to endotoxin exposure in vivo.

Studies in rats showed that when administered together, recombinant interleukin-1 and tumor necrosis factor can induce tolerance to lethal pulmonary O_2 toxicity in a similar fashion to injected endotoxin. With the available doses of cytokines used in our initial studies (10 μg of each), neither IL-1 nor TNF alone induced measurable protection. Tolerance to hyperoxia increased with increasing amounts of injected interleukin-1 in combination with a fixed amount of TNF. Heat-inactivated cytokines did not provide protection, suggesting that the minute amounts of contaminating endotoxin were not playing a major role in conferring tolerance (White et al., 1987). With the availability of larger quantities of recombinant proteins, our more recent studies have shown that interleukin-1 alone, but not tumor necrosis factor, when injected parenterally can provide partial protection relative to that which we initially described with the two cytokines combined (C. W. White, unpublished observations). Others have shown that tumor necrosis factor or interleukin-1 alone, when administered via the airway, also can provide protection against pulmonary oxygen toxicity (Tsan, 1990, 1991). Certainly TNF can induce IL-1 production (Dinarello et al., 1986a; Libby et al., 1986; Bachwich et al., 1986) as well as IL-1 receptors (Naworth et al., 1986), and thus both cytokines may be playing a role when protection is provided by locally administered TNF. When not confined to the airway, the toxic potential of TNF may be enhanced. Its ability to alter endothelial permeability directly, increase neutrophil adherence and oxidant and protease release, and cause multiple organ damage are well documented (Sato et al., 1986; Stolpen et al., 1986; Horvath, et al., 1988; Royall et al., 1989; Tracey et al., 1986; Stephens et al.,

1988; Remick et al., 1987). Indeed, lethal systemic inflammatory illness and shock are induced by TNF alone or in synergy with interleukin-1 (Mathison et al., 1988; Okusawa et al., 1988; Dinarello et al., 1986a, b). However, even though IL-1 can increase endothelial permeability (Royall et al., 1989), lethality due to IL-1 alone does not appear to occur in nonadrenalectomized rodents at any achievable dose (Bertini et al., 1988).

Protection against pulmonary oxygen toxicity by cytokines is associated with decreased ultrastructural evidence of lung damage, pulmonary hypertension, pleural fluid accumulation and hemoconcentration, and lethality. At a time when these differences were observed, however, lung antioxidant enzyme activities, including total superoxide dismutase, glucose-6 phosphate dehydrogenase, glutathione reductase and peroxidase, and catalase, were not different in cytokine- and saline-pretreated rats. Nonetheless, accumulation of oxidized glutathione was markedly decreased and reduced/oxidized glutathione (GSH/ GSSG) ratios were greatly increased in cytokine-pretreated compared to saline-pretreated animals. This suggested that the oxidant/antioxidant balance was altered. This could be the result of decreased oxidant production (Freeman and Crapo, 1982; Ischiropoulos et al., 1989), increased antioxidant defenses, or both.

In continued investigations we studied the effects of cytokine treatment on rat lung antioxidant enzyme activities after continuous oxygen exposure for various intervals. Significant but relatively unimpressive increases in lung glucose-6-phosphate dehydrogenase and glutathione reductase, but not total superoxide dismutase, catalase, or glutathione peroxidase, activities occurred after 4 and 16 h of oxygen exposure following cytokine treatment. However, impressive two- to sixfold increases in the lung activities of each of these five enzymes occurred in rats exposed to hyperoxia for 72 h following cytokine treatment (White et al., 1989). All saline-treated control animals were no longer surviving at this time. The timing and magnitude of the increases in lung antioxidant enzyme activities in these animals were similar to those observed in endotoxin-treated rats exposed to hyperoxia (Frank et al., 1980). However, the changes in antioxidant enzyme activities that we found did not appear to explain the differences in GSSG accumulation and reduced/oxidized glutathione ratios between cytokine- and saline-treated rats which were present after 52 h of oxygen exposure.

The work of Berg and co-workers supports the notion that cytokines play a role in causing endotoxin-mediated tolerance to hyperoxic lung injury. They demonstrated passive transfer of factors causing protection against hyperoxia using serum from endotoxin-treated donor rats. The degree of protection observed was similar to that seen in endotoxin-treated rats exposed simultaneously to hyperoxia. They demonstrated elevated levels of both interleukin-1 and tumor necrosis factor in the transferred serum but excluded the possibility that transfer of residual endotoxin caused the observed protection by using the *Limulus* amebocyte lysate assay. While these workers demonstrated increased lung total superoxide dismutase and catalase activities in endotoxin-treated, oxygen-exposed rats, such increases were not present in the serum-treated animals following oxygen exposures at 60 h (Berg et al., 1990). Thus an earlier difference in lung oxidant/antioxidant balance again is suggested.

IV. Role of Manganese SOD in Cytokine-Induced Tolerance to Oxidants

A plausible explanation for this early change in lung oxidant/antioxidant balance in lungs from cytokine-treated rats was suggested by the work of Wong and Goeddel (Wong and Goeddel, 1988). They found that both interleukins 1 and tumor necrosis factors (both α and β) induce manganese (mitochondrial) SOD mRNA and activity in the human A549 lung carcinoma cell line and in a variety of other cell lines. TNF α also was found to induce MnSOD mRNA in normal cells in vitro and in a variety or organs (kidney, thymus, bone marrow, and spleen) in mice in vivo. Other mitochondrial marker enzymes, such as cytochrome oxidase, were not increased by cytokine exposure. Interferons, IL-2, IL-6, TGF β, phorbol myristate acetate plus bacterial lipopolysaccharide, and hydrogen peroxide all failed to induce MnSOD mRNA in their system. Other antioxidant enzyme mRNAs, including those for copper,zinc SOD, glutathione peroxidase, and catalase, were not induced by TNF α. These studies were extended elegantly when it was shown in two different tumor cell lines that overexpression of MnSOD confers increased resistance to killing by tumor necrosis factor plus cycloheximide, whereas expression of antisense MnSOD RNA renders the cells sensitive to TNF killing even in the absence of cycloheximide (Wong et al., 1989). More recently, exogenously administered copper,zinc superoxide dismutase was found to decrease TNF toxicity in mice, whereas glutathione depletion, via inhibition of its synthesis with buthionine sulfoximine, enhanced toxicity (Hauser et al., 1990). Thus mitochondrially generated superoxide is implicated as an important component of TNF-mediated tumor cell killing, and superoxide may be implicated in systemic toxicity of TNF. Whether or not and how this hypothetical mitochondrial superoxide overproduction might be linked to MnSOD overexpression and antioxidant protection in vivo is an unresolved question.

In studies focusing on interleukin-1, Masuda and co-workers found that IL-1 induced MnSOD protein in human melanoma A375 cells and in normal human skin fibroblasts and peripheral blood mononuclear cells. At comparable concentrations, IL-1 is cytotoxic in A375 cells, whereas it stimulates growth of both of the normal cell types (Masuda et al., 1988). This demonstrated that cytokines capable of pleiotropic effects induce MnSOD in a common fashion. A link between IL-1 and increased superoxide production has been suggested in endothelial cells (Matsubara and Ziff, 1986), and this work was extended by others. In studies reported by Meier and co-workers, IL-1 and TNF were found to increase superoxide production by human fibroblasts as detected with nitroblue tetrazolium, ferricytochrome *c,* and by electron spin resonance using DMPO as a spin trap. IL-1 and TNF also increased hydrogen peroxide released from cells as measured by peroxidase-mediated oxidation of scopoletin. Other possible indicators of increased free-radical activity following cytokine administration included increased low-level chemiluminescence and liberation of ethane. None of these indicators was inhibited or enhanced by addition of xanthine, allopurinol, azide, cyanide, or rotenone, although the signal was enhanced both by NADH and NADPH (Meier et al, 1989).

Rat pulmonary epithelial-like cells (L2 cells line) also are induced to increase MnSOD, but not Cu,Zn SOD, mRNA by LPS, IL-1, and TNF. Concomitant exposure to a hyperoxic environment was not required for increased MnSOD mRNA expression, although MnSOD mRNA induction by LPS appeared to be increased somewhat by hyperoxia in most cases. Cytokine (TNF)-mediated MnSOD induction was potentiated more greatly by hyperoxia. Over 2 to 24 h, mRNA for neither SOD was induced by hyperoxia alone. As expected, actinomycin D, an RNA synthesis inhibitor, completely inhibited MnSOD mRNA induction by LPS. Cycloheximide alone also induced MnSOD mRNA equivalent to the induction by endotoxin (bacterial lipopolysaccharide, LPS). Cycloheximide plus LPS caused a superinduction of MnSOD mRNA (Visner et al., 1990). Cycloheximide-dependent superinduction of IL-1, c-*fos,* and c-*myc* also have been described. This superinduction suggests either that these cells constitutively produce a tonic labile repressor of transcription of MnSOD cDNA and/or an RNase protein which acts on MnSOD mRNA. IL-1 and/or TNF may not play an important role in mediating LPS-induced MnSOD mRNA increases in this cell line.

Earlier studies also have shown that LPS induces immunoreactive MnSOD, but not Cu,Zn SOD, protein in human monocytes (Asayama et al., 1985). In more recent studies, bovine pulmonary artery endothelial cells increased immunoreactive MnSOD, but not Cu,Zn SOD, in response to LPS. The activities of mitochondrial marker enzymes (cytochrome *c* oxidase and fumarase) and other antioxidant enzymes (glutathione peroxidase and catalase) were not increased by LPS (Shiki et al., 1987). Thus MnSOD induction by LPS, IL-1, and TNF has been demonstrated in a variety of malignant and normal cells. Cu,Zn SOD mRNA has not been found to be induced in these studies. In preliminary experiments, we have observed increases in rat lung MnSOD, but not

Cu,Zn SOD, mRNAs and activity in response to LPS, IL-1, TNF, and TNF+IL-1 at early time points at which we have not observed increases in total lung superoxide dismutase activity (Lewis-Molock and White, unpublished observations). Others have suggested that rat lung MnSOD activity is increased at much later time points (72 to 96 h after cytokine injection) by both endotoxin and TNFα. In contrast, TNFα alone decreased lung Cu,Zn SOD activity, whereas this activity was unchanged by endotoxin (Green et al., 1990). Taken together, these studies may suggest a final common pathway for MnSOD induction which can be activated by LPS, IL-1, and TNF. That such an increase in MnSOD could be protective against oxidative injury is suggested by studies in which TNFα was used to induce increases in MnSOD mRNA and activity in a pulmonary adenocarcinoma cell line, NCI-H820. Loss of cell viability due to paraquat, an intracellular generator of superoxide ($O_2^{\bar{\bullet}}$), was decreased following TNFα treatment of cells (Warner et al., 1991).

In in vivo studies it was shown that aerosol TNF achieves lung levels comparable to lethal TNF doses given intravenously. However, plasma levels were several thousandfold lower after aerosol administration. Aerosolized cytokines did not induce lung edema or inflammation of airways or alveoli. Nonetheless, pulmonary leukostasis (1 day after administration) and focal pulmonary hemorrhage (5 days after administration) resulted from aerosolized TNF or TNF plus interferon gamma administration. Either cytokine enhanced both pulmonary and systemic monocyte function, and together they gave additive or synergistic effects (Debs et al., 1988). In subsequent elegant studies, Tsan and co-workers observed that lung MnSOD activity increases following intratracheal administration of TNF and IL-1 in association with protection against hyperoxic lung injury. At a time shortly before onset of mortality of control rats, IL-1-injected, but not saline-injected, rats showed increased lung activities of MnSOD (Tsan et al, 1990, 1991). However, in recently reported studies in sheep, both oxygen alone and endotoxin plus oxygen induced similar increases in MnSOD in lung (Kobayashi et al., 1991). In addition, in vivo studies have not shown increased survival of transgenic mice with increased lung activities of MnSOD (Ho and Crapo, 1990). This discrepant effect compared to the apparent association of increased lung MnSOD activity and cytokine treatment in rats may be related to species differences or to other effects of cytokines. Further studies of this phenomenon are needed, and are hampered primarily by various types of interference that occur with most of the commonly used assays for MnSOD activity in crude lung homogenates and cell extracts (Beyer and Fridovich, 1987; Spitz and Oberley, 1989; Iqbal and Whitney, 1991). That Cu,Zn SOD may also be induced in vivo in rats by endotoxin plus oxygen, and in later stages of O_2 exposure in cytokine-treated rats, again suggests that superoxide itself could be at the center of a common mechanism for transcription of these two genetically unrelated dismutases. However, such a possibility remains unconfirmed at present.

Parallels may exist between tolerance produced by endotoxin, cytokines, and hypoxia. Preexposure to hypoxia induces a remarkable tolerance to hyperoxic lung injury in vivo and to oxidative lung injury in vitro. In our experience, this tolerance has been greater than that afforded by prexposure to endotoxin, interleukin-1, and/or tumor necrosis factor, sublethal hyperoxia, or following administration of exogenous antioxidants. Sjostrom and Crapo (1983) showed that MnSOD, but not Cu,Zn SOD, activity is increased in lungs of rats preexposed to hypoxia. We found that lung activities of the glutathione redox cycle and of glucose-6-phosphate dehydrogenase were also increased in hypoxia- compared to air-preexposed rats (White et al., 1988). To determine whether cytokine induction by hypoxia could be involved in tolerance induced by that stimulus, we exposed human peripheral blood mononuclear cells to normoxia or hypoxia, and to endotoxin or no additional stimulus. In the absence of endotoxin, cells exposed to normoxia or hypoxia did not produce detectable TNF, IL-1α, or IL-1β. However, in the presence of minute amounts of endotoxin (1 ng/mL), all three cytokines were induced and the levels of each were approximately 2.5-fold increased in those cells exposed to severe hypoxia (pO_2 approximately 10 torr) over 24 h compared to those exposed to normoxia. However, mRNA for IL-1 was not changed in hypoxia compared to normoxia in the presence (or absence) of endotoxin. Thus the increases in immunoreactive cytokine induced by hypoxia in the presence of endotoxin do not occur at the mRNA level (Ghezzi et al., 1991). On this basis, it does not appear that increases in MnSOD or other antioxidant enzymes induced by preexposure to hypoxia are necessarily related to cytokine production.

V. Potential Effects of Cytokines on Oxidant Production

Infusion of endotoxin also attenuates O_2 toxicity in newborn lambs. Although GSH/GSSG ratios were increased in lungs of endotoxin-treated compared to saline-treated lambs, there were no changed in lung antioxidant enzyme (total SOD, CAT, GR, or GPX) activities. Although GSSG accumulation was decreased in endotoxin-treated lambs, the increase in GSH/GSSG ratios in endotoxin-treated lambs occurred on the basis of more impressive increases in GSH relative to both saline-treated oxygen- and air-exposed controls (Hazinski, et al., 1988). A possibility which has received less attention than that of increased antioxidants induced by endotoxin is that toxic oxygen metabolites are produced in lesser quantities in lungs of endotoxin- or cytokine-treated rats relative to controls during exposure to hyperoxia. Such a possibility does not exclude antioxidant enzyme increases to enhance tolerance, but such a process could function in additive or synergistic fashion with increased antioxidant enzymes. The potential importance of such a mechanism recently was suggested by studies of spontaneously developing O_2 tolerance in newborn rats (Ischiropoulos et al., 1989).

Inhibition of cytochrome P450 in the lung could decrease microsomal production of toxic oxygen radicals, thereby contributing to a more favorable oxidant–antioxidant balance. Endotoxin, IL-1, and TNF can decrease hepatic cytochrome P450–dependent enzyme activities and may have similar effects in the lung (Sonowane et al., 1982; Falzon et al., 1984; Ghezzi et al., 1986). Inhibitors of cytochrome P450 activity, such as cimetidine, also may have a palliative effect on pulmonary O_2 toxicity (Hazinski et al., 1989). Inducers of interferons, which, like interleukin-1 and tumor necrosis factor, decrease cytochrome P450 activity in liver and lung, also cause reduction of pulmonary oxygen toxicity (Kikkawa et al., 1984). In addition, mice with genetically determined decreased cytochrome P450 inducibility show longer survival during exposure to hyperoxia (Gonder et al., 1985). However, not all investigators have observed a parallel effect. For example, pharmacologic induction of cytochrome P450 may afford protection against oxygen toxicity to the lung in some models (Mansour et al., 1988a, b). Thus the effects of cytochrome P450 induction/inhibition are not entirely clear-cut and may vary with species, strain, timing of dosage and types of inducers or inhibitors administered, and age of the animal. Whether or not such mechanisms may be involved in cytokine- or endotoxin-mediated oxygen tolerance remains to be shown.

VI. Potential Role of Arachidonate Metabolites and Other Inflammatory Mediators in Cytokine-Induced Oxidant Tolerance

It has been suggested that inhibitors of arachidonate metabolism can prevent endotoxin-induced protection of rats against hyperoxic lung injury (Klein and Trouwborst, 1985; Klein et al., 1987). Virtually all of the products of arachidonate metabolism have been implicated in at least some of the actions of endotoxin and/or the cytokines IL-1 and TNF (Wise et al., 1980; Snapper et al., 1983; Dinarello et al., 1983; Rossi et al., 1985; Dayer et al., 1985; Dinarello et al., 1986a, b; Chang et al., 1987; Bussolino et al., 1988; Camussi et al., 1987). Indeed, the production of IL-1 induced by LPS and by IL-1 itself, as well as TNF production, may be regulated by prostaglandins or other arachidonate products (Dinarello et al., 1984; Bachwich et al., 1986; Kunkel et al., 1986, 1988; Knudsen et al, 1986; Endres et al., 1989). Salicylic acid inhibits the endotoxin-induced protection of rats against lethal hyperoxic lung injury (Klein et al., 1987). We have found a similar inhibition of cytokine-induced protection by aspirin in the rat model (White and Ghezzi, 1989). Ibuprofen caused a less impressive inhibition of protection. Indomethacin could not be adequately tested because adequate inhibitory doses caused severe toxicity to the gastrointestinal tract. At this time the role of arachidonate products in inducing the protective effects of endotoxin and cytokines against pulmonary oxygen toxicity remains unresolved. It is known, however, that certain important enzymes involved in arachidonate metabolism (lipoxygenase, prostaglandin synthetase) can be activated by lipid peroxides produced via oxygen radical reactions (Hemler et al., 1979; Taylor et al., 1983; Chakraborti et al., 1989). Similarly, free radicals can be generated through the actions of other arachidonate-metabolizing enzymes such as cyclooxygenase (Kontos et al., 1985). Thus several possibilities exist by which interactions between cytokines and oxygen radicals could involve arachidonate metabolism.

Several investigators have suggested that initial actions of both endotoxin and cytokines may lead to subsequent relative inhibition of oxidative metabolism and protease release by neutrophils. Indeed, prior exposure to TNF attenuates subsequent airways injury in a neutrophil-dependent model (Gordon et al., 1987). To the extent that neutrophils could compound lung injury during prolonged exposure to hyperoxia, such a mechanism could contribute to protection by endotoxin or cytokines.

Multiple antiproteolytic acute-phase proteins as well as some with antioxidant effects, such as ceruloplasmin, are induced by interleukin-1 directly, as well as indirectly by endotoxin, primarily through IL-1 and IL-6. Endotoxin induces a large increase in lung proteins to an extent exceeding that of Cu,Zn SOD, and these proteins are incompletely characterized. Such actions could have additional protective effects beyond those provided by induction of lung superoxide dismutase and other antioxidant enzymes (Pohlman and Harlan, 1989; Harlan et al., 1983). Endotoxin, and possibly cytokines induced by LPS, could have mitogenic effects either directly or through induction of growth factors (Koizumi et al., 1985; Albelda et al., 1989). Stimulators of lung growth have been implicated in some models of tolerance (Thet et al., 1984; Tierney and Hacker, 1989).

VII. Summary

Cytokines have multiple complex interactions systemically and in the lung. As a rule, lung antioxidant enzymes appear to increase in tolerance to hyperoxia induced by cytokines, although large increases are slow to develop in vivo.

Rapid, early induction of manganese superoxide dismutase occurs in vitro in a variety of normal and malignant cells, and available data suggest that such an effect occurs in the lung in vivo as well. copper,zinc superoxide dismutase increases in lungs in vitro and in vivo upon exposure to endotoxin *and* hyperoxia are reported by one group. Such an effect on Cu,Zn SOD has not been observed following administration of TNF and/or IL-1.

Alterations in oxidant formation within the lung that may be produced by exposure to endotoxin and cytokines are not well characterized. Passive serum transfer from endotoxin-injected rats has suggested that cytokines contribute to endotoxin-induced tolerance. A clearer cause-and-effect relationship between endotoxin- and cytokine-induced tolerance and associated changes in various lung proteins, independent of oxygen-induced effects, needs to be established. This might occur if simplified in vitro models, in which such protein changes *and* hyperoxic cell injury can be studied simultaneously, become available. Such models would allow application of contemporary molecular tools to resolve these questions. It is likely that a better understanding of the mechanism and signal transduction involved in this protective process will be required for effective therapies to be developed. Nonetheless, recent studies have shown that as with animals (Debs et al., 1988), humans can be treated safely with cytokines such as γ-interferon via the aerosol route with minimal systemic toxicity but with ample local effect (Jaffe et al., 1991). Even with local therapy, administration of cytokines such as IL-1 and TNF to patients with inflammatory lung disorders would have to be considered with extreme caution because systemic absorption of even very small doses of these agents has the potential for causing disastrous complications, including severe hypotension, renal insufficiency, and myocardial infarction (Smith et al., 1990).

Note Added in Proof: New information in this area is provided by two carefully performed, current studies: (1) Gibbs, L. S., Del Vecchio, P. J., and Shaffer, J. B. Mn and Cu,Zn SOD expression in cells from LPS-sensitive and LPS-resistant mice. Free Radical Biol. Med. **12:**107–111; and (2) Melendez, J. A., and C. Baglioni. Reduced expression of manganese superoxide dismutase in cells resistant to cytolysis by tumor necrosis factor. Free Radical Biol. Med. **12:**151–159, 1992.

Acknowledgments

This work was done during the tenure of an Established Investigatorship from the American Heart Association and was also supported by a Grant-in-Aid from the American Heart Association to Dr. White. Additional research support was provided by National Jewish Center for Immunology and Respiratory Medicine, the C. Henry Kempe Research Center for the Children's Hospital of Denver,

Ronald McDonald Children's Charities, and NIH SCOR 1-P50-HL46481. The author is grateful to Ms. Dawnett Marples for secretarial assistance.

References

Albelda, S. M., Elias, J. A., Levine, E. M., and Kern, J. A. (1989). Endotoxin stimulates platelet-derived growth factor production from cultured human pulmonary endothelial cells. *Am. J. Physiol.,* **257:**L65–L70.

Alexander, H. R., Sheppard, B. C., Jensen, J. C., Langstein, H. N., Buresh, C. M., Venzon, D., Walker, E. C., Fraker, D. L., Stovroff, M. C., and Norton, J. A. (1991). Treatment with recombinant human tumor necrosis factor-alpha protects rats against the lethality, hypotension, and hypothermia of gram-negative sepsis. *J. Clin. Invest.* **88:**34–39.

Asayama, K., Janco, R. L., and Burr, I. M. (1985). Selective induction of manganous superoxide dismutase in human monocytes. *Am. J. Physiol.* **249:**C393–C397.

Bachwich, P. R., Chensue, S. W., Larrick, J. W., and Kunkel, S. L. (1986). Tumor necrosis factor stimulates interleukin 1 and prostaglandin E_2 production in resting macrophages. *Biochem. Biophys. Res. Commun.* **136:**94–101.

Berg, J. T., Allison, R. C., Prasad, V. R., and Taylor, A. E. (1990). Endotoxin protection of rats from pulmonary oxygen toxicity: Possible cytokine involvement. *J. Appl. Physiol.* **68:**549–553.

Berkow, R. L., Wang, D., Larrick, J. W., Dodson, R. W., and Howard, T. H. (1987). Enhancement of neutrophil superoxide production by preincubation with recombinant human tumor necrosis factor. *J. Immunol.* **139:**3783–3791.

Bertini, R., Bianchi, M., and Ghezzi, P. (1988). Adrenalectomy sensitizes mice to the lethal effects of interleukin-1 and tumor necrosis factor. *J. Exp. Med.* **167:** 1708–1712.

Beutler, B., and Cerami, A. (1987). Cachectin: More than a tumor necrosis factor. *N. Engl. J. Med.* **316:**379–385.

Bevilacqua, M. P., Pober, J. S., Wheeler, M. E., Cotran, R. A., and Gimbrone, M. A. (1985). Interleukin-1 acts on cultured human vascular endothelium to increase the adhesion of polymorphonuclear leukocytes, monocytes and related leukocyte cell lines. *J. Clin. Invest.* **76:**2003–2011.

Beyer, W. F., and Fridovich, I. (1987). Assaying for superoxide dismutase activity: Some large consequences of minor changes in conditions. *Anal. Biochem.* **161:**559–566.

Block, E. R. (1983). Endotoxin protects against hyperoxic alterations in lung endothelial cell metabolism. *J. Appl. Physiol.* **54:**24–30.

Brigham, K. L., Meyrick, B., Berry, L. C., Jr., and Repine, J. E. (1987). Antioxidants protect cultured bovine drug endothelial cells from injury by endotoxin. *J. Appl. Physiol.* **63:**840–850.

Bussolino, F., Camussi, G., and Baglioni, C. (1988). Synthesis and release of platelet-activating factor by human vascular endothelial cells treated with tumor necrosis factor or interleukin 1α. *J. Biol. Chem.* **263:**11856–11861.

Camussi, G., Bussolino, F., Salvidio, G., and Baglioni, C. (1987). Tumor necrosis factor/cachectin stimulates peritoneal macrophages, polymorphonuclear neutrophils, and vascular endothelial cells to synthesize and release platelet-activating factor. *J. Exp. Med.* **166:**1390–1404.

Chakraborti, S., Gurtner, G. H., and Michael, J. R. (1989). Oxidant-mediated activation of phospholipase A_2 in pulmonary endothelium. *J. Appl. Physiol.* **257:**L430–L437.

Chang, S.-W., Feddersen, C. O., Henson, P. M., and Voelkel, N. F. (1987). Platelet-activating factor mediates hemodynamic changes and lung injury in endotoxin-treated rats. *J. Clin. Invest.* **79:**1498–1509.

Chang, S.-W., Lauterburg, B. H., and Voelkel, N. F. (1988). Endotoxin causes neutrophil-independent oxidative stress in rats. *J. Appl. Physiol.* **65:**358–367.

Chang, S.-W., Westcott, J. Y., Pickett, W. C., Murphy, R. C., and Voelkel, N. F. (1989). Endotoxin-induced lung injury in rats: Role of eicosanoids. *J. Appl. Physiol.* **66:**2407–2418.

Dayer, J. M., Beutler, B., and Cerami, A. (1985). Cachectin/tumor necrosis factor stimulates collagenase and prostaglandin E_2 production by human synovial cells and dermal fibroblasts. *J. Exp. Med.* **162:**2163–2168.

Debs, R. J., Fuchs, H. J., Philip, R., Montgomery, A. B., Brunette, E. N., Liggitt, D., Patton, J. S., and Shellito, J. E. (1988). Lung-specific delivery of cytokines induces sustained pulmonary and systemic immunomodulation in rats. *J. Immunol.* **140:**3482–3488.

Dinarello, C. A. (1984). Interleukin-1. *Rev. Infect. Dis.* **6:**51–95.

Dinarello, C. A. (1988). Biology of interleukin 1. *FASEB J.* **2:**108–115.

Dinarello, C. A., Marnoy, S. I., and Rosenwasser, L. J. (1983). The role of arachidonate metabolism in the immunoregulatory function of human leukocytic pyrogen/lymphocyte activating factor/interleukin-1. *J. Immunol.* **130:**890–895.

Dinarello, C. A., Bishai, I., Rosenwasser, L. J., and Coceani, F. (1984). The influence of lipoxygenase inhibitors on the in vitro production of human leukocytic pyrogen and lymphocyte activating factor (interleukin-1). *Int. J. Immunopharmacol.* **6:**43.

Dinarello, C. A., Cannon, J. G., Wolff, S. M., Bernheim, H. A., Beutler, B., Cerami, A., Palladino, M. A., Jr., and O'Connor, J. V. (1986a). Tumor necrosis factor (cachectin) is an endogenous pyrogen and induces production of interleukin-1. *J. Exp. Med.* **163:**1433–1450.

Dinarello, C. A., Cannon, J. G., Mier, J. W. Bernheim, H. A., LoPreste, G., Lynn, D. L., Love, R. N., Webb, C., Auron, P. E., Reuben, R. C., Rich, A., Wolf, S. M., and Putney, S. D. (1986b). Multiple biological activities of human recombinant interleukin 1. *J. Clin. Invest.* **77:**1734–1739.

Endres, S., Ghorbani, R., Kelley, V. E., Georgilis, K., Lonnemann, G., van der Meer, J. W. M., Cannon, J. G., Rogers, T. S., Klempner, M. S., Weber, P. C., Schaefer, E. J., Wolff, S. M., and Dinarello, C. A. (1989). The effect of dietary supplementation with n-3 polyunsaturated fatty acids on the synthesis of interleukin-1 and tumor necrosis factor by mononuclear cells. *N. Engl. J. Med.* **320:**265–271.

Falzon, M., Milton, A. S., and Burke, M. D. (1984). Are the decreases in hepatic cytochrome P-450 and other drug-metabolising enzymes caused by indomethacin in vivo mediated by intestinal bacterial endotoxins? *Biochem. Pharmacol.* **33:**1285–1292.

Frank, L. (1982). Protection from O_2 toxicity by preexposure to hypoxia: Lung antioxidant enzyme role. *J. Appl. Physiol.* **53:**475–482.

Frank, L. (1985). Effects of oxygen on the newborn. *Fed. Proc.* **44:**2328–2334.

Frank, L., Yam, J., and Roberts, R. (1978). The role of endotoxin in protection of adult rats from high oxygen toxicity. *J. Clin. Invest.* **61:**269–275.

Frank, L., Summerville, J., and Massaro, D. (1980). Protection from oxygen toxicity with endotoxin: Role of the endogenous antioxidant enzymes of the lung. *J. Clin. Invest.* **65:**1104–1110.

Freeman, B. A., and Crapo, J. D. (1982). Biology of disease. Free radicals and tissue injury. *Lab. Invest.* **47:**412–426.

Ghezzi, P., Saccardo, B., and Bianchi, M. (1986a). Recombinant tumor necrosis factor depresses cytochrome P-450-dependent microsomal drug metabolism in mice. *Biochem. Biophys. Res. Commun.* **136:**316–321.

Ghezzi, P., Saccardo, B., Villa, P., Rossi, V., Bianchi, M., and Dinarello, C. A. (1986b). Role of interleukin-1 in the depression of liver drug metabolism by endotoxin. *Infect. Immun.* **54:**837–840.

Ghezzi, P., Dinarello, C. A., Bianchi, M., Rosandich, M. E., Repine, J. E., and White, C. W. (1991). Hypoxia increases production of cytokines IL-1 and TNF by human mononuclear cells. *Cytokine.* **3:**189–194.

Goldblum, S. E., Cohen, D. A., Gillespie, M. N., and McClain, C. J. (1987a). Interleukin-1-induced granulocytopenia and pulmonary leukostasis in rabbits. *J. Appl. Physiol.* **62:**122–128.

Goldblum, S. E., Jay, M., Yoneda, K., Cohen, D. A., McClain, C. J., and Gillespie, M. N. (1987b). Monokine-induced acute lung injury in rabbits. *J. Appl. Physiol.* **63:**2093–2100.

Gonder, J. C., Proctor, R. A., and Will, J. A. (1985). Genetic differences in oxygen toxicity are correlated with cytochrome P-450 inducibility. *Proc. Natl. Acad. Sci. USA* **82:**6315–6319.

Gordon, T., Milligan, S. A., Levin, J., Thompson, J. E., Fine, J. M., and Sheppard, D. (1987). Apparent effect of catalase on airway edema in guinea pigs: Role of endotoxin contamination. *Am. Rev. Respir. Dis.* **135:**854–859.

Green, D. W., Burhans, M. S., and Wispé, J. R. (1990). Endotoxin and TNF-a have different effects on lung SOD. *Pediatr. Res.* **27**(4;part 2):304 (abstract #1804).

Guthrie, L. A., McPhail, L. C., Henson, P. M., and Johnston, R. B., Jr., (1984). The priming of neutrophils for enhanced release of oxygen metabolites by bacterial lipopolysaccharide: Evidence for increased activity of the superoxide-producing enzyme. *J. Exp. Med.* **160:**1656–1671.

Harlan, J. M., Harker, L. A., Reidy, M. A., Gajdusek, C. M., Schwartz, S. M., and Striker, G. E. (1983). Lipopolysaccharide-mediated bovine endothelial cell injury in vitro. *Lab. Invest.* **48:**269–274.

Hass, M. A., Frank, L., and Massaro, D. (1982). The effect of bacterial endotoxin on synthesis of (Cu,Zn) superoxide dismutase in lungs of oxygen-exposed rats. *J. Biol. Chem.* **257:**9379–9383.

Hass, M. A., Iqbal, J., Clerch, L. B., Frank, L., and Massaro, D. (1989). Rat lung Cu,Zn superoxide dismutase. Isolation and sequence of a full-length cDNA and studies of enzyme induction. *J. Clin. Invest.* **83:**1241–1246.

Hauser, G. J., McIntosh, J. K., Travis, W. D., and Rosenberg, S. A. (1990). Manipulation of oxygen radical-scavenging capacity in mice alters host sensitivity to tumor necrosis factor toxicity but does not interfere with its antitumor efficacy. *Cancer Res.* **50:**3503–3508.

Hazinski, T. A., Kennedy, K. A., France, M. L., and Hansen, T. N. (1988). Pulmonary O_2 toxicity in lambs: Physiological and biochemical effects of endotoxin infusion. *J. Appl. Physiol.* **65:**1579–1585.

Hazinski, T. A., France, M., Kennedy, K. A., and Hansen, T. N. (1989). Cimetidine reduces hyperoxic lung injury in lambs. *J. Appl. Physiol.* **67:**2586–2592.

Hemler, M. E., Cook, H. W., and Lands, W. E. M. (1979). Prostaglandin biosynthesis can be triggered by lipid peroxides. *Arch. Biochem. Biophys.* **193:**340–345.

Ho, Y.-S., and Crapo, J. D. (1990). Establishment of transgenic mice expressing human manganese-containing superoxide dismutase in the lungs. *Am. Rev. Respir. Dis.* **141**(4;part 2):A819 (abstract).

Horvath, C. J., Ferro, T. J., Jesmols, G., and Malik, A. B. (1988). Recombinant tumor necrosis factor increases pulmonary vascular permeability independent of neutrophils. *Proc. Natl. Acad. Sci. USA* **85:**9219–9223.

Iqbal, J., and Whitney, P. (1991). Use of cyanide and diethyldithiocarbamate in the assay of superoxide dismutases. *Free Radic. Biol. Med.* **10:**69–77.

Iqbal, J., Clerch, L. B., Hass, M. A., Frank, L., and Massaro, D. (1989). Endotoxin increases lung Cu,Zn superoxide dismutase mRNA:O_2 raises enzyme synthesis. *Am. J. Physiol.* **257:**L61–L64.

Ischiropoulos, H., Nadziejko, C. E., Kumae, T., and Kikkawa, Y. (1989). Oxygen tolerance in neonatal rats: Role of subcellular superoxide generation. *Am. J. Physiol.* **257:**L411–L420.

Jaffe, H. A., Buhl, R., Mastrangeli, A., Holroyd, K. J., Saltini, C., Czerski, D., Jaffe, H. S., Kramer, S., Sherwin, S., and Crystal, R. G. (1991). Organ specific cytokine therapy. Local activation of mononuclear phagocytes by delivery of an aerosol of recombinant interferon-γ to the human lung. *J. Clin. Invest.* **88:**297–302.

Kettelhut, I. C., Fiers, W., and Goldberg, A. L. (1987). The toxic effects of tumor necrosis factor in vivo and their prevention by cyclooxygenase inhibitors. *Proc. Natl. Acad. Sci. USA* **84:**4273–4277.

Kikkawa, Y., Yano, S., and Skoza, L. (1984). Protective effect of interferon inducers against hyperoxic pulmonary damage. *Lab. Invest.* **50:**62–71.

Klebanoff, S. J., Vads, M. A., Harlan, J. M., Sparks, L. H., Gamble, J. R., Agosti, J. M., and Waltersdorph, A. M. (1986). Stimulation of neutrophils by tumor necrosis factor. *J. Immunol.* **136:**4220–4225.

Klein, J., and Trouwborst, A. (1985). Endotoxin protection against oxygen toxicity and its reversal by salicylate. *Adv. Exp. Med. Biol.* **191:**655–659.

Klein, J., Trouwborst, A., and Erdmann, W. (1987). Endotoxin protection against pulmonary oxygen toxicity and plasma prostaglandin levels in the rat. *Adv. Exp. Biol. Med.* **215:**355–358.

Knudsen, P. J., Dinarello, C. A., and Strom, T. B. (1986). Prostaglandins posttranscriptionally inhibit monocyte expression of interleukin 1 activity by increasing intracellular cyclic adenosine monophosphate. *J. Immunol.* **137:**3189–3194.

Kobayashi, T., Shiki, Y., Meyrick, B., Burr, I. M., and Newman, J. H. (1991). Simultaneous exposure of sheep to endotoxin and 100% oxygen. *Am. Rev. Respir. Dis.* **144:**600–605.

Koizumi, M., Frank, L., and Massaro, D. (1985). Mitogenic effect of endotoxin on lung and tolerance of rats to hyperoxia. *J. Appl. Physiol.* **59:**315–319.

Kontos, H. A., Wei, E. P., Ellis, E. F., Jenkins, L. W., Povlishock, J. T., Rowe, G. T., and Hess, M. L. (1985). Appearance of superoxide anion radical in cerebral extracellular space during increased prostaglandin synthesis in cats. *Circ. Res.* **57:**142–151.

Kunkel, S. L., Chensue, S. W., and Phan, S. H. (1986). Prostaglandins as endogenous mediators of interleukin 1 production. *J. Immunol.* **136:**186.

Kunkel, S. L., Spengler, M., May, M. A., Spengler, R., Larrick, J., and Remick, D. (1988). Prostaglandin, E_2 regulates macrophage-derived tumor necrosis factor gene expression. *J. Biol. Chem.* **263:**5380–5384.

Larrick, J. W., Graham, D., Toy, K., Lin, L., Senyk, G., and Fendly, B. M. (1987). Recombinant tumor necrosis factor causes activation of human granulocytes. *Blood* **69:**640–644.

Libby, P., Ordovas, J. M., Auger, K. R., Robbins, A. H., Birinyi, L. K., and Dinarello, C. A. (1986). Endotoxin and tumor necrosis factor induce interleukin-1 gene expression in adult human vascular endothelial cells. *Am. J. Pathol* **124:**179.

Madonna, G. S., Peterson, J. E., Ribi, E. E., and Vogel, S. N. (1986). Early-phase endotoxin tolerance: Induction by a detoxified lipid A derivative, monophosphoryl lipid A. *Infect. Immun.* **52:**6–11.

Mansour, H., Levacher, M., Azoulay-Dupuis, E., Moreau, J., Marquetty, A. C., and Gougerot-Pocidalo, M. A. (1988a). Genetic differences in response to pulmonary cytochrome P-450 inducers and oxygen toxicity. *J. Appl. Physiol.* **64:**1376–1381.

Mansour, H., Brun-Pascuad, H., Marquetty, C., Gougerot-Pocidalo, M. A., Hakim, J., and Pocidalo, J. J. (1988b). Protection of rat from oxygen toxicity by inducers of cytochrome P-450 system. *Am. Rev. Respir. Dis.* **137:**688–694.

Masuda, A., Longo, D. L., Kobayashi, Y., Appella, E., Oppenheim, J. J., and Matsushima, K. (1988). Induction of mitochondrial manganese superoxide dismutase by interleukin 1. *FASEB J.* **2:**3087–3091.

Mathison, J. C., Wolfson, E., and Ulevitch, R. J. (1988). Participation of tumor necrosis factor in the mediation of gram negative bacterial lipopolysaccharide-induced injury in rabbits. *J. Clin. Invest.* **81:**1925–1937.

Matsubara, T., and Ziff, M. (1986). Increased superoxide anion release from human endothelial cells in response to cytokines. *J. Immunol.* **137:**3295–3298.

Matthews, N. (1981). Tumor necrosis factor from the rabbit. V. Synthesis in vitro by mononuclear phagocytes from various tissues of normal and BCG-injected rabbits. *Br. J. Cancer,* **44:**418–424.

Matthews, N., Neale, M. L., Jackson, S. K., and Stark, J. M. (1987). Tumour cell killing by tumour necrosis factor: Inhibition by anaerobic conditions, free-radical scavengers and inhibitors of arachidonate metabolism. *Immunology,* **62:**153–155.

Meier, B., Radeke, H. H., Selle, S., Younes, M., Sies, H., Resch, K., and Habermehl, G. G. (1989). Human fibroblasts release reactive oxygen species in response to interleukin-1 or tumor necrosis factor-α. *Biochem. J.* **263:**539–545.

Michie, H. R., Manogue, K. R., Spriggs, D. R., Revhaug, A., O'Dwyer, S., Dinarello, C. A., Cerami, A., Wolff, S. M., and Willmore, D. W. (1988). Detection of circulating tumor necrosis factor after endotoxin administration. *N. Eng. J. Med.* **318:** 1481–1486.

Movat, H. Z., Cybulsky, M. I., Colditz, I. G., Chan, M. K. W., and Dinarello, C. A. (1987). Acute inflammation in gram negative infection: Endotoxin, interleukin-1, tumor necrosis factor and neutrophils. *Fed. Proc.* **46:**97–104.

Nawroth, P. P., Bank, I., Handley, D., Cassimeris, J., Chess, L., and Stern, D. (1986). Tumor necrosis factor/cachectin interacts with endothelial cell receptors to induce release of interleukin 1. *J. Exp. Med.* **163:**1363–1375.

Neta, R., Douches, S., and Oppenheimer, J. J. (1986). Interleukin-1 is a radioprotector. *J. Immunol.* **136:**2483–2485.

Neta, R., Sztein, M. B., Oppenheim, J. J., Gillis, S., and Douches, S. D. (1987). The in vivo effects of interleukin 1. I. Bone marrow cells are induced to cycle after administration of interleukin 1. *J. Immunol.* **139:**1861–1866.

Okusawa, S., Gelfand, J. A., Ikejima, T., Connolly, R. J., and Dinarello, C. A. (1988). Interleukin 1 induces a shock-like state in rabbits. Synergism with tumor necrosis factor and the effect of cyclooxygenase inhibition. *J. Clin. Invest.* **81:**1162–1172.

Ozaki, Y., Ohashi, T., Minami, A., and Nakamura, S. A. (1987). Enhanced resistance of mice to bacterial infection induced by recombinant human interleukin 1α. *Infect. Immun.* **55:**1436–1440.

Patton, J. S., Peters, P. M., McCabe, J., Crase, D., Hansen, S., Chen, A. B., and Liggitt, D. (1987). Development of partial tolerance to the gastrointestinal effects of high doses of recombinant tumor necrosis factor-α in rodents. *J. Clin. Invest.* **80:** 1587–1596.

Pohlman, T. H., and Harlan, J. M. (1989). Human endothelial cell response to lipopolysaccharide, interleukin-1, and tumor necrosis factor is regulated by protein synthesis. *Cell. Immunol.* **119:**41–52.

Pohlman, T. H., Stanness, K. A., Beatty, P. G., Ochs, H. D., and Harlan, J. M. (1986). An endothelial cell surface factor(s) induced in vitro by lipopolysaccharide, interleukin 1, and tumor necrosis factor-alpha increases neutrophil adherence by a CDw18-dependent mechanism. *J. Immunol.* **136:**4548–4553.

Remick, D. G., Kunkel, R. G., Larrick, J. W., and Kunkel, S. L. (1987). Acute in vivo effects of human recombinant tumor necrosis factor. *Lab. Invest.* **56:**583–590.

Rossi, V., Breviario, F., Ghezzi, P., Dejana, E., and Mantovani, A. (1985). Prostaglandin synthesis induced in vascular cells by interleukin-1. *Science* **229:**174.

Royall, J. A., Berkow, R. L., Beckman, J. S., Cunningham, M. K., Matalon, S., and Freeman, B. A. (1989). Tumor necrosis factor and interleukin 1α increase vascular endothelial permeability. *Am. J. Physiol.* **257:**L399–L410.

Sato, N., Goto, T., Haranaka, K., Satomi, N., Nariuchi, H., Mano-Hirano, Y., and Sawasaki, Y. (1986). Actions of tumor necrosis factor on cultured vascular endothelial cells: Morphologic modulation, growth inhibition, and cytotoxicity. *J. Natl. Cancer Inst.* **76:**1113–1118.

Shiki, Y., Meyrick, B. O., Brigham, K. L., and Burger, I. M. (1987). Endotoxin increases superoxide dismutase in cultured bovine pulmonary endothelial cells. *Am. J. Physiol.* **252:**C436–C440.

Sjostrom, K., and Crapo, J. D. (1983). Structural and biochemical adaptive changes in rat lungs after exposure to hypoxia. *Lab. Invest.* **48:**68–79.

Smedley, L. A., Tonnesen, M. G., Snadhaus, R. A., Haslett, C., Guthrie, L. A., Johnston, R. B. Jr., Henson, P. M., and Worthen, G. S. (1986). Neutrophil-mediated injury to endothelial cells: Enhancement by endotoxin and essential role of neutrophil elastase. *J. Clin. Invest.* **77:**1233–1242.

Smith, W. W., Alderman, I. M., and Gillespie, R. F. (1958). Hematopoietic recovery induced by bacterial endotoxin in irradiated mice. *Am. J. Phys.* **192:**549.

Smith, C. W., Marlin, S. D., Rothlein, R., Toman, C., and Anderson, D. C. (1989). Cooperative interactions of LFA-1 and Mac-1 with intercellular adhesion molecule 1 in facilitating adherence and transendothelial migration of human neutrophils in vitro. *J. Clin. Invest.* **83:**2008–2017.

Smith, J., II, Urba, W., Steis, R., Janik, J., Fenton, B., Sharfman, W., Conlon, K., Sznol, M., Creekmore, S., Wells, N., Elwood, L., Keller, J., Hestdal, K., Ewel, C., Rossio, J., Kopp, W., Shimuzu, M., Oppenheim, J., and Longo, D. (1990). A phase I trial of interleukin-1 alpha (IL-1α) alone and in combination with indomethacin. *Lymphokine Res.* *9:*568 (abstract S5.3).

Snapper, J. R., Hutchison, A. A., and Ogletree, M. L. (1983). Effects of cyclooxygenase inhibitors on the alterations in lung mechanics caused by endotoxemia in the unanesthetized sheep. *J. Clin. Invest.* **72:**63–76.

Sonowane, B. R., Yaffe, S. J., Witmer, C. M. (1982). Effects of endotoxin upon rat hepatic microsomal drug metabolism in vivo and in vitro. *Xenobiotica* **12:**303–313.

Spitz, D. R., and Oberley, L. W. (1989). An assay of superoxide dismutase activity in mammalian tissue homogenates. *Anal. Biochem.* **179:**8–18.

Stephens, K. E., Ishizaka, A., Larrick, J. W., and Raffin, T. A. (1988). Tumor necrosis factor causes increased pulmonary permeability and edema. *Am. Rev. Respir. Dis.* **137:**1364–1370.

Stolpen, A. H., Guinan, E. C., Fiers, W., and Pober, J. S. (1986). Recombinant tumor necrosis factor and immune interferon act singly and in combination to reorganize human vascular endothelial cell monolayers. *Am. J. Pathol.* **123:**16–24.

Stork, L., Barczuk, L., Kissinger, M., and Robinson, W. (1989). Interleukin-1 accelerates murine granulocyte recovery following treatment with cyclophosphamide. *Blood* **73:**938–944.

Suffys, P., Beyoert, R., Van Roy, R., and Fiers, W. (1987). Reduced tumor necrosis factor-induced cytotoxicity by inhibitors of the arachidonic acid metabolism. *Biochem. Biophys. Rs. Commun.* **149:**735–743.

Sun, X. M., and Hsueh, W. (1988). Bowel necrosis induced by tumor necrosis factor in rats is mediated by platelet-activating factor. *J. Clin. Invest.* **81:**1328–1331.

Taylor, L., Menconi, M. J., and Polgar, P. (1983). The participation of hydroperoxides and oxygen radicals in the control of prostaglandin synthesis. *J. Biol. Chem.* **258:**6855–6857.

Thet, L. A., Parra, S. C., and Shelburne, J. D. (1984). Repair of oxygen-induced lung injury in adult rats. The role of ornithine decarboxylase and polyamines. *Am. Rev. Respir. Dis.* **129:**174–181.

Tierney, D. F., and Hacker, A. D. (1989). Polyamines, DNA synthesis, and tolerance to hyperoxia of mice and rats. *Am. Rev. Respir. Dis.* **139:**387–392.

Tracey, K. J., Beutler, B., Lowry, S. F., Merryweather, J., Wolpe, S., Milsark, I. W., Hariri, R. J., Fahey, T. J., III, Zentella, A., Albert, J. D., Shires, G. T., and Cerami, A. (1986). Shock and tissue injury induced by human recombinant cachectin. *Science* **234:**470–474.

Tsan, M. F., White, J. E., Santana, T. A., and Lee, C. Y. (1990). Tracheal insufflation of tumor necrosis factor protects rats against oxygen toxicity. *J. Appl. Physiol.* **68:**1211–1219.

Tsan, M. F., Lee, C. Y., and White, J. E. (1991). Interleukin 1 protects rats against oxygen toxicity. *J. Appl. Physiol.* **71:**688–697.

Tsujimoto, M., Yokota, S., Vilcek, J., and Weissman, G. (1986). Tumor necrosis factor provokes superoxide anion generation from neutrophils. *Biochem. Biophys. Res. Commun.* **137:**1094–1100.

Urban, J. L., Shephard, H. M., Rothstein, J. L., Sugarman, B. J., and Schreiber, H. (1986). Tumor necrosis factor: A potent effector molecule for tumor cell killing by activated macrophages. *Proc. Natl. Acad. Sci. USA* **83:**5233–5237.

Van der Meer, J. W. M., Barza, M., Wolff, S. M., and Dinarello, C. A. (1988). A low dose of recombinant interleukin 1 protects granulocytopenic mice from lethal gram-negative infection. *Proc. Natl. Acad. Sci. USA* **85:**1620–1623.

Visner, G. A., Dougall, W. C., Wilson, J. M., Burr, I. A., and Nick, H. S. (1990). Regulation of manganese superoxide dismutase by lipopolysaccharide, interleukin-1, and tumor necrosis factor. Role in the acute inflammatory response. *J. Biol. Chem.* **265:**2856–2864.

Vogel, S. N., Kaufman, E. N., Tate, M. D., and Neta, R. (1988). Recombinant interleukin-1α and recombinant tumor necrosis factor α synergize in vivo to induce early endotoxin tolerance and associated hematopoietic changes. *Infect. Immun.* **56:** 2650–2657.

Warner, B. B., Burhans, M. S., Clark, J. C., and Wispé, J. R. (1991). Tumor necrosis factor-α increases Mn-SOD expression: Protection against oxidant injury. *Am. J. Physiol.* **260:**L296–L301.

White, C. W., and Ghezzi, P. (1989). Protection against pulmonary oxygen toxicity by interleukin-1 and tumor necrosis factor: Role of antioxidant enzymes and effect of cyclooxygenase inhibitors. *Biotherapy* **1:**361–367.

White, C. W., Ghezzi, P., Dinarello, C. A., Caldwell, S. A., McMurtry, I. F., and Repine, J. E. (1987). Recombinant tumor necrosis factor/cachectin and interleukin 1 pretreatment decreases lung oxidized glutathione accumulation, lung injury, and mortality in rats exposed to hyperoxia. *J. Clin. Invest.* **79:**1868–1873.

White, C. W., Jackson, J. H., McMurty, I. F., and Repine, J. E. (1988). Hypoxia increases glutathione redox cycle and protects rat lungs against oxidants. *J. Appl. Physiol.* **65:**2605–2616.

White, C. W., Ghezzi, P., McMahon, S., Dinarello, C. A., and Repine, J. E. (1989).

Cytokines increase rat lung antioxidant enzymes during exposure to hyperoxia. *J. Appl. Physiol.* **66:**1003–1007.

White, C. W., Avraham, K. B., Shanley, P. F., and Groner, Y. (1991). Transgenic mice with expression of elevated levels of copper,zinc superoxide dismutase in the lungs are resistant to pulmonary oxygen toxicity. *J. Clin. Invest.* **87:**2162–2168.

Wise, W. C., Cook, J. A., Eller, T., and Halushka, P. V. (1980). Ibuprofen improves survival from endotoxin shock in the rat. *J. Pharmacol. Exp. Ther.* **215:**160–164.

Wong, G. H. W., and Goeddel, D. V. (1988). Induction of manganous superoxide dismutase by tumor necrosis factor: Possible protective mechanism. *Science* **242:** 941–944.

Wong, G. H. W., Elwell, J. H., Oberley, L. W., and Goeddel, D. V. (1989). Manganous superoxide dismutase is essential for cellular resistance to cytotoxicity of tumor necrosis factor. *Cell* **58:**923–931.

Yamauchi, N., Kuriyama, H., Watanabe, N., Neda, H., Maeda, M., and Niitsu, Y. (1989). Intracellular hydroxyl radical production induced by recombinant human tumor necrosis factor and its implication in the killing of tumor cells in vitro. *Cancer Res.* **49:**1671–1675.

Zimmerman, R. J., Chan, A., and Leadon, S. A. (1989). Oxidative damage in murine tumor cells treated in vitro be recombinant human tumor necrosis factor. *Cancer Res.* **49:**1644–1648.

8

Endothelial Cell–Derived Novel Chemotactic Cytokines

STEVEN L. KUNKEL, THEODORE STANDIFORD, ANDREW P. METINKO, and ROBERT M. STREITER

University of Michigan Medical School
Ann Arbor, Michigan

I. Introduction

Like many of the individual events that occur during inflammation, the recruitment of inflammatory cells is dictated by a cascade of specific reactions. For the chemotactic response to occur successfully, each of these reactions must occur in a concordant manner. Interestingly, each step appears to contain unique induction and suppression mechanisms which can effectively modulate the movement of inflammatory cells. Although individual aspects of the chemotactic response are well understood, the entire process remains an enigma. The importance of the chemotactic response is underscored by the redundancy that is inherent in this system. For example, a number of protein and lipid compounds are known to possess chemotactic activity for inflammatory cells. Historically, a variety of peptide, protein, and lipid mediators, with different chemical structures, have been identified that possess similar recruitment activities (Table 1). These chemotactic factors have been identified from sources ranging from bacteria (FMLP) to cells (LTB_4 and PAF) to serum proteins (split product of the fifth component of complement, C5a). As shown in Fig. 1, these mediators can interact via individual receptors and activate a number of granulocyte functions in addition to chemotaxis, including secretion of enzymes and release of oxygen metabolites.

Table 1 Mediators That Have Been Identified As Possessing Chemotactic Activity for Various Inflammatory Cells

C5a	Interleukin-8 (IL-8)
Leukotriene B_4 (LTB_4)	Neutrophil activating factor-2 (NAP-2)
Platelet activating factor (PAF)	GRO
f-met-leu-phe (FMLP)	Monocyte chemotactic protein (MCP)
Transforming growth factor (TGFβ)	

II. Initiation of Cell Movement

The sequence of events that results in the recruitment of inflammatory cells from the peripheral blood to a site of tissue injury is complex. While the vasculature is undergoing a number of physical changes, such as vasoconstriction or vasodilation, the inflammatory cells must adhere to the endothelium, recognize a chemotactic signal, and then undergo directed movement to an area of inflammation (Brown et al., 1989; Hoffstein et al., 1982; Snyderman and Pike, 1984). The importance of the chemotactic response is underscored by the fact that this process can occur in a normal manner even in the presence of altered vessel hemostasis. The cascade of cellular events, which leads to the successful elicitation of inflammatory cells, is influenced by the induction and subsequent regulation of signals that modulate this dynamic recruitment process. As shown by the electron micrograph in Fig. 2, circulating granulocytes in the lumen of a vessel must travel through the endothelium and basement membrane and transverse the interstitium in order for these cells to participate in an inflammatory response. The movement of these cells is fundamental to the entire process of inflammation.

As discussed previously, the importance of a successful chemotactic response during inflammation is accentuated by the large number of different chemotactic factors that may be generated during an immune response. Many of these chemotaxins are structurally unrelated and possess unique receptors, yet, all induce the directed migration of inflammatory cells. While a number of different soluble signals may be available to interact with granulocytes during the recruitment process, the cellular interactions involved in chemotaxis are more limited. A good example is the interactions that lead to the adherence between leukocytes and endothelial cells. This event is required for the initiation of in vivo chemotaxis. The expression of adherence proteins on the surface of endothelial cells, which binds peripheral blood leukocytes to the vascular wall, is one of the first characterized events of an elicitation response. These endothelial cell-derived proteins include intercellular adhesion molecule-1 (ICAM) (Roth-

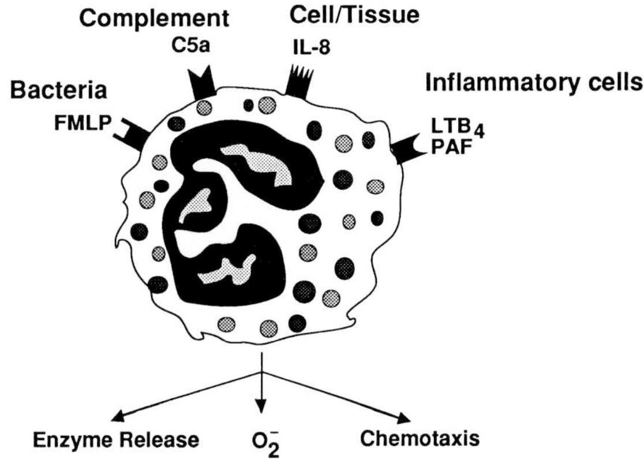

Figure 1 Stimulation of neutrophils can occur via a number of inflammatory mediators that bind unique receptors. Although neutrophils can bind to a number of different receptors, the neutrophil activation events are relatively the same.

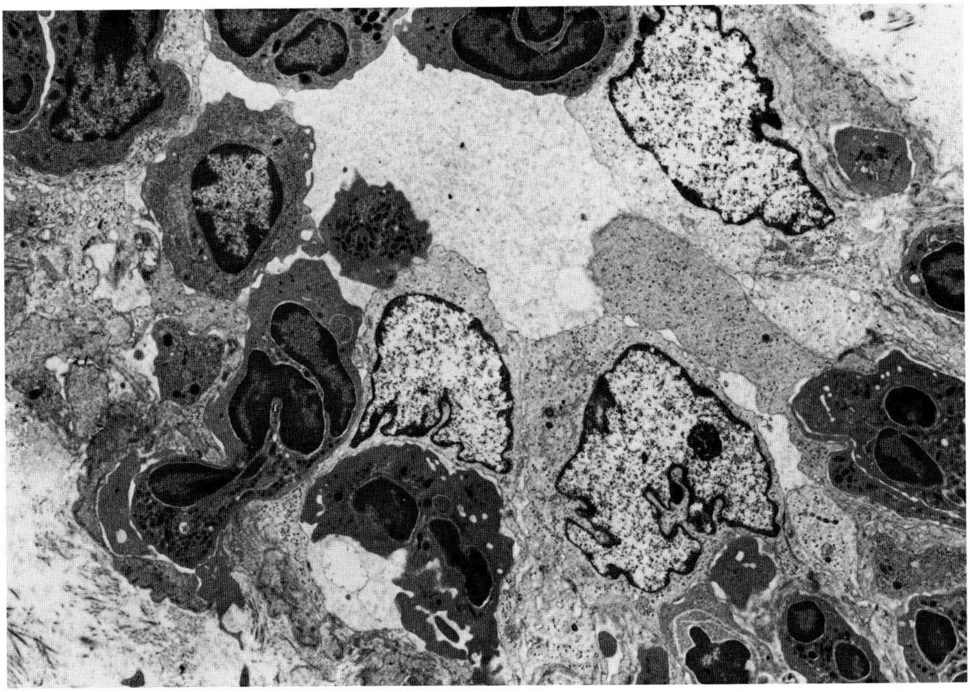

Figure 2 Electron micrograph of the chemotactic response of neutrophils moving from the lumen of a vessel into an interstitial area of inflammation.

lein et al., 1986) and endothelial leukocyte adhesion molecule (ELAM) (Bevilacqua et al., 1989). The expression of the adherence proteins above appear to be driven by specific cytokines, including interleukin-1 (IL-1) and tumor necrosis factor-α (TNF) (Pohlman et al., 1986; Schleimer and Rutledge 1986). As shown schematically in Fig. 3, IL-1 and TNF are cytokines that have a potent effect on the expression of ICAM and ELAM. It is apparent that either IL-1 or TNF may be expressed early during inflammation and set the stage for subsequent events. Although alterations in the vasculature, such as changes in blood pH or oxygenation, may be a more proximal event and important in priming the inflammatory system, little is known regarding the role of physical alterations and the initiation of inflammation, albeit these changes could be the mechanism that induces IL-1 and TNF gene expression. An interesting aspect of the adherence phenomenon is that for leukocytes to migrate out of the confines of the vessel, the binding of leukocytes and endothelial cells must be reversible. The binding interaction must be engaged to localize the cells to an inflammatory area, yet in a temporal sequence, the cells must be released to continue their directed movement. The events that initiate and regulate the expression of these endothelial cell-derived proteins have received much attention, as these mediators represent an intricate mechanism for the successful movement of cells from the vascular lumen to the interstitium.

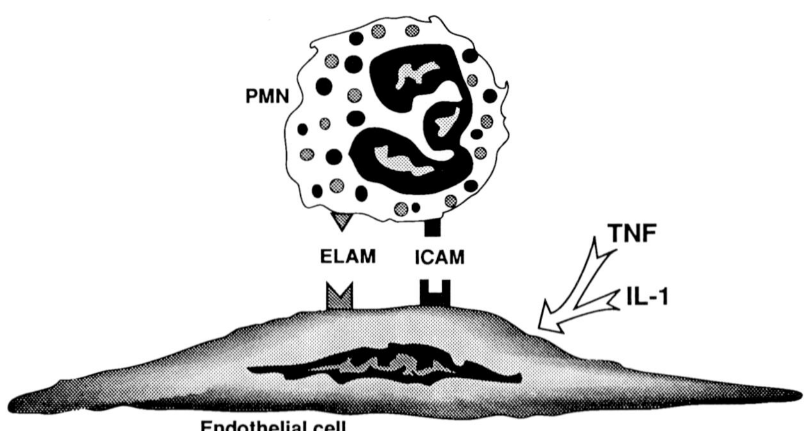

Figure 3 The stimulation of endothelial cells by IL-1 and/or TNF results in the expression of specific adherence proteins ICAM and ELAM on the surface of endothelial cells.

III. Chemotactic Cytokines: Interleukin-8/Neutrophil Activating Protein (IL-8) and Monocyte Chemotactic Protein (MCP)

There is little doubt that many of the mediators above play an important role in the recruitment of inflammatory cells, but recent studies have provided evidence that additional chemotactic proteins are important for the successful elicitation of cells (Baggiolini et al., 1989; Larsen et al., 1989; Robinson et al., 1989; Schroeder et al., 1987; Yoshimura et al., 1987, 1989a). The identification of a family of chemotactic cytokines synthesized from both immune and nonimmune cells has renewed interest in the mechanism of the recruitment process (Anisowicz et al., 1987; Brown et al., 1989; Strieter et al., 1989a, b, c; Thornton et al., 1990). As shown in Table 2, a family of structurally related proteins have been identified with chemotactic activity for various inflammatory cells. These polypeptides belong to a novel supergene family of chemotactic cytokines and share a high degree of homology at the nucleotide level (Brown et al., 1989; Matsushima and Oppenheim, 1989). This family can be further subdivided according to their amino acid sequence. Specifically, the position of the four cysteine residues can be used to categorize these proteins as members of a C–X–C family, where the first pair of cysteines are separated by one amino acid, and the C–C family, where the first pair of cysteines are in juxtaposition to each other. A number of proteins have been isolated, sequenced, and cloned that belong to either the C–X–C or C–C supergene family (Table 2). The chemotactic cytokine that possess activity for neutrophils (IL-8) belongs to the C–X–C family, while the monocyte chemotactic protein (MCP) is a member of the C–C family. All of the neutrophil activating proteins share the C–X–C configuration, including IL-8, NAP-2, and GRO (Matsushima and Oppenheim, 1989). Investigations have assessed the granulocyte activating potential of all three of these related proteins

Table 2 Representative Members of the Chemotactic Cytokine Supergene Family That Belong to C–X–C or C–C Subgroup

C–X–C	C–C
Interleukin-8 (IL-8)	Monocyte chemotactic protein (MCP)
GRO	JE
NAP-2	RANTES
Platelet factor 4	MIP-1
Platelet basic protein	TCA-3
β-Thromboglobulin	

Table 3 In Vitro and In Vivo Effects of IL-8, NAP-2, and GRO on Neutrophil Function

	IL-8	NAP-2	GRO
CA^{2+}	++++	+++	+++
Enzyme release	+++	+++	+++
Respiratory burst	++	+	+
Chemotaxis	++++	+++	+++
Infiltration in vivo	+++	+++	+++

and have found them to induce a number of in vitro and in vivo events (Table 3). The most active member of the supergene family appears to be IL-8, as this protein can fully activate neutrophils in vitro and induce neutrophil movement in vivo. The chemotactic activity of IL-8 for neutrophils is as potent as other well-characterized chemotaxins, such as C5a and FMLP. As shown in Fig. 4, IL-8 can induce the directed movement of neutrophils in vitro, using a modified Boyden chamber, in a dose-dependent manner. Concentrations of IL-8 between 1.0 and 10 ng/mL significantly increased the movement of human neutrophils in vitro. The chemotactic response of neutrophils to IL-8 reached a plateau at concentrations above 10 ng/mL. Peripheral blood monocytes did not demonstrate directed migration to IL-8 over a wide dose–response range.

Interestingly, fibroblasts (Strieter et al., 1989b), epithelial cells (Elner et al., 1990), hepatocytes (Thornton et al., 1990), and endothelial cells (Strieter et al., 1989a) are all important cellular sources of these chemotactic cytokines. The expression of polypeptide mediators by these cells is an important consideration, as these participants must now be recognized as important effector cells during an inflammatory response. There is little doubt that investigations into the expression of these factors by nonimmune cells represent a new avenue of study regarding mechanisms that regulate the chemotactic response.

IV. Interleukin-8 Gene Expression by Endothelial Cells

A number of investigations have now identified endothelial cells as an important source for the production of many different inflammatory mediators (Table 4). Of particular interest is the expression of cytokines with diverse activities. These cytokines include members of the interleukin family (IL-1, IL-6, IL-8) (Miossec et al., 1986), chemotactic factors (Strieter et al., 1989a), and growth factors (Di Carleto and Bowen-Pope, 1983). The production of chemotactic cytokines by endothelial cells is of particular interest, as these cells are anatomically located

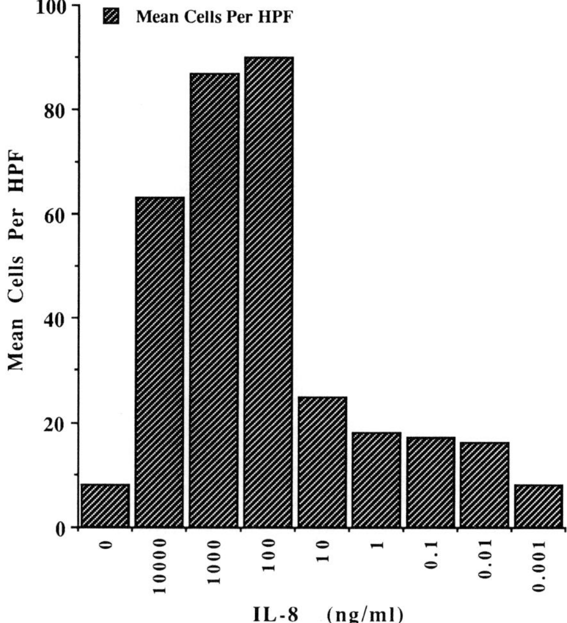

Figure 4 Dose-dependent increase in the directed migration of neutrophils in response to human interleukin-8.

to provide a communication link between cells in the lumen of a vessel and the interstitium. Initial studies from our laboratories demonstrated that IL-8 gene expression could be induced by both exogenous signals, such as bacteria-derived endotoxin (lipopolysaccharide) or endogenous, host-derived mediators. Both IL-1 and TNF are endogenous signals that possess potent activity for the induction of endothelial cell IL-8 bioactivity. Endothelial cells stimulated with as little as 100 pg/mL of IL-1 beta could synthesize IL-8, while undectable levels were observed in a resting state. Either IL-1 beta or TNF could induce a time-depen-

Table 4 Inflammatory Mediators Derived from Endothelial Cells

Interleukin-1α, β	Transforming growth factor-β
Interleukin-6	MHC I, II
Interleukin-8	Arginine metabolites
Monocyte chemotactic protein	Arachidonate metabolites
Tissue factor	Oxygen metabolites

dent increase in endothelial cell-derived IL-8 mRNA. By 0.5 h post IL-1 beta challenge, human endothelial cells were found to express IL8 mRNA. (Fig. 5). Similar results were observed using LPS as the stimulus. This expression persisted for longer than 24 h, as long as the stimulus remained in the media. Washout experiments demonstrated that the half-live of IL-8 mRNA is less than 1 h, suggesting that stimulated cells are constantly transcribing new mRNA for IL-8 and not stabilizing a pool of intracellular mRNA.

To further address the molecular level of IL-8 regulation, endothelial cells were treated with cycloheximide (5 μg/mL) concomitantly with either IL-1β or TNF. These studies demonstrated that cycloheximide alone was relatively ineffective in causing an induction of IL-8 mRNA, but the combination of IL-1β or TNF resulted in a superinduction of IL-8 mRNA. These data support the view that either IL-1β or TNF can serve as primary inducers of IL-8 gene expression. That is, de novo protein synthesis is not needed in order for IL-1β or TNF to serve as a stimulus for the expression of IL-8 mRNA. In addition, the augmentation of IL-8 mRNA by cycloheximide plus IL-1β or TNF suggests that IL-8 gene expression is regulated by a intracellular repressor protein(s) that may be involved in IL-8 mRNA degradation or instability. A physiologic correlate that appears to mimic some of the stabilizing effects of cycloheximide on augmenting endothelial cell-derived IL-8 mRNA is gamma interferon. The addition of low levels of human recombinant gamma interferon to human endothelial cells resulted in a threefold increase in IL-1β- or TNF-induced IL-8 mRNA. Gamma

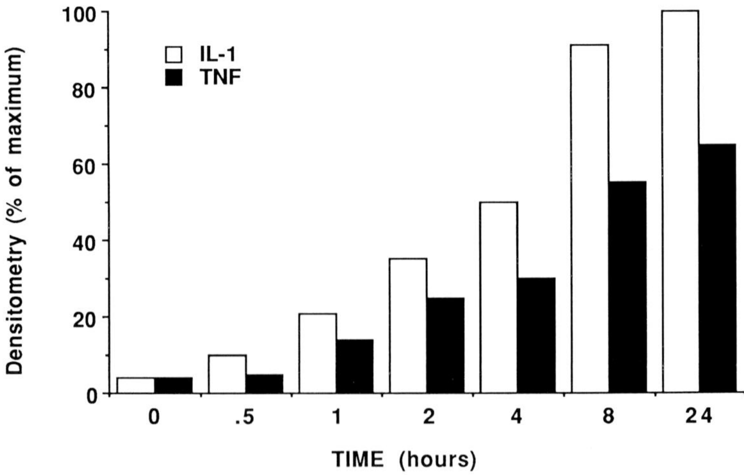

Figure 5 Kinetic analysis of IL-1β- or TNF-induced IL-8 gene expression by human endothelial cells. The bar graphs represent laser densitometer analysis of the autoradiographs of various Northern blots.

interferon alone did not result in the expression of endothelial cell IL-8. These observations are quite interesting, as gamma interferon has been demonstrated to increase the expression of TNF mRNA by LPS-triggered macrophages (Collart et al., 1986). In the latter studies, gamma interferon was shown to stabilize the pool of macrophage TNF mRNA. Thus there are similarities between the molecular mechanism(s) of IL-8 gene expression by endothelial cells and the expression of certain macrophage-derived cytokines.

Further studies from our laboratory have also attempted to assess the events that lead to suppression of IL-8 mRNA expression by endothelial cells. Dexamethasone, prostaglandin E_2, and interleukin-4 (IL-4) were studied for their ability to reduce the expression of IL-8 mRNA. These compounds were chosen as they have been identified as regulating the expression of different cytokines (Kunkel et al., 1988; Remick et al., 1989; Standiford et al., 1990). For example, IL-4 has been shown to suppress the accumulation of IL-1, TNF, and IL-8 mRNA expression from LPS-stimulated human blood monocytes (Hart et al., 1989; Standiford et al., 1990). In our studies the addition of either IL-4, dexamethasone, or PGE_2 in the presence of LPS did not reduce the expression of human endothelial cell–derived IL-8 mRNA. As shown by the densitometer scan of the Northern blot in Fig. 6, neither IL-4, PGE, nor dexamethasone altered the expression of IL-8 mRNA. The studies above demonstrate that endothelial cells are a rich source of IL-8 and the expression of this chemotactic cytokine is not easily regulated.

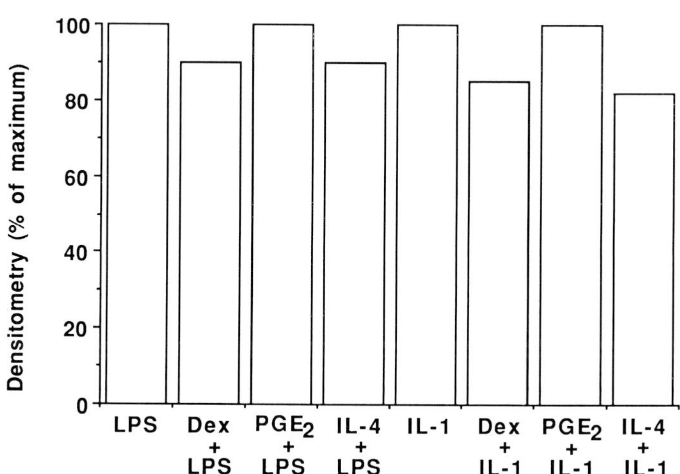

Figure 6 Inability of dexamethasone (10 n*M*), prostaglandin E_2 (100 n*M*), or interleukin-4 (1 ng/mL) to regulate interleukin-8 gene expression. Bar graphs represent laser densitometer analysis of the autoradiographs of the specific Northern blots.

V. Monocyte Chemotactic Protein (MCP) Expression by Endothelial Cells

An additional chemotactic cytokine that has generated a great deal of interest is monocyte chemotactic protein (MCP). This chemotactic cytokine was originally isolated and cloned from a human glioma cell line (Yoshimura et al., 1989b). MCP is actually two proteins, MCPα and MCPβ (Leonard and Yoshimura, 1990). The two proteins appear to be due to posttranscriptional modification of a single gene product, as the amino acid composition of the two proteins is nearly identical. As a chemotactic factor, MCP possesses the unique attribute of eliciting only peripheral blood monocytes. Yet chemotaxis is not the only activity of this protein. Recent studies have identified MCP as a mononuclear phagocytic cell activating factor. The addition of MCP to cocultures of monocytes and tumor cells resulted in the inhibition of the growth of the tumor cells.

Our studies have focused on the expression of MCP mRNA by various cells. As with IL-8, MCP is a product of many cells. Epithelial cells, fibroblasts, and endothelial cells (Strieter et al., 1989c) are all capable of synthesizing MCP. Of particular interest is the expression of MCP mRNA by human endothelial cells. In response to a wide dose range of TNF (20 pg/mL to 20 ng/mL), endothelial cells were shown to express increasing levels of MCP mRNA. Laser densitometer of Northern blot analysis has shown that significant expression of endothelial cell MCP mRNA was observed at 200 pg/mL of TNF, while a plateau in MCP mRNA was reached at 20 ng/mL (Fig. 7). Addition studies demonstrated that MCP mRNA expression was induced in a time-dependent manner by either IL-1β-, TNF-, or LPS-stimulated endothelial cells. Each of the agents above was capable of inducing MCP mRNA production by 30 min post stimulation. By Northern blot analysis, MCP and IL-8 were identified as 0.7 and 1.8 kb mRNA species, respectively. Endothelial cells in the unstimulated state did not constitutively express MCP mRNA. Endothelial cells were unique with respect to the expression of IL-8 and MCP by nonimmune cells in that these cells respond to LPS, as well as host-derived cytokines. Epithelial cells and fibroblasts could generate IL-8 and MCP mRNA, but only to IL-1β and TNF. Thus epithelial cells and fibroblast expression of chemotactic cytokines is dependent on a host response that generates specific inducing cytokines, such as IL-1 and TNF. The latter phenomenon is indicative of cytokine networking, whereby a primary signal causes the synthesis of proximal cytokines (IL-1 or TNF), which in turn can induce the production of additional cytokines (IL-8 or MCP). This cascade of events is responsible for the controlled production of specific mediators which are needed to initiate, maintain, and finally, resolve an inflammatory response.

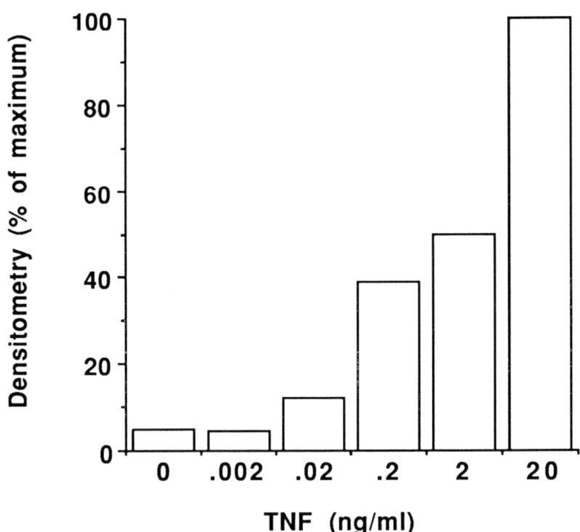

Figure 7 Expression of endothelial cell MCP mRNA in response to graded doses of TNF. The bar graphs represent laser densitometer of the specific Northern blots for the MCP mRNA.

Recent studies have proposed alternate roles for endothelial cell derived chemotactic cytokines. For example, Gimbrone et al. (1989) have described a endothelial cell-derived IL-8 as a leukocyte adhesion inhibitor factor. The predominate IL-8 species identified by this group of investigators has 77 amino acids compared to the predominate 72 amino acid species isolated from monocytes. In provocative studies using the 77 amino acid species of endothelial cell–derived IL-8, the addition of IL-8 to IL-1 activated endothelial cells attenuated the normal adhesion of neutrophils (Gimbrone et al., 1989). These investigations suggest that IL-8 may possess activities far removed from its chemotactic activity. This observation may be explained by the potential of IL-8 to modulate the adherence phenomenon. For example, IL-8 may play a key role in reversing the adherence of granulocytes to the endothelium. Other studies provide data that IL-8 may have immuno-enhancing activities (Matsushima and Oppenheim, 1989). This hypothesis is based on data demonstrating that IL-8 can induce a profound neutrophilia when administered in vivo. In addition, the high concentration and relatively widespread synthesis of IL-8 by a variety of cells suggests that these chemotactic cytokines may have alternative activities. The expression of IL-8 by noninflammatory cells raises the speculation that these factors may be involved in collagen deposition and fibrotic responses. Further analyses are clearly needed to understand more fully the role of these cytokines in health and disease.

Acknowledgments

The authors wish to thank the secretarial support of Peggy Otto. This work was supported in part by NIH Grants HL-31693, HL-35276, HL-02401, and DK-38149. Additional support was provided by the Council on Tobacco Research, American Lung Association. Dr. Strieter is a RJR Nabisco Research Scholar.

References

Anisowicz, A., Bardwell, L., and Sager, R. (1987). Constitutive overexpression of a growth-related gene in transformed Chinese hamster and human cells. *Proc. Natl. Acad. Sci. USA* **84:**7188–7192.

Baggiolini, M., Walz, A., and Kunkel, S. L. (1989). Neutrophil-activating peptide-1/interleukin 8, a novel cytokine that activates neutrophils. *J. Clin. Invest.* **84:**1045–1049.

Bevilacqua, M. P., Stengelin, S., Gimbrone, M. A., and Seed, B., (1989). Endothelial-leukocyte adhesion molecule-1: An inducible receptor for neutrophils related to complement regulatory proteins and lectins. *Science* **243:**1160–1165.

Brown, K. D., Zurawski, S. M., Mosmann, T. R., and Zurawski, G. (1989). A family of small inducible proteins secreted by leukocytes are members of a new super family that includes leukocyte and fibroblast-derived inflammatory agents, growth factors, and indicators of various activation processes. *J. Immunol.* **142:**679–687.

Charo, I. F., Yuen, C., Perez, H. D., Goldstein, I. M., (1986). Chemotactic peptides modulate adherence of human polymorphonuclear leukocytes to monolayers of cultured endothelial cells. *J. Immunol.* **136:**3412–3419.

Collart, M. A., Belin, D., Vassalli, J., DeKossodo, S., and Vassalli, D., (1986). Gamma interferon enhances macrophage transcription of the tumor necrosis factor/cachectin, interleukin-1, and urokinase genes, which are controlled by short-lived repression. *J. Exp. Med.* **164:**2113–2119.

Di Carleto, P. E., Bowen-Pope, D. F. (1983). Cultured endothelial cells produce a platelet-derived growth factor-like protein. *Proc. Natl. Acad. Sci. USA* **80:**1919–1924.

Elner, V. M., Strieter, R. M., Elner, S. G., Baggiolini, M., Lindley, I., and Kunkel, S. L. (1990). Neutrophil chemotactic factor (IL-8) expression by cytokine treated retinal pigmented epithelial cells. *Am. J. Pathol.* **136:**745–750.

Gimbrone, M. A., Obin, M. S., Brock, A. F., Luis, E. A., Hass, P. E., Hebert, C. A., Yip, Y. K., Leung, D. W., Lowe, D. G., Kohr, W. J., Darbonne, W. C., Bechtol, K. B., and Baker, J. B. (1989). Endothelial Interleukin-8: A novel inhibitor of leukocyte–endothelial interactions. *Science* **246:**1601–1603.

Hart, P. H., Vitti, G. F., Burgess, D. R., Whitty, G. A., Piccoli, D. S., and Hamilton, J. H. (1989). Potential antiinflammatory effects of IL-4: Suppression of human monocyte tumor necrosis factor, interleukin-1, and prostaglandin E. *Proc. Natl. Acad. Sci. USA* **86:**3803–3810.

Hoffstein, S. T., Friedman, R. S., and Weissmann, G. (1982). Degranulation, membrane addition, and shape change during chemotactic factor-induced aggregation of human neutrophils. *J. Cell Biol.* **95:**234–244.

Kunkel, S. L., Spengler, M., May, M. A., Spengler, R., Larrick, J., and Remick, D. G. (1988). Prostaglandin E regulates macrophage-derived tumor necrosis factor gene expression. *J. Biol. Chem.* **263:**5380–5384.

Larsen, C. G., Anderson, A. O., Appella, E., Oppenheim, J. J., and Matsushima, K. (1989). The neutrophil-activating protein (NAP-1) is also chemotactic for T lymphocytes. *Science* **243:**1464–1466.

Leonard, E. J., and Yoshimura, T. (1990). Human monocyte chemoattractant protein-1 (MCP-1). *Immunol. Today* **11:**97–100.

Matsushima, K., and Oppenheim, J. J. (1989). Interleukin 8 and MCAF: Novel inflammatory cytokines inducible by IL-1 and TNF. *Cytokine* **1:**2–13.

Miossec, P., Cavender, D., and Ziff, M. (1986). Production of interleukin-1 by human endothelial cells. *J. Immunol.* **136:**2486–2495.

Pohlman, T. H., Stanness, K. A., Beatty, P. G., Ochs, H. D., and Harlan, J. M. (1986). An endothelial cell surface factor(s) induced in vitro by lipopolysaccharide, interleukin-1, and tumor necrosis factor-alpha increases neutrophil adherence by a CDw18-dependent mechanism. *J. Immunol.* **136:**4548–4553.

Remick, D. G., Strieter, R. M., Lynch, J. P., Nguyen, D., Eskandari, M., and Kunkel, S. L. (1989). In vivo dynamics of murine tumor necrosis factor gene expression. Kinetics of dexamethasone-induced suppression. *Lab. Invest.* **60:**766–771.

Robinson, E. A., Yoshimura, T., Leonard, E. J., Tanaka, S., Griffin, P. R., Shabanowitz, J., Hunt, D. F., and Appella, E. (1989). Complete amino acid sequence of a human monocyte chemoattractant, a putative mediator of cellular immune reactions. *Proc. Natl. Acad. Sci. USA* **86:**1850–1854.

Rothlein, R., Dustin, M. L., Marlin, S. D., Springer, T. A. (1986). An intercellular adhesion molecule (ICAM-1) distinct from LFA-1. *J. Immunol.* **138:**4298–4302.

Schleimer, R. P., and Rutledge, B. K. (1986). Cultured human vascular endothelial cells acquire adhesiveness for neutrophils after stimulation with interleukin 1, endotoxin, and tumor-promoting phorbol esters. *J. Immunol.* **136:**649–654.

Schroeder, J., Mrowietz, U., Morita, E., and Christophers, E. (1987). Purification and partial biochemical characterization of a human monocyte-derived, neutrophil-activating peptide that lacks interleukin-1 activity. *J. Immunol.* **139:**3474–3483.

Snyderman, R., and Pike, M. C. (1984). Chemoattractant receptors on phagocytic cells. *Annu. Rev. Immunol.* **2:**257–281.

Standiford, T. J., Strieter, R. M., Chensue, S. W., Westwick, J., Kasahara, K., and Kunkel, S. L. (1990). IL-4 inhibits the expression of IL-8 from stimulated human monocytes *J. Immunol.* **145:**1435–1439.

Strieter, R. M., Kunkel, S. L., Showell, H. J., Remick, D. G., Phan, S. H., Ward, P. A., and Marks, R. M. (1989a). Endothelial cell gene expression of a neutrophil chemotactic factor by TNF, LPS, and IL-1. *Science* **243:**1467–1469.

Strieter, R. M., Phan, S. H., Showell, H. J., Remick, D. G., Marks, R. M., and Kunkel, S. L. (1989b). Monokine-induced neutrophil chemotactic factor gene expression in human fibroblasts. *J. Biol. Chem.* **264:**10621–10626.

Strieter, R. M., Wiggins, R., Phan, S. H., Warram, B. L., Showell, H. J., Remick, D. G., Chensue, S. W., and Kunkel, S. L. (1989c). Monocyte chemotactic protein gene expression by cytokine treated human fibroblasts and endothelial cells. **162:** 694–700.

Thornton, A. J., Strieter, R. M., Lindley, I., Baggiolini, M., and Kunkel, S. L. (1990). Cytokine-induced gene expression of a neutrophil chemotactic factor/IL-8 in human hepatocytes. *J. Immunol.* **144:**2609–2613.

Yoshimura, T., Matsushima, K., Tanaka, S., Robinson, E. A., Appella, E., Oppenheim, J. J., and Leonard, E. J. (1987). Purification of a human monocyte-derived neutrophil chemotactic factor that has peptide sequence similarity to other host defense cytokines. *Proc. Natl. Acad. Sci. USA* **84:**9233–9237.

Yoshimura, T., Robinson, E. A., Appella, E., Matsushima, K., Showaiter, S. D., Skeel, A., and Leonard, E. J. (1989a). Three forms of monocyte-derived neutrophil chemotactic factor distinguished by different lengths of the amino-acid terminal sequence. *Mol. Immunol.* **26:**87–93.

Yoshimura, T., Robinson, E. A., Tanaka, S., Eppella, E., Kuratsu, J. I., and Leonard, E. J. (1989b). Purification and amino acid analysis of two human glio-derived monocyte chemoattractants. *J. Exp. Med.* **169:**1449–1459.

9

Impaired Pulmonary Vascular Smooth Muscle Function in Lung Injury

C. SUBAH PACKER and RODNEY A. RHOADES

Indiana University School of Medicine
Indianapolis, Indiana

I. Introduction

With the advances in the last decade, it is increasingly apparent that pulmonary circulation is not merely a passive conduit involved in gas exchange, but is a complex system composed of highly differentiated cells with specialized functions that play key roles in health and disease. The endothelial cells that line the pulmonary vessels have received much attention in this regard and have been reviewed in previous chapters. However, smooth muscle is by far the most numerous cell type in the pulmonary vessel, yet its functional properties are the least well understood. This is particularly important since smooth muscle in pulmonary vessels often responds differently than does smooth muscle of the systemic vasculature to agonists and to other bloodborne signals.

How pulmonary arterial smooth muscle (PASM) is altered with lung injury is even less well understood. Since the lung receives all of the cardiac output and is the only organ literally exposed to the external environment, the endothelial/smooth muscle cells are especially susceptible to injury. The effects of lung injury on PASM can occur directly from bloodborne signals, environmental oxidants, altered endothelial-derived signals, or from a combination of these factors. In this chapter we examine recent findings of the effects of lung injury on PASM function. The focus is on four of the more prominent types of injury:

altered oxygen tension (chronic-hypoxia and hyperoxia), oxygen radicals, ischemia-reperfusion, and inflammation.

II. Chronic Hypoxia-Induced Pulmonary Hypertension

Chronic hypoxia affects pulmonary and systemic circulation oppositely, eliciting pulmonary vasoconstriction while relaxing systemic vascular smooth muscle (Fishman, 1976; Heath and Williams, 1981). Chronic hypoxia is one of the principal stimuli to evoke pulmonary hypertension while having no effect on systemic blood pressures. Chronic hypoxia-induced hypertension can result from either of two mechanisms. One is chronic airway obstruction (e.g., chronic bronchitis or cystic fibrosis), and the other is exposure to lower ambient $P0_2$ levels (i.e., living at high altitude). In either case pulmonary hypertension occurs when P_AO_2 remains less than 75 torr (Reeves and Grover, 1984). This level of hypoxia corresponds to an altitude of about 2100 m.

Normal pulmonary arterial mean pressure in humans is 14 mm Hg. Pulmonary hypertension is defined as having sustained mean pressure greater than 18 mmHg (Reeves and Grover, 1975). Pulmonary hypertension causes right ventricular hypertrophy and is often associated with cor pulmonale, which, in turn, generally leads to recurrent heart failure (especially with chronic obstructive disorders). However, it should be pointed out that millions of people who live at high altitude have pulmonary hypertension, live normal, active lives, and are free of any signs of heart failure. In fact, these individuals have pulmonary arterial pressures comparable to those of individuals with chronic obstructive lung disease.

The pulmonary circulation, which is characterized as a low-resistance, high-compliance system, is markedly altered with chronic hypoxia. Structural remodeling involves thickening of the blood vessel walls by hypertrophy and hyperplasia of PASM and deposition of excessive connective tissue (Reeves and Grover, 1984; Jones et al., 1985a). Several specific changes occur in arterial structure. First, the large cross-sectional area of the arterial tree, which is normally an area of low resistance, is significantly reduced (Meyrick and Reid, 1980). Second, there is wall thickening (especially thickening of the adventitia) and a reduced lumen that can be seen from pulmonary arteriograms of the large arteries (Jones et al., 1985a). Vessel remnants are not observed, suggesting that the reduction in arterial/alveolar density is due to functional narrowing of vessels rather than to vessel obliteration (Fried and Reid, 1984). Third, smooth muscle appears in the walls of arteries that are not normally muscular, and the walls of previously muscular arteries become abnormally thick (Jones et al., 1985b; Heath and Smith, 1983). Fourth, there is a significant loss of small pulmonary arterioles (Hislop and Reid, 1976). Finally, there is a selective increase in collagen and elastin deposition (Meyrick and Reid, 1980; Hislop and Reid, 1976; Kerr, et al., 1984 and 1987).

While much has been learned from extensive investigations of the structural properties of the pulmonary vascular walls, it has only been recently that functional properties of PASM have been examined. Some studies of PASM reactivity and responsiveness have been carried out on preparations from animals with pulmonary hypertension. McMurty et al. (1978) showed an increase in reactivity to angiotensin and prostaglandin $F_{2\alpha}$ in rat lung. Paterson et al. (1988) also showed an increased reactivity to leukotrienes (LTD_{4}) in the rat pulmonary artery with chronic hypoxia. However, Tozzi et al. (1989) reported no change in reactivity to prostaglandin $F_{2\alpha}$, while reactivity to angiotensin II, norepinephrine, and high KCl was decreased in rat lungs exposed to chronic hypoxia. Additionally, Porcelli and Bergman (1983) reported that hypoxia converts vasoconstriction in response to histamine and norepinephrine to vasodilation. There is some evidence to suggest that this change in response to norepinephrine is due to an effect of pulmonary PO_2 on receptors (Cutaia and Friedrich, 1987).

Given the demonstrated importance of smooth muscle in the control of pulmonary vascular tone, we chose to investigate both the biochemical and mechanical properties of PASM (Roepke et al., 1988, 1991; Griffith et al., 1990). Male Sprague-Dawley rats were exposed to 10% oxygen for 2 weeks (controls breathed room air). Hypoxia-induced pulmonary hypertension was verified by a significant increase in right-to-left ventricular weight ratios (0.40 vs. 0.25) and significantly elevated right ventricular pressure (16 vs. 10 mmHg). To verify that pulmonary arterial smooth muscle from hypoxia-induced pulmonary hypertensive is less reactive than controls, active force development in response to a range of norepinephrine doses (10^{-10} to 5×10^{-5} *M)* was measured. Isolated pulmonary arterial segments (1.5 to 2.0 mm in diameter and 2 to 2.5 mm in length) cut from the main pulmonary arteries were placed in tissue baths containing 10 mL of Earle's balanced salt solution (EBSS) gassed with 95% 0_2–5% CO_2 (37°C, pH 7.4). Each arterial ring was connected to a force transducer and isometric tension was recorded as a function of time. Each ring was equilibrated 1 hr at the mean optimal resting tension for maximal active tension development in response to 80 m*M* KCl (P_o), and all subsequent active responses were expressed as a percent of P_o. Each preparation was then stimulated to contract with cumulative doses of norepinephrine (NE) and mean NE dose–response curves for hypertensive and control arterial rings were generated. As seen from Fig. 1, there was a downward shift in the hypertensive dose–response curve. Similar experiments were then performed with other vascular smooth muscle agonists, such as serotonin and angiotensin II. Results support the idea that hypoxia-induced pulmonary hypertension causes a decrease in reactivity.

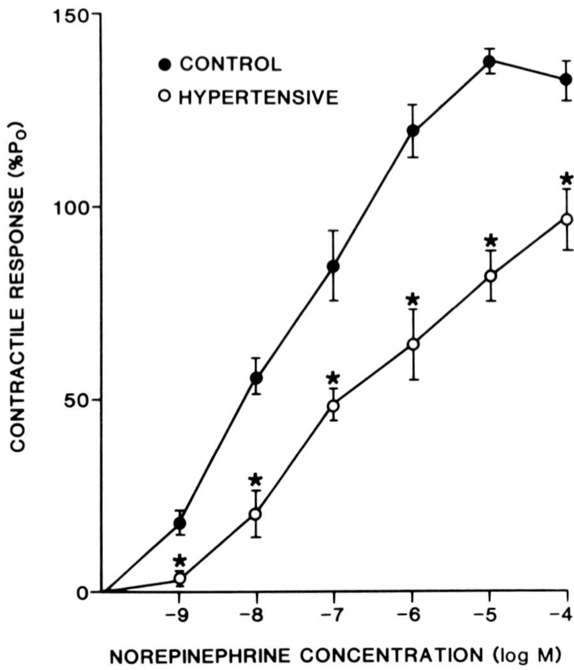

Figure 1 Mean NE dose–response curves for control ($n = 9$) and hypoxia-induced pulmonary hypertensive ($n = 6$) arterial rings. There is a downward shift in the hypertensive curve, indicating decreased reactivity ($p < 0.01$).

A general decrease in reactivity to a variety of agonists implies that the contractile apparatus, rather than membrane receptors, is altered. If, indeed, the hypertensive pulmonary arterial muscle contractility is decreased, measurements of active force-producing ability and/or velocity of shortening would provide evidence of impaired contractile function. Therefore, a second series of experiments were carried out to examine the mechanical properties. Pulmonary rings (2 to 3 mm in length) were cut and mounted onto a sensitive photoelectric force transducer and a movable support allowing small, calibrated lengthening steps. The PASM rings were maintained in a 37°C muscle bath of Krebs–Henseleit bicarbonate solution gassed with 95% O_2–5% CO_2. Supramaximal electrical field stimulation (45 V, 60 Hz, 10 s) was administered through platinum electrodes mounted parallel to the vertically mounted rings (Fig. 2). Each preparation was subjected to manual (passive) 0.2-mm lengthening steps and stimulated to contract isometrically at each length, beginning at that length which caused a measurable passive force and proceeding until maximal isometric force production (P_o) occurred or until the tissue yielded. Measurements of the resting force

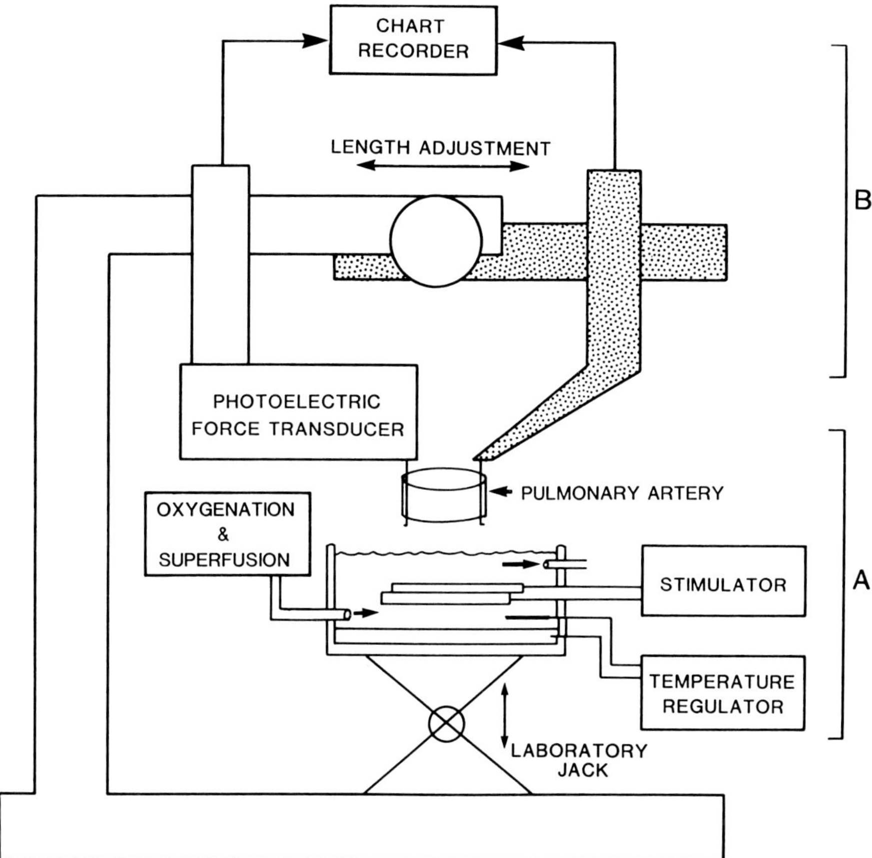

Figure 2 Schematic of experimental system. The conditions in which the PASM rings were maintained and stimulated to contract include a 37°C-regulated water bath, platinum electrodes and a square-wave stimulator, an oxygenator (95% O_2–5% CO_2), and a superfusion system distal from the water bath chamber (A). The apparatus for data collection included a photoelectric force transducer with a fine stainless steel wire for ring mounting and a movable rigid assembly allowing calibrated length changes (B). The data from both the calibrated force transducer and calibrated length changes were recorded on a Gould chart recorder.

and the peak of the active isometric force were normalized to tissue cross-sectional area (CSA). Mean passive and active length–tension (L–T) curves were constructed for both the hypertensive and control groups. The mean passive hypertensive L–T curve was elevated above the mean control curve, indicating that the hypertensive tissue was less compliant (Fig. 3). The mean active hyperten-

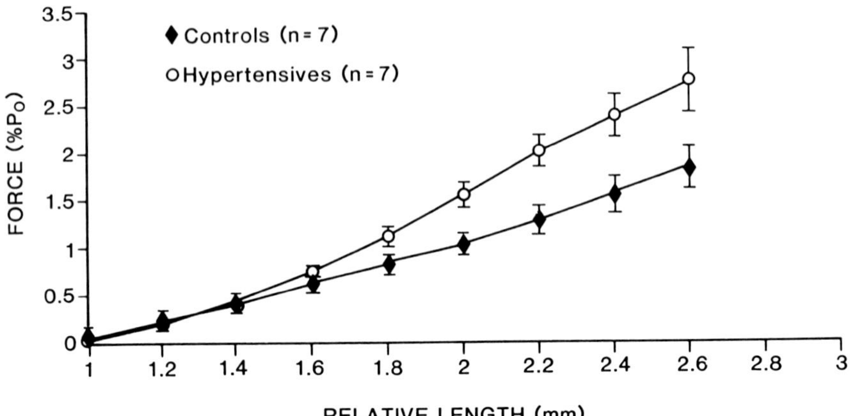

Figure 3 Passive length–tension curves. PASM rings were subjected to passive lengthening steps, beginning at a length (l_i) that showed an initial measurable force. The mean hypertensive L–T curve is elevated above the mean control curve, indicating less tissue compliance and an increased stiffness.

sive L–T curve was shifted to the left and was narrower than the mean control curve (Fig. 4). The steeper rise and sharper decline might be explained by the increased passive stiffness of the hypertensive tissue. Absolute optimal resting tensions (RP_o) were not different. However, when normalized for cross-sectional area, the hypertensive PASM RP_o was significantly less ($p < 0.05$) than the control RP_o, providing functional evidence for wall thickening. P_o normalized for CSA was not different for hypertensive or control PASM. Since P_o/CSA was not different but RP_o/CSA was decreased in hypertensive PASM, the wall thickening at this stage of hypertension is probably due to a proportional increase in actin and myosin relative to connective tissue.

PASM relaxation rates from control and pulmonary hypertensive rats were also compared. The rationale for measuring relaxation rates is based on the observation that slower arterial smooth muscle relaxation has been reported to be a possible causative mechanism of systemic arterial essential hypertension. Slower vascular muscle relaxation would result in prolonged wall stiffening and/or lumen narrowing (Cohen and Berkowitz, 1976; Shibata and Cheng, 1977; Packer and Stephens, 1985, 1987). All experiments were conducted at each PA ring's optimal resting length (l_o) for maximum isometric force production (P_o). PA rings were contracted isometrically or isotonically by applying a range of afterloads (i.e., load clamping) from P_o to optimal resting tension (RP_o) and even below RP_o. Load clamps below RP_o were achieved by a quick-release method which resulted in an instantaneous release of the elastic components followed by

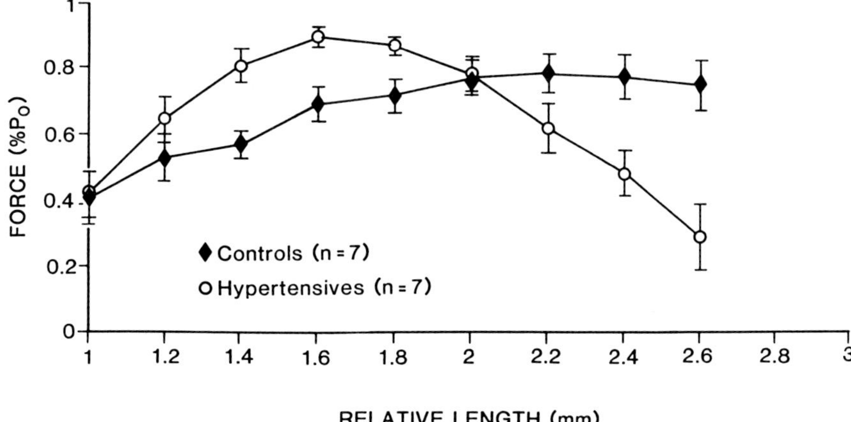

Figure 4 Active length–tension curves. PASM rings were stimulated to contract isometrically at various resting lengths. The mean control L–T curve increases to the maximum active force (P_o) and plateaus at this force. In contrast, the mean hypertensive L–T curve has a steeper rise to P_o (peak) and then declines markedly. This indicates increased tissue stiffness.

active shortening at each new low load. Isometric and isotonic relaxation were evaluated by (1) the measurement of relaxation half-times ($t_{1/2}$) and (2) rate constant (k) analysis. The relaxation $t_{1/2}$ was defined as the time (s) to reach one-half of 0.90 P_o or 0.90 ΔL for isometric and isotonic relaxation phases, respectively. Ninety percent of P_o (or ΔL) was chosen as the point of commencement of relaxation because it is difficult to define the precise point in time at which the onset of the relaxation phase occurs. Instantaneous data points from the relaxation phase of either the force curve (i.e., isometric) or the ΔL curve (i.e., isotonic) were taken at 0.04-s intervals between 90% and 10% of P_o or ΔL_{max}, respectively. These data were transformed by taking the natural logarithm of each point and performing a linear regression (mean $r^2 = 0.929 \pm 0.038$) to compute the slope (i.e., the rate constant, k) of the defined regression line. This method of analysis is important since the rate constant is independent of starting lengths, degree of active shortening, or the amount of force developed. In addition to the measured $t_{1/2}$ values and the k values, $t_{1/2}$ values were also computed from the equation $t_{1/2} = \ln 2/\text{-}k$, which is typical of first-order kinetics. Mean $t_{1/2}$ versus afterload (normalized as a percentage of the relative maximum force developed, $\%P_o$) curves were generated for the isotonic contractions. Finally, $t_{1/2}$ values were plotted as a function of the ratios of the afterload/optimal resting tension. All mean data are presented as mean values ± SEM.

Both relaxation half-times ($t_{1/2}$) and rate constants (k) of isometric and variously afterloaded isotonic relaxation phases of hypertensive PASM were compared with those of control PASM. Neither the relaxation rate nor the relaxation $t_{1/2}$ were different for hypertensive and control PASM operating in isometric mode ($p > 0.05$). As seen in Fig. 5, the mean hypertensive and control $t_{1/2}$ values as a function of afterload/optimal resting tension shifted the mean hypertensive curve to the right ($p < 0.04$). The mean measured $t_{1/2}$ values for preloaded

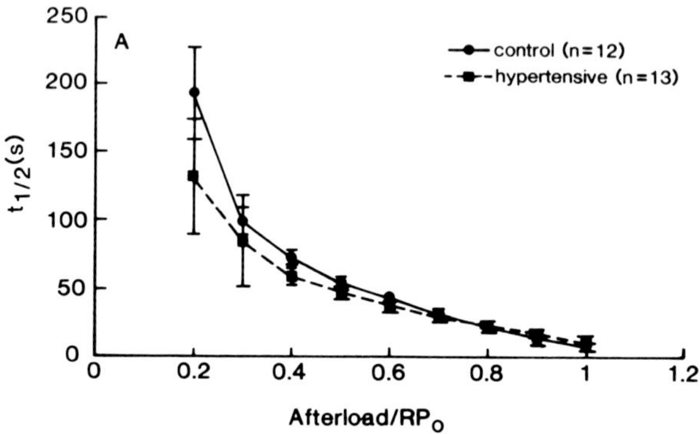

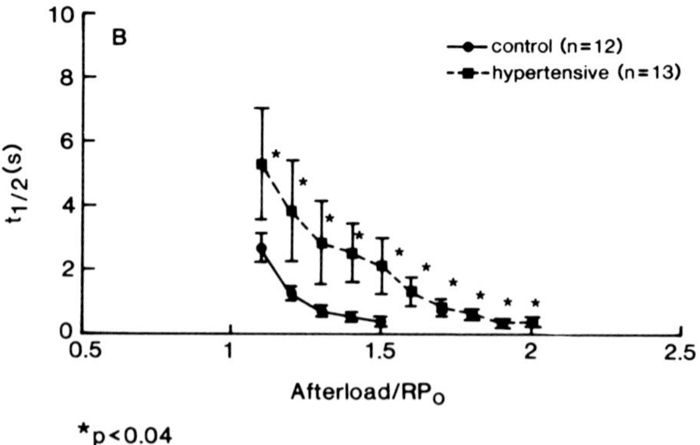

Figure 5 Isotonic relaxation of pulmonary arterial rings expressed as a function of afterload (P) relative to optimal resting tension (RP_o). Panel A shows afterload values below resting tension, and panel B shows afterload values above resting tension. In the case of afterloads above resting tension, the mean curve for the hypertensive group is shifted above and to the right of the mean curve for the control group. This indicates a greater half-time for any given relative afterload (P/RP_o) and thus a slower relaxation rate for the hypertensive group.

isotonically relaxing hypertensive PASM were also greater than the mean control $t_{1/2}$ values ($p < 0.02$), supporting the latter finding that relaxation rates (k) are slower for the hypertensive vascular tissue (Table 1). These results suggest that any apparent decrease in relaxation rate of isotonically contracted hypertensive pulmonary arteries is due to differences in the proportion of muscle to connective tissue rather than to differences in either smooth muscle Ca^{2+} resequestration or myosin dephosphorylation rates. Prolonged narrowing due to the structural changes in the pulmonary arterial wall may contribute to some degree to the maintenance but not to the development of hypoxia-induced pulmonary hypertension, since structural changes in the vessel are probably responsible and therefore precede the changes in relaxation rate.

Since changes in myosin heavy-chain (MHC) isoforms correlate with changes in contractility in striated muscles, a third series of experiments was carried out to determine whether MHC isoforms shift in hypertensive PASM. MHC isoform content and the relative proportions of MHC isoforms were determined by quantitative sodium dodecyl sulfate polyacrylamide gel electrophoresis, using bovine serum albumin as the standard. A total of 500 μg of pulmonary arterial tissue (which had previously been frozen with liquid N_2, pulverized, acetone-dried, desiccated with a low vacuum and stored at –70°C) was dissolved in 100 μL of sodium dodecyl sulfate (SDS) gel dissociation medium (200 m*M* Tris, pH 8.0, 3% SDS, 10 m*M* DTT, and 0.1% bromophenol blue). The material was heated to 100°C for 30 min, sedimented (Eppendorf centrifuge), and the supernatant applied to 5% acrylamide/0.75% bis slab gels using the buffer system of Porzio and Pearson (1977). Bovine serum albumin (BSA) standards were concurrently subjected to electrophoresis, and gels were stained in Coomassie blue. For separation of the various MHC isoforms, gels were subjected to electrophoresis for about 5.5 h, 4°C at 300 V, constant voltage. Myosin content was determined by quantitative densitometric scanning. Two different smooth muscle MHC isoforms (204- and 200-kD proteins) and a nonmuscle MHC isoform (196 or 198 kD) have been reported for a variety of smooth muscles. Interestingly, the rat PASM myosin consists of four MHC

Table 1 Relaxation Rate Constants of Preloaded Isotonic Contractions

	Rate (mm/s) calculated from measured $t_{1/2}$ values	Rate (mm/s) from k analysis
Control PA	0.299	0.144
(n = 12)	±0.030	±0.022
Hypertensive PA	0.022	0.089
(n = 13)	±0.037	±0.010
p-value	0.047	0.037

isoforms, corresponding in molecular weight to 204, 200, 196, and 190 kD (Fig. 6). Four isoforms, two smooth muscle and two nonmuscle, have been reported to occur in guinea pig and rat uterine and aortic muscle also (Eddinger, 1991). Therefore, the 190-kD isoform does not appear to be unique to PASM. Hypertensive and control isoform peak areas were compared (Table 2). The MHC_{200}/MHC_{204} ratios were not different. However, the mean $MHC_{190+196}/MHC_{200} + MHC_{204}$ ratio was greater in the hypertensive than in the control muscle. The data suggest the possibility of a change from contractile to synthetic

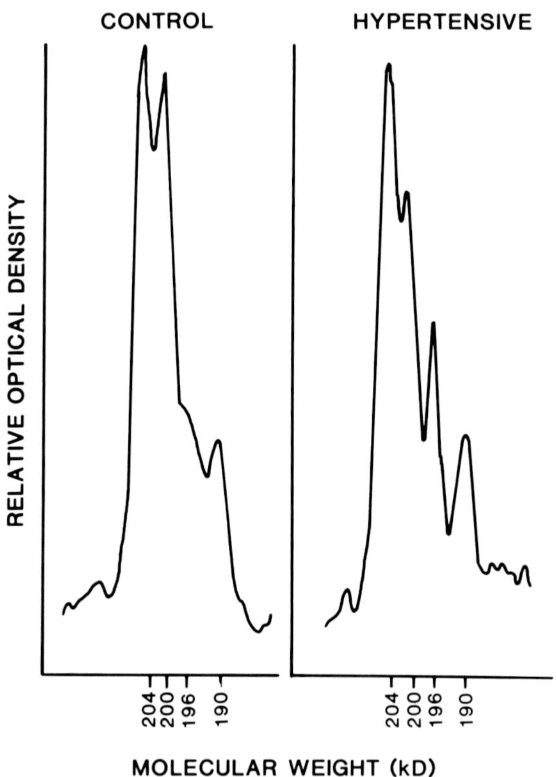

Figure 6 Densitometric scans representative of those obtained from sodium dodecyl sulfate 1.5% bis polyacrylamide gels for pulmonary arterial smooth muscle in the region corresponding to myosin heavy chains. The majority of reports indicate that most smooth muscle types contain only the muscle MHC isoforms (i.e., MHC_{200} and MHC_{204}), while a few smooth muscle types, mostly vascular, contain varying amounts of MHC_{198} or MHC_{196} (i.e., the nonmuscle forms) in addition to the MHC_{200} and MHC_{204}. The pulmonary arterial muscle may be somewhat unique in clearly separating into four MHC isoforms.

Table 2 Comparison of Pulmonary Arterial MHC Isoform Concentrations

	Ratio of peak areas	
	Hypertensives	Controls
MHC_{200}/MHC_{204}	0.987 ± 0.417 ($n = 4$)	1.134 ± 0.229 ($n = 8$)
$MHC_{(196+190)}/MHC_{(204+200)}$	*0.339 ± 0.041 ($n = 4$)	0.136 ± 0.068 ($n = 4$)
$MHC_{196}/MHC_{(204+200)}$	**0.256 ± 0.0322 ($n = 8$)	0.178 ± 0.032 ($n = 8$)

*$p < 0.00002$.
**$p < 0.02$.

smooth muscle phenotype with hypoxia-induced pulmonary hypertension. Such a phentotypic change would explain the decreased reactivity of the hypertensive PASM. In addition, conversion from the contractile to the synthetic state would not be surprising given that (1) there is significant smooth muscle hypertrophy and hyperplasia with pulmonary hypertension, and (2) phenotypic change is typical of hyperplastic smooth muscles in a variety of models, such as cell culture (Chambley-Campbell et al., 1979), and in atherosclerotic plaque (Ross et al., 1982). This speculation and the results of the myosin isoform experiments are further supported by a study of actin isoforms in hypoxia-induced hypertensive pulmonary arterial smooth muscle (Betty M. Twarog et al., personal communication). Apparently, there is an increase in the nonmuscle form of actin relative to the muscle actin isoforms just as is the case for myosin.

III. Hyperoxia-Induced Pulmonary Hypertension

Breathing a high concentration of oxygen ($F_IO_2 > 0.8$) can also lead to pulmonary hypertension (Wagenvoort and Wagenvoort, 1977). The potential toxic nature of hyperoxia on the lung is well documented (Crapo, 1986; Denke and Fanburg, 1980). Although pulmonary hypertension is common to both hypoxia and hyperoxia, the early events leading to hypertrophy and hypertension are quite different. Necrosis is an important initiating event with hyperoxic injury, while vasoconstriction has no role in hyperoxia-induced pulmonary hypertension (Kaplan et al., 1969; Crapo, 1986). The major phases, including initiation, inflammatory, destructive, proliferative, and fibrotic phases, associated with hyperoxic lung injury appear to be very similar in all animal models studied (Reid, 1990; Crapo, 1986; Jones et al., 1984). During the initiation phase hyperoxia damages alveolar macrophages which release factors that attract neurtrophils to the lung (Bowman et al., 1983; Adams and Hamilton, 1984). These neutrophils, in turn, adhere and release oxygen radicals and proteases (Harlan, 1985; Ward et al., 1983). The latter injures endothelial cells and reduces the integrity of the alveolar capillary membrane. The migration, adherence, and activation of neutrophils constitute the inflammatory phase. During the inflammatory phase pulmonary edema occurs. Pulmonary pressure does not rise in this early phase but increases only after small vessels are obliterated during the destructive phase. This is quite different from the scenario of events in hypoxia-induced pulmonary hypertension, in which pulmonary pressure rises immediately with hypoxia due to vasoconstriction. Other important differences occur during vascular restructuring. Hyperoxia causes restructuring of both pulmonary arteries and veins. However, with hypoxia-induced hypertension restructuring occurs almost exclusively on the arterial side (Reid, 1990). In addition, there is no smooth muscle phenotypic change with the vascular restructuring process with hyperoxia as there is with hypoxia. It is only when the lung is exposed to ambient O_2 levels again (i.e., relative hypoxia) that a phenotypic change occurs (Jones et al., 1984; Reid, 1990). Finally, the mechanism by which pulmonary hypertension is maintained once the stimulus is removed differs. The drop from high oxygen to normoxia in the presence of pulmonary edema causes alveolar hypoxia. Thus the return of the hyperoxic lung to air leads to vasoconstriction (i.e., analogous at this stage to hypoxic vasoconstriction), which in turn causes further resistance and more restructuring. This latter restructuring involves smooth muscle phenotypic changes and a disproportionate increase in connective tissue as is seen with hypoxia-induced pulmonary hypertension (Tozzi et al., 1989; Mecham et al., 1987; Stenmark et al., 1987).

The mechanical properties of hyperoxia-induced pulmonary hypertensive arterial tissue appear to be similar (Coflesky et al., 1987; Coflesky and Evans, 1988) to those of hypoxia-induced hypertensive arterial tissue. Evans et al. have shown that pulmonary hypertension in rats exposed to hyperoxia (21 days of 87% O_2) is not explained by an increase in maximal contractile capabilities of the vascular muscle but rather by a combination of vessel obliteration and increased resting stiffness. While hypoxia does not involve vessel obliteration, decreased arterial tissue compliance is a common factor to both hyperoxia- and hypoxia-induced pulmonary hypertension.

IV. Reactive Oxygen Species–Mediated Injury

A biological paradox has long been recognized in nature, but only recently fully understood: Although O_2 is essential for life, too much or inappropriate metabolism of O_2 becomes toxic to cells. Under most conditions, almost all O_2 consumed (about 98%) enters the mitochondria, where it is utilized in the production of cellular ATP. The utilization of O_2 in this process involves four electron reductions of O_2 to form water by the electron transport system. However, during the course of normal oxidative metabolism, O_2 can accept fewer than four electrons, to form important by-products known as reactive oxygen species: the superoxide ion (O_2^-), hydrogen peroxide (H_2O_2), and the hydroxyl radical (•OH). Reactive oxygen species can be produced outside the mitochondria as well; these important extramitochondrial sources of oxygen radical by-products include enzymes associated with arachidonate metabolism, such as cyclooxygenase, lipoxgenase, and cytochrome P450 (Table 3). In addition, the endothelial lining of the vasculature, especially in the pulmonary circulation, contains xanthine oxidase which can generate superoxide anions and other reactive oxygen species in the presence of hypoxanthine or xanthine (Granger, 1988).

Under normal physiological conditions these reactive oxygen species are either scavenged or catalyzed, which prevents cytotoxic effects. Superoxide ions are catalyzed by superoxide dismutase and H_2O_2 is scavenged by catalase or by peroxidases. Other nonenzymatic antioxidant defenses include vitamin E, glutathione, and cysteamine. However, under pathophysiological conditions reactive oxygen species overwhelm the antioxidant defense system and cause cellular damage. Several pathophysiological conditions that can generate reactive oxygen species include activation of neutrophils and alveolar macrophages, hyperoxia, and exposure to the herbicide paraquat, ozone, NO_2, or α-naphthylthiourea (Table 3).

Reactive metabolities derived from the reduction of molecular oxygen can alter vascular tone and blood flow and cause arterial damage (Hammond et al., 1983; Rubanyi, 1988). The lung is a primary site of oxygen radical generation and such generation has been linked to inflammation, oxygen toxicity, acute hypertension (Fridovich, 1983; Hammond et al., 1983), and ischemia-reperfusion injury (Koyama et al., 1987). In isolated perfused lung preparations, reactive oxygen species have been shown to cause increased pulmonary arterial pressure (Barnard et al., 1989) and a loss of vascular reactivity (Archer et al., 1989). In vascular tissue, exposure to a superoxide source induces a contractile response

Table 3 Sources of Reactive Oxygen Species

Normal	Pathological
Oxidative metabolism	Neutrophil activation, alveolar macrophage activation
Lipoxygenase	Hyperoxia
Cyclooxygenase	Paraquat
Cytochrome P450	Nitrogen dioxide
Flavin enzymes	Ozone
Xanthine oxidase	α-Naphthylthiourea

(Heinle, 1984). Rosenblum (1983) showed that the addition of an acetaldehyde/xanthine oxidase system to the perfusate of an in vivo mouse pial arteriole system will cause dilation at low concentration and constriction followed by dilation at high concentration, the varying responses being attributed to stimulation and/or inhibition of dilator and constrictor prostaglandin synthesis. Recent evidence presented by Gryglewski et al. (1986) indicates that superoxide ions contribute significantly to the breakdown of endothelial-derived vascular relaxing factor. This might account for the initial constrictor effect seen by Rosenblum (1983) at high superoxide-generator concentrations. However, the direct effects of reactive oxygen species on pulmonary arterial smooth muscle have been studied only sparingly.

Superoxide anions have been reported to cause contraction of vascular smooth muscle (Katusic and Vanhoutte, 1989). Burke and Wolin (1987) have reported that H_2O_2 caused relaxation of precontracted isolated bovine intrapulmonary arterial rings that was independent of endothelial or prostaglandin mediators. However, at higher concentrations (> 10^{-4}M), H_2O_2 contracted the pulmonary artery and vein (Wolin et al., 1985). Thus there are conflicting reports regarding the action of reactive oxygen metabolites on pulmonary arterial smooth muscle. Recently, our laboratory has reported that relatively higher doses of reactive oxygen species causes reversible endothelial-independent contraction of rat pulmonary arterial smooth muscle (Rhoades et al., 1988, 1990; Jin et al., 1991). This contractile response was accompanied by some damage to the vascular muscle, since subsequent force-developing ability was diminished. While the cellular damage could be completely prevented by pretreatment with superoxide dismutase and catalase, the initial contractile response could be completely blocked with catalase alone but not with superoxide dismutase alone. Thus the smooth muscle damage appears to be a result of exposure to superoxide anions and H_2O_2, while the contractile response appears to be initiated by H_2O_2. The contractile response and subsequent decreased responsiveness of the isolated pulmonary artery assumes functional importance, since the lung is a major site of production and a primary target organ of O_2 radicals that cause vasoconstriction and vascular injury (Archer et al., 1989; Sutko et al., 1985; Tate et al., 1982; Wei et al., 1985). The mechanism by which reactive oxygen species (H_2O_2 specifically) induce contractile activity in pulmonary arterial muscle is unknown.

According to current knowledge of cellular and molecular physiology, there are at least four or five possible pathways by which a stimulus can result in vascular smooth muscle contraction. First, cell membrane depolarization (by high extracellular potassium, for example) activates voltage-gated Ca^{2+} channels, resulting in Ca^{2+} influx (Meisheri et al., 1981). A second mechanism of increasing arterial smooth muscle intracellular Ca^{2+} is by membrane receptor binding and activation of ligand-gated Ca^{2+} channels (Bolton 1979). This also results in

Ca^{2+} influx. A third and perhaps the more common physiological method of raising intracellular Ca^{2+} in arterial muscle is via the second messenger inositol trisphosphate (IP_3) and subsequent release of Ca^{2+} from the sarcoplasmic reticulum (SR) into the cytosol (Berridge and Irvine, 1984). Some agonist–receptor interactions, such as norepinephrine binding to α_1 receptors, results in simultaneous opening of ligand-gated channels and IP_3 production by phospholipase C activation. Fourth, phospholipase C activity results not only in IP_3 production but also in a concomitant rise in diacylglycerol (DAG; Berridge, 1984). DAG results in activation of protein kinase C (PKC). PKC can either phosphorylate myosin directly or produce an actin and myosin interaction without requiring the Ca^{2+}–calmodulin–myosin light-chain kinase cascade, thus producing cross-bridge activity perhaps even in the absence of increased cytosolic Ca^{2+} (Chatterjee and Foster, 1987). Finally, it is possible for some agents, such as caffeine or carbachol, to increase the level of cytosolic Ca^{2+} by direct release of stored Ca^{2+} from the SR without involving the IP_3–second messenger system (Tetsuhiro and Takayanagi, 1988).

The xanthine oxidase (XO) reaction generates superoxide anions and H_2O_2 (Fridovich, 1970), while the glucose oxidase (GO) reaction generates only H_2O_2 (Nilsson et al., 1969). Isolated pulmonary arterial rings develop active isometric forces of similar magnitude when exposed either to 2 m*M* xanthine and 0.4 U/mL xanthine oxidase or to 0.4 U/mL glucose oxidase (Fig. 7; and Jin et al., 1991). These reactive oxygen species–induced contractions are independent of the endothelium and of extracellular calcium (Fig. 8; Rhoades et al., 1990; Jin et al., 1991). Therefore, the PASM contractile response to the reactive oxygen species appears to be a direct effect and not mediated by any endothelial-derived contracting factor. Nor does this PASM contractile response require Ca^{2+} influx. One might then suspect that the contractile activity is mediated through release of Ca^{2+} from the intracellular stores. However, results of experiments with ryanodine, a sarcoplasmic reticulum Ca^{2+} depleter, do not support this idea. Ryanodine has no more effect on the reactive oxygen species–mediated contraction than do Ca^{2+}-channel blockers (verapamil) or Ca^{2+} free, 0.1% EGTA media (Fig. 9; Jin et al., 1991). Given this information it is probably no surprise then that the α_1- and β-receptor blockers, phentolamine and propranolol, also have no effect on the XO-mediated PASM contractions. (It may be recalled that α_1-receptor activation of smooth muscle contraction is transduced primarily through the IP_3-intracellular Ca^{2+} release pathway.)

The mechanism appears to be an enigma. Yet there are some logical possibilities that should be explored. Only the H_2O_2 scavenger, catalase, has been found to abolish completely the contractile response to H_2O_2, XO, or GO. Superoxide dismutase only reduces the response; mannitol and deferoxamine (scavenger and inhibitor of formation of hydroxyl radicals, respectively) have no

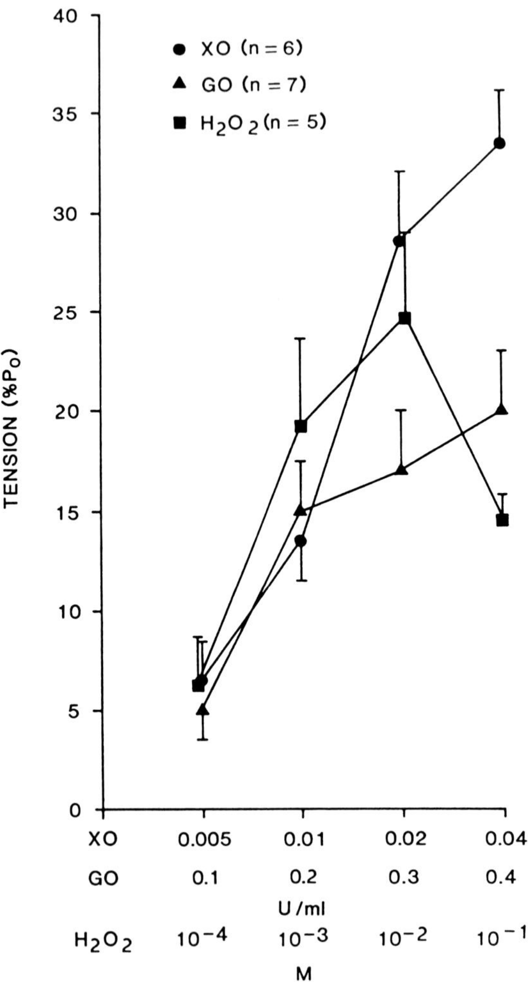

Figure 7 Mean responses of rat pulmonary arterial smooth muscle to a variety of concentrations of xanthine oxidase (XO), glucose oxidase (GO), and hydrogen peroxide (H_2O_2). Active tension is expressed as a percentage of maximum tension developed ($\%P_o \pm$ SE) in response to 80 m*M* KCL. The magnitude of the reactive oxygen–mediated contractions is concentration dependent. (From Rhoades et al., 1990).

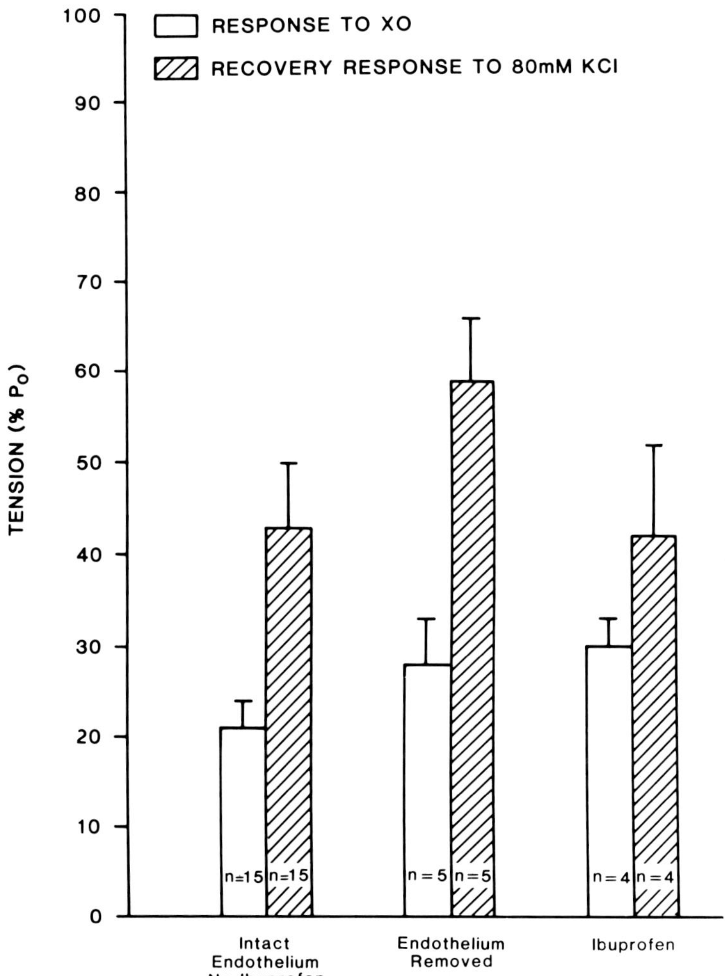

Figure 8 Effect of reactive oxygen species on contractile properties of pulmonary artery. Mean responses ± SE (%P_o) to XO are compared for vessels with and without endothelium and in the presence and absence of ibuprofen, a cyclooxygenase inhibitor. Mean recovery responses (responses to 80 m*M* KCL) following complete relaxation of XO-induced contraction are also compared for vessels under these same treatments (i.e., with and without endothelium and in the presence or absence of ibuprofen). Neither endothelium removal nor ibuprofen treatment has any affect on the XO-induced contractions or the recovery responses. (From Rhoades et al., 1990.)

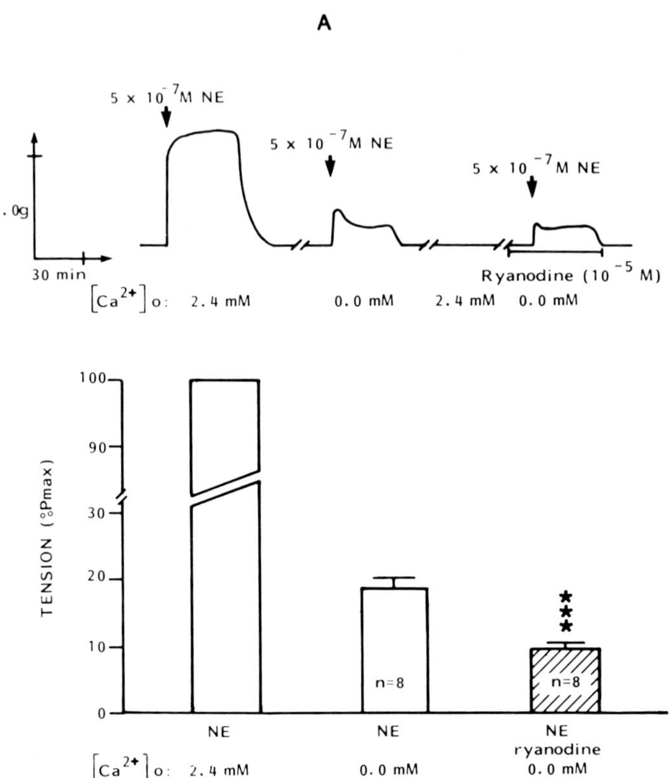

Figure 9 Upper panels: Typical tension trace showing the effect of extracellular Ca^{2+} and the effect of ryanodine, a sarcoplasmic reticulum Ca^{2+} depleter, on the contractile response of rat pulmonary arterial muscle to 5×10^{-7} *M* NE. Eliminating extracellular Ca^{2+} reduced the responses to NE, and addition of ryanodine resulted in a further reduction of the contractile response to NE (A). The response to XO was not inhibited by ryanodine treatment in Ca^{2+}-free solution (B). Lower panels: Comparison of the mean SE active responses to NE in 2.4 m*M* extracellular Ca^{2}, 0.0 m*M* extracellular Ca^{2+}, and in Ca^{2+}-free solution containing ryanodine (A) and of the responses to XO in 0.0 m*M* Ca^{2+} solution in the absence and in the presence of ryanodine (B). The maximum active tension developed in response to 5×10^{-7}*M* NE in 2.4 m*M* Ca^{2+} -containing media was defined as P_{max} and the mean values are presented as $\%P_{max}$. The mean response of vessels in Ca^{2+} -free solution was significantly reduced from the response in 2.4 m*M* Ca^{2+}-solution ($p < 0.05$). The mean active tension developed in Ca^{2+}-free solution with ryanodine was significantly lower than the mean tension developed in Ca^{2+}-free solution in the absence of ryanodine ($p < 0.001$). There was no difference between the mean responses to XO in the absence or in the presence of ryanodine in Ca^{2+}-free media ($p < 0.05$). (From Jin et al., 1991.)

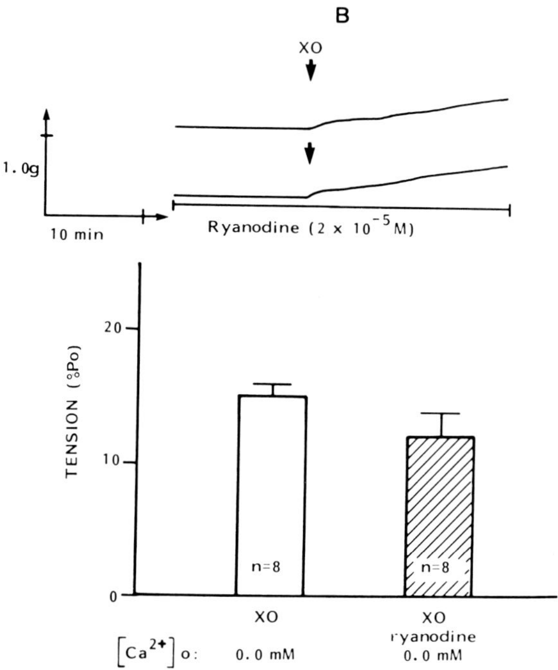

effect. Therefore, H_2O_2 is implicated as causative of the contractions. H_2O_2 is known to penetrate the cell (Hammond et al., 1983) and could elicit a contraction by changing transmembrane Ca^{2+} flux (Rasmussen et al., 1986). This is an unlikely causative given the findings that verapamil or Ca^{2+}-free and EGTA-containing media had no effect. Alternatively, H_2O_2 can stimulate IP_3 production (Henson and Johnston, 1987), resulting in intracellular Ca^{2+} release and contraction. However, this is also unlikely given that ryanodine had no effect on the response. A third possibility is that H_2O_2 stimulates protein kinase C (PKC), which is known to cause phosphorylation of myosin light chains, leading to smooth muscle contraction without a significant increase in intracellular free Ca^{2+}. Interestingly, H7 (a PKC inhibitor) significantly reduces the PASM response to xanthine oxidase as shown in Fig. 10 (Jin et al., 1991). But one must keep in mind that PKC inhibitors are nonspecific. Indeed, staurosporine (another commonly utilized PKC inhibitor) is more potent in phosphorylating myosin light-chain kinase (MLCK) than in inhibiting PKC activity, and H7 is also

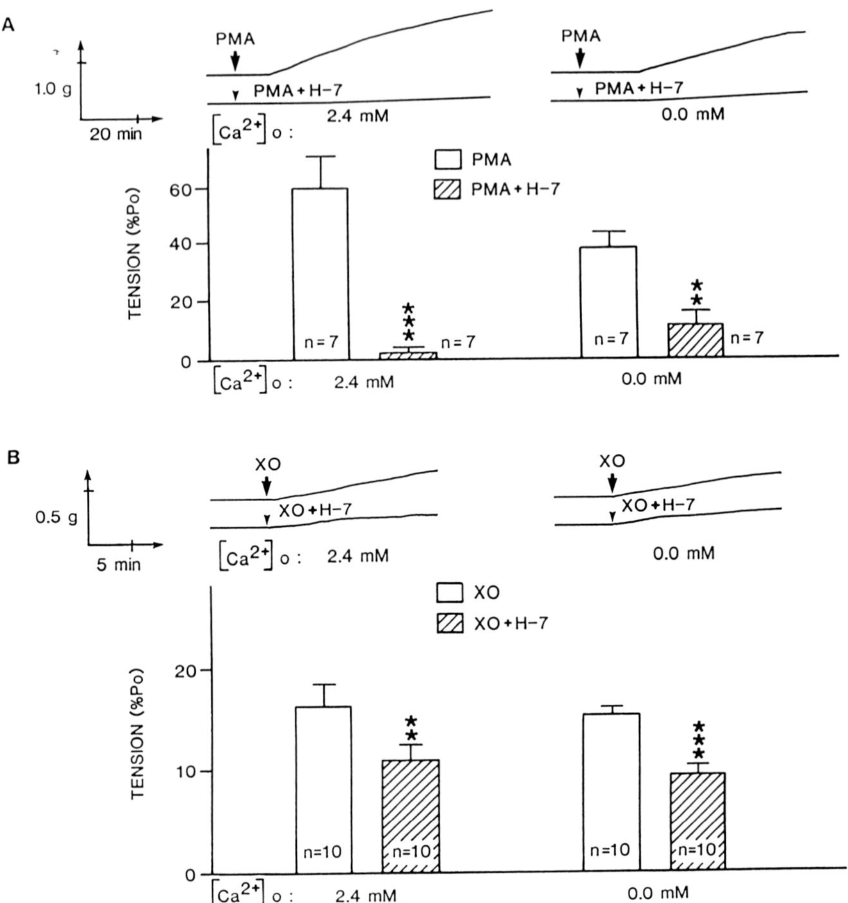

Figure 10 Upper panels: Typical tracings of tension produced in response to XO in the absence or presence of H7 in 2.4 m*M* Ca^{2+} media (left-hand tracings) or in 0.0 m*M* Ca^{2+} media (right-hand tracings). H7 reduced the response to XO regardless of the extracellular Ca^{2+} concentration. Lower panels: Comparison of the mean ± SE active tension developed ($\%P_o$) in response to XO in the absence of H7 and in the presence of H7 in 2.4 m*M* extracellular Ca^{2+} solution and to XO in the absence and in the presence of H7 in 0.0 m*M* extracellular Ca^{2+} solution. H7 significantly reduced the response to XO in the 2.4 m*M* Ca^{2+} media ($p < 0.01$). Similarly, H7 reduced the response to XO in the Ca^{2+}-free media ($p < 0.001$). (From Jin et al., 1991).

known to inhibit MLCK. Phosphorylation of MLCK renders it inactive (Adelstein et al., 1978), thus preventing muscle contraction by the currently accepted more usual physiological mechanism of MLCK-catalyzed phosphorylation of myosin. The possibility exists that the H7 reduction of the reactive oxygen species–induced PASM contraction may indicate that H_2O_2 is activating MLCK without raising intracellular Ca^{2+} or activating PKC. A change in the Ca^{2+} sensitivity of the regulatory and/or contractile proteins may be the key. On the other hand, Harold Davis has shown that H7 is more potent in inhibiting nonmuscle PKC (from bovine pulmonary arterial endothelial cells) than in inhibiting MLCK (from bovine platelets), as shown in Fig. 11 (personal communication). Others have reported that the K_i value of H7 for smooth muscle MLCK is 97 μM for PKC (Hidaka et al., 1984; Saitoh et al., 1986, 1987). Therefore, PKC may be correctly implicated as the second messenger of the reactive oxygen–mediated pulmonary arterial smooth muscle contraction after all.

While vasoconstriction in response to reactive oxygen species may play a role in the etiology of various forms of lung injury, the concomitant damage of pulmonary arterial smooth muscle due to reactive oxygen species exposure must

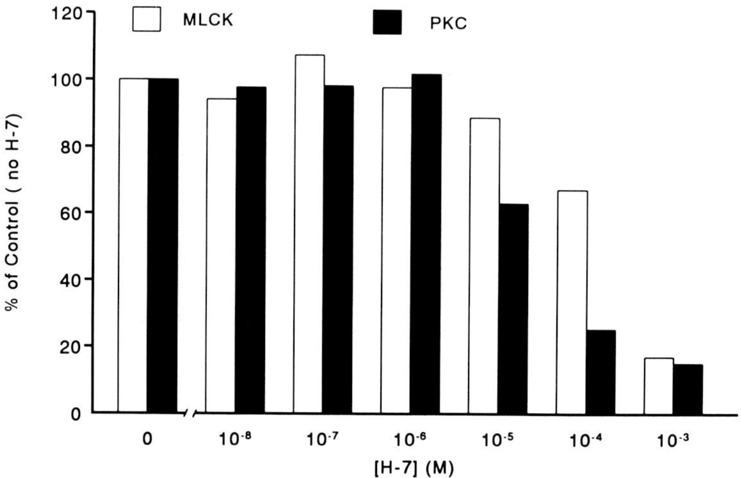

Figure 11 Effect of the kinase inhibitor, H7, on myosin light-chain kinase and protein kinase C activities. Bovine platelet myosin light-chain kinase activity was determined as described hy Hathway and Adelstein (1979) and bovine pulmonary artery endothelial cell protein kinase activity was measured according to the method of Myers et al. (1989). (Courtesy of Harold Davis, Ph.D., Dept. of Medicine, Indiana University School of Medicine.)

not be overlooked. The pulmonary arterial smooth muscle contractile function is impaired subsequent to exposure to reactive oxygen species and the acute initial vasoconstriction. The responsiveness of the pulmonary arterial smooth muscle to high K^+ membrane depolarization is decreased following exposure to reactive oxygen species (Fig. 12). The observations that treatment with either superoxide dismutase alone or catalase alone reduces this loss of pulmonary arterial responsiveness and that SOD plus CAT offer complete protection against reduced responsiveness suggest that the superoxide ion and H_2O_2 may both have deleterious effects on the subsequent responsiveness of the pulmonary arterial muscle. The additive protective effect of catalase and superoxide dismutase may be due to a reduction of the total concentration of damaging oxygen radicals irrespective of species. This explanation is strengthened by the fact that increas-

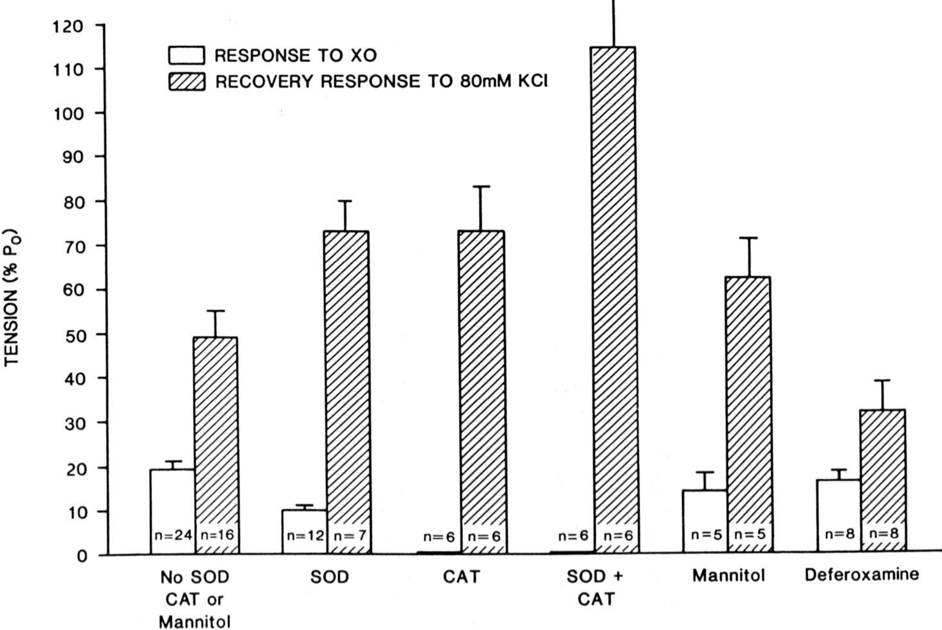

Figure 12 Effect of O_2-derived radical scavengers on rat pulmonary arterial muscle exposed to XO. Mean responses ± SE (%P_o) of arterial rings pretreated with superoxide dismutase (SOD) alone, catalase (CAT) alone, or CAT plus SOD, mannitol, or deferoxamine and then exposed to 0.02 U/mL XO. Similarly, mean recovery responses (i.e., subsequent responses to 80 m*M* KCL) for the various treatments are also compared. SOD alone or CAT alone decreases the XO-induced contraction and increases the recovery responses. SOD and CAT together abolish the effects of XO exposure, while mannitol or deferoxamine does not alter the XO effects. (From Rhoades et al., 1990.)

ing concentration of either XO, GO, or H_2O_2 results in concomitant decreases in arterial muscle responsiveness (Rhoades et al., 1990).

Vascular responsiveness in cerebral vessels has also been reported to be lost following exposure to reactive oxygen species, and this was attributed to endothelial damage (Wei et al., 1985). However, the decreased responsiveness of the pulmonary arterial muscle is neither enhanced nor prevented by cyclooxygenase inhibition or by endothelial removal (Rhoades et al., 1990). Since H_2O_2 is cell membrane soluble, it is plausible that H_2O_2 could either damage smooth muscle cell membranes or alter smooth muscle contractile activity by direct action on the regulatory or contractile apparatus. O_2 radicals are known to cause cell damage (Heinle, 1984), and more specifically, XO has been shown to alter myofibrillar sulfhydryl content and ATPase activity in vitro (Ventura et al., 1985). Such changes would be expected to decrease contractility in the intact muscle.

V. Ischemia-Reperfusion

Ischemia-reperfusion (I-R) injury occurs in a number of organs, including the lung (Rubanyi, 1988). Cardiopulmonary bypass and lung transplantation are two obvious examples where blood flow is interrupted and ischemia-reperfusion injury can occur in the lung (Braude et al., 1986; Stuart et al., 1985). Removal of a thrombotic obstruction in a major pulmonary vessel is another example of I-R in lung (Martin et al., 1983; Moser et al., 1983). Ischemia-reperfusion injury can also occur in reexpanding an edematous lung or a pneumothorax (Sprung et al., 1981). Finally, some investigators contend that I-R injury occurs in adult respiratory distress syndrome after vascular thrombosis has been resolved (Tomashefski et al., 1983).

Regardless of the different clinical situations in which I-R can occur, vascular injury resulting in increased miscrovascular permeability and pulmonary edema appears to be common to all (Baire et al., 1981; Johnson et al., 1981). The vascular injury is thought to occur mostly during the reperfusion phase rather than during the ischemic phase. However, since metabolic acidosis and Ca^{2+} reallocation occur during ischemia (Vandeplassche and Borges, 1990), additional studies will be required to rule out injury during this phase. Reperfusion injury occurs in two stages. The initial insult appears to be xanthine-oxidase mediated (Granger, 1988). During ischemia, when high-energy purine nucleotides are dephosphorylated, hypoxanthine accumulates. Then, during reperfusion, the accumulated pool of hypoxanthine is rapidly catalyzed in the presence of oxygen by xanthine oxidase, which is present in the pulmonary endothelium, to produce toxic reactive oxygen species. The secondary insult is often associated with neutrophil recruitment. The neutrophils adhere as a result of lipid peroxidation and leukotriene release, become activated, and in turn release toxic reactive oxygen species and proteases (Inauen et al., 1989). Although increased pulmonary vascular permeability has received extensive investigation, very little is known about the effect of I-R injury on vascular smooth muscle function. Accordingly, our laboratory investigated the effect of I-R on both pulmonary arterial and venous smooth muscle reactivity and responsiveness. (Jin et al., 1989).

The main pulmonary artery to the left lower lobe of anesthetized dogs was isolated and occluded by a parallel-jawed spring clip (Baxter Healthcare Co. Irvine, CA). The left chest was then closed and the dogs were maintained with the left lobe artery occluded for 48 h. Then a second surgery was performed to return blood flow to the previously occluded artery by removing the clip (i.e, reperfusion). Animals were ventilated and anesthetized by giving pentobarbital at intervals during 4 h of reperfusion. Lungs were then removed and lung wet weight/dry weight ratios were measured. Contralateral lobes from ischemia reperfused dogs and left lower lobes from nonoperated dogs served as controls.

Intrapulmonary arterial and venous rings (1.5 to 2.5 mm in diameter and 2.5 to 3.0 mm long) were placed in muscle chambers and connected to force transducers. Dose–response curves to norepinephrine were generated and the dose that resulted in a half maximum response (ED_{50}) to NE was identified. In other experiments, the maximum responses to serotonin (5HT) were compared. In a final series of experiments, the magnitude of ACh-induced relaxation and relaxation half-times ($t_{1/2}$) were compared. At the end of each experiment, the length, width, and weight of each ring was measured and tissue cross-sectional areas were calculated. Force production was normalized in grams per cross-sectional area of tissue (g/cm^2).

Ischemia-reperfusion of the left lower lobe (LL, n=8) resulted in a significant increase in lung wet/dry weight ratios. The water content (percent wet weight of lung) from LL was 85.0 ± 0.9%, while the percentages of water in the contralateral lobe (RL), right upper lobe (RU), and the left upper lobe (LU) were 78.7 ± 1.1, 77.5 ± 1.6, and 79.1 ± 2.2%, respectively ($p < 0.05$ for each group compared with the mean LL value). Pulmonary edema was considered an index of ischemia-reperfusion vascular injury.

The maximum force-generating ability of pulmonary arteries from nonoperated dogs in response to 80 mM KCL or to 0.1 μM NE was not different from the contralateral arteries (RL) from dogs in which the left lower lobes had been ischemic and reperfused (Table 4). However, pulmonary arteries of ischemia-reperfused left lower lobes produced significantly lower force than those of the contralateral vessels in response to these same respective agonists. Is-

Table 4 Effect of Ischemia-Reperfusion on Force Generation of Pulmonary Arteries ($n = 8$) to Various Agonists

	Force (g/cm^2)		
Agonist	Nonoperated	Contralateral	Ischemia-reperfused[a]
80 m*M* KCl	348 ± 26	351 ± 40	250 ± 42
100 μ*M* NE	211 ± 47	277 ± 40	148 ± 23
10 μ*M* 5HT	356 ± 45	355 ± 50	248 ± 44

[a]Ischemia-reperfusion preparations produced less force than was produced with contralateral preparations ($p < 0.05$).

chemia-reperfusion caused a similar decrease in force generation of pulmonary veins to that seen in arteries.

Both dose–response curves of ischemia-reperfused pulmonary arteries and veins show a rightward shift compared with the respective control curves (Fig. 13). Figure 13 also shows that the maximum response to NE decreased significantly following ischemia-reperfusion. Maximum contraction of pulmonary veins in response to NE occurred at 10 μ*M*, while maximum contraction of pulmonary arteries in response to NE occurred on the average at 100 μ*M*. The doses required to produce a half maximal response to NE (ED_{50}) in contralateral arteries and veins were 0.73 ± 0.09 μM and 0.33 ± 0.08 μM, respectively. Ischemia-reperfusion caused a downward shift in the sensitivity of both arteries and veins. A twofold-higher concentration was required to produce half-maximal response in the ischemia-reperfused vessels.

Ischemia-reperfusion did not alter the endothelium-dependent relaxation responses of the canine pulmonary artery to ACh. The magnitude of relaxation is ischemic-reperfused arterial rings was 59.3 ± 4.7% P_{NE} (i.e., percent of maximum response to 0.5 μ*M* NE), and this was not different from the contralateral arterial relaxation (61.7 ± 5.3% P_{NE}; $p > 0.05$). The relaxation half-time ($t_{1/2}$) in ischemic-reperfused arterial rings was also not different from that of the contralateral arterial preparations. In contrast to the pulmonary artery, precontracted pulmonary veins responded to ACh with additional force production rather than with relaxation. 5μ*M* ACh caused 133.9 ± 14.8 g/cm^2 of additional force (in addition to the NE-induced precontractile force) in contralateral veins and 96.6 ± 25.1 g/cm^2 in ischemic-reperfused veins ($p > 0.05$).

These studies show that lung I-R causes pulmonary edema and decreased reactivity and responsiveness of smooth muscle in the pulmonary artery and vein. However, I-R endothelial-dependent arterial relaxation does not appear to be altered following I-R injury.

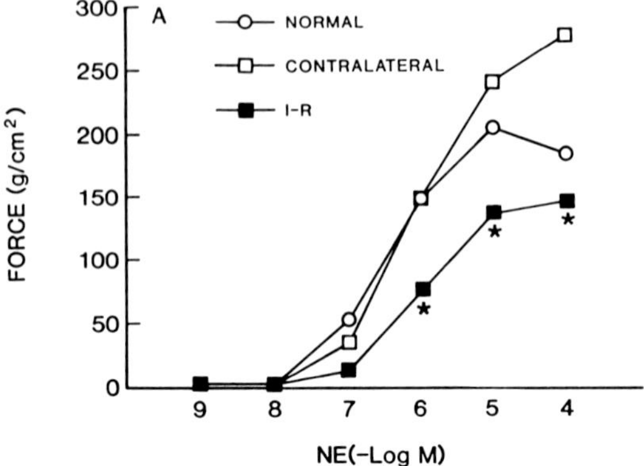

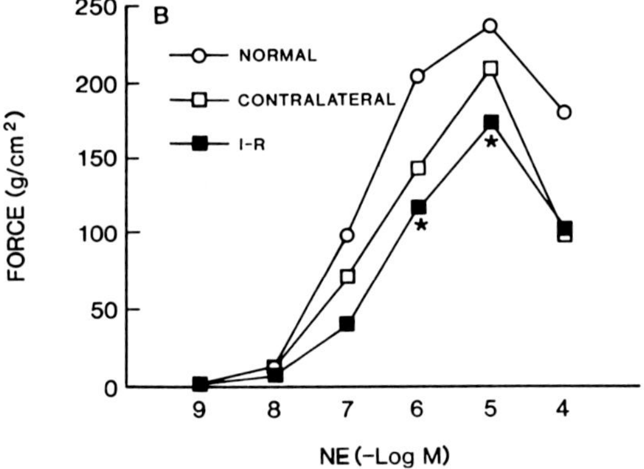

Figure 13 NE dose–response curves of vessels from ischemia-reperfused and controllobes. Ischemia-reperfusion caused a rightward shift of dose–response curves for both the artery ($n = 8$; panel A) and vein ($n = 5$; panel B), indicating a decreased sensitivity. *$p < 0.05$ for ischemia-reperfusion curves compared with contralateral curves.

VI. Neutrophil Injury

Inflammatory lung injury involves the sequestration and activation of polymorphonuclear neutrophils (PMN) and is characterized by elevated perfusion pressures and edema (Brigham and Meyrick, 1984; Repine et al., 1985; Harlan, 1985; Warshawski et al., 1986; Lee et al., 1981). Neutrophils have been shown to cause both hemodynamic effects and increased permeability in isolated blood-free perfused lungs (Shasby et al., 1982, 1983; Carpenter et al., 1987; Patterson et al., 1989). Since neutrophils have been implicated in I-R injury, another series of experiments was carried out to examine the direct interaction of neutrophils on pulmonary vascular rings (Patterson et al., in press). In this study right and left extralobar rat pulmonary arterial rings were utilized. In some arterial rings the endothelium was removed mechanically. Intact rings responded to norepinephrine with 40 to 60% of the initial contraction to KCl (described below). This norepinephrine-induced contraction was reversed by addition of acetylcholine. Rings mechanically denuded of endothelium showed no tendency to relax to acetylcholine. Each arterial segment (intact or denuded) was placed in a glass muscle chamber and isometric tensions were recorded. Each vessel was equilibrated for 1 h at the optimum resting tension (0.9 g) for maximum active tension development in response to KCl depolarization (P_o). Active tensions developed with subsequent treatments were expressed as percentages of the maximal active tension development in response to 80 m*M* KCl ($\%P_o$). Subsequent treatments included exposure to nonactivated neutrophils, PMA, FMLP, or neutrophils activated with either PMA or FMLP. Results of this study demonstrate that activated neutrophils cause both acute contraction in pulmonary arterial smooth muscle and a decreased ability of the vessel to contract in response to subsequent depolarization, as shown in Fig. 14. The acute contraction and subsequent decrease in contractility appear to be due to different activated neutrophil products.

When activated, neutrophils produce a wide array of products, including free radicals, bioactive arachidonate metabolites, and degradative enzymes. Although reactive oxygen species have been shown to cause contraction in isolated rat pulmonary arterial segments (Rhoades et al., 1990; Jin et al., 1991), tension development in response to activated neutrophils was not inhibited by free-radical scavenging enzymes nor was the contraction decreased by suppression of the neutrophil superoxide release after PMA pretreatment.

The contractile response to activated neutrophils in this study probably involves cyclooxygenase products, since neutrophil-induced active tension development in the arterial rings was inhibited by direct addition of anti-inflammatory drugs to the muscle bath and by aspirin pretreatment of the neutrophils, as shown in Fig. 15. The cyclooxygenase products may be released directly by the activated neutrophils and/or possibly by the endothelium responding to activated neutrophils.

Since the acute contraction due to neutrophil activation in this study was also shown to be dependent on the presence of intact endothelium, it may be that thromboxane and/or other cyclooxygenase products act on the endothelium, which subsequently releases a secondary contractile factor (possibly EDCF) to the underlying smooth muscle. If contraction occurs downstream from the

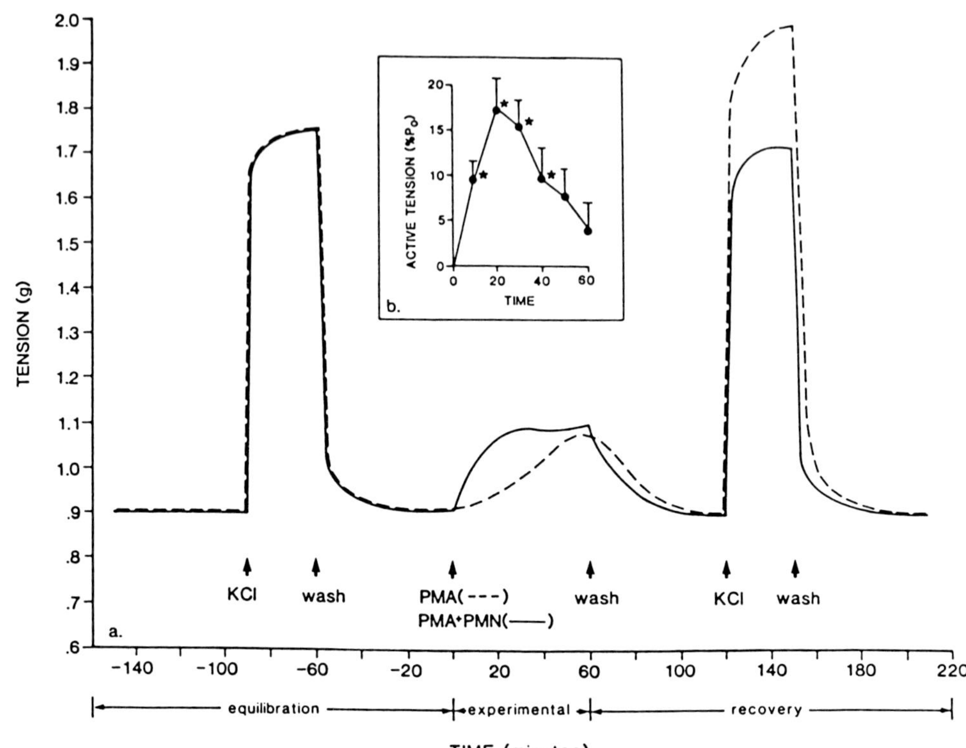

Figure 14 Activated neutrophil-induced tension development in pulmonary arterial rings. Representative time course illustrating protocol and tension development. After 1 h equilibration in Earle's balanced salt solution bubbled with 95% O_2–5% CO_2, arterial rings were contracted with 80 m*M* KCL. Rings were than washed, allowed to relax, and then treated at time 0 with either phorbol myristate acetate (PMA; 10 ng/mL) or neutrophils (PMN; 20 million) activated by subsequent addition of PMA for 1 h. During the experimental period, 25 m*M* HEPES buffer was substituted for the bicarbonate buffer and the solution was gases at the surface with 100% O_2. At the end of the treatment period, the arterial rings were washed and bubbling was resumed before being recontracted with KCL. Inset: Net contraction due to activated neutrophils. Active tension development expressed as a percentage of the initial KCL contraction (P_o) due specifically to the activated neutrophils was calculated for paired vessels by subtraction of the tension in PMA alone vessels from the tension in the PMN + PMA vessels at each time point ($n = 17$). An asterisk indicates a significant difference from PMA alone, $p < 0.05$. (From Patterson et al., in press.)

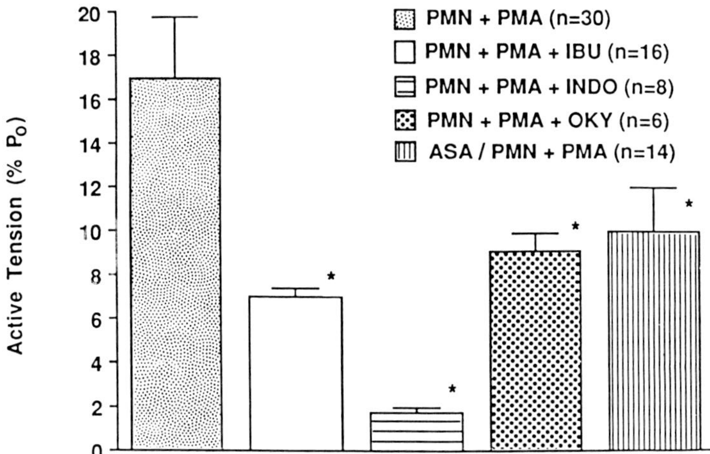

Figure 15 Effect of cyclooxygenase and thromboxane inhibitors on PMA-activated neutrophil-mediated contraction. First bar represents pulmonary arterial ring contraction at 20 min in PMN + PMA group ($n = 30$). Second bar is PMN + PMA-mediated contraction in the presence of 2.4×10^{-4} *M* ibuprofen (IBU, $n = 16$). Third bar is contraction in the presence of 10 μ*M* indomethacin (INDO, $n = 8$). Fourth bar is the contraction in the presence of 10 n*M* OKY-04f6 (OKY, $n = 6$). Fifth bar represents contraction due to neutrophils that had been pretreated for 10 min with aspirin (250 μg/mL), centrifuged, resuspended immediately prior to addition to the arterial rings, and then activated with PMA ($n = 14$). An asterisk indicates a significant difference from PMA alone in paired vessels, $p < 0.05$. (From Patterson et al., in press.)

arterial bed such that there is a resistance increase in the microvascular bed or venoconstriction, it is possible that microvascular pressure would be elevated. An increase in microvascular pressure would play an important role in determining the rate of edema formation due to concomitant changes in alveolar capillary permeability resulting from neutrophil activation, as has been shown in intact lung (Patterson et al., 1989).

The activated neutrophil-induced decline in contractile ability of the arterial rings following the initial acute contraction was not altered by the presence of the anti-inflammatory drugs and is therefore probably not related to cyclooxygenase products. Damage to the smooth muscle by reactive oxygen species generated by activated neutrophils might be responsible for the decreased recovery contraction, based on our previous finding that exposure of pulmonary arterial rings to xanthine oxidase–generated products produced a similar decline in subsequent contractile force (Rhoades et al., 1990; Jin et al., 1991). However, the inability of catalase and superoxide dismutase to prevent the decline after neutrophil exposure and the failure of PMA pretreatment of the neutrophils, which greatly decreased superoxide release, to alter the decline in recovery suggest that superoxide and hydrogen peroxide are not involved. A third possible mechanism that might be responsible for this effect is release of proteases by the activated neutrophils. However, a mixture of antiproteases also failed to protect the smooth muscle contractile function. Although the neutrophil product causing this effect has not been identified, it is known to be relatively stable, filterable, and not dependent on the presence of an intact functional endothelium (Patterson et al., in press).

Acknowledgment

We gratefully acknowledge the skillful assistance of Ms. Marlene King in the preparation of this manuscript.

References

Adams, D. O., and Hamilton, T. A. (1984). The cell biology of macrophage activation. *Annu. Rev. Immunol.* **2:**283–318.

Adelstein, R. S., Conti, M. A., Hathaway, D. K., and Klee, C. B. (1978). Phosphorylation of smooth muscle myosin light chain kinase by the catalytic subunit of adenosine 3′-5′ monophosphate-dependent protein binase. *J. Biol. Chem.* **253:**8347–8350.

Archer, S. L., Peterson, D., Nelson, D. P., DeMaster, E. G., Kelly, B., Eaton, J. W., and Weir, E. K. (1989). Oxygen radicals and antioxidant enzymes alter pulmonary vascular reactivity in the rat lung. *J. Appl. Physiol.* **66:**102–111.

Barie, P. S., Hakim, T. S., and Malik, A. B. (1981). Effect of pulmonary artery occlusion and reperfusion on extravascular fluid accumulation. *J. Appl. Physiol.* **50:**102–106.

Barnard, J. W., Patterson, C. E., Hull, M. T., Wagner, W. W., Jr., and Rhoades, R. A. (1989). Role of microvascular pressure in reactive oxygen-induced lung edema. *J. Appl. Physiol.* **66:**1486–1493.

Berridge, M. J. (1984). Inositol trisphosphate and diacylglycerol as second messengers. *Biochem. J.* **220:**345–360.

Berridge, M. J., and Irvine, R. (1984). Inositol trisphosphate, a novel second messenger in cellular signal transduction. *Nature (Lond.)* **321:**315–321.

Bolton, T. B. (1979). Mechanism of action of transmitters and other substances on smooth muscle. *Physiol. Rev.* **59:**606–718.

Bowman, C. M., Harada, R. N., and Repine, J. E. (1983). Hyperoxia stimulated alveolar macrophages to produce and release a factor which increases neutrophil adherence. *Inflammation* **7:**331–338.

Bruade, S., Nolop, K. B., Flemming, J. S., Krausz, T., Taylor, K. M., and Royston, D. (1986). Increased pulmonary transvascular protein flux after canine cardiopulmonary bypass. *Am. Rev. Respir. Dis.* **135:**463–481.

Brigham, K. L., and Meyrick, B. (1984). Interaction of granulocytes with the lungs. *Circ. Res.* **54:**623–645.

Burke, T. M., and Wolin, M. S. (1987). Hydrogen peroxide elicits pulmonary arterial relaxation and guanylate cyclase activation. *Am. J. Physiol.* **21:**H721–H732.

Carpenter, L. J., Johnson, K. L., Kunkel, R. G., and Roth, R. A. (1987). Phorbol myristate acetate produces injury to isolated rat lungs in the presence and absence of perfused neutrophils. *Toxicol. Appl. Pharmacol.* **91:**22–32.

Chambley-Campbell, J., Campbell, G. R., and Ross, R. (1979). The smooth muscle cell in culture. *Physiol. Rev.* **59:**1–61.

Chatterjee, M., and Foster, C. (1987). Activation of protein kinase C and contraction in skinned muscle. In *Regulation and Contraction of Smooth Muscle.* Edited by M. J. Siegman, A. P. Somlyo, and N. L. Stephens. Alan R. Liss, New York, pp. 219–231.

Coflesky, J. T., and Evans, J. N. (1988). Pharmacologic properties of isolated proximal pulmonary arteries after seven-day exposure to in vitro hyperoxia. *Am. Rev. Respir. Dis.* **138:**945–951.

Coflesky, J. T., Jones, P. C., Reid, L. M., and Evans, J. N. (1987). Mechanical properties and structure of isolated pulmonary arteries remodeled by chronic hyperoxia. *Am. Rev. Respir. Dis.* **136:**388–394.

Cohen, M. L., and Berkowitz, B. A. (1976). Decreased vascular relaxation in hypertension. *J. Pharmacol. Exp. Ther.* **196**(2):396–406.

Crapo, J. D. (1986). Morphologic changes in pulmonary oxygen toxicity. *Annu. Rev. Physiol.* **48:**721–731.

Cutaia, M., and Friedrich, P. (1987). Hypoxia-induced alterations of norepinephrine vascular reactivity in isolated perfused cat lung. *J. Appl. Physiol.* **63:**982–987.

Deneke, S. M., and Fanburg, B. L. (1980). Normobaric oxygen toxicity of the lung. *N. Engl. J. Med.* **303**(2):76–86.

Eddinger, T. J., (1991). Gel electrophoretic resolution of a possible fourth myosin heavy chain in smooth muscle tissues. *Biophys. J.* **59:**437a.

Fishman, A. P. (1976). Hypoxia on the pulmonary circulation. How and where it acts. *Circ. Res.* **38:**221–231.

Fridovich, I. (1970). Quantitative aspects of the production of superoxide anion radical by milk xanthine oxidase. *J. Biol. Chem.* **245:**4053–4057.

Fridovich, I. (1983). Superoxide radical: an endogenous toxicant. *Ann. Rev. Pharm.* **23:**239–257.

Fried, R., and Reid, L. (1984). Early recovery from hypoxic pulmonary hypertension. *J. Appl. Physiol.* **57:**1246–1253.

Granger, D. N. (1988). Role of xanthine oxidase and granulocytes in ischemia-reperfusion injury. *Am. J. Physiol.* **255:**H1269–H1275.

Griffith, S. L., Packer, C. S., Meiss, R. A., and Rhoades, R. A. (1990). Length-tension characteristics of pulmonary arterial smooth muscle from hypoxia-induced pulmonary hypertensive rats. *FASEB J.***4:**A575.

Gryglewski, R. J., Palmer, R. M. J., and Moncada, S. (1986). Superoxide anion is involved in the breakdown of endothelium-derived vascular relaxing factor. *Nature* **320:**454–456.

Hammond, B., Kontos, H. A., and Hess, M. L. (1983). Oxygen radicals in the adult respiratory distress syndrome, in myocardiol ischemia and reperfusion injury and in cerebral vascular damage. *Can. J. Physiol. Pharmacol.* **63:**173–187.

Harlan, J. M. (1985). Leukocyte-endothelial interactions. *Blood* **65:**513–525.

Hathaway, D. R., and Adelstein, R. S. (1979). Human platelet myosin light chain kinase requires the calcium-binding protein calmodulin for activity. *Proc. Natl. Acad. Sci.* **76:**1653–1657.

Heath, D., and Smith, P. (1983). Electron microscopy of hypertensive pulmonary vascular disease. *Br. J. Dis. Chest* **77:**1–13.

Heath, D., and Williams, D. R. (1981). *Man at High Altitude: The Pathophysiology of Acclimatization and Adaptation,* 2nd ed. Churchill Livingstone, New York.

Heinle, H. (1984). Vasoconstriction of carotid artery induced by hydrogen peroxides. *Arch. Int. Physiol. Biochim.* **92:**1–5.

Henson, P. M., and Johnston, R. B. Jr. (1987). Tissue injury in inflammation. *J. Clin. Invest.* **79:**669–674.

Hidaka, H., Inagaki, M., Kawamoto, S., and Sasaki, Y. (1984). Isoquinolinesulfonamides, novel and potent inhibitors of cyclic nucleotide dependent proten kinase and protein kinase C. *Biochemistry* **23:**5036.

Hislop, A., and Reid, L. (1976). New findings in pulmonary arteries of rats with hypoxia-induced pulmonary hypertension. *Br. J. Exp. Pathol.* **57:**542–554.

Inauen, W., Suzuki, M., and Granger, D. N. (1989). Mechanisms of cellular injury: Potential sources of oxygen free radicals in ischemia reperfusion. *Microcirc. Endothelium Lymphatics* **5:**143–155.

Jin, N., Packer, C. S., Lloyd, T. C., and Rhoades, R. A. (1989). Ischemia reperfusion injury does not alter canine pulmonary arterial smooth muscle reactivity. *Physiologist* **32:**196.

Jin, N., Packer, C. S., and Rhoades, R. A. (1991). Reactive oxygen-mediated contraction in pulmonary arterial smooth muscle: cellular mechanisms. *Can. J. Physiol. Pharmacol.* **69:**383–388.

Johnson, R. L., Cassidy, S. S., Haynes, M., Reynolds, R. L., and Schulz, W. (1981). Microvascular injury distal to unilateral pulmonary artery occlusion. *J. Appl. Physiol.* **51:**845–851.

Jones, R., Zapol, W. M., and Reid, L. (1984). Pulmonary artery remodeling and pulmonary hypertension after exposure to hyperoxia for 7 days: A morphometric and hemodynamic study. *Am. J. Pathol.* **117:**273–285.

Jones, R., Langleben, D., and Reid, L. M. (1985a). Patterns of remodeling of the pulmonary circulation in acute and subacute lung injury. In *The Pulmonary Circulation and Acute Lung Injury.* Edited by S. I. Said. Futura Publishing Co., Mount Kisco, N. Y., pp. 137–188.

Jones, R., Zapol, W. M., and Reid, L. (1985b). Oxygen toxicity and restructuring of pulmonary arteries a morphometric study, the response to 4 weeks exposure to hyperoxia and return to breathing air. *Am. J. Pathol.* **121:**221–223.

Kaplan, H. P., Fobinson, F. R., Kapanci, Y., and Weibel, E. R. (1969). Pathogenesis and reversibility of pulmonary lesions of oxygen toxicity in monkeys. *Lab. Invest.* **20:**94–100.

Katusic, Z. S., and Vanhoutte, P. M. (1989). Superoxide anion is an endothelium-derived contracting factor. *Am. J. Physiol.* **257:**H33–H37.

Kerr, J. S., Riley, D. J., Frank, M. M., Trelstad, R. L., and Frankel, H. M. (1984). Reduction of chronic hypoxic pulmonary hypertension in the rat by B-aminopropionitrile. *J. Appl. Physiol.* **57:**1760–1766.

Kerr, J. S., Ruppert, C. L., Tozzi, C. A., Neubauer, J. A., Frankel, H. M., Yu, S. Y., and Riley, D. J. (1987). Reduction of chronic hypoxic pulmonary hypertension in the rat by an inhibitor of collagen production. *Am. Rev. Respir. Dis.* **135:**300–305.

Koyama, I., Toung, T. J. K., Rogers, M. C., Guntner, G. H., and Traystman, R. J. (1987). O_2 radicals mediate reperfusion lung injury in ischemia O_2-ventilated canine pulmonary lobe. *J. Appl. Physiol.* **63:**111–115.

Lee, C. T., Fein, A. M., Lippman, M., Holtzman, H., Kimbel, P., and Weinbaum, G. (1981). Elastolytic activity in pulmonary lavage fluid from patients with adult respiratory distress syndrome. *N. Eng. J. Med.* **304:**192–196.

Martin, R. J., Sandblom, R. L., and Johnson, R. J. (1983). Adult respiratory distress syndrome following thrombolytic therapy for pulmonary embolism. *Chest* **1:** 151–153.

McMurty, I. F., Petrun, D. M., and Reeves, J. T. (1978). Lungs from chronic hypoxia rats have decreased presser response to acute hypoxia. *Am. J. Physiol.* **235** (*Heart Circ. Physiol.*):H104–H109.

Mecham, R. P., Whitehouse, L. A., Wrenn, D. S., Park, W. C., Griffin, G. L., Senoir, R. M., Crouch, E. C., Stenmark, K. R., and Voelkel, N. F. (1987). Smooth muscle-mediated connective tissue remodeling in pulmonary hypertension. *Science* **237:**423–426.

Meisheri, K. D., Hwang, O., and Van Breeman, C. (1981). Evidence for two separate Ca^{2+} pathways in smooth muscle plasmalemma. *J. Membr. Biol.* **59:**19–25.

Meyrick, B., and Reid, L. (1980). Hypoxia-induced structural changes in the media and adventitia of the rat hilar pulmonary artery and their regression. *Am. J. Physiol.* **100**:151–178.

Moser, K. M., Spragy, R. G., Utley, J., and Dailey, P. O. (1983). Chronic thrombotic obstruction of major pulmonary arteries. *Ann. Intern. Med.* **99:**299–305.

Myers, C. L., Lazo, J. C., and Pitt, B. R. (1989). Translocation of protein kinase C is associated with inhibition of 5-HT uptake by cultured endothelial cells. *Am. J. Physiol.* **257:**L253–L258.

Nilsson, R. F., Dick, M., and Bray, R. C. (1969). ESR studies on reduction of oxygen to superoxide by some biochemical systems. *Biochim. Biophys. Acta* **192:**145–148.

Packer, C. S., and Stephens, N. L. (1985). Mechanics of caudal artery relaxation in control and hypertensive rats. *Can. J. Physiol. Pharmacol.* **63:**209–213.

Packer, C. S., and Stephens, N. L. (1987). Prolonged isobaric relaxation time in small mesenteric arteries of the spontaneously hypertensive rat. *Can. J. Physiol. Pharmacol.* **65:**230–235.

Paterson, N. A. M., Hamilton, J. T., Yaghi, A., and Miller, D. S. (1988). Effect of hypoxia on responses of respiratory smooth muscle to histamine and LTD_4. *J. Appl. Physiol.* **64:**435–440.

Patterson, C. E., Barnard, J. W., Lafuze, J. E., Hull, M. T., Baldwin, S. J., and Rhoades, R. A. (1989). The role of activation of neutrophils and microvascular pressure in acute pulmonary edema. *Am. Rev. Respir. Dis.* **140:**1052–1062.

Patterson, C. E., Jin, N., Packer, C. S., and Rhoades, R. A. Activated neutrophils alter contractile properties of the pulmonary artery. *Am. J. Respir. Cell Mol. Biol.* (in press).

Porcelli, R. S., and Bergman, M. J. (1983). Effects of chronic hypoxia on pulmonary vascular response to biogenic amines. *J. Appl. Physiol.* **55**(C2):534–540.

Porzio, M. A., and Pearson, A. M. (1977). Improved resolution of myofibrillar proteins with sodium dodecyl sulfate–polyacrylamide gel electrophoreis. *Biochem. Biophys. Acta* **490:**27–34.

Reeves, J. T., and Grover, R. F. (1975). High altitude pulmonary hypertension and pulmonary edema, In *Progress in Cardiology,* Vol. 4. Edited by P. N. Yu and J. F. Goodwin. Lea & Febiger, Philadelphia, pp. 99–118.

Rasmussen H., Kojima, I., and Barrett, P. (1986). Information flow in the calcium messenger system. In *Insights into Cell and Membrane Transport Processes.* Edited by G. Poste and S. T. Crooke. Plenum Press, New York, pp. 145–174.

Reeves, J. T., and Grover, B. M. (1984). Approach to the patient with pulmonary hypertension. In *Pulmonary Hypertension.* Edited by E. K. Weir, and J. T. Reeves. Futura Publishing Co., Mount Kisco, N. Y., pp. 1–44.

Reid, L. M. (1990). Vascular remodeling. In *The Pulmonary Circulation: Normals and Abnormals.* Edited by A. P. Fishman. University of Pennsylvania Press, Philadelphia, pp. 259–282.

Repine, J. E., Bowman, C. W., and Tate, R. M. (1985). Neutrophils and lung edema. *Chest* **81S:**47–50.

Rhoades, R. A., Packer, C. S., and Meiss, R. A. (1988). Pulmonary vascular smooth muscle: Effect of free radicals. *Chest* **93**(Suppl.):945–955.

Rhoades, R. A., Packer, C. S., Roepke, D. A., Jin, N., and Meiss, R. A. (1990). Reactive oxygen species after contractile properties of pulmonary arterial smooth muscle. *Can. J. Physiol. Pharmacol.* **68:**1581–1589.

Roepke, J. E., Packer, C. S., Meiss, R. A., and Rhoades, R. A. (1988). Effect of pulmonary hypertension on the sensitivity and reactivity of pulmonary arterial smooth muscle to norepinephrine. *FASEB J.* **2:**1182.

Roepke, J. E., Packer, C. S., and Rhoades, R. A. (1991). Arterial smooth myosin heavy chain isoform shifts are not primary in the etiology of hypoxia-induced pulmonary hypertension. *FASEB J.* **5:**A403.

Rosenbaum, W. I. (1983). Effects of free radical generation on mouse pial arterioles: Probable role of hydroxyl radicals. *Am. J. Physiol.* **245** (*Heart Circ. Physiol.* **14**):H139–H142.

Ross, R., Raines, E., and Bowen-Pope, D. (1982). Growth factores from platelets, monocytes and endothelium: Their role in proliferation. *Ann. N. Y. Acad. Sci.* **397:**18–24.

Rubanyi, G. M. (1988). Vascular effects of oxygen-derived free radicals. *Free Radic. Biol. Med.* **4:**107–120.

Saitoh, M., Naka, N., and Hidaka, H. (1986). The modulatory role of myosin light chain phosphorylation in human platelet activation. *Biochem. Biophys. Res. Commun.* **140:**280.

Saitoh, M., Ishikawa, T., Matsushima, S., Naka, M., and Hidaka, H. (1987). Selective inhibition of catalytic activity of smooth muscle myosin light chain kinase. *J. Biol. Chem.* **262:**7796.

Shasby, D. M., Vanbenthuysen, K. M., Tate, R. M., Shasby, S. S., McMurtry, I., and Repine, J. E. (1982). Granulocytes mediate acute adematous lung injury in rabbits and in isolated rabbit lung perfused with phorbol myristate acetate: Role of oxygen radicals. *Am. Rev. Respir. Dis.* **125:**443–447.

Shasby, D. M., Shasby, S. S., and Peach, M. J. (1983). Granulocyte and phorbol myristate acetate increase permeability to albumin of cultured endothelial monolayers and isolated perfused lungs. *Am. Rev. Respir. Dis.* **127:**72–76.

Shibata, S., and Cheng, J. R. (1977). Relaxation of vascular smooth muscle in spontaneously hypertensive rats. *Blood Vessels* **14:**247–248.

Sprung, C. L., Leowenherz, J. W., Baier, H., and Hauser, M. J. (1981). Evidence of increased permeability in reexpansion pulmonary edema. *Am. J. Med.* **71:**497–500.

Stenmark, K. R., Orton, E. C., Reeves, J. T., Voelkel, N. F., Crouch, E. P., and Mecham, R. P. (1987). Vascular smooth muscle controls elastin production in pulmonary hypertension arteriopathy of the new born calf. *Am. Rev. Respir. Dis.* **135:**A129.

Stuart, R. S., Baumgartner, W. A., Berkon, A. M., Bulkley, G. B., Brown, J. D., Del monte, S. M., Hutchin, G. M., and Reitz, B. A. (1985). Five hour hypothermic lung preservation with oxygen free radical scavenger. *Transplant. Proc.* **17:**1454–1456.

Sutko, J. L., Ito, K., and Kenyon, J. L. (1985). Ryanodine: a modifier of sarcoplasmic reticulum calcium release in striated muscle. *Fed. Proc. Am. Soc. Exp. Biol.* **44:**2984–2988.

Tate, R. M., Vanbenthuysen, K. M., Shasby, D. M., McMurty, I. F., and Repine, J. E. (1982). Oxygen radical mediated permeability, edema and vasoconstriction in isolated perfused rabbit lungs. *Am. Rev. Respir. Dis.* **126:**802–806.

Tetsuhiro, H., and Takayanagi, I. (1988). Ryanodine: its possible mechanism of action in the caffeine-sensitive calcium store of smooth muscle. *Pflugers Arch.* **412:** 376–381.

Tomashefski, J. F., Jr., Davier, P., Boggin, C., Green, R., Zapol, W. M., and Reid, L. M. C. (1983). The pulmonary vascular lesion of the adult respiratory distress syndrome. *Am. J. Pathol.* **112:**112–126.

Tozzi, C. A., Poinani, G. J., Edelman, N. H., and Riley, D. J. (1989). Vascular collagen affects reactivity of hypertensive pulmonary arteries of the rat. *J. Appl. Physiol.* **66:**1730–1735.

Vandeplassche, G., and Borges, M. (1990). Ultrastructure and Ca^{2+} reallocation during ischemia: The calcium paradox and metabolic acidosis. *Cell. Biol. Int. Rep.* **14:**317–334.

Ventura, C., Guarnieri, C., and Calderesa, C. M. (1985). Inhibitory effects of superoxide radicals and cardiac myofibrilar ATPase activity. *Ital. J. Biochem.* **34:**267–274.

Wagenvoort, C. A., and Wagenvoort, A. (1977). *Pathology of Pulmonary Hypertension.* Wiley, New York, pp. 9–16.

Ward, P. A., Till, G. O., Kunkel, R., and Beauchamp, G. (1983). Evidence for the role of hydroxyl radicals in compliment and neutrophil-dependent tissue injury. *J. Clin. Invest.* **72:**789–801.

Warshawski, F. J., Sibbald, W. J., Driedger, A. A., and Cheung, H. (1986). Abnormal neutrophil-pulmonary interaction in the adult respiratory distress syndrome. *Am. Rev. Respir. Dis.* **133:**797–804.

Wei, E. P., Christman, C. W., Kontos, H. A., and Povlishock, J. T. (1985). Effects of oxygen radicals and cerebral arterioles. *Am. J. Physiol.* **248:**H157–H162.

Wolin, M. S., Rodriques, A. M., and Yu, J. M. (1985). Peroxides causes dose-dependent relaxant and constrictor responses in isolated bovine intrapulmonary arterial and venous rings. *Fed. Proc. Am. Soc. Exp. Biol.* **44:**821.

10

Eosinophils, Mast Cells, and Basophils: Cellular Mechanisms Contributing to Lung Microvascular Injury

FRANKLIN CERASOLI, JR.

Sandoz Research Institute
East Hanover, New Jersey

ALASDAIR M. GILFILLAN and WILLIAM M. SELIG

Hoffmann–La Roche
Nutley, New Jersey

I. Introduction

Lung microvascular injury is exhibited in clinical and experimental pulmonary diseases such as adult respiratory distress syndrome (ARDS) and asthma. In the case of ARDS, the pulmonary microvasculature is altered to allow the escape of fluid and plasma proteins into the perivascular spaces, pulmonary interstitium, and alveoli. In asthma, the bronchial (and possibly the pulmonary) circulation is altered, leading to tissue edema. Lung microvascular injury may be produced by several mechanisms, including the activation of phagocytic leukocytes.

The theory that activated leukocytes contribute to increased pulmonary microvascular permeability is substantiated by clinical and experimental data (Bachofen and Weibel, 1977; Tate and Repine, 1983). Neutrophils apparently play a major role in the increase of pulmonary microvascular permeability. These cells adhere to the pulmonary microvascular endothelium that forms the major barrier to transvascular fluid and protein flux (Bachofen and Weibel, 1977, 1982). Once adherent, neutrophils become activated to degranulate (Harlan et al., 1985; Lee et al., 1981), produce chemotactic eicosanoids (Liles et al., 1987), and release toxic oxygen radicals (Sacks et al., 1978; Till et al., 1982) in a ''frustrated'' attempt to phagocytize the large endothelial surface (Henson, 1971). The highly deleterious microenvironment that forms between neutrophils and endothelial cells damages or kills endothelial cells, permitting fluid and protein exudation from the microvasculature.

Other leukocytes may also play a significant role in increasing lung microvascular permeability. Eosinophils, another phagocytic cell type, are capable of the same bactericidal properties as neutrophils; therefore, they may produce lung microvasculature injury in a manner analogous to neutrophils. Although eosinophils are presently overlooked as important effector cells of increased microvascular permeability, increasing evidence suggests that they do contribute to the destruction of the microvasculature (Hoidal, 1990). In fact, eosinophils are currently viewed as a critical link in the inflammatory component of asthma in which lung microvascular injury and plasma exudation are present. Mast cells and basophils are also viewed as important effector cells in asthma since both cells release inflammatory mediators that can injure the lung microvasculature. Following antigen challenge, mast cell degranulation may directly contribute to increased airway microvascular permeability and mucosal edema formation (Didier et al., 1990; Sertl et al., 1988). Alternatively, mast cells and basophils may also indirectly contribute to lung microvascular injury by communicating with other cells (including eosinophils and neutrophils).

In this chapter we present the current evidence supporting a role for eosinophils, mast cells, and basophils in lung microvascular injury. We also describe the intercellular communications between these cells that may contribute to lung microvascular injury and the intracellular mechanisms regulating various functions of these cells. To introduce these topics, the morphological and functional characteristics of these cell types are discussed.

II. Location, Morphology, and Function of Eosinophils, Basophils, and Mast Cells

In this section, we present briefly the characteristics of eosinophils, mast cells, and basophils. Readers are also directed to more detailed reviews discussing eosinophils (Bainton, 1988; Gleich and Adolphson, 1986; Spry, 1985), mast cells (Galli, 1990; Siraganian, 1988), and basophils (Siraganian, 1988).

A. Eosinophils

Eosinophils originate in bone marrow, enter the circulation, and then become tissue-dwelling cells. Eosinophils develop within the bone marrow, from multipotential precursors to mature cells, over the course of 5 to 6 days (Beeson and Bass, 1977; Spry, 1971a). The final maturation of eosinophils may occur in either the spleen (in rats; Spry, 1971b) or in the bone marrow (in guinea pigs;

Hudson, 1963, 1968). In guinea pigs, mature eosinophils comprise up to 75% of the eosinophilic cells in bone marrow, suggesting a large "marrow reserve" of mature eosinophils (Hudson, 1963, 1968). Similarly, a marrow storage pool for eosinophils is also present in humans and may represent a 5- to 6-day supply of usable eosinophils (Parwaresch et al., 1976). Eosinophils, marginated along the vascular endothelium in rats, may also represent a readily available storage pool (Archer, 1968), although the number of marginated eosinophils is not precisely known. Once eosinophils enter the peripheral blood, their circulating half-life is from 3 to 8 h in humans (Parwaresch et al., 1976) and 6.5 to 10.5 h in rats (Cohen et al. 1967; Foot, 1965; Spry, 1972). In humans, eosinophils are normally only a small percentage (1 to 3%) of the total circulating leukocytes. Eosinophils depart the circulation, via diapedesis through the vascular endothelium, and subsequently take up residence in tissues. Approximately 100 tissue eosinophils are present for every circulating eosinophil in humans (Stryckmans et al., 1968). Eosinophils are found primarily in the tissues of organs with epithelial surfaces, such as the gut, the lower urinary tract, and the lung (Archer, 1963; Bainton, 1988). Interestingly, eosinophils and mast cells are often found together in these tissues. In rats, eosinophils are prevalent in the perivascular and peribronchial spaces (Gleich, 1988). The tissue half-life of rat eosinophils is approximately 22 to 48 h (Cohen et al. 1967; Foot, 1965).

Eosinophils are phagocytic cells approximately 9.0 to 15.0 μm in diameter that possess a bilobate nucleus and cytoplasmic granules (Bloom and Fawcett, 1975; Weller, 1989). The nucleus is centrally located and the ratio of nuclear volume to cytoplasmic volume is low (Zucker-Franklin, 1974). The cytoplasmic granules stain red with Wright's stain, indicating a high content of basic proteins housed within these granules. Mature eosinophils possess both small and specific (or secondary) granules. Small granules primarily contain acid phosphatase and arylsulfatase B. Specific granules contain various arginine-containing basic proteins, including major basic protein (MBP), eosinophil cationic protein (ECP), and eosinophil-derived neurotoxin (EDN). MBP comprises the cystalloid core of specific granules (Peters et al., 1986) and 50 to 60% of the total protein content of the granule (Gleich et al., 1973). ECP is found in the amorphous matrix surrounding the crystalloid core (Peters et al., 1986) and is estimated to be less than 2% of the MBP content (Ackerman et al., 1983). Eosinophil peroxidase (EPO) and catalase are also found in specific granules, suggesting that the granules are true peroxisomes (Iozzo et al., 1982; Yokota et al., 1984). The amount of EPO in the granule is only 10 to 20% that of MBP (Klebanoff et al., 1989). EPO, catalase, collagenase, and alkaline phosphatase are all found in the granule matrix (Peters et al., 1986). A small population of primary granules, associated with the eosinophil plasma membrane, contains a protein that possesses lysophospholipase activity (Dvorak et al., 1988, 1990). This activity is responsible for the presence of hexagonal, bipyramidal Charcot–Leyden crystals often found in body fluids and tissues that are eosinophilic (Weller et al., 1982, 1984). A membrane-bound phospholipase D also appears to be present in rat and human eosinophils (Kater et al., 1976; Lempereur et al., 1980).

Eosinophils, from humans and experimental animals, have several densities (dependent on eosinophil mass and/or size) when isolated on density step gradients. Normodense eosinophils are isolated from the blood of normal humans; however, both normodense and hypodense eosinophils are isolated from patients with hypereosinophilic syndrome or atopy (Fukuda et al., 1985). In guinea pigs, eosinophils of several densities are isolated from the airways (Cerasoli et al., 1991; Hirata et al., 1989; Sun et al., 1989). The origin of hypodense eosinophils is controversial. They may be immature eosinophilic myeolocytes released from bone marrow during disease states (Olofsson et al., 1980). Alternatively, they may be activated normodense eosinophils since hypodense eosinophils have enhanced cytotoxicity and fewer granules (Butterworth et al., 1975; De Simone et al., 1982; Prin et al., 1983, 1984). Stimulation of normodense eosinophils in vitro converts these cells from normodense to hypodense eosinophils (Kloprogge et al., 1989a). Evidence suggests that the conversion may be due to increased water content of the granules, leading to vacuolation rather than degranulation (Spry, 1985).

Several eosinophil functions enable these cells to execute their parasitidal role in host defense. Irreversible adherence of eosinophils to parasites is the initial step in their cytotoxic activity (Butterworth et al., 1979). Since eosinophils have Fc and C3b receptors on their membranes, adherence is most effective when it is complement- or antibody-mediated (Ottesen et al., 1977). Once adherent, eosinophils attempt to phagocytize the organism. Eosinophils are poor phagocytes (compared to neutrophils); however, phagocytosis is enhanced by coating parasites with IgG and IgE antibodies (Beeson and Bass, 1977; Grover et al., 1978). This enhancement is probably due to an increase in adherence rather than an actual increase in the ability of eosinophils to phagocytize.

Eosinophils release granule contents and toxic oxygen radicals during parasitidal activity. MBP, released from specific granules, is intrinsically cytotoxic (Butterworth et al., 1979). The exact mechanisms by which MBP kills parasites is unclear; however, this cationic protein may interact with anionic parasite membrane proteins, alter ion fluxes, and disturb osmotic homeostasis (Brandt and Freeman, 1967; Quinton and Philpott, 1973). ECP is also deleterious to parasites and is estimated to be 10 times more potent than MBP, although it may contribute less to cytoxicity due to its relatively small quantities (Ackerman et al., 1985). EPO, released from specific granules, aids in the generation of hypohalus acids that are 10- to 100-fold more toxic than the basic proteins (Klebanoff et al., 1989). Hypohalus acid formation occurs when EPO catalyzes the oxidation of halides (particularly Br^-) by H_2O_2. H_2O_2 and other toxic oxygen radicals, such as superoxide anion, are formed at the eosinophil membrane (Klebanoff, 1988). Superoxide anion release from eosinophils occurs at a greater rate than release from neutrophils (Petreccia et al., 1987; Sedgwick et al., 1988). However, this observation is dependent not only on the stimulating agent for radical release but also on the source of the eosinophils (i.e., normal volunteers versus hypereosinophilic patients; Tauber et al., 1979).

Finally, several lipid mediators are produced by eosinophils through phospholipase A_2, cyclooxygenase, and lipoxygenase activation. Leukotriene C_4 (Kajita et al., 1985) or B_4 (Henderson et al., 1984; Hirata et al., 1989), 5- or 15-hydroxyeicosatetraneoic acid (Goetzl et al., 1980; Henderson et al., 1984), lipoxin A (Steinhilber and Roth, 1989), thromboxane B_2 (Sun et al., 1989), platelet activating factor (PAF), and prostaglandins (D_2, $F_{2\alpha}$, and E_2; Giembycz et al., 1990; Lee et al., 1984) can all be produced from eosinophils (depending on the species examined). These mediators may play regulatory roles in leukocyte activation by modulating the function of other leukocytes, such as neutrophils, in an area of inflammation (Kloprogge et al., 1989b).

In summary, eosinophil function significantly contributes to host defense through parasitidal activity. However, the release of cytotoxic and pro-inflammatory mediators from eosinophils may also contribute to the pathophysiological events leading to lung microvascular injury. Some of these mechanisms of eosinophil-induced lung microvascular injury are discussed below (see Section V).

B. Mast Cells and Basophils

Mast cells and basophils differ in their distribution in the body (Siraganian, 1988). Mast cells are associated with connective tissue compartments. In the lung, approximately half of the mast cells are found in airway connective tissue; the remainder are associated with peripheral lung tissues (Friedman and Kaliner, 1987). Airway mast cells are most abundant beneath the basement membrane, in close proximity to small blood vessels in the submucosa (Agius et al., 1986; Friedman and Kaliner, 1987). They are also found adjacent to submucus glands, in the intraalveolar septa (Casale and Marom, 1983), and in the airway lumen between the epithelial cells (Agius et al., 1986). In contrast to mast cells, basophils circulate within the vasculature.

Although they are ontologically related, mast cells and basophils are morphologically distinct. Mast cells and basophils originate in bone marrow and may develop from the same progenitor cell (Galli et al., 1984; Zucker-Franklin, 1980). However, mast cells remain as mononuclear leukocytes, while basophils mature into polymorphonuclear granulocytes (Galli et al., 1984). The diameter of mast cells ranges between 5 and 7 μm; that of basophils is 6 to 12 μm (Galli,

1990). The pseudopodia of mast cells are elongated and uniformly distributed. In contrast, the pseudopodia of basophils are short, blunt, and irregularly dispersed (Galli et al., 1984). The granules associated with mast cells are smaller and more numerous than those of basophils, although both cell types possess a similar collection of mediators within their granules.

Two major categories of inflammatory mediators are released from stimulated mast cells and basophils:

1. *Presynthesized mediators*: These mediators include bioactive amines (i.e., histamine and 5-hydroxytryptamine), proteolytic and hydrolytic enzymes (i.e., chymase and tryptase), and a chemotactic factor for eosinophils (ECF; Bryant et al., 1977). Presynthesized mediators are stored in secretory granules and released during degranulation.
2. De novo-*synthesized mediators*: These mediators include prostaglandins, leukotrienes, platelet activating factor (PAF), and adenosine. De novo-synthesized mediators are produced and released into the extracellular space in response to mast cell and basophil stimulation.

Mast cells and basophils also synthesize and secrete several cytokines, including interleukins (ILs) 3 to 6 (Plaut et al., 1989; Wodnar-Filipowicz et al., 1989), tumor necrosis factor (TNF; Gordon and Galli, 1990; Ohno et al., 1990; Steffen et al., 1989), and granulocyte/macrophage-colony stimulating factor (GM-CSF; Wodnar-Filipowicz et al., 1989). These cytokines play regulatory roles in the proliferation, differentiation, and function of eosinophils, mast cells, basophils, and other leukocytes (see Section IV). Therefore, cytokine production and release from mast cells and basophils, may constitute a mechanism for the modification of leukocyte function.

The initiating event for the release of inflammatory mediators and cytokines from mast cells and basophils generally involves the cross-bridging of receptor-bound IgE by specific antigens. Several other endogenous mediators can also elicit mediator release, including adenosine (Church et al., 1983; Gilfillan et al., 1990b; Holgate et al., 1980; Lohse et al., 1987; Marqaurdt et al., 1978; Peachell et al., 1988), neurotensin (Foreman et al., 1982), complement components C3a and C5a (Hartman and Glovsky, 1981; Hook et al., 1975; Johnson et al., 1975; Regal et al., 1983), substance P (Foreman et al., 1982; Piotrowski and Foreman, 1985; Piotrowski et al., 1987), ILs 3 to 5 (Morita et al., 1987; Schleimer et al., 1989; Subramanian and Bray, 1987; Valent et al., 1989), TNF (Schleimer et al., 1981), and GM-CSF (Haak-Frendscho et al., 1988). Mediator release from mast cells and basophils is induced by several factors, including cytokines, released from other inflammatory cells, such as eosinophils (see Section IV), neutrophils (White et al., 1986), and macrophages (Liu et al., 1986).

III. Signal Transduction Mechanisms in Eosinophils, Mast Cells, and Basophils

Signal transduction mechanisms in eosinophils are not adequately characterized. Since eosinophils and neutrophils respond in a similar manner to the same stimulating agents, it is likely that signal transduction mechanisms in eosinophils are similar to those in neutrophils. For this reason, readers are directed toward several excellent reviews and original works describing signal transduction in neutrophils (Omann et al., 1987; Sanborg and Smolen, 1988). Signal transduction pathways in mast cells and basophils are better characterized (Beaven and Cunha-Melo, 1988; Oliver et al., 1988; Pecht and Corcia, 1987). The purpose of this section is to present a brief overview of these mechanisms.

A. G Proteins

The term *G protein* describes a family of GTP-binding proteins that act functionally as transmembrane couplers between cell-surface receptors and ionic channels or enzymes that regulate cell function (Gilman, 1987). G proteins can be experimentally manipulated by several approaches. Activation is produced by the introduction of stable analogs, such as GTPγS and GPP(NH)P, into permeabilized cells or by the addition of cholera toxin, which activates specific G proteins (e.g., G_s and G_t proteins) as a consequence of ADP ribosylation. Inhibition is produced by the addition of GDPβS, which competes with GTP for the GTP binding site, or by the addition of pertussis toxin, which inhibits the actions of specific G proteins (e.g., G_i and G_p proteins) by ADP ribosylation.

The functional evidence for a role for G proteins in mast cell mediator release comes from studies demonstrating degranulation in response to GTPγS and GPP(NH)P (Gomperts et al., 1987; Howell et al., 1987; Narasimhan et al., 1990; Wilson et al., 1989; Woldemussie et al., 1987). In addition, cholera toxin potentiates IgE-dependent mediator release from a rat mast cell line (RBL 2H3) by mechanisms that appear to involve G protein–mediated enhancement of IP_3 release and/or elevated calcium influx (McCloskey, 1988; Narasimhan et al., 1988). The strongest evidence supporting a role for G proteins in IgE-dependent mediator release from mast cells and basophils comes from studies demonstrating that GDPβS blocks IgE-dependent mediator release (Penner, 1988). Additionally, myclophenic acid, which depletes intracellular gaunine nucleotides, suppresses antigen-dependent responses in RBL 2H3 cells (Wilson et al., 1989). Finally, an RBL 2H3 variant, which is unresponsive to activators of G proteins, is also unresponsive to antigen (Woldemussie et al., 1987). In contrast to the observations above, pertussis toxin fails to inhibit IgE-dependent histamine release in several mast cell and basophil models (Ali et al., 1990; Gilfillan et al., 1990b; Saito et al., 1987; Warner et al., 1987). This lack of inhibition occurs despite the ability of pertussis toxin to inhibit mediator release in response to agents, such as compound 48/80 (Nakamura and Ui, 1985; Saito et al., 1987), GPP(NH)P (Nakamura and Ui, 1984), thrombin (Saito et al., 1987). C5a (Warner et al., 1987), and adenosine P_l purinoceptor agonists (Ali et al., 1990; Gilfillan et al., 1990b). Although the majority of evidence suggests that G proteins influence mediator release from mast cells and basophils, the exact role of G proteins in IgE-dependent mediator release remains to be fully established.

B. Inositol Trisphosphate and Intracellular Calcium

In response to cross-bridging of IgE receptors (Cunha-Melo et al., 1987; Maeyama et al., 1988) or to other stimuli, such as GTP analogs (Woldemussie et al., 1987) and adenosine analogs (Ali et al., 1990), inositol phosphate levels rapidly increase in mast cells and basophils. This increase closely correlates to the extent of mediator release from RBL 2H3 cells (Maeyama et al., 1988). Inositol trisphosphate (IP_3), together with diacylglycerol (DAG), is produced by the phospholipase C–catalyzed breakdown of phosphatidylinositol 4,5-bisphosphate (Berridge, 1987). The major function of IP_3 in cells appears to be the liberation of calcium from intracellular storage sites, primarily the endoplasmic reticulum (Berridge, 1987). Cross-bridging of IgE receptors on the surface of mast cells and basophils results in a rapid and prolonged increase in cytosolic free calcium ($[Ca^{2+}]_i$; Ali et al., 1989; Beaven et al., 1987; Crews et al., 1981). The initial rapid increase in $[Ca^{2+}]_i$ appears to be dependent on IP_3-induced release of Ca^{2+} from intracellular stores, whereas the sustained elevation appears to be due to the interaction of a cAMP and Ca^{2+}- activated chloride current with IP_3-dependent Ca^{2+} influx (Penner et al., 1988). Other stimuli for mast cells degranulation, including adenosine analogs (Ali et al., 1990; Miller et al., 1990), thrombin (Miller et al., 1990), and prostaglandin D_2 (Miller et al., 1990), also increase $[Ca^{2+}]_i$, although they produce a more rapid and transient calcium response. Calcium ionophores, such as A23187 and ionomycin, also result in a rapid increase in $[Ca^{2+}]_i$ (Lo et al., 1987) and release both histamine (Crews et al., 1981; Gilfillan et al., 1990a; Lo et al., 1987) and arachidonic acid metabolites (Crews et al., 1981; Gilfillan et al., 1990a) from mast cells.

The IgE-dependent increase in $[Ca^{2+}]_i$ (Beaven et al., 1984) and release of histamine (Beaven et al., 1984; Foreman et al., 1973) are blocked by the addition of the extracellular calcium chelator, EGTA. This demonstrates a requirement for extracellular calcium in the $[Ca^{2+}]_i$ increase and mediator release. Extracellular calcium is also required for GTPγS-dependent mast cell degranulation (Koopman and Jackson, 1990). Despite the presence of extracellular calcium, GTPγS- (Penner and Neher, 1988) or antigen-dependent (P. Lin and A. M. Gilfillan, unpublished observations) mast cell degranulation is inhibited by the intracellular chelator BAPTA, demonstrating that the release of mediators is directly influenced by $[Ca^{2+}]_i$.

C. Diacylglycerol Production and Protein Kinase C Activation

As discussed earlier, diacylglycerol (DAG) levels are rapidly elevated in activated mast cells (Gruchalla et al., 1990; Kennerly, 1987; 1990; Kennerly et al., 1979; Lin et al., 1991). Intracellular DAG regulates the activation of protein kinase C (PKC; Berridge, 1987). A role for PKC activation in inflammatory mediator release from mast cells and basophils is suggested by several studies. Activation of PKC by 12-*O*-tetradecanoyl phorbol-13-acetate (PMA) induces degranulation (Cantwell and Foreman, 1986, 1987; Katakami et al., 1984; Sagi-Eisenberg and Pecht, 1984, Sagi-Eisenberg et al., 1985; Schleimer et al., 1981) and arachidonic acid release (Jacobsen et al., 1987) from several mast cell and basophil models, although in some studies, these effects are observed only in conjunction with other stimuli such as A23187. PKC activation involves translocation from the cytosol to the membrane. In rat peritoneal mast cells, PKC translocation occurs in response to stimuli that induce mast cell mediator release, including PMA, compound 48/80, and concanavalin A (Nagao et al., 1987). PKC translocation also results from treatment of mast cells with antigen (White et al., 1984).

PKC inhibitors, including staurosporine and K252a, inhibit IgE-dependent degranulation of arachidonic acid release from mast cells (White et al., 1984), basophils (Morita et al., 1988; Warner and MacGlashan, 1990), and RBL 2H3 cells (Gilfillan et al., 1990a). These results suggest that PKC activation may be a pivotal step in mediator release from mast cells and basophils, although PKC activation may not be selectively inhibited by these agents. In contrast, staurosporine does not inhibit degranulation in response to GTPγS and Ca^{2+} despite inhibiting the degranulating effect of PMA (Koopman and Jackson, 1990). This suggests that the sensitivity of mast cells to stimuli can be altered by PKC-catalyzed phosphorylation events, although PKC activation may not be required for exocytosis to occur (Koopman and Jackson, 1990).

The extent to which PIP_2 hydrolysis influences intracellular DAG levels and subsequent PKC activation has recently been questioned. For example, when mass is taken into consideration during cell activation, the amount of DAG formed is in excess of that which can be accounted for by hydrolysis of PIP_2 alone (Kennerly, 1990). In addition, in mast cells, the fatty acid composition of DAG shows greater similarity to phosphatidylcholine (PC) than to phosphatidylinositol (PI) (Kennerly, 1990). Activation of PC-specific phospholipase D (PC-PLD) may explain these discrepancies (Gruchalla et al., 1990; Lin et al., 1991). PC-PLD cleaves PC to yield phosphatidic acid (PA), which is subsequently dephosphorylated by PA phosphohydrolase (PAPase) to form DAG.

PC-PLD activation, in mast cells and basophils, may be a possible unifying mechanism for degranulation and release of de novo synthesized arachidonic acid metabolites (Lin et al., 1991). The precise role that PC-PLD plays in degranulation is unclear; however, the increase in DAG levels and PKC activation in stimulated mast cells may be initiated by PLC activation. The subsequent maintenance of elevated DAG levels and PKC activation, which is necessary for degranulation, may be dependent on PKC-mediated PC-PLD activation (Lin et al., 1991).

D. Adenylate Cyclase

Aggregation of IgE receptors on the surface of mast cells and basophils results in a rapid and biphasic increase in intracellular cAMP (Ishizaka et al., 1981; Lewis et al., 1979; Sullivan et al., 1976). The role of cAMP in signal transduction, in mast cells, is unclear; however, the elevation of cAMP may inhibit mediator release. For example, agents that elevate intracellular cAMP, including cAMP analogs (Winslow and Austen, 1984), forskolin (Marone et al., 1987), and β_2 agonists (Undem et al., 1988), prevent IgE-dependent degranulation and release of de novo synthesized mediators. The degree of inhibition correlates with cAMP levels (Sullivan et al., 1976), inhibition of $^{45}Ca^{2+}$ flux (Teshima et al., 1984), activation of cAMP-dependent protein kinase, and results in increased protein phosphorylation (see below).

E. Protein Phosphorylation

Phosphorylation of specific intracellular proteins results from activation of protein kinases, including PKC, the Ca^{2+}/calmodulin-dependent protein kinase, and cAMP-dependent protein kinase. Phorbol myristate acetate (PMA)-dependent PKC activation results in the phosphorylation of 48,000-, 55,000-, 59,000-, and 78,000-kD proteins (Heiman and Crews, 1985). The most notable change occurs in the 48,000-kD band. The relevance of phosphorylation of these proteins is unknown; however, the phosphorylation of 78,000-kD protein may act as an ''off switch'' for histamine release (Theoharides et al., 1980; Wells and Mann, 1983). The phosphorylation of this protein is believed to be one of the mechanisms by which the antiasthmatic compound cromolyn induces its effect (Theoharides et al., 1980; Wells and Mann, 1983). The extent of protein phosphorylation also correlates with the inhibitory effects of cAMP on antigen-induced histamine release (Winslow and Austen, 1984). The phosphorylation of several proteins is associated with IgE-dependent activation of RBL 2H3 cells (Hattori and Siraganian, 1987; Ludowyke et al., 1989; Marone et al., 1987; Teshima et al., 1984; Undem et al., 1988). The identity and function of these proteins remain to be fully established; however, the β subunit of the IgE receptor (Teshima et al., 1984) and myosin light and heavy chains (Ludowyke et al., 1989) are some of the phosphorylated proteins. Therefore, protein phosphorylation may influence mast cell mediator release by influencing several different processes within mast cells.

IV. Interrelationship Between Eosinophils, Mast Cells, and Basophils

Mediators released from leukocytes are capable of influencing the function of their respective cell types as well as other cell types. For example, eosinophil-derived mediators are capable of inducing mast cell and basophil degranulation. Mast cell- and basophil-derived mediators can activate eosinophils. Mediators released from mast cells and basophils can also stimulate or, in certain circumstances, inhibit the activation of other mast cells and basophils. Therefore, mediators released from these cell types may provide mechanisms of communication that alter leukocyte responses, leading to altered lung microvascular permeability.

A. Eosinophil Mediators That Affect Mast Cells and Basophils

Mediators, released from the granules of activated eosinophils, can produce activation of mast cells, basophils, and other leukocytes. When applied in submicromolar and micromolar concentrations, MBP produces a dose-dependent increase in histamine release from mast cells and basophils (O'Donnell et al., 1983; Zheutlin et al., 1984). The histamine release from basophils occurs for up to 40 min, while release from mast cells is complete in 1 min. Since MBP is actively phagocytized by mast cells (Butterfield et al., 1990), MBP may increase histamine release from phagocytizing mast cells to a greater extent than nonphagocytizing mast cells. MBP also produces superoxide anion release and degranulation from neutrophils and enhances fMLP- or PAF-induced superoxide anion release (Moy et al., 1990). Therefore, MBP stimulates and enhances mast cell and basophil (and possibly other leukocyte) function.

In the presence of H_2O_2 and halide, EPO produces mast cell degranulation (Henderson et al., 1980a) through either cytotoxic or noncytotoxic mechanisms (Chi and Henderson, 1984). Furthermore, EPO's bactericidal activity may be enhanced through binding to extracellular mast cells granules (Fig. 1; Henderson et al., 1980b). This suggests that eosinophil activity can be regulated through the influence of eosinophils on other cell types. In addition, EPO may alter the effects of activated inflammatory leukocytes by altering the activity of pro-inflammatory mediators released from these leukocytes. For example, EPO decreases the smooth muscle–contracting activity of leukotrienes C_4 and D_4 and the

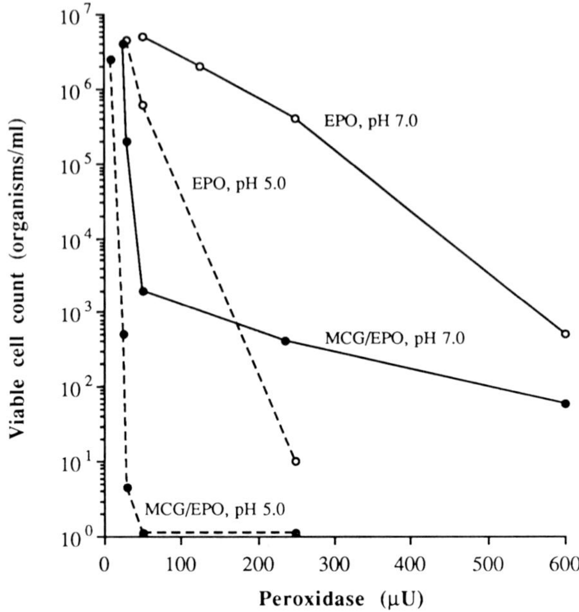

Figure 1 Enhancement of eosinophil peroxidase (EPO)-induced bacterial cytotoxicity by mast cell granules (MCG). EPO is purified from peritoneal eosinophils of Hartley guinea pigs and MCG is purified from peritoneal mast cells of Sprague–Dawley rats. EPO/MCG complexes are made prior to their use in the assay. *Escherichia coli* cytotoxicity assays are conducted in 0.05 *M* sodium phosphate at pH 5.0 or 7.0. Assay mixtures contain 5×10^6 *E. coli*, 10μ*M* H_2O_2, 0.1 m*M* NaI, and EPO or EPO/MCG. Mixtures are incubated for 60 min at 37°C. Equal amounts of EPO activity (gauiacol units) are present in each condition. The results indicate that bactericidal activity of EPO is augmented when it is complexed to MCG. (Adapted from Henderson et al., 1980b.)

chemoattractant activity of leukotriene B_4 (Henderson et al., 1982). Possibly, EPO has undefined potentiating effects on other pro-inflammatory mediators. Therefore, mediators released from eosinophils may influence other leukocytes ultimately to potentiate their contribution to the development of increased microvascular permeability.

B. Mast Cell and Basophil Mediators That Affect Eosinophils

Mediators released from mast cells and basophils can influence the activity of eosinophils. Cytokines, including granulocyte-macrophage colony stimulating factor (GM-CSF), interleukins 3 to 6 (IL), and tumor necrosis factor (TNF), are all released from mast cells and basophils. GM-CSF induces eosinophil colony formation (Metcalf et al., 1986) and enhances several eosinophil functions, such as ionophore-induced LTC_4 release (Howell et al., 1989; Owen et al., 1987), antibody-dependent cytoxicity, fMLP- and C3b-induced degranulation and toxic oxygen radical release (Dessein et al., 1982; Lopez et al., 1986), and IgGFc receptor expression (Dessein et al., 1982). IL-3 enhances eosinophil phagocytosis, toxic oxygen radical release, and antibody-dependent cytotoxicity (Lopez et al., 1987). IL-3 also contributes to the formation of hypodense eosinophils and increases eosinophil viability (Rothenberg et al., 1988). IL-5, along with G-CSF, produces eosinophil colony formation (Enokihara et al., 1988; Yamaguchi et al., 1988). IL-5 also elicits eosinophil phagocytosis, membrane receptor expression, and toxic oxygen radical release (Lopez et al., 1988), and is a specific chemoattractant for eosinophils (Wang et al., 1989). Finally, TNF enhances toxic oxygen radical release (Slungaard et al., 1990) and sulfidopeptide leukotriene release (Roubin et al., 1987). TNF may also directly cause eosinophils to adhere to endothelial cells, as it does for neutrophils (Gamble et al., 1985). Alternatively, TNF may indirectly induce eosinophil adherence by enhancing the expression of adherence proteins on microvascular endothelium (Gamble et al., 1985). Cytokines, released from mast cells and basophils, may directly or indirectly affect eosinophil function to increase lung microvascular permeability.

Other mediators, released from mast cells and basophils, recruit eosinophils into local sites of inflammation. 12-HETES, PGD_2, and LTB_4 are all released from mast cells after antigen challenge and induce eosinophil chemokinesis and chemotaxis (Goetzl, 1976; Goetzl and Gorman, 1978). PAF is also highly chemotactic for eosinophils (Tamura et al., 1987; Wardlaw et al., 1986) and produces airway eosinophilia when aerosolized into guinea pig airways (Sanjar et al., 1990). Eosinophil chemotactic factor of anaphylaxis (ECF-A) may also be released from mast cells in response to IgE challenge of guinea pig and human lung tissue (Kay et al., 1971). ECF-A is a strong chemotactic agent for eosinophils and produces selective eosinophil accumulation in vivo (Bryant et al., 1977).

In addition to being potent chemoattractants, these mediators also affect eosinophil function. Leukotriene B_4 enhances toxic oxygen radical release and parasite cytotoxicity (Moqbel et al., 1983). ECF-A enhances C3bi and IgGFc receptor expression (Capron et al., 1981); therefore, it may enhance other eosinophil functions, such as phagocytosis or cytotoxicity. PAF directly induces toxic oxygen radical release, eosinophil degranulation (Kroegel et al., 1989a,b), LTC_4 (Bruijnzeel et al., 1987), TxB_2, and PGE_1/E_2 (Giembycz et al., 1990) release from human and guinea pig eosinophils. PAF also enhances Ca^{2+} ionophore-, zymosan-, and arachidonic acid–induced LTC_4 release (Bruijnzeel et al., 1987). Furthermore, PAF appears to convert normodense eosinophils into hypodense eosinophils (Yukawa et al., 1989), a process thought to be associated with eosinophil activation. Histamine enhances C3bi (Anwar and Kay, 1978; Capron et al., 1981) and IgGFc receptor (Anwar and Kay, 1978) expression, as well as toxic oxygen radical release (Pincus et al., 1982) from eosinophils.

Mediators, released from mast cells and basophils, may have an autoregulatory function since they can modulate the activity of the cells that release them or of other mast cells and basophils in close proximity. In this context, histamine inhibits the IgE-dependent degranulation of human basophils (Bourne et al., 1971). In contrast to this inhibitory activity, arachidonic acid metabolites (Chi et al., 1982; Marone et al., 1979; Sullivan and Parker, 1979), and cytokines (Haak-Frendscho et al., 1988; Morita et al., 1987; Schleimer et al., 1981, 1989; Subramanian and Bray, 1987; Valent et al., 1989) result in the degranulation of mast cells and basophils.

In summary, activated mast cells and basophils produce mediators that may elicit increased eosinophil production, accumulation of eosinophils at sites of inflammation, and eosinophil activation. Under appropriate conditions, communications between mast cells, basophils, and eosinophils may contribute to the propagation of events that lead to increased lung microvascular permeability.

V. Contribution of Eosinophils, Mast Cells, and Basophils to Lung Microvascular Injury

A. Eosinophils

Clinical studies suggest that eosinophils contribute to the pathophysiology associated with acute lung injury. Bronchoalveolar lavage fluid and serum, removed from patients at risk for or exhibition adult respiratory distress syndrome, contain elevated levels of eosinophil cationic protein (Hälgren et al., 1984, 1987; Modig and Hälgren, 1986; Modig et al., 1986). This finding suggests that eosinophils release granule enzymes and/or have a high turnover rate in patients with adult respiratory distress syndrome (Hälgren et al., 1987). Although the clinical evidence implies that eosinophils are activated in conditions associated with acute lung injury, the precise role of eosinophils in lung microvascular injury remains unclear.

Experimental studies, conducted in isolated-perfused rat lungs, suggest that eosinophils may directly contribute to acute lung injury. The coadministration of isolated human eosinophils and phorbol myristate acetate (PMA) into the pulmonary artery of rat lungs, but not eosinophils or PMA alone, causes a three- to fourfold increase in lung weight (Rowen et al., 1990). The increase in lung weight may be due to eosinophil aggregation within venules (Fig. 2A) and/or endothelial cell damage (Fig. 2B). These events can lead to increased fluid and protein flux from the microvasculature. In addition to endothelial cell injury,

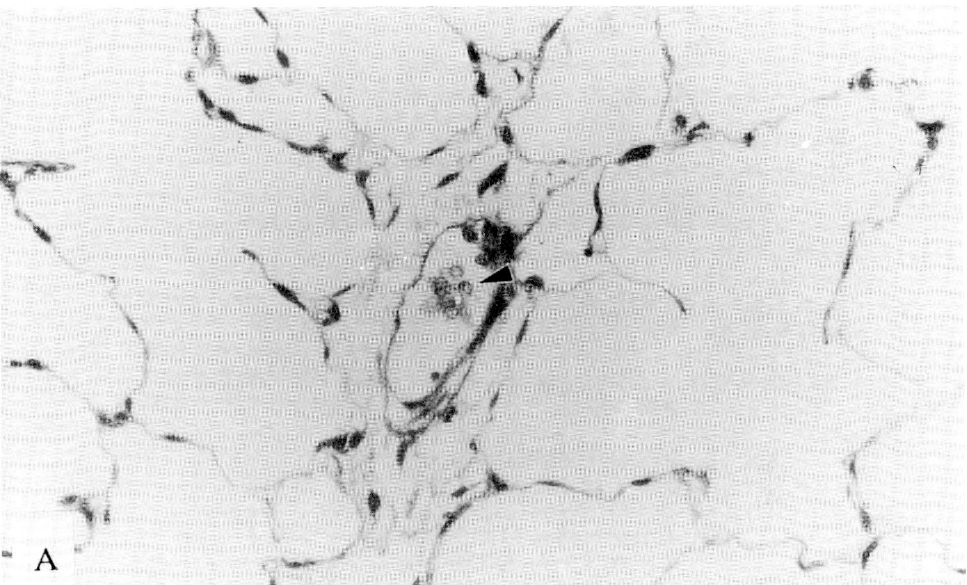

Figure 2 Micrographs of pulmonary tissues in isolated perfused rat lungs infused with eosinophils and PMA. (A) A light micrograph illustrating eosinophil aggregation (arrow) within a pulmonary venule and suggesting that eosinophil aggregates within the pulmonary microvasculature may contribute to edema formation in these lungs. (B) A transmission electron micrograph of an eosinophil (E), closely approximated to an endothelial cell (En), in an intraalveolar septal capillary. The endothelial cell exhibits vesicles and membrane damage, suggesting that eosinophils may be deleterious to the endothelial cells, compromise the integrity of the microvascular barrier, and lead to protein-rich edema formation. (Adapted from Rowen et al., 1990.)

epithelial cell damage is also observed (Rowen et al., 1990). The eosinophil-induced increase in lung weight is inhibited by the presence of catalase, suggesting that toxic oxygen species contribute to the formation of lung edema. In a similar type of experiment, administration of PMA-stimulated rat eosinophils into the pulmonary artery of isolated-perfused rat lungs elicits pulmonary vasoconstriction, bronchoconstriction, and increases the capillary fluid filtration coefficient (Fig. 3; Fujimoto et al., 1990). The increased filtration coefficient, an index of vascular integrity, suggests that increased lung weight may result from increased microvascular permeability. In our laboratory, coinjection of guinea pig eosinophils and antigen (ovalbumin) into the pulmonary artery of sensitized, isolated-perfused guinea pig lungs produces enhancement of the antigen-induced

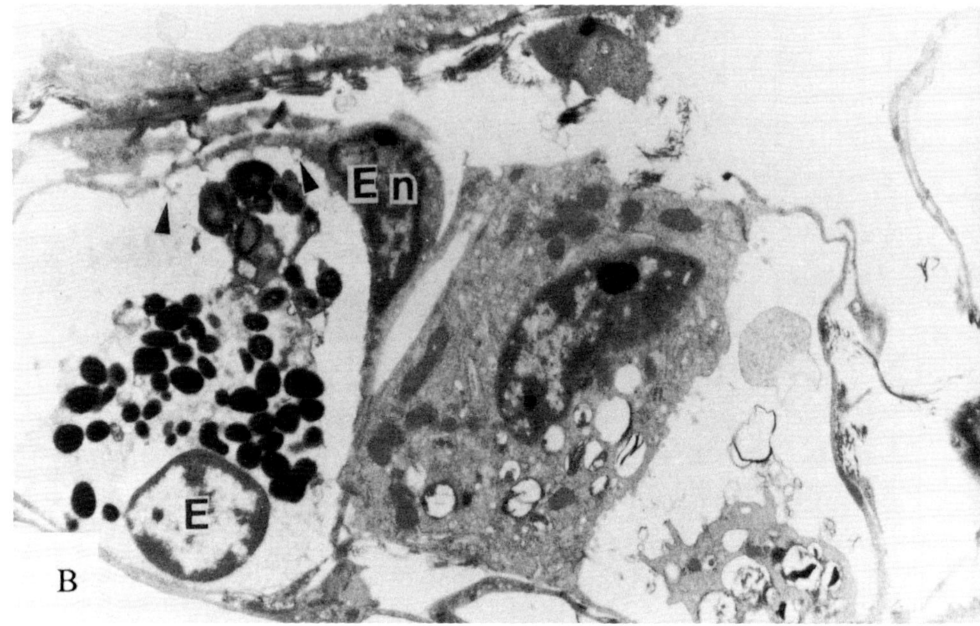

Figure 2 (*Continued*)

edema formation (Fig. 4; Selig et al., 1991). In this study, the presence of eosinophils produces a 2.5-fold increase in lung weight change. The increase in lung weight change, in the presence of eosinophils, suggests that these cells may contribute to edema formation in vivo during antigen challenge of sensitized guinea pigs or possibly in atopic asthmatics. Interestingly, the presence of eosinophils produces no enhancement of antigen-induced increases in pulmonary arterial pressure or intratracheal pressure. Eosinophils or antigen alone produce no changes in lung weight, pulmonary arterial pressure, or intratracheal pressure in unsensitized lungs (data not shown). The data above suggest that activated eosinophils may contribute to pulmonary edema formation, possibly by increasing microvascular permeability. Eosinophils, through the release of granule contents and/or toxic oxygen radicals, may produce this pathophysiologic effect by altering the microvascular endothelium.

Adherence of eosinophils to the endothelium may be the first step in their contribution to microvascular injury. Close association of eosinophils to the endothelium can create a microenvironment that effectively increases the concentration of deleterious mediators released from eosinophils. In sensitized guinea pigs, eosinophils marginate in capillaries and venules of bronchi, bronchioles, and alveoli within 8 min following antigen challenge (Dunn et al., 1988). Eosinophils avidly adhere to human umbilical vein endothelial cells under

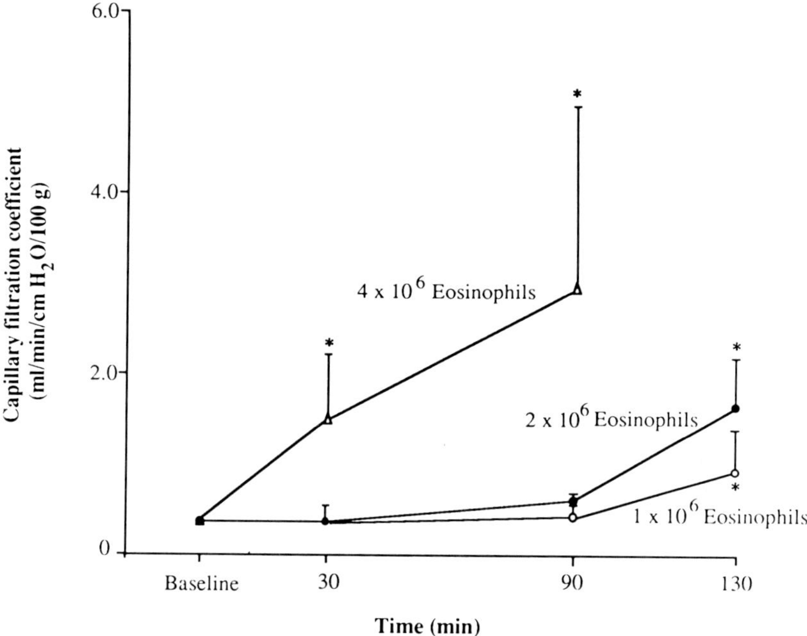

Figure 3 Eosinophil-induced increase in the capillary filtration coefficient of isolated-perfused rat lungs. Eosinophils are activated by incubation with 10 μg/mL PMA for 30 min, centrifuged, and resuspended in 50 μL of the remaining supernatant. Eosinophils are then infused into the pulmonary artery and capillary filtration coefficients are measured at various times. These data illustrate that eosinophils produce a dose-dependent increase in the pulmonary capillary filtration coefficient. Eosinophil numbers of 1 and 2×10^6 produce a three- to fivefold increase (respectively) in the capillary filtration coefficient between 90 and 130 min after initial injection. Higher eosinophil numbers (4×10^6 produce a ninefold increase in the capillary filtration coefficient within 30 min after initial injection. Unactivated eosinophils or PMA alone produce no increases in the capillary filtration coefficient (data not shown). An asterisk represents $p < 0.05$ as assessed by one-way analysis of variance and Newman–Keuls multiple range testing. Mean ± SD. These data suggest that activated eosinophils can increase microvascular permeability in isolated perfused lungs. (Adapted from Fujimoto et al., 1990.)

in vitro conditions (Kimani et al., 1988; Lamas et al., 1988). Adherence may occur by two methods: activation of eosinophils by circulating factors such as PAF or bacterial products (as suggested through the use of fMLP; Kimani et al., 1988; Lamas et al., 1988) and/or activation of endothelial cells by circulating factors such as cytokines (TNF or IL-1) or bacterial products (endotoxin) to attract eosinophils for adherence (Lamas et al., 1988). The dependency of eosinophil adherence on endothelial cell activation is illustrated in vivo by eosinophil

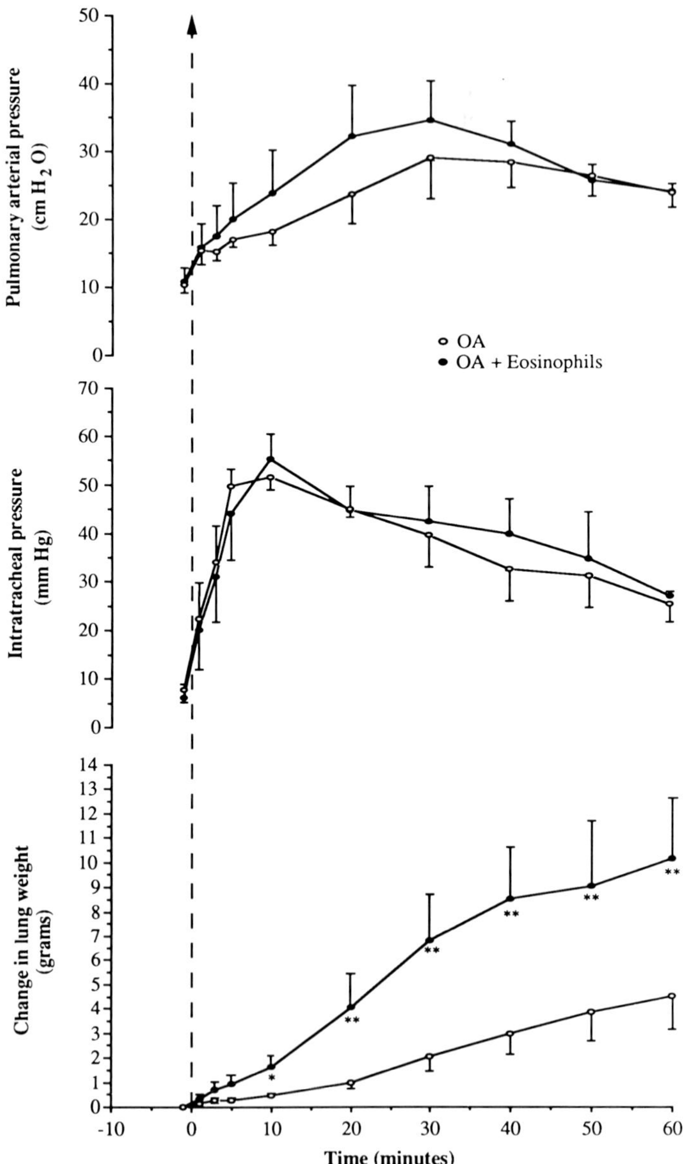
Pulmonary arterial pressure (cm H_2O)
Intratracheal pressure (mm Hg)
Change in lung weight (grams)
Time (minutes)
OA
OA + Eosinophils
*
**

accumulation in the interstitium and lumen of airways after *Ascaris suum* challenge of sensitized monkeys (Wegner et al., 1990). This eosinophil accumulation appears to be associated with airway hyperreactivity. Eosinophil adherence is dependent on enhanced expression of intercellular adhesion molecule-1 (ICAM-1), which is present on vascular endothelium and the basolateral epithelium of the airway. Blocking the function of ICAM-1 with a monoclonal antibody against ICAM-1 (MAb R6.5) attenuates eosinophil influx and inhibits the increase in airway responsiveness (Wegner et al., 1990). Therefore, eosinophil adherence may be a critical step in microvascular injury and airway responsiveness in this model, and may result from eosinophil or endothelial cell activation, or a combination of both.

Once adherent to the endothelium, eosinophils may quickly migrate through the endothelial layer. Accumulation of eosinophils in the interstitial space occurs within 30 min following antigen challenge of sensitized guinea pigs (Dunn et al., 1988). Eosinophil influx into the airways is evident 6 to 24 h following antigen challenge and persists for several days (Dunn et al., 1988; Selig et al., 1990). Clinically, this influx is associated with the presence of protein in the airway (Fick et al., 1987; Lam et al., 1987).

Release of toxic oxygen radicals and peroxidatic enzymes, under in vitro conditions, suggests these mediators may contribute to changes in lung microvascular permeability in vivo. The contribution of oxygen radicals, released from activated neutrophils, to lung microvascular injury is well documented. Neutrophil-derived toxic oxygen radicals alter endothelial cells in isolated-perfused lungs (Shasby et al., 1982, 1983); endothelial monolayers (Shasby et al., 1983), and in vivo (Gee et al., 1986; Shasby et al., 1982; Till et al., 1982),

---

Figure 4 Changes in pulmonary arterial pressure, intratracheal pressure, and lung weight in response to antigen challenge alone (ovalbumin, OA) and antigen challenge in the presence of eosinophils (OA + eosinophils) in isolated, perfused, sensitized guinea pig lungs. Guinea pigs were sensitized over a 2-week period by two subcutaneous injections of 10.0 μg of ovalbumin and 1.0 mg of $Al(OH)_3$ in 0.5 ml. One week after the last injection, guinea pigs were anesthetized and the heart and lungs were removed *en bloc* and perfused. After lung equilibration and baseline measurements, antigen (ovalbumin, 30 μg in saline) or antigen and isolated guinea pig eosinophils (2×10^7) were injected into the pulmonary artery (dashed arrow). Eosinophils produce no alterations of the antigen induced increase in pulmonary arterial pressure or intratracheal pressure. However, eosinophils significantly enhance the antigen-induced increase in lung weight. Eosinophils alone produce no alterations from baseline in any of the variables measured (data not shown). Mean ± SEM, $n = 4$. Asterisk and double asterisk ($p < 0.05$ and $p < 0.01$, respectively), represent significance as assessed by one- way analysis of variance and Dunnett's test for multiple comparisons.

thereby increasing permeability across the endothelial barrier. The contribution of toxic oxygen radicals, released from activated eosinophils, is less defined. Toxic oxygen radicals are released from eosinophils, stimulated in vitro with fMLP (Sedgwick et al., 1988), opsonized zymosan (Pincus, 1983; Sedgwick et al., 1988), PAF (Kroegel et al., 1989a,b), PMA (Cerasoli et al., 1991; Kroegel et al., 1989a; Pincus, 1983; Sedgwick et al., 1988), and recombinant TNF (Slungaard et al., 1990). Toxic oxygen radicals, released from TNF-stimulated eosinophils, are believed to contribute to the release of ^{51}Cr from human umbilical vein endothelial cells, suggesting endothelial cell death (Slungaard et al., 1990). EPO contributes to this endothelial cell cytotoxicity since Br^-, which is preferentially oxidized by eosinophil peroxidase, significantly enhances ^{51}Cr release (Fig. 5). The radical–peroxidase–halide system also contributes to human nasal and pulmonary epithelial cell death in vitro (Ayars et al., 1985, 1989). As discussed earlier, peroxidase activity is enhanced in vitro by the presence of extracellular mast cell granules (Fig. 1). Similar mast cell granule–mediated enhancement of EPO cytotoxicity may occur in inflammatory areas within the lung, where activated mast cells and eosinophils are present, to increase microvascular permeability.

Changes in the ability of airway eosinophils to release superoxide anion in vivo are estimated in vitro (Cerasoli et al., 1991). Airway eosinophils, collected from sensitized guinea pigs 24 h after in vivo aerosolized antigen challenge, spontaneously release six- to sevenfold more superoxide anion than normal airway eosinophils (Fig. 6). Eosinophils also release two- to sixfold more superoxide anion when stimulated with low doses of PMA (10^{-11} or 10^{-9} *M*); however, release is similar to control when eosinophils are stimulated with a maximal dose of PMA (10^{-7} *M*, data not shown). The presence of enhanced superoxide anion release is concomitant with airway hyperreactivity (Selig et al., 1990) and the presence of eosinophil peroxidase within the airway (see below). This enhancement of superoxide anion release, from airway eosinophils, may result from exposure of the eosinophils to humoral mediators or cytokines. f-Methionine-leucine-phenylalanine (fMLP)-stimulated superoxide anion release, from human blood eosinophils, is enhanced 1.5- to 1.8-fold by prior incubation with nonactivating concentrations of PAF (Zoratti et al., 1990). This enhancement is associated with reduced eosinophil density and increased expression of membrane CR3 receptors induced by the nonactivating doses of PAF. Several eosinophil functions are also enhanced by cytokines (see Section IV.B). These data suggest that eosinophils may be activated in vivo, possibly by humoral mediator and/or cytokine release, to produce toxic oxygen radicals and release peroxidatic enzymes.

Another indication of eosinophil activation in vivo is increased eosinophil peroxidase in guinea pig airways after antigen challenge (F. Cerasoli, J. Tocker,

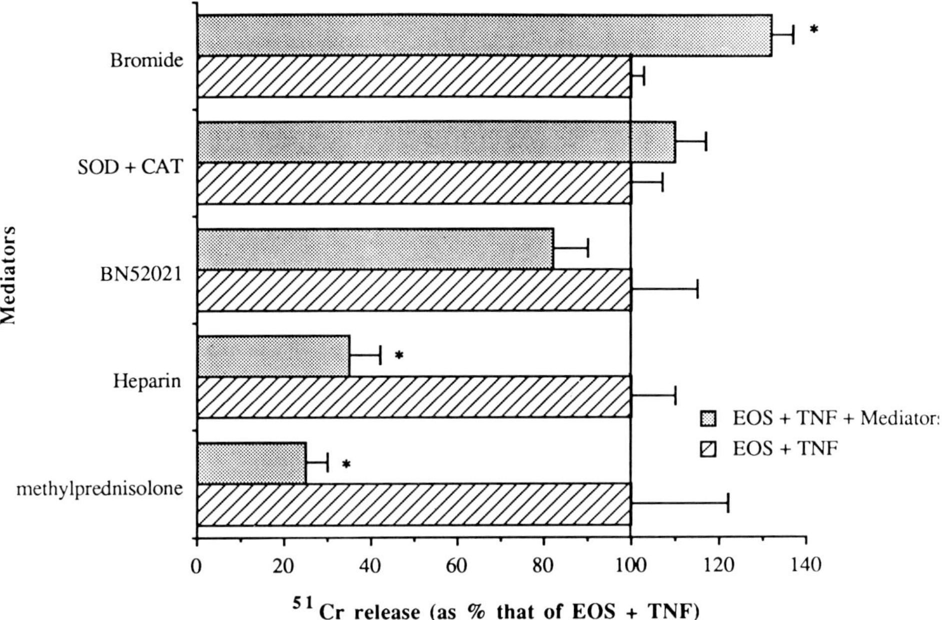

Figure 5 Cytotoxicity of endothelial cells by isolated eosinophils. Human umbilical vein endothelial cells, in monolayers, are loaded with ^{51}Cr. Isolated blood eosinophils are applied to the monolayers in a ratio of 20 to 25 eosinophils /endothelial cell. After a 16-h incubation, cell-free ^{51}Cr in the supernatant (indicating endothelial cell cytotoxicity) is measured by gamma counting. Unstimulated eosinophils alone induce the release into the supernatant of $10.8 \pm 12.1\%$ (standard deviation) of the total ^{51}Cr, while TNF-stimulated eosinophils induce the release of $21.4 \pm 15.6\%$. Bromide (100 μ*M* NaBr) enhances ^{51}Cr release, suggesting a role for both eosinophil peroxidase and toxic oxygen radicals in eosinophil-dependent endothelial cell cytoxicity. Superoxide dismutase (SOD, 100 μg/mL) and catalase (CAT, 100 μg/ml) provide no endothelial cell protection. Although this may suggest that toxic oxygen radicals play no role in cytoxicity, Slungaard et al. (1990) believe that these proteins are too large to gain access and be effective in the microenvironment produced by eosinophil–endothelial cell contact. BN52021 (200 μ*M*), a PAF antagonist, tends to afford only a 20% protection against endothelial cell cytoxicity. Heparin (10 U/mL) affords 70% protection, suggesting that cationic proteins, released by eosinophils, contribute to endothelial cell cytotoxicity. Finally, methylprednisolone (10 μg/mL), a lucocorticoid with anti-inflammatory activity, also affords 70 to 80% protection. These data suggest that activated eosinophils, through the release of toxic oxygen radicals, peroxidatic enzymes, and cationic proteins, produce cyto- toxic effects on endothelial cells. Mean ± SEM, $n = 3$ *to* 9 for each mediator. An asterisk represent significance ($p < 0.05$) as assessed by Student's *t*-test. (Adapted from Slungaard et al., 1990.)

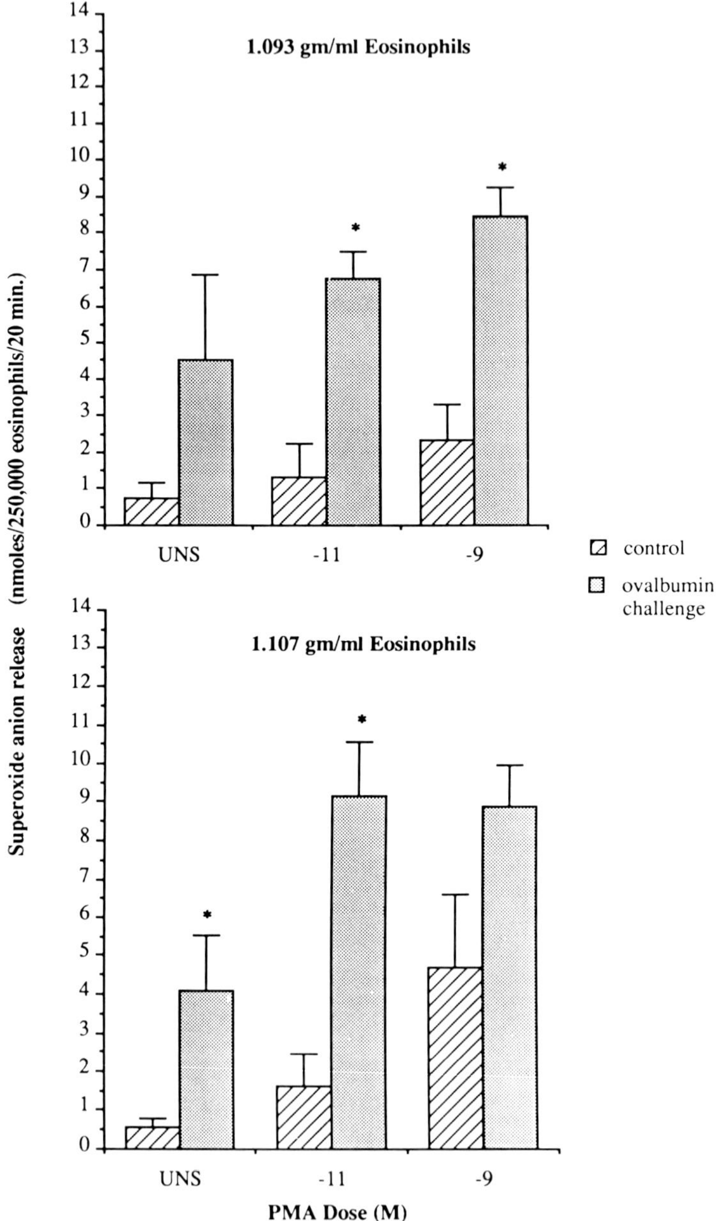
1.093 gm/ml Eosinophils
1.107 gm/ml Eosinophils
Superoxide anion release (nmoles/250,000 eosinophils/20 min.)
0
1
2
3
4
5
6
7
8
9
10
11
12
13
14
UNS
-11
-9
PMA Dose (M)
control
ovalbumin challenge
*

and W. M. Selig, unpublished observation). Eosinophil peroxidase, measured in cell-free bronchoalveolar lavage fluid 24 h after aerosolized antigen challenge of sensitized guinea pigs, is increased threefold (Fig. 7). The peroxidase may come from actively degranulating eosinophils and/or dead eosinophils that lyse within the airways. Collectively, the data above suggest that the release of toxic oxygen radicals and peroxidatic enzymes is deleterious to endothelial and epithelial cells in vitro, occurs in vivo, and can be enhanced in pulmonary pathophysiological conditions. Eosinophil activation in vivo, resulting in toxic oxygen radical and peroxidatic enzyme release, may elicit endothelial cell (and epithelial cell) damage and promote increases in lung microvascular or airway epithelial permeability.

Cationic proteins, released from eosinophils, may also be instrumental in producing lung microvascular permeability. Several exogenous cationic substances produce pulmonary hypertension and edema formation in rats (Fairman et al., 1987) as well as increase pulmonary microvascular permeability in rats (Chang et al., 1987; DeVries et al., 1953; Vehaskari et al., 1984) and conscious sheep (Toyofuku et al., 1989). These microvascular changes, which lead to increased transudation of anionic plasma proteins, are believed to result from neutralization of the negative charge that is characteristic of the endothelial barrier that lines the microvascular lumen (Skutelsky et al., 1975). Cationic substances, including neutrophil-derived cationic protein (NCP), elastase, and protamine, also increase the permeability of porcine pulmonary artery endothelial cell monolayers in vitro (Peterson et al., 1987). The cationic nature of NCP and elastase, rather than their enzymatic properties, may be responsible for increased permeability since heating the proteins also increases permeability. Elastase apparently leads to increased permeability by causing endothelial cell death; however, NCP or protamine may increase permeability by mechanisms

---

Figure 6 Superoxide anion release from airway eosinophils collected from control guinea pigs (control) or sensitized guinea pigs (as described in Fig. 4) 24 h after ovalbumin challenge (ovalbumin challenge, 0.1% in sterile saline, and aerosolized for 30 min). Two eosinophils populations are collected based on their density in a Percoll-plasma discontinuous density gradient (1.093 and 1.107 g/mL). Superoxide anion release is measured from eosinophils (either unstimulated [UNS] or stimulated with 10^{-11} *M* [-11] or 10^{-9} *M* [-9] PMA) in microtiter wells by the reduction of ferricytochrome *c*. Superoxide anion release from eosinophils collected 24 h after ovalbumin challenge is enhanced, suggesting that these eosinophils may be activated to produce toxic oxygen radicals in vivo. Superoxide anion release is unaffected by the sensitization procedure or by aerosolized saline challenge of sensitized guinea pigs (data not shown). Maximal superoxide anion release, elicited with 10^{-7} *M* PMA, is unaffected by antigen challenge (data not shown). Mean ± SEM, $n = 4$ each. An asterisk represents statistical significance ($p < 0.05$) as assessed by unpaired *t*-tests. (Adapted from Cerasoli et al., 1991.)

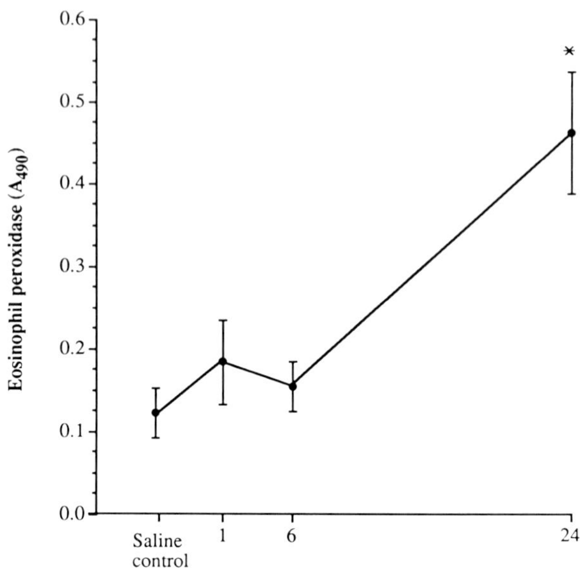

Figure 7 Eosinophil peroxidase activity in cell-free bronchoalveolar lavage fluid in response to antigen challenge of sensitized guinea pigs. Guinea pigs are sensitized as described in Fig. 4 and challenged as described in Fig. 6. At various times after challenge, guinea pigs are lavaged with 5.0 mL of Hank's balanced salt solution which is centrifuged at 900*g* for 15 min to pellet suspended cells. Eosinophil peroxidase is measured by modifications of previously described methods using *o*-phenylenediamine dihydrochloride (Strath et al., 1985). Eosinophil peroxidase in lavage fluid collected 1 h and 6 h after ovalbumin challenge is the same as in lavage fluid collected from control guinea pigs. Twenty-four hours after ovalbumin challenge, eosinophil peroxidase activity is increased fourfold. This suggests that eosinophils, present in the airway 24 h after antigen challenge, are activated to release eosinophil peroxidase. Alternatively, eosinophil peroxidase may come from eosinophils that are dead and lysed within the airways. Mean ± SEM, $n = 3$. An asterisk represents statistical significance as assessed by one-way analysis of variance with Dunnett's multiple comparison test.

other than endothelial cell death (Peterson et al., 1987). Major basic protein, isolated from guinea pig eosinophils, produces porcine aortic endothelial cell death (Gleich et al., 1979; Kierszenbaum et al., 1982) and pulmonary epithelial cell death in vitro (Ayars et al., 1985). MBP, ECP, and EDN are found in areas of cardiac muscle damage associated with endomyocardial fibrosis in humans (Tai et al., 1987), suggesting a role for eosinophil-derived cationic proteins in host tissue damage. In addition, supernatants from eosinophil cultures, presumably containing eosinophil-derived mediators, produces disruption of myocardial cell membranes, intercellular gap formation, and myocardial cell death in vitro (Shay et al., 1990). ECP may be capable of producing these morphologic findings since this protein causes transmembrane pore formation and cell death (Young et al., 1986). Cationic protein-induced endothelial cell cytotoxicity, measured in vitro, is decreased by the presence of heparin (Fig. 5; Slungaard et al., 1990), which may be due to the anionic properties of heparin. These anionic properties may neutralize the cationic proteins, rendering them harmless (Kieszenbaum et al., 1982). These data suggest that cationic proteins, released from activated eosinophils, may produce the destruction of endothelial barrier integrity and increase lung microvascular permeability.

In addition to their direct physical effect in the microvasculature, cationic substances may stimulate release of vasoactive mediators that in turn affect the vasculature. Synthetic polycations (Suzuki-Nushimura et al., 1989), polymyxin B (an antibacterial cation) (Peachell and Pearce, 1984), and MBP (O'Donnell et al., 1983; Zheutlin et al., 1984) induce the release of histamine from mast cells, which consequently increases lung microvascular permeability (see Section V.B). Therefore, cationic substances, released from eosinophils, may affect lung microvasculature through indirect mechanisms, such as mast cell activation.

B. Mast Cells and Basophils

Mast cells and basophils may contribute to lung microvascular injury, in several pathophysiological conditions, by several different mechanisms. The high concentration of mast cells in tissues surrounding blood vessels places them at a critical site for contributing to increased microvascular permeability. Mast cell secretagogues elicit rapid formation of protein-rich pulmonary edema fluid in several species (Persson, 1987; Saria et al., 1983). Inhibitors of mast cell function, such as the mast cell stabilizing agent nedocromil sodium, can reduce the increased airway microvascular permeability following antigen challenge (Evans et al., 1988b). The contribution of mast cells and basophils is twofold: (1) direct, by the release of inflammatory mediators which act on the lung microvasculature and induce edema formation, and (2) indirect, by the release of chemotactic factors for other cell types, including eosinophils (Bryant et al., 1977; Goetzl and Gorman, 1978; Tamura et al., 1987), macrophages (Friedman and Kaliner, 1987), and neutrophils (Friedman and Kaliner, 1987; Goetzl and Pickett, 1980; Klickstein et al., 1980), which contribute to microvascular injury.

Mediators, released from mast cells and basophils, directly increase lung microvascular permeability. Histamine contributes to antigen-induced increases in tracheal and bronchial (but not intrapulmonary airway) microvascular permeability in sensitized guinea pigs (Evans et al., 1988b). Histamine elicits the contraction of venule endothelial cells (Persson, 1987) that leads to widened intraendothelial junctions (Majno et al., 1969) and increased fluid leakage from the microvasculature (Persson, 1987; Saria et al., 1983). Histamine also increases the permeability of bovine pulmonary artery explants in vitro (Meyrick and Brigham, 1983) and the pulmonary microvasculature in vivo when it is infused into the pulmonary or bronchial artery of sheep (Brigham and Owen, 1975a; Nakahara et al., 1979). Serotonin, another mast cell granule–associated bioactive amine, produces increased microvascular permeability in guinea pig airways (Saria et. al., 1983). Serotonin infusion into conscious sheep increases pulmonary venous pressure, capillary pressure, and lung water (Brigham and Owen, 1975b; Demling, 1985). This results in a ''high-pressure'' form of pulmonary edema (Brigham and Owen, 1975b; Demling, 1985). Serotonin-induced high-pressure edema also occurs in dog lungs (Rippe et al., 1984) and isolated-perfused guinea pig lungs (Selig et al., 1988). Therefore, histamine and serotonin can increase lung microvascular permeability and/or edema formation through their direct effects on components in the microvasculature.

De novo synthesized mediators, released from mast cells and basophils (and other leukocytes, including eosinophils), profoundly influence microvascular permeability. Leukotrienes C_4, D_4, and E_4, instilled into the trachea of guinea pig lungs, increase the permeability of the airway microvasculature (Woodward et al., 1983) with a potency about 100 to 1000 times that of histamine (Dahlén, 1981; Woodward et al., 1983). The increased permeability of the microvasculature may be a consequence of postcapillary venule endothelial cell contraction (Dahlén, 1981). In contrast to the sulfidopeptide leukotrienes, LTB_4 appears to produce less of an increase in microvascular permeability than histamine (Woodward et al., 1983). Leukotrienes appear to induce increases in microvascular permeability in all airway generations, whereas histamine appears to have localized actions on the microvasculature of trachea and the bronchi (Evans et al., 1988a,b). PAF, another de novo synthesized mediator, is one of the most potent agents that increases the permeability of both the pulmonary (Burhop et al., 1986; Mojarad et al., 1983) and the tracheobronchial microvasculature (Evans et al., 1987; O'Donnell and Barnett, 1987). In the tracheobronchial circulation, intravenous PAF increases microvascular permeability by a mechanism independent of PAF-induced arachidonic acid metabolite production (Evans et al., 1987). However, compared to leukotrienes, PAF appears to play less of a role in antigen-induced increases in permeability of tracheobronchial microvasculature (Evans et al., 1988b).

Several inhibitors and antagonists of mast cell mediators reduce the increases in lung microvascular permeability following antigen challenge. Nedocromil sodium inhibits increases in microvascular permeability in the tracheobronchial circulation as well as the circulation of the central and peripheral intrapulmonary airways (Evans et al., 1988b). Nedocromil sodium also inhibits the release of prostaglandin D_2, histamine, and leukotriene C_4 from mast cells in vitro (Eady et al., 1985). Taken together, these data suggest that mast cells directly contribute to lung microvascular permeability. The histamine H1 antagonist, chlorpheniramine, and the H2 antagonist, cimetidine, both inhibit antigen-induced increases in permeability of the tracheobronchial microvasculature but not the central and peripheral intrapulmonary airway microvasculature (Evans et al., 1988b). The sulfidopeptide leukotriene antagonist, FPL 55712, and the dual cyclooxygenase-lipoxygenase inhibitor, BW 755c, also reduce tracheobronchial microvascular permeability by approximately 50%. In contrast, indomethacin, the cyclooxygenase inhibitor, produces no reduction in the permeability of the tracheobronchial or the central and peripheral intrapulmonary airways microvasculature (Evans et al., 1988b). The PAF antagonist, BN 52063, produces no reduction in antigen-induced microvascular permeability (Evans et al., 1988b) as it does when intravenous PAF is used to increase permeability (Evans et al., 1987). The data above suggest that mast cells, through the release of histamine and lipoxygenase products, contribute to lung microvascular permeability induced by antigen challenge.

VI. Conclusions

In summary, through a coherent review of the literature, evidence is provided demonstrating that eosinophils, mast cells, and basophils contribute to lung microvascular injury in disease states such as adult respiratory distress syndrome and asthma. These cells are capable of directly affecting the lung microvasculature to produce edema formation and increased permeability. Furthermore, they can communicate with each other to regulate, and possibly potentiate, each others' contribution to lung microvascular injury.

Certainly, the eosinophils possess an adequate armamentarium to produce lung microvascular injury. Additionally, eosinophil products are elevated in blood and bronchoalveolar lavage fluid of patients with adult respiratory distress syndrome and asthma. Eosinophils (1) can directly contribute to pulmonary edema in vivo, (2) may be in an activated state in vivo during pathophysiologic conditions, and (3) elicit endothelial and epithelial cell death in vitro. Several mediators, such as MBP and EPO, are released from eosinophils and affect mast cell (and other leukocyte) function. Eosinophils can also be influenced by ECF, IL 3-6, GM-CSF, and leukotrienes released from mast cells and basophils. These mediators can recruit eosinophils into a site of inflammation and potentiate the eosinophil's contribution to lung microvascular injury.

Mast cells and basophils may also contribute to lung microvascular injury. They are located in strategic areas to affect the microvasculature. Upon activation, mast cells and basophils can release several vasoactive and permeability-inducing mediators, including histamine, serotonin, PAF, and leukotrienes. Mast cells can also potentiate eosinophil (and other leukocyte) function as mentioned above through the release of cytokines and other mediators. Therefore, mast cells and basophils may also play as very active role in the development of lung microvascular injury, especially in asthma.

Acknowledgment

The authors wish to express their thanks to David L. Shrier for his assistance in the preparation of this manuscript.

References

Ackerman, S. J., Loegering, D. A., Venge, P., Olsson, I., Harley, J. B., Fauci, A. S., and Gleich, G. J. (1983). Distinctive cationic proteins of the human eosinophil granule: Major basic protein, eosinophil cationic protein, and eosinophil derived neuroxin. *J. Immunol.* **131:**2977–2982.

Ackerman, S. J., Gleich, G. J., Loegering, D. A., Richardson, B. A., and Butterworth, A. E. (1985). Comparative toxicity of purified human eosinophil cationic patients for schistosomula of *Schistosomula mansoni. Am. J. Trop. Med. Hyg.* **34:**735–745.

Agius, R. M., Howarth, P. H., Church, M. K., Robinson, C., and Holgate, S. T. (1986). Luminal mast cells of the human respiratory tract. In *Mast Cell Differentiation and Heterogeneity.* Edited by A. Befus, J., Bienenstock, and J. A. Denborg. Raven Press, New York, pp. 277–288.

Ali, H., Collado-Escobar, D. M., and Beaven, M. A. (1989). The rise in concentration of free Ca^{2+} and of pH provides sequential synergistic signals for secretion in antigen-stimulated rat basophilic leukemia (RBL-2H3) cells. *J. Immunol.* **143:**2626–2633.

Ali, H., Cunha-Melo, J. R., Saul, W. F., and Beaven, M. A. (1990). Activation of phospholipase C via adenosine receptors provides synergistic signals for secretion in antigen-stimulated RBL-2H3 cells, *J. Biol. Chem.* **265:**745–753.

Anwar, A. R. E., and Kay, A. B. (1978). Enhancement of human eosinophil complement receptors by pharmacologic mediators. *J. Immunol.* **121:**1245–1250.

Archer, R. K. (1963). *The Eosinophil Leukocytes.* Blackwell Scientific, Oxford, pp. 5–7.

Archer, R. K. (1968). The eosinophil leukocyte. *Ser. Hematol.* **1:**3–22.

Ayars, G. H., Altman, L. C., Gleich, G. J., Loegering, D. A., and Baker, C. B. (1985). Eosinophil and eosinophil-granule mediated pneumocyte injury. *J. Allergy Clin. Immunol.* **76:**595–604.

Ayars, G. H., Altman, L. C., McManus, M. M., Agosti, J. M., Baker, C., Luchtel, D. L., Loegering, D. A., and Gleich, G. J. (1989). Injurious effect of the eosinophil peroxide-hydrogen peroxide-halide system and major basic protein on human nasal epithelium in vitro. *Am. Rev. Respir. Dis.* **140:**125–131.

Bachofen, M., and Weibel, E. R. (1977). Alterations of the gas exchange apparatus in adult respiratory insufficiency associated with septicemia. *Am. Rev. Respir. Dis.* **116:**589–615.

Bachofen, M., and Weibel, E. R. (1982). Structural alteration of lung parenchyma in the adult respiratory distress syndrome. In *Clinics in Chest Medicine.* Edited by R. Bone. W. B. Saunders, Philadelphia, pp. 35–56.

Bainton, D. F. (1988). Phagocytic cells: developmental biology of neutrophils and eosinophils. In *Inflammation: Basic Principles and Clinical Correlates.* Edited by J. I. Gallin, I. M. Goldstein, and R. Snyderman. Raven Press, New York, pp. 265–280.

Beaven, M. A., and Cunha-Melo, J. R. (1988). Membrane phosphoinositide-activated signals in mast cells and basophils. *Prog. Allergy* **42:**123–184.

Beaven, M. A., Rogers, J., Moore, J. P., Hesketh, T. R., Smith, G. A., and Metcalfe, J. D. (1984). The mechanism of the calcium signal and correlation with histamine release in 2H3 cells. *J. Biol. Chem.* **259:**7129–7136.

Beaven, M. A., Guthrie, D. F., Moore, J. P., Smith, G. A., Hesketh, T. R., and Metcalfe, J. C. (1987). Synergistic signals in the mechanism of antigen-induced exocytosis in 2H3 cells: Evidence for an unidentified signal required for histamine release. *J. Cell Biol.* **105:**1129–1136.

Beeson, P. B., and Bass, D. A. (1977). *The Eosinophil.* W. B. Saunders, Philadelphia, pp. 46–49.

Berridge, M. J. (1987). Inositol triphosphate and diacylglycerol: Two interacting second messengers. *Annu. Rev. Biochem.* **56:**159–193.

Bloom, W., and Fawcett, D. W. (1975). *Textbook of Histology*, 10th ed. W. B. Saunders, Philadelphia, pp. 145–147.

Bourne, H. R., Melmon, K. L., and Lichtenstein, L. M. (1971). Histamine augments leukocyte adenosine 3′,5′-monophosphate and blocks antigenic histamine release. *Science* **20:**743–745.

Brandt, P. W., and Freeman, A. R. (1967). Plasma membrane: Substructural changes correlated with electrical resistance and pinocytosis. *Science* **155:**582–585.

Brigham, K. L., and Owen, P. J. (1975a). Increased sheep lung vascular permeability caused by histamine. *Circ. Res.* **37:**647–657.

Brigham, K. L., and Owen, P. J. (1975b). Mechanisms of serotonin effect on lung transvascular fluid and protein management in awake sheep. *Circ. Res.* **36:** 761–770.

Bruijnzeel, P. L. B., Kok, P. T. M., Hamelink, M. L., Kijne, A. M., and Verhagen, J. (1987). Platelet-activating factor induces leukotriene C_4 synthesis by purified human eosinophils. *Prostaglandins* **34:**205–214.

Bryant, D. H., Turnbull, L. W., and Kay, A. B. (1977). Eosinophil chemotaxis to an ECF-A tetrapeptide and histamine: The response in various disease states. *Clin. Allergy* **7:**219–226.

Burhop, K. E., Garcia, J. G. N., Selig, W. M., Lo, S. K., van der Zee, H., Kaplan, J. E., and Malik, A. B. (1986). Platelet-activating factor increases lung vascular permeability to protein. *J. Appl. Physiol.* **61:**2210–2217.

Butterfield, J. H., Weiler, D., Peterson, E. A., Gleich, G. J., and Leiferman, K. M. (1990). Sequestration of eosinophil major basic protein in human mast cells. *Lab. Invest.* **62:**77–86.

Butterworth, A. E., Sturrock, R. F., Houha, V., Sher, A., and Rees, P. K. (1975). Eosinophils as mediators of antibody-dependent damage to schistosomula. *Nature* **256:**727–729.

Butterworth, A. E., Wasson, D. C., Gleich, G. J., Loegering, D. A., and David, J. R. (1979). Damage to schistosomula of *Schistosoma mansoni* induced directly by eosinophil major basic protein. *J. Immunol.* **122:**221–229.

Cantwell, M. E., and Foreman, J. C. (1986). Characteristics of the effects of phorbol ester on rat mast cells: Interaction with anti-IgE. *Agents Actions* **18:**77–80.

Cantwell, M. E., and Foreman, J. C. (1987). Phorbol esters induce a slow non-cytoxic release of histamine from rat peritoneal mast cells. *Agents Actions* **20:**165–168.

Capron, M., Capron, A., Goetzl, E. J., and Austen, K. F. (1981). Tetrapeptides of the eosinophil chemotactic factor of anaphylaxis (ECF-A) enhance eosinophil F_c receptors. *Nature (Lond.)* **289:**71–73.

Casale, T. B., and Marom, Z. (1983). Mast cells and asthma. The role of mast cell mediators in the pathogenesis of allergic asthma. *Ann. Allergy* **51:**2–6.

Cerasoli, F., Jr., Tocker, J., and Selig, W. M. (1991). Airway eosinophils from actively sensitized guinea pigs exhibit enhanced superoxide anion release in response to antigen challenge. *Am. J. Respir. Cell Mol. Biol.* **4:**355–363.

Chang, S. W., Wescott, J. Y., Henson, J. E., and Voelkel, N. F. (1987). Pulmonary vascular injury by polycations in perfused at lungs. *J. Appl. Physiol.* **62:**363–1367.

Chi, E. Y., and Henderson, W. R. (1984). Ultrastructure of mast cell degranulation induced by eosinophil peroxidase: Use of diaminobenzidine cytochemistry by scanning electron microscopy. *J. Histochem. Cytochem.* **32:**332–341.

Chi, E. Y., Henderson, W. R., and Klebanoff, S. J. (1982). Phospholipase A_2-induced rat mast cell secretion: Role of arachidonic acid metabolites. *Lab. Invest.* **47:**579–585.

Church, M. K., Holgate, S. T., and Hughes, P. J. (1983). Adenosine inhibits and potentiates IgE-dependent histamine release from human basophils by an A2-receptor mediated mechanism. *Br. J. Pharmacol.* **80:**719–726.

Cohen, N. S., LoBue, J., and Gordon, A. S. (1967). Mechanisms of leukocyte production and release. VIII. Eosinophil and neutrophil kinetics in rats. *Scand. J. Haematol.* **4:**339–350.

Crews, F. T., Morita, Y., McGivney, A., Hirata, F., Siraganian, R. P., and Axelrod, J. (1981). IgE-mediated histamine release in rat basophilic leukemia cells: Receptor activation, phospholipid methylation, Ca^{2+} flux, and release of arachidonic acid. *Arch. Biochem. Biophys.* **212:**561–571.

Cunha-Melo, J. R., Dean, N. M., Moyer, J. D., Maeyama, K., and Beaven, M. A. (1987). The kinetics of phosphoinositide hydrolysis in rat basophilic leukemia (RBL-2H3) cells varies with the type of IgE receptor cross-linking agent used. *J. Biol. Chem.* **262:**11455–11463.

Dahlén, S. E. (1981). Leukotrienes promote plasma leakage and leukocyte adhesion in postcapillary venules: In vivo effects with relevance to the acute inflammatory response. *Proc. Natl. Acad. Sci. USA* **78:**3887–3891.

Demling, R. H. (1985). Mechanisms of pulmonary vascular injury in sepsis. In *The Pulmonary Circulation and Acute Lung Injury.* Edited by S. Said. Futura Publishing Co., Mount Kisco, N.Y., pp. 403–427.

De Simone, C., Donelli, G., Meli, D., Rosati, F., and Sorici, F. (1982). Human eosinophils and parasitic diseases. II. Characterization of two cell fractions isolated at different densities. *Clin. Exp. Immunol.* **48:**249–255.

Dessein, A. J., Vadas, M. A., Nicola, N. A., Metcalf, D., and David, J. R. (1982). Enhancement of human blood eosinophil cytotoxicity by semi-purified eosinophil colony stimulating factor(s). *J. Exp. Med.* **156:**90–103.

DeVries, A., Feldman, J. O., Stein, O., Stein, Y., and Katchalski, E. (1953). Effects of intravenously administered poly-D-C-lysine in rats. *Proc. Soc. Exp. Biol. Med.* **82:**237–240.

Didier, A., Kowalski, M. L., Jay, J., and Kaliner, M. A. (1990). Neurogenic inflammation, vascular permeability, and mast cells: Capsaicin desensitization fails to influence IgE-anti-DNP induced vascular permeability in rat airways. *Am. Rev. Respir. Dis.* **141:**398–406.

Dunn, C. J., Elliot, G. A., Oostveen, J. A., and Richards, I. M. (1988). Development of a prolonged eosinophil-rich inflammatory leukocyte infiltration in the guinea pig asthmatic response to ovalbumin inhalation. *Am. Rev. Respir. Dis.* **137:**541–547.

Dvorak, A. M., Letourneau, L., Login, G. R., Weller, P. F., and Ackerman, S. J. (1988). Ultrastructural localization of the Charcot–Leyden crystal protein (lysophospholipase) to a distinct crystalloid-free granule population in mature human eosinophils. *Blood* **72:**150–157.

Dvorak, A. M., Weller, P. F., Monahan-Earley, R. A., Letourneau, L., and Ackerman, S. J. (1990). Ultrastructural localization of Charcot–Leyden crystal protein (lysophospholipase) and peroxidase in macrophages, eosinophils, and extracellular matrix of the skin in hypereosinophilic syndrome. *Lab. Invest.* **62:**590–607.

Eady, R. P., Greenwood, B., Jackson, D. M., Orr, T. S. C., and Wells, E. (1985). The effect of nedocromil sodium and sodium cromoglycate on antigen-induced bronchoconstriction in the *Ascaris*-sensitive monkey. *Br. J. Pharmacol.* **85:**323–325.

Enokihara, H., Nagashima, S., Noma, T., Kajitani, H., Hamaguchi, H., Saito, K., Furusawa, S., Shishido, H., and Honjo, T. (1988). Effect of human recombinant interleukin 5 and G-CSF on eosinophil colony formation. *Immunol. Lett.* **18:** 73–76.

Evans, T. M., Rogers, D. F., Aursudkij, B., Chung, K. F., and Barnes, P. J. (1988a). Differential effect of inflammatory mediators on microvascular permeability in different parts of the guinea pig airways. *Clin. Sci.* **74:**46 (abstract).

Evans, T. W., Rogers, D., Boonrut, A., Chung, K. F., and Barnes, P. J. (1988b). Inflammatory mediators involved in antigen-induced airway microvascular leakage in guinea pigs. *Am. Rev. Respir. Dis.* **138:**395–399.

Evans, T. W., Chung, K. F., Rogers, D. F., and Barnes, P. J. (1987). Effect of platelet activating factor on airway vascular permeability: Possible mechanisms. *J. Appl. Physiol.* **63:**479–484.

Fairman, R. P., Sessler, C. N., Bierman, M., and Glauser, F. L. (1987). Protamine sulfate causes pulmonary hypertension and edema in rat lungs. *J. Appl. Physiol.* **62:**1363–1367.

Fick, R. B., Jr., Metzger, W. J., Richerson, H. B., Zavala, D. C., Moseley, P. L., Schoderbek, W. E., and Hunninghake, G. W. (1987). Increased bronchoalveolar permeability after allergen exposure in sensitive asthmatics. *J. Appl. Physiol.* **63:**1147–1155.

Foot, E. C. (1965). Eosinophil turnover in the normal rat. *Br. J. Hematol.* **11:**439–445.

Foreman, J. C., Mongar, J. L., and Gomperts, B. D. (1973). Calcium ionophores and movement of calcium ions following the physiological stimulus to a secretory process. *Nature* **245:**249–251.

Foreman, J. C., Jordan, C. C., and Piotrowski, W. (1982). Interaction of neurotensin with the substance P receptor mediating histamine release from rat mast cells and the flare in human skin. *Br. J. Pharmacol.* **77:**531–539.

Friedman, M. M., and Kaliner, M. A. (1987). Human mast cells and asthma. *Am. Rev. Respir. Dis.* **135:**1157–1164.

Fujimoto, K., Parker, J. C., and Kayes, S. G. (1990). Effect of activated eosinophils on isolated perfused rat lungs. *Am. Rev. Respir. Dis.* **142:**1414–1421.

Fukuda, T., Dunnette, S. L., Reed, C. E., Ackerman, S. J., Peters, M. S., and Gleich, G. J. (1985). Increased numbers of hypodense eosinophils in the blood of patients with bronchial asthma. *Am. Rev. Respir. Dis.* **132:**981–985.

Galli, S. J. (1990). Biology of disease. New insights into "the riddle of mast cells": Microenvironmental regulation of mast cell development and phenotypic heterogeneity. *Lab. Invest.* **62:**5–33.

Galli, S. J., Dvorak, A. M., and Dvorak, H. F. (1984). Basophils and mast cells: Morphologic insights into their biology, secretory patterns, and function. *Prog. Allergy* **34:**1–118.

Gamble, J. R., Harlan, J. M., Klebanoff, S. J., and Vadas, M. A. (1985). Stimulation of the adherence of neutrophils to umbilical vein endothelium by human recombinant tumor necrosis factor. *Proc. Natl. Acad. Sci. USA* **82:**8664–8671.

Gee, M. H., Margiotta, M., Tahamont, M. V., and Flynn, J. T. (1986). Free-radical generation in complement-induced pulmonary dysfunction. In *Physiology of Oxygen Radicals.* Edited by A. E. Taylor, S. Matalon, and P. Ward. American Physiology Society, Bethesda, Md., pp. 187–197.

Giembycz, M. A., Kroegel, C., and Barnes, P. J. (1990). Platelet activating factor stimulates cyclo-oxygenase activity in guinea pig eosinophils. *J. Immunol.* **144:** 3489–3497.

Gilfillan, A. M., Wiggan, G. A., and Welton, A. F. (1990a). The effects of the protein kinase C inhibitors staurosporine and H7 on the IgE dependent mediator release from RBL 2H3 cells. *Agents Actions* **30:**418–425.

Gilfillan, A. M., Wiggan, G. A., and Welton, A. F. (1990b). Pertussis toxin pretreatment reveals differential effects of adenosine analogs on IgE-dependent histamine and peptidoleukotriene release form RBL-2H3 cells. *Biochem. Biophys. Acta* **1052:**467–474.

Gilman, A. G. (1987). G proteins: Transducers of receptor-generated signals. *Annu. Rev. Biochem.* **56:**615–649.

Gleich, G. J. (1988). Current understanding of eosinophil function. *Hosp. Pract.* **23:** 97–120.

Gleich, G. J., and Adolphson, C. R. (1986). The eosinophilic leukocyte: Structure and function. *Adv. Immunol.* **39:**177–253.

Gleich, G. J., Loegering, D. A., and Maldonado, J. E. (1973). Identification of major basic protein in guinea pig eosinophil granules. *J. Exp. Med.* **137:**1459–1471.

Gleich, G. J., Frigas, E., Loegering, D. A., Wassom, D. L., and Steinmuller, D. (1979). Cytotoxic properties of the eosinophil major basic protein. *J. Immunol.* **123:**2925–2927.

Goetzl, E. J. (1976). Modulation of human eosinophil polymorphonuclear leukocyte migration and function. *Am. J. Pathol.* **85:**419–436.

Goetzl, E. J., and Gorman, R. R. (1978). Chemotactic and chemokinetic stimulation of human eosinophil and neutrophil polymorphonuclear leukocytes by 12-L-hydroxy-5,8,10 heptadecatrienoic acid (HHT). *J. Immunol.* **120:**526–531.

Goetzl, E. J., and Pickett, W. C. (1980). The human PMN leukocyte activity of complex hydroxyeicosatetraenoic acids (HETEs). *J. Immunol.* **125:**1789–1794.

Goetzl, E. J., Weller, P. H., and Sun, F. F. (1980). Regulation of human eosinophil function by endogenous mono-hydroxyeicosatetraenoic acids (HETEs). *J. Immunol.* **124:**926–933.

Gomperts, B. D., Cockcroft, S., Howell, T. W., Nusse, O., and Tatham, P. E. R. (1987). The dual effector system for exocytosis in mast cells: Obligatory requirement for both Ca^{2+} and GTP. *Biosci. Rep.* **7:**369–381.

Gordon, J. R., and Galli, S. J. (1990). Mast cells as a source of both performed and immunologically inducible TNF-α/cachectin. *Nature* **346:**274–276.

Grover, W. H., Winkler, H. H., and Normansell, D. E. (1978). Phagocytic properties of isolated human eosinophils. *J. Immunol.* **121**:718–725.

Gruchalla, R. S., Dinh, T. T., and Kennerly, D. A. (1990). An indirect pathway of receptor-mediated 1,2-diacylglycerol formation in mast cells. *J. Immunol.* **144:**2334–2342.

Haak-Frendscho, M., Arai, N., Baeza, M. L., Finn, A., and Kaplan, A. P. (1988). Human recombinant granulocyte macrophage colony-stimulating factor and interleukin-3 cause basophil histamine release. *J. Clin. Invest.* **82:**17–20.

Hälgren, R., Borg, T., Venge, P., and Modig, J. (1984). Signs of neutrophil and eosinophil activation in adult respiratory distress syndrome. *Crit. Care Med.* **12:**14–18.

Hälgren, R., Samuelsson, T., Venge, P., and Modig, J. (1987). Eosinophil activation in the lung is related to lung damage in adult respiratory distress syndrome. *Am. Rev. Respir. Dis.* **135:**639–642.

Harlan, J. M., Schwartz, B. R., Reidy, M. A., Schwartz, S. M., Ochs, H. D., and Harker, L. A. (1985). Activated neutrophils disrupt endothelial monolayer integrity by an oxygen radical-independent mechanism. *Lab. Invest.* **52:**141–150.

Hartman, C. T., Jr., and Glovsky, M. M. (1981). Complement activation requirements for histamine release from human leukocytes: Influence of purified $C3a_{hu}$ and $C5a_{hu}$ on histamine release. *Int. Arch. Allergy Appl. Immunol.* **66:**274–281.

Hattori, Y., and Siraganian, R. P. (1987). Rapid phosphorylation of a 92,000 MW protein on activation of rat basophilic leukaemia cells for histamine release. *Immunology* **60:**573–578.

Heiman, A. S., and Crews, F. T. (1985). Characterization of the effects of phorbol esters on rat mast cell secretion. *J. Immunol.* **134:**548–555.

Henderson, W. R., Chi, E. Y., and Klebanoff, S. J. (1980a). Eosinophil peroxidase-induced mast cell secretion. *J. Exp. Med.* **152:**265–279.

Henderson, W. R., Jong, E. C., and Klebanoff, S. J. (1980b). Binding of eosinophil peroxidase to mast cell granules with retention of peroxidatic activity. *J. Immunol.* **124:**1383–1388.

Henderson, W. R., Jorg, A., and Klebanoff, S. J. (1982). Eosinophil peroxidase mediated inactivation of leukotrienes B_4, C_4, and D_4. *J. Immunol.* **128:**2609–2613.

Henderson, W. R., Harley, J. B., and Fauci, A. S. (1984). Arachidonic acid metabolism in normal and hypereosinophilic syndrome eosinophils: Generation of leukotriene B_4, C_4, D_4 and 15-lipoxygenase products. *Immunology* **51:**679–686.

Henson, P. M. (1971). The immunologic release of constituents from neutrophil leukocytes. II. Mechanisms of release during phagocytosis and adherence to non-phagocytosable surfaces. *J. Immunol.* **107:**1547–1557.

Hirata, K., Pele, J. P., Robidoux, C., and Sirois, P. (1989). Guinea pig lung eosinophils: Purification and prostaglandin production. *J. Leukocyte Biol.* **45:**523–528.

Hoidal, J. R. (1990). The eosinophil and acute lung injury. *Am. Rev. Respir. Dis.* **142:**1245–1246.

Holgate, S. T., Lewis, R. A., and Austen, K. F. (1980). Role of adenylate cyclase in immunologic release of mediators from rat mast cells: Agonist and antagonist effects of purine- and ribose-modified adenosine analogs. *Proc. Natl. Acad. Sci. USA* **77:**6800–6804.

Hook, W. A., Siraganian, R. P., and Wahl, S. M. (1975). Complement-induced histamine release from human basophils. I. Generation of activity in human serum. *J. Immunol.* **114:**1185–1190.

Howell, T. W., Cockcroft, S., and Gomperts, B. D. (1987). Essential synergy between Ca^{2+} and guanine nucleotides in exocytotic secretion from permeabilized rat mast cells. *J. Cell Biol.* **105:**191–197.

Howell, C. J., Pujol, J. L., Crea, A. E. G., Davidson, R., Gearing, A. J. H., Godard, P. H., and Lee, T. H. (1989). Identification of alveolar macrophage-derived activity in bronchial asthma that enhances leukotriene C4 generation by human eosinophils stimulated with ionophore A23187 as granulocyte-macrophage colony stimulating factor. *Am. Rev. Respir. Dis.* **140:**1340–1347.

Hudson, G. (1963). Changes in the marrow reserve of eosinophil following re-exposure to foreign antigen. *Br. J. Haematol.* **9:**446–455.

Hudson, G. (1968). Quantitative study of the eosinophil granulocytes. *Semin. Hematol.* **5:**166–186.

Iozzo, R. V., MacDonald, G. H., and Wright, T. N. (1982). Immunoelectron microscopic localization of catalase in human eosinophilic leukocytes. *J. Histochem. Cytochem.* **30:**697–701.

Ishizaka, T., Hirata, F., Sterk, A. R., Ishizaka, K., and Axelrod, J. A. (1981). Bridging of IgE receptor activates phospholipid methylation and adenylate cyclase in mast cell plasma membranes. *Proc. Natl. Acad. Sci. USA* **78:**6812–6816.

Jacobsen, S., Hansen, H. S., and Jensen, B. (1987). Synergism between thapsigargin and the phorbol ester 12-*O*-tetradecanoylphorbol 13-acetate on the release of [^{14}C]arachidonic acid and histamine from rat peritoneal mast cells. *Biochem. Pharmacol.* **36:**621–626.

Johnson, A. R., Hugli, T. E., and Müller-Eberhard, H. J. (1975). Release of histamine from rat mast cells by complement peptides C3a and C5a. *Immunology* **28:**1067–1080.

Kajita, T., Yui, Y., Mita, H., Tamaguchi, N., Saito, H., Mishima, T., and Shida, T. (1985). Release of leukotriene C_4 from human eosinophils and its relationship to cell density. *Int. Arch. Appl. Immunol.* **78:**406–410.

Katakami, Y., Kaibuchi, K., Sawamura, M., Takai, Y., and Nishizuka, Y. (1984). Synergistic action of protein kinase C and calcium for histamine release from rat peritoneal mast cells. *Biochem. Biophys. Res. Commun.* **121:**573–578.

Kater, L. A., Goetzl, E. J., and Austen, K. F. (1976). Isolation of human eosinophil phospholipase D. *J. Clin. Invest.* **57:**1173–1180.

Kay, A. B., Stechschulte, D. J., and Austen, K. F. (1971). An eosinophil leukocyte chemotactic factor of anaphylaxis. *J. Exp. Med.* **133:**602–619.

Kennerly, D. A. (1987). Diacylglycerol metabolism on mast cells: Analysis of lipid metabolic pathways using molecular species analysis of intermediaries. *J. Biol. Chem.* **262:**16305–16313.

Kennerly, D. A. (1990). Phosphatidylcholine is a quantitatively more important source of increased 1,2-diacylglcerol than is phosphatidylinositol in mast cells. *J. Immunol.* **144:**3912–3919.

Kennerly, D. A., Sullivan, T. J., Sylvester, P., and Parker, C. W. (1979). Diacylglycerol metabolism in mast cells: A potential role in membrane fusion and arachidonic acid release. *J. Exp. Med.* **150:**1039–1044.

Kierszenbaum, F., Ackerman, S. J., and Gleich, G. J. (1982). Inhibition of antibody dependent eosinophil-mediated cytotoxicity by heparin. *J. Immunol.* **128:**515–521.

Kimani, G., Tonnesen, M. G., and Henson, P. M. (1988). Stimulation of eosinophil adherence to human vascular endothelial cells in vitro by platelet activating factor. *J. Immunol.* **140:**3161–3166.

Klebanoff, S. J. (1988). Phagocytic cells: Products of oxygen metabolism. In *Inflammation: Basic Principles and Clinical Correlates.* Edited by J. I. Gallin, I. M. Goldstein, and R. Snyderman. Raven Press, New York, pp. 391–444.

Klebanoff, S. J., Agosti, J. M., Jorg, A., and Waltersdorf, A. M. (1989). Comparative toxicity of horse eosinophil peroxidase–H_2O_2–halide system and granule basic proteins. *J. Immunol.* **143:**239–244.

Klickstein, L. B., Shapleigh, C., and Goetzl, E. J. (1980). Lipoxygenation of arachidonic acid as a source of polymorphonuclear leukocyte chemotactic factors in synovial fluid and tissue in rheumatoid arthritis and spondyloarthritis. *J. Clin. Invest.* **66:**606–616.

Kloprogge, E., de Leeuw, A. J., de Monchy, J. G. R., and Kauffman, H. F. (1989a). Cellular communication in leukotriene C_4 production between eosinophils and neutrophils. *Int. Arch. Allergy Appl. Immunol.* **90:**20–23.

Kloprogge, E., de Leeuw, A. J., de Monchy, J. G. R., and Kauffman, H. F. (1989b). Hypodense eosinophilic granulocytes in normal individuals and patients with asthma: Generation of hypodense cell populations in vitro. *J. Allergy Clin. Immunol.* **83:**393–400.

Koopman, W. R., Jr., and Jackson, R. C. (1990). Calcium- and guanine-nucleotide-dependent exocytosis in permeabilized rat mast cells: Modulation by protein kinase C. *Biochem. J.* **265:**365–373.

Kroegel, C., Yukawa, T., Dent, G., Venge, P., Chung, K. F., and Barnes, P. J. (1989a). Stimulation of degranulation from human eosinophils by platelet activating factor. *J. Immunol.* **142:**3518–3526.

Kroegel, C., Yukawa, T., Westwick, J., and Barnes, P. J. (1989b). Evidence for two platelet activating factor receptors on eosinophils: Dissociation between PAF-induced calcium mobilization, degranulation, and superoxide anion generation in eosinophils. *Biochem. Biophys. Res. Commun.* **162:**511–521.

Lam, S., LeRiche, J., Phillips, D., and Chan-Yeung, M. (1987). Cellular and protein changes in bronchial lavage fluid after late asthmatic reaction in patients with red cedar asthma. *J. Allergy. Clin. Immunol.* **80:**44–50.

Lamas, A. M., Mulroney, C. M., and Schleimer, R. P. (1988). Studies on the adhesive interaction between purified human eosinophils and cultured vascular endothelial cells. *J. Immunol.* **140:**1500–1505.

Lee, T. C., Fein, A. M., Lippman, M., Holtzman, H., Kimbel, P., and Weinbaum, G. (1981). Elastolytic activity in pulmonary lavage fluid from patients with adult respiratory distress syndrome. *N. Engl. J. Med.* **304:**192–196.

Lee, T. C., Lenihan, D. J., Malone, B., Roddy, L. L., and Wasserman, S. I. (1984). Increased biosynthesis of platelet activating factor in activated human eosinophils. *J. Biol. Chem.* **259:**5526–5530.

Lempereur, C., Capron, M., and Capron, A. (1980). Identification and measurement of rat eosinophil phospholipase D. Its activity of schistosomula phospholipids. *J. Immunol. Methods* **33:**249–260.

Lewis, R. A., Holgate, S. T., Roberts, J. J., Maguire, J. F. Oates, J. A., and Austen, K. F. (1979). Effects of indomethacin on cyclic nucleotide levels and histamine release from rat serosal mast cells. *J. Immunol.* **123:**1663–1668.

Liles, W. C., Meier, K. E., and Henderson, W. R. (1987). Phorbol myristate acetate and calcium ionophore A23187 synergistically induce release of LTB_4 by human neutrophils: Involvement of protein kinase C activation in the regulation of 5-lipoxygenase pathway. *J. Immunol.* **138:**3396–3402.

Lin, P., Wiggan, G. A., and Gilfillan, A. M. (1991). Activation of phospholipase D in a rat mast (RBL 2H3) cell line: A possible unifying mechanism for IgE-dependent degranulation and arachidonic acid metabolite release. *J. Immunol.* **146:**1609–1616.

Liu, M. C., Proud, D., Lichtenstein, L. M., MacGlashan, R. P., Schleimer, N. F., Adkinson, N. F., Kagey-Sobotka, A., Schulman, E. S., and Plaut, M. (1986). Human lung derived histamine-releasing activity is due to IgE dependent factors. *J. Immunol.* **136:**2588–2595.

Lo, T. N., Saul, W., and Beaven, M. A. (1987). The actions of Ca^{2+} ionophores on rat basophilic (2H3) cells are dependent on cellular ATP and hydrolysis of inositol phospholipids. *J. Biol. Chem.* **262:**4141–4145.

Lohse, M. J., Maurer, K., Gensheimer, H. P., and Shwabe, U. (1987). Dual actions of adenosine on rat peritoneal mast cells. *Arch. Pharmacol.* **335:**555–560.

Lopez, A. F., Williamson, D. J., Gamble, J. R., Begley, C. G., Harlan, J. M., Klebanoff, S. J., Waltersdorph, A., Wong, G., Clark, S. C., and Vadas, M. A. (1986). Recombinant human granulocyte colony-stimulating factor stimulates in vitro mature human neutrophil and eosinophil function, surface receptor expression, and survival. *J. Clin. Invest.* **78:**1220–1228.

Lopez, A. F., To, L. B., Yang, Y. C., Gamble, J. R., Shannon, M. F., Burns, G. F., Dyson, P. G., Juttner, C. A., Clark, S., and Vadas, M. A. (1987). Stimulation of proliferation, differentiation, and function of human cells by primate interleukin 3. *Proc. Natl. Acad. Sci. USA* **84:**2761–2765.

Lopez, A. F., Sanderson, C. J., Gamble, J. R., Campbell, H. D., Young, I. G., and Vadas, M. A. (1988). Recombinant human interleukin 5 is a selective activator of human eosinophil function. *J. Exp. Med.* **167:**219–224.

Ludowyke, R. I., Peleg, I., Beaven, M. A., and Adelstein, R. S. (1989). Antigen-induced secretion of histamine and the phosphorylation of myosin by protein kinase C in rat basophilic leukemia cells. *J. Biol. Chem.* **264:**12492–12501.

Maeyama, K., Hohman, R. J., Ali, H., Cunha-Melo, J. R., and Beaven, M. A. (1988). Assessment of IgE-receptor function through measurement of hydrolysis of membrane inositol phospholipids. *J. Immunol.* **140:**3919–3927.

Majno, G., Shea, S. M., and Levanthal, M. M. (1969). Endothelial contraction induced by histamine-type mediators: An electron microscopic study. *J. Cell Biol.* **42:**647–672.

Marone, G., Kagey-Sobotka, A., and Lichtenstein, L. M. (1979). Effects of arachidonic acid and its metabolites on antigen-induced histamine release from human basophils. *J. Immunol.* **123:**1669–1677.

Marone, G., Colombo, M., Triggiani, M., Cirillo, R., Genovese, A., and Formisano, S. (1987). Inhibition of IgE-mediated release of histamine and peptide leukotriene from human basophils and mast cells by forskolin. *Biochem. Pharmacol.* **36:**13–20.

Marqaurdt, D. L., Parker, C. W., and Sullivan, T. J. (1978). Potentiation of mast cell mediator release by adenosine. *J. Immunol.* **120:**871–878.

McCloskey, M. A. (1988). Cholera toxin potentiates IgE-coupled inositol phospholipid hydrolysis and mediator secretion by RBL-2H3 cells. *Proc. Natl. Acad. Sci. USA* **85:**7260–7264.

Metcalf, D., Begley, C. G., Johnson, G. R., Nicola, N. A., Vadas, M. A., Lopez, A. F., Williamson, D. J., Wong, G. G., Clark, S. C., and Wang, E. A. (1986). Biologic properties in vitro of a recombinant human granulocyte-macrophage colony-stimulating factor. *Blood* **67:**37–45.

Meyrick, B., and Brigham, K. L. (1983). Increased permeability of bovine pulmonary artery intimal explants caused by histamine structure and function. *Fed. Proc.* **42:**3650A.

Miller, L., Alber, G., Varin-Blank, N., Ludowyke, R., and Metzger, H. (1990). Transmembrane signaling in P815 mastocytoma cells by transfected IgE receptors. *J. Biol. Chem.* **265:**12444–12453.

Modig, J., and Hälgren, R. (1986). Lethal adult respiratory distress syndrome after meningococcal septicemia. Biochemical markers in bronchoalveolar lavage fluid. *Resuscitation* **13:**159–163.

Modig, J., Samuelson, T., and Hälgren, R. (1986). The predictive and discriminative value of biologically active products of eosinophils, neutrophils, and complement in bronchoalveolar lavage and blood in patients with adult respiratory distress syndrome. *Resuscitation* **14:**121–134.

Mojarad, M., Hamasaki, Y., and Said, S. I. (1983). Platelet-activating factor increases pulmonary microvascular permeability and induces pulmonary edema. A preliminary report. *Bull. Eur. Physiopathol. Resp.* **19:**253–256.

Moqbel, R., Sass-Kuhn, S. P., Goetzl, E. J., and Kay, A. B. (1983). Enhancement of neutrophil and eosinophil-mediated complement-dependent killing of schistosomula of *Schistosoma mansoni* in vitro by leukotriene B_4. *Clin. Exp. Immunol.* **52:**519–527.

Morita, Y., Goto, M., and Miyamoto, T. (1987). Effect of interleukin on basophil histamine release. *Allergy* **42:**104–108.

Morita, Y., Takaishi, T., Honda, Z., and Miyamoto, T. (1988). Role of protein kinase C in histamine release from human basophils. *Allergy* **43:**100–104.

Moy, J. N., Gleich, G. J., and Thomas, L. L. (1990). Noncytotoxic activation of neutrophils by eosinophil granule major basic protein. Effect on superoxide anion generation and lysozomal enzyme release. *J. Immunol.* **145:**2626–2632.

Nagao, S., Nagata, K., Kohmura, Y., Ishizuka, T., and Nozowa, Y. (1987). Redistribution of phospholipid/Ca^{++} dependent protein kinase in mast cells activated by various agonists. *Biochem. Biophys. Res. Commun.* **142:**645–653.

Nakahara, K., Ohkuda, K., and Staub, N. C. (1979). Effect of infusing histamine into pulmonary or bronchial artery on sheep pulmonary fluid balance. *Am. Rev. Respir. Dis.* **20:**875–882.

Nakamura, T., and Ui, M. (1984). Islet-activating protein, pertussis toxin, inhibits Ca^{2+}-induced and guanine nucleotide-dependent releases of histamine and arachidonic acid from rat mast cells. *FEBS Lett.* **173:**414–418.

Nakamura, T., and Ui, M. (1985). Simultaneous inhibitions of inositol phospholipid breakdown, arachidonic acid release and histamine secretion in mast cells by islet-activating protein, pertussis toxin. A possible involvement of the toxin-specific substrate in the Ca^{++} mobilizing receptor-mediated biosignaling system. *J. Biol. Chem.* **260:**3584–3593.

Narasimhan, V., Holowka, D., Fewtrell, C., and Baird, B. (1988). Cholera toxin increases the rate of antigen-stimulated calcium influx in rat basophilic leukemia cells. *J. Biol. Chem.* **263:**19626–19632.

Narasimhan, V., Holowka, D., and Baird, B. (1990). Microfilaments regulate the rate of exocytosis in rat basophilic leukemia cells. *Biochem. Biophys. Res. Commun.* **171:**222–229.

O'Donnell, S. R., and Barnett, C. J. K. (1987). Microvascular leakage to platelet activating factor in guinea pig trachea and bronchi. *Eur. J. Pharmacol.* **138:**385–396.

O'Donnell, M. C., Ackerman, S. J., Gleich, G. J., and Thomas, L. L. (1983). Activation of basophil and mast cell histamine release by eosinophil granule major basic protein. *J. Exp. Med.* **157:**1981–1991.

Ohno, I., Yamauchi, K., and Takishima, T. (1990). Gene expression and production of tumor necrosis factor by a rat basophilic leukaemia cell line (RBL-2H3) with IgE receptor triggering. *Immunology* **70:**88–93.

Oliver, J. M., Seagrave, J. C., Stump, R. F., Pfeiffer, J. M., and Deanin, G. G. (1988). Signal transduction and cellular response in RBL-2H3 mast cells. *Prog. Allergy* **42:**185–245.

Olofsson, T., Gartner, I., and Olsson, I. (1980). Separation of human bone marrow cells in density gradients of polyvinylpyrrolidone coated silica beads (Percoll). *Scand. J. Hematol.* **24:**254–262.

Omann, G. M., Allen, R. A., Bokoch, G. M., Painter, R. G., Traynor, A. E., and Skar, L. A. (1987). Signal trandsduction and cytoskeletal activation in the neutrophil. *Pharmacol. Rev.* **67:**285–322.

Ottesen, E. A., Stanley, A. M., Gelfland, J. A., Gadek, J. E., Frank, M. M., Nash, T. E., and Cheever, A. W. (1977). Immunoglobulin and complement receptors on human eosinophils and their role in cellular adherence to schistosomules. *Am. J. Trop. Med. Hyg.* **26:**134–141.

Owen, W. F., Rothenberg, M. E., Silberstein, D. R., Gasson, J. C., Stevens, R. L., Austen, K. F., and Soberman, R. J. (1987). Regulation of human eosinophil viability. Density and function by granulocyte-macrophage colony stimulating factor in the presence of 3T3 fibroblasts. *J. Exp. Med.* **166:**

Parwaresch, M. R., Walle, A. J., and Arndt, D. (1976). The peripheral kinetics of human radiolabelled eosinophils. *Virchow Arch.* (*Cell Pathol.*) **21:**57–66.

Peachell, P. J., and Pearce, F. L. (1984). Some studies on the release of histamine from mast cells treated with polymyxin. *Agents Actions* **14:**379–385.

Peachell, P. T., Columbo, M., Kagey-Sobotka, A., Lichtenstein, L. M., and Marone, G. (1988). Adenosine potentiates mediator release from human lung mast cells. *Am. Rev. Respir. Dis.* **138:**1143–1151.

Pecht, I., and Corcia, A. (1987). Stimulus-secretion coupling mechanisms in mast cells. *Biophys. Chem.* **26:**291–301.

Penner, R. (1988). Multiple signaling pathways control stimulus–secretion coupling in rat peritoneal mast cells. *Proc. Natl. Acad. Sci. USA* **85:**9856–9860.

Penner, R., and Neher, E. (1988). Secretory responses of rat peritoneal mast cells to high intracellular calcium. *FEBS Lett.* **226:**307–313.

Penner, R., Matthews, G., and Neher, E. (1988). Regulation of calcium influx by second messengers in rat mast cells. *Nature* **334:**499–503.

Persson, C. (1987). Cromoglicate, plasma exudation and asthma. *Trends Pharmacol. Sci.* **8:**202–203.

Peters, M. S., Rodriguez, M., and Gleich, G. J. (1986). Localization of human eosinophil granule basic proteins, eosinophil cationic protein, and eosinophil-derived neurotoxin by immunoelectron microscopy. *Lab. Invest.* **65:**656–662.

Peterson, M. W., Stone, P., and Shasby, D. M. (1987). Cationic neutrophil proteins increase transendothelial albumin movement. *J. Appl. Physiol.* **62:**1521–1530.

Petreccia, D., Nauseef, W. M., and Clark, R. A. (1987). Respiratory burst of normal human eosinophils. *J. Leukocyte Biol.* **41:**283–288.

Pincus, S. H. (1983). Hydrogen peroxide release from eosinophils: Quantitative comparative studies of human and guinea pig eosinophils. *J. Lab. Invest. Dermatol.* **80:**278–281.

Pincus, S. H., Di Napoli, A. M., and Schooley, W. R. (1982). Superoxide production by eosinophils: Activation by histamine. *J. Invest. Dermatol.* **79:**53–57.

Piotrowski, W., and Foreman, J. C. (1985). On the actions of substance P, somatostatin and vasoactive intestinal polypeptide on rat peritoneal mast cells and in human skin. *Arch. Pharmacol.* **331:**364–368.

Piotrowski, W., Mead, M., and Foreman, J. C. (1987). Action of the $SP_{2\text{-}11}$ fragments of substance P on rat peritoneal mast cells. *Agents Actions* **20:**178–180.

Plaut, M., Pierce, J. H., Watson, C., Hanley-Hyde, J., Nordan, R. P., and Paul, W. E. (1989). Mast cell lines produce lymphokines in response to cross-linkage of $Fc_{\varepsilon}RI$ or to calcium ionophores. *Nature* **339:**64–67.

Prin, L., Capron, M., Tonnel, A. B., Bletry, O., and Capron, A. (1983). Heterogeneity of human peripheral blood eosinophils: variability in cell density and cytotoxic ability in relation to the level and origin of eosinophilia. *Int. Arch. Allergy Appl. Immunol.* **72:**236–246.

Prin, L., Charon, J., Capron, M., Gosset, P., Taelman, H., Tonnel, A. B., and Capron, A. (1984). Heterogeneity of human eosinophils. II. Variability of the respiratory burst activity related to cell density. *Clin. Exp. Immunol.* **57:**735–742.

Quinton, P. M., and Philpott, C. W. (1973). A role for anionic sites in epithelial architecture. Effects of cationic polymers on cell membrane structures. *J. Cell Biol.* **56:**787–796.

Regal, J. F., Hardy, T. M., Casey, F. B., and Chakrin, L. W. (1983). C5a induced histamine release; species specificity. *Int. Arch. Allergy Appl. Immunol.* **72:**362–365.

Rippe, B., Allison, R. C., Parker, J. C., and Taylor, A. E. (1984). Effects of histamine, serotonin, and norepinephrine on the circulation of dog lungs. *J. Appl. Physiol.* **57:**223–232.

Rothenberg, M. E., Owen, W. F., Jr., Silberstein, D. S., Woods, J., Soberman, R. J., Austen, K. F., and Stevens, R. L. (1988). Human eosinophils have prolonged survival, enhanced functional properties, and become hypodense when exposed to human interleukin 3. *J. Clin. Invest.* **81:**1986–1992.

Roubin, R., Elias, P. P., Fiers, W., and Dessein, D. J. (1987). Recombinant tumor necrosis factor (rTNF) enhances leukotriene biosynthesis in neutrophils and eosinophils stimulated with Ca^{++} ionophore A23187. *Clin. Exp. Immunol.* **70:**484–490.

Rowen, J., Hyde, D. M., and McDonald, R. J. (1990). Eosinophils cause acute edematous injury in isolated perfused rat lungs. *Am. Rev. Respir. Dis.* **142:**215–220.

Sacks, T., Moldow, C. F., Craddock, P. R., Bowers, T. K., and Jacob, H. S. (1978). Oxygen radicals mediate endothelial damage by complement stimulated granulocytes. An in vivo model of immune vascular damage. *J. Clin. Invest.* **61:**1161–1167.

Sagi-Eisenberg, R., and Pecht, I. (1984). Protein kinase C, a coupling element between stimulus and secretion of basophils. *Immunol. Lett.* **8:**237–243.

Sagi-Eisenberg, R., Foreman, J. C., and Shelley, R. I. (1985). Histamine release induced by histone and phorbol ester from rat peritoneal mast cells. *Eur. J. Pharmacol.* **113:**11–17.

Saito, H., Okajima, F., Molski, T. F., Sha'afri, R. I., Ui, M., and Ishizaka, T. (1987). Effects of ADP-ribosylation of GTP-binding protein by pertussis toxin on immunoglobulin E-dependent and -independent histamine release from mast cells and basophils. *J. Immunol.* **138:**3927–3934.

Sanborg, R. R., and Smolen, J. E. (1988). Biology of disease: Early biochemical events in leukocyte activation. *Lab. Invest.* **59:**300–320.

Sanjar, S., Acki, S., Boubekar, K., Smith, D., Kings, M. A., and Morley, J. (1990). Eosinophil accumulation in pulmonary airways of guinea pigs induced by exposure to an aerosol of platelet activating factor: Effects of anti-asthma drugs. *Br. J. Pharmacol.* **99:**267–272.

Saria, A., Lundberg, J. M., Skofitsch, G., and Lembeck, F. (1983). Vascular protein leakage in various tissues is induced by substance P, capsaicin, bradykinin, serotonin, histamine, and by antigen challenge. *Arch. Pharmacol.* **324:**212–218.

Schleimer, R. P., Gillespie, E., and Lichtenstein, L. M. (1981). Release of histamine from human leukocytes stimulated with the tumor-promoting phorbol diesters. I. Characterization of the response. *J. Immunol.* **126:**570–574).

Schleimer, R. P., Derse, C. P., Friedman, B., Gillis, S., Plaut, M., Lichtenstein, L. M., and MacGlashan, D. W., Jr. (1989). Regulation of human basophil mediator release by cytokines. I. Interaction with antiinflammatory steroids. *J. Immunol.* **143:** 1310–1317.

Sedgwick, J. B., Vrtis, R. F., Goveley, M. F., and Busse, W. W. (1988). Stimulus-dependent differences in superoxide anion generation by normal human eosinophils and neutrophils. *J. Allergy Clin. Immunol.* **81:**876–873.

Selig, W. M., Bloomquist, M. A., Cohen, M. L., and Fleisch, J. H. (1988). Serotonin-induced pulmonary responses in the perfused guinea pig lung: evidence for $5HT_2$ receptor-mediated pulmonary vascular and airway smooth muscle contraction. *Pulmonary Pharmacol.* **1:**93–99.

Selig, W. M., Cerasoli, F., Jr., Welton, A., Durham, S., and Tocker, J. (1990). Substance P-induced airway reactivity following low dose antigen challenge in the guinea pig. *FASEB J.* **4:**A613 (abstract).

Selig, W. M., Tocker, J., and Cerasoli, F., Jr. (1991). Eosinophils exacerbate antigen-induced edema formation in the perfused guinea pig lung. *FASEB J.* (abstract) **5**(5):A1243.

Sertl, K., Kowalski, M. L., Slater, J., and Kaliner, M. A. (1988). Passive sensitization and antigen challenge increase vascular permeability in rat airways. *Am. Rev. Respir. Dis.* **138:**1295–1299.

Shasby, D. M., Vanbenthuysen, K. M., Tate, R. M., Shasby, S. S., McMurtry, I., and Repine, J. E. (1982). Granulocytes mediate acute edematous lung injury in rabbits and in isolated rabbit lungs perfused with phorbol myristate acetate: Role of oxygen radicals. *Am. Rev. Respir. Dis.* **125:**443–447.

Shasby, D. M., Shasby, S. S., and Peach, M. J. (1983). Granulocytes and phorbol myristate acetate increase permeability to albumin of cultured endothelial monolayers and isolated perfused lungs: Role of oxygen radicals and granulocyte adherence. *Am. Rev. Respir. Dis.* **127:**72–76.

Shay, A. M., Brutsaert, D. L., Meulemans, A. L., Andries, L. J., and Capron, M. (1990). Eosinophils from hypereosinophilic patients damage endocardium of isolated feline heart muscle preparations. *Circulation* **81:**1081–1088.

Siraganian, R. P. (1988). Mast cells and basophils. In *Inflammation: Basic Principles and Clinical Correlates.* Edited by J. I. Gallin, I. M. Goldstein, and R. Snyderman. Raven Press, New York, pp. 513–542.

Skutelsky, E., Rudich, Z., and Danon, D. (1975). Surface charge properties of the luminal front of blood vessel walls: An electron microscopical analysis. *Thromb. Res.* **7:**623–634.

Slungaard, A., Vercellotti, G. M., Walker, G., Nelson, R. D., and Jacob, H. S. (1990). Tumor necrosis factor α/cachectin stimulates eosinophil oxidant production and toxicity towards human endothelium. *J. Exp. Med.* **171:**2025–2041.

Spry, C. J. F. (1971a). Mechanisms of eosinophilia. V. Kinetics of normal and accelerated eosinopoiesis. *Cell Tissue Kin.* **4:**351–364.

Spry, C. J. F. (1971b). Mechanisms of eosinophilia. VI. Eosinophil mobilization. *Cell Tissue Kinet.* **4:**365–374.

Spry, C. J. F. (1972). Mechanisms of eosinophilia. VII. Eosinophilia in rats with lymphoma. *Br. J. Haematol.* **22:**407–413.

Spry, C. J. F. (1985). Synthesis and secretion of eosinophil granule substances. *Immunol. Today* **6:**332–335.

Steffen, M., Aboud, M., Potter, G. K., Yung, Y. P., and Moore, A. S. (1989). Presence of tumor necrosis factor or a related factor in human basophil/mast cells. *Immunology* **66:**445–450.

Steinhilber, D., and Roth, H. J. (1989). New series of lipoxins isolated from human eosinophils. *FEBS Lett.* **255:**143–148.

Strath, M., Warren, D. J., and Sanderson, C. J. (1985). Detection of eosinophils using an eosinophil peroxidase assay. Its use as an assay for eosinophil differentiation factors. *J. Immunol. Methods* **83:**209–215.

Stryckmans, P. A., Cronkite, E. P., Greenberg, M. L., and Schiffer, L. M. (1968). Kinetics of eosinophil proliferation in man. In *Proceedings of the 12th Congress of the International Society of Hematology.* International Society of Hematology, New York, p. F19.

Subramanian, N., and Bray, M. A. (1987). Interleukin 1 releases histamine from human basophils and mast cells in vitro. *J. Immunol.* **138:**271–275.

Sullivan, T. J., and Parker, C. W. (1979). Possible role of arachidonic acid and its metabolites in mediator release from rat mast cells. *J. Immunol.* **122:**431–436.

Sullivan, T. J., Parker, K. L., Kulcycki, A., and Parker, C. W. (1976). Modulation of cyclic AMP in purified rat mast cells III. Studies on the effect of concanavalin A and anti-IgE on cyclic AMP concentration during histamine release. *J. Immunol.* **117:**713.

Sun, F. F., Czuk, C. I., and Taylor, B. M. (1989). Arachidonic acid metabolism in guinea pig eosinophils: Synthesis of thromboxane B_2 and leukotriene B_4 in response to soluble or particulate activators. *J. Leukocyte Biol.* **46:**152–160.

Suzuki-Nushimura, T., Sekino, H., Yoshino, Y., Nagaya, K., Oku, N., Nanago, M., and Uchida, M. K. (1989). Synthetic polycations, polyethylenimines, and polyallylamines release histamine from rat mast cells. *Jpn. J. Pharmacol.* **51:**279–290.

Tai, P. C., Ackerman, S. J., Spry, C. J. F., Dunnette, S., Olssen, E. G. J., and Gleich, G. J. (1987). Deposits of eosinophil granule proteins in cardiac tissues of patients with eosinophilic endomyocardial disease. *Lancet* **1:**643–647.

Tamura, N., Agrawal, B. K., Suliaman, F. A., and Townley, R. G. (1987). Effects of platelet-activating factor eosinophil on the chemotaxis of normodense eosinophils from normal subjects. *Biochem. Biophys. Res. Commun.* **142:**638–643.

Tate, R. M., and Repine, J. E. (1983). Neutrophils and adult respiratory distress syndrome. *Am. Rev. Respir. Dis.* **128:**552–559.

Tauber, A. L., Goetzl, E. J., and Babior, B. M. (1979). Unique characteristics of superoxide production by eosinophils in eosinophilic states. *Inflammation* **3:**261–267.

Teshima, R., Ikebuchi, H., and Terao, T. (1984). Ca^{2+}-dependent and phorbol ester activating phosphorylation of a 36k-dalton protein of rat basophilic leukemia cell membranes and immunoprecipitation of the phosphorylated protein with IgE-anti IgE system. *Biochem. Biophys. Res. Commun.* **125:**867–874.

Theoharides, T. C., Siegart, W., Greengard, P., and Douglas, W. W. (1980). Antiallergic drug cromolyn may inhibit histamine secretion by regulating phosphorylation of a mast cell protein. *Science* **207:**80–82.

Till, G. O., Johnson, K. J., Kunkel, R., and Ward, P. A. (1982). Intravascular activation of complement and acute lung injury. Dependence on neutrophil and toxic oxygen metabolites. *J. Clin. Invest.* **69:**1126–1135.

Toyofuku, T., Koyama, S., Kobayashi, T., Kusama, S., and Ueda, G. (1989). Effects of polycations on pulmonary vascular permeability in conscious sheep. *J. Clin. Invest.* **83:**2063–2069.

Undem, B. J., Peachell, P. T., and Lichtenstein, L. M. (1988). Isoproterenol-induced inhibition of immunoglobulin E-mediated release of histamine and arachidonic acid metabolites from the human lung mast cell. *J. Pharmacol. Exp. Ther.* **247:**209–217.

Valent, P., Besemer, J., Muhm, M., Majdic, O., Lechner, K., and Bettleheim, P. (1989). Interleukin 3 activates human blood basophils via high-affinity binding sites. *Proc. Natl. Acad. Sci. USA* **86:**5542–5546.

Vehaskari, V. M., Chang, C. T., Stevens, J. K., and Robson, A. M. (1984). The effects of polycations on vascular permeability in the rat. *J. Clin. Invest.* **73:**1053–1061.

Wang, J. M., Rambaldi, A., Blondi, A., Chen, Z. G., Sanderson, C. J., and Mantovani, A. (1989). Recombinant human interleukin 5 is a selective eosinophil chemoattractant. *Eur. J. Immunol.* **19:**701–705.

Wardlaw, A. J., Moqbel, R., Cromwell, O., and Kay, A. B. (1986). Platelet-activating factor. A potent chemotactic and chemokinetic factor for eosinophils. *J. Clin. Invest.* **78:**1701–1706.

Warner, J. A., and MacGlashan, D. W. (1990). Signal transduction in human basophils:

A comparative study of the role of protein kinase C in basophils activated by anti-IgE antibody and formyl-methionyl-leucyl phenylalanine. *J. Immunol.* **145:**1897–1905.

Warner, J. A., Yancey, K. B., and MacGlashin, D. W. (1987). The effect of pertussis toxin on mediator release from human basophils. *J. Immunol.* **139:**161–165.

Wegner, C. D., Gundel, R. H., Reilly, P., Haynes, N., Letts, L. G., and Rothlein, R. (1990). Intracellular adhesion molecule-1 (ICAM-1) in the pathogenesis of asthma. *Science* **24:**456–459.

Weller, P. F. (1989). Eosinophil structure and function. In *Arthritis and Allied Conditions: A Textbook of Rheumatology*. Edited by D. McCarty. Lea & Febiger, Philadelphia, pp. 366–374.

Weller, P. F., Bach, D., and Austen, K. F. (1982). Human eosinophil phospholipase: The sole protein component of Charcot–Leyden crystals. *J. Immunol.* **128:**1346–1349.

Weller, P. F., Bach, D. S., and Austen, K. F. (1984). Biochemical characterization of human eosinophil Charcot–Leyden crystal protein (lysophospholipase). *J. Biol. Chem.* **259:**15100–15105.

Wells, E., and Mann, J. (1983). Phosphorylation of a mast cell protein in response to treatment with anti-allergic compounds. Implications for the mode of action of sodium cromoglycate. *Biochem. Pharmacol.* **32:**837–842.

White, J. R., Ishizaka, K., Ishizaka, T., and Sha'afi, R. (1984). Direct demonstration of increased intracellular concentration of free calcium as measured by Quin-2 in stimulated rat peritoneal mast cell. *Proc. Natl. Acad. Sci. USA* **81:**3978–3982.

White, M. V., Kaliner, M. A., and Baer, H. (1986). Stimulated neutrophils release a histamine releasing factor. *J. Allergy Clin. Immunol.* **133:**2100–2185.

Wilson, B. S., Deanin, G. G., Standefer, J. C., Vanderjagt, D., and Oliver, J. M. (1989). Depletion of guanine nucleotides with mycophenolic acid suppresses IgEr receptor-mediated degranulation in rat basophilic leukemia cells. *J. Immunol.* **143:**259–265.

Winslow, C. M., and Austen, K. F. (1984). Role of cyclic nucleotides in the activation secretion response. *Prog. Allergy* **34:**236–270.

Wodnar-Filipowicz, A., Heusser, C. H., and Moroni, C. (1989). Production of the haemopoietic growth factors GM-CSF and interleukin-3 by mast cells in response to IgE receptor-mediated activation. *Nature* **339:**

Woldemussie, E., Ali, H., Takaishi, T., Siraganian, R. P., and Beaven, M. A. (1987). Identification of variants of the basophilic leukemia (RBL-2H3) cells that have defective phosphoinositide responses to antigen and stimulants of guanine 5′-triphosphate-regulatory proteins. *J. Immunol.* **139:**2431–2438.

Woodward, D. F., Weichman, B. M., Gill, C. A., and Wasserman, M. A. (1983). The effect of synthetic leukotrienes on tracheal microvascular permeability. *Prostaglandins* **25:**131–142.

Yamaguchi, T., Suda, T., Suda, J., Eguchi, M., Miura, Y., Harada, N., Tominaga, A., and Takatsu, K. (1988). Purified interleukin 5 supports the terminal differentiation and proliferation of murine eosinophilic precursors. *J. Exp. Med.* **167:**43–48.

Yokota, S., Deimann, W., Hasimoto, T., and Fahimi, H. D. (1984). Specific granules of rat eosinophils contain peroxisomal acyl-CoA oxidase: Possible involvement in production of H_2O_2. *Histochem. J.* **16:**573–577.

Young, J. D., Peterson, C. G. B., Venge, P., and Cohn, Z. A. (1986). Mechanism of membrane damage mediated by human eosinophils. *Nature* **321:**613–616.

Yukawa, T., Kroegel, C., Evans, P., Fukuda, T., Chung, K. F., and Barnes, P. J. (1989). Density heterogeneity of eosinophil leucocytes: Induction of hypodense eosinophils by platelet-activating factor. *Immunology* **68:**143–149.

Zheutlin, L. M., Ackerman, S. J., Gleich, G. J., and Thomas, L. L. (1984). Stimulation of basophil and rat mast cell histamine release by eosinophil-granule derived cationic proteins. *J. Immunol.* **133:**2180–2185.

Zoratti, E. M., Geiger, K., Bates, M. E., Sedgwick, J. B., and Busse, W. W. (1990). Platelet activating factor (PAF) primes human eosinophil (EOS) function. *J. Allergy Clin. Immunol.* **85:**261 (abstract).

Zucker-Franklin, D. (1974). Eosinophil function and disorders. *Adv. Intern. Med.* **19:** 1–26.

Zucker-Franklin, D. (1980). Ultrastructural evidence for the common origin of human mast cells and basophils. *Blood* **56:**534–540.

11

Thrombin-Induced Platelet Adhesion to the Pulmonary Vasculature

CATHERINE M. VENTURINI

Wellcome Research Laboratories
Beckenham, Kent, England

JOHN E. KAPLAN

Albany Medical College
Albany, New York

I. Introduction

The pulmonary endothelium provides the lung with a nonthrombogenic surface, over which blood flows freely. Maintenance of vascular patency by endothelium is not a passive process, and much has been discovered about how endothelial cells create this unique antiadhesive barrier. Injury and inflammation can lead to altered endothelial function or endothelial dysfunction, and intravascular thrombosis can occur.

Platelet adhesion to subendothelial matrix has been studied extensively. When endothelial cells are removed from the vessel wall, platelets adhere readily and aggregates form (for a review, see Turitto and Baumgartner, 1987). It is only now becoming clear that the endothelial barrier is not passively antithrombotic. Antithrombosis results from a series of ongoing processes and properties. The endothelium can lose its ability to repel blood cells. Platelets can adhere directly to these altered endothelial cells (Venturini and Kaplan, 1991).

In this chapter the role of platelet adhesion to the endothelium in the development of pulmonary dysfunction is examined. In particular, we describe current results obtained from the study of thrombin-induced platelet adhesion to pulmonary endothelium and the endothelial mediators that regulate this pathological event.

II. Pathophysiology of Pulmonary Thrombosis

The endothelium is not an inert lining of the blood vessel wall. Rather, the nonthrombogenic nature of the endothelial cell is dynamic and can be modulated. Endothelial cells are potently antithrombotic. However, after injury or trauma, platelets adhere to the subendothelium and may also adhere directly to endothelial cells. Pulmonary embolism, acute respiratory distress syndrome (ARDS), and disseminated intravascular coagulation (DIC) may involve altered platelet reactivity with the pulmonary vessel wall.

The contribution of platelets to pulmonary embolism has been reviewed (Kaplan and Malik, 1991). Pulmonary embolism involves two very different thrombotic events. Ninety-five percent of pulmonary emboli arise from deep vein thrombosis (Moser, 1991). The cause of deep vein thrombosis is not clear. Malone (1977) suggested that stasis or reduced blood flow may lead to metabolic deprivation of venous endothelium and that white blood cells and platelets could adhere to these damaged cells. Alternatively, Kakkar and Day (1983) suggested a model of deep vein thrombosis in which endothelial cell contraction leads to the exposure of extracellular matrix upon which platelets adhere. Secondary thrombosis can occur at the site of the occlusive emboli and further obstruct pulmonary blood flow.

A second type of pulmonary embolism involves microemboli, which may develop in the lung in response to injury, sepsis, and with various pathologies that lead to the initiation of disseminated thrombosis. These microemboli are frequently associated with pulmonary dysfunction. ARDS is a form of respiratory failure affecting many seriously ill patients of various etiologies. Early in the progression of the disease, increased permeability of the alveolar–capillary barrier leads to pulmonary edema (Dal Nogare, 1989). Diffuse thrombosis of small and large pulmonary arteries is common. Prominent accumulation of platelets is unusual, but thrombi composed of platelets, fibrin, and polymorphonuclear cells can be seen in the lungs of these patients.

ARDS is associated with pulmonary platelet sequestration (Orell, 1971) and thrombocytopenia (Hill et al., 1975). Many animal models of acute pulmonary dysfunction have been associated with thrombocytopenia or pulmonary sequestration of platelets (reviewed in Kaplan and Malik, 1991). Platelets are implicated in the induction of endothelial injury and increased vascular permeability. Platelet release products increase albumin accumulation in rabbit skin (Mustard et al., 1965; Nachman, 1978) and in synovial vessels (Bignold, 1980).

Disseminated intravascular coagulation is a condition where the clotting mechanism becomes activated in widespread areas of the circulation. Frequently, the clots are small but numerous. This is a heterogeneous group of disorders and can be manifested by a wide range of hemorrhagic and thrombotic pathologies. Some examples are obstetric accidents, intravascular hemolysis, bacteremia, viremia, disseminated malignancy, burn, trauma, and vascular disease (Bick, 1988). The manifestations of these disorders result, in part, from thrombin formation (Marder et al., 1987).

III. Thrombin-Induced Platelet Adhesion to Pulmonary Endothelium

The antithrombotic properties of endothelial cells can be compromised by several types of insults. Platelets adhere to endothelium after exposure to altered flow conditions (Lough and Moore, 1975), injury without detachment (Booyse et al., 1975), oxygen free radicals (Shatos et al., 1991), chemotherapy (Bertomeu et al., 1990), tumor cell adhesion (Mondhiry and McGarvey, 1987), viral infection (Curwen et al., 1980; Vercellotti, 1990), *Trypanosoma cruzi* infection (Tanowitz et al., 1990), and thrombin (Rafelson et al., 1973).

Thrombin induces platelet adhesion directly to confluent endothelial cell monolayers (Czervionke et al., 1978). This effect is reversed by heparin (Essien et al., 1978). Thrombin is a product of prothrombin cleavage and is an essential component of coagulation. Plasma contains sufficient prothrombin to generate 150,000 U of thrombin per liter (Walz et al., 1986). Its function in coagulation is the enzymatic cleavage of fibrinopeptides A and B of fibrinogen. These fibrin monomers spontaneously polymerize and, in the presence of activated factor XIII, are cross-linked to form the fibrin clot. Thrombin is a selective serine protease (Gladner and Laki, 1956; Fenton et al., 1991) and, like trypsin, cleaves peptides at arginine residues. Thrombin also has substrate binding sites, which lends specificity to the enzyme (Fenton et al., 1988). Thrombin binding to fibrinogen is essential for cleavage to fibrin. Both platelets and endothelial cells express receptors to thrombin.

In our laboratories we have developed two models of thrombin-induced platelet adhesion to pulmonary endothelium. In a system developed by Kaplan et al. (1989), confluent monolayers of sheep pulmonary artery endothelial cells were incubated with isolated radiolabeled sheep platelets. After incubation, the monolayers were washed with buffer and lysed. The lysate was counted and the percentage of adherent platelets determined.

Few platelets adhered to untreated endothelial cells. The addition of thrombin to the incubation mixture significantly increased adhesion. Further, thrombin-pretreated endothelial cells supported platelet adhesion, even after the removal of fluid-phase thrombin. Electron microscopy revealed that platelets and platelet aggregates were adherent to the confluent monolayer (Fig. 1).

A second model was developed to examine the effect of flow on platelet adhesion to the endothelium (Venturini et al., 1989a). Isolated rat lungs were perfused ex vivo with buffer and respirated to provide oxygenation. Radiolabeled rat platelets were circulated through the lungs, followed by a buffer rinse. The percentage of platelet adhesion was assessed by counting the radioactivity of the lung at the end of the perfusion.

Few platelets adhered to perfused lungs under control conditions. However, when thrombin was recirculated through the lungs, followed by a washout of fluid phase thrombin, a significant increase in platelet adherence occurred. Electron microscopy revealed that single platelets were adherent to the confluent pulmonary microcirculatory endothelium (Fig. 2).

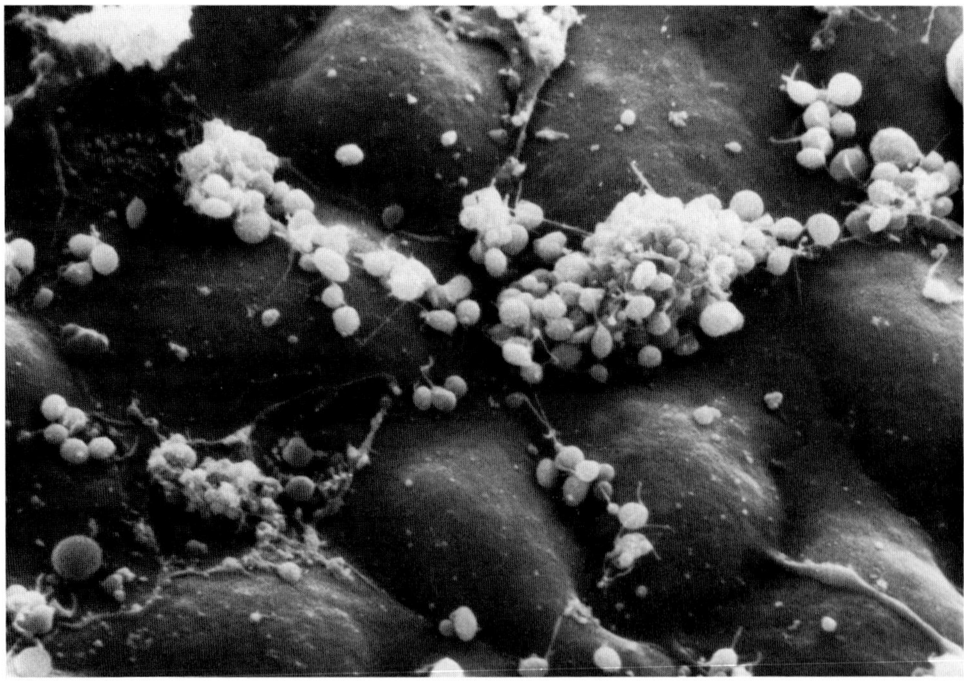

Figure 1 Scanning electron micrograph of a platelet aggregate adherent to a confluent monolayer of sheep pulmonary artery endothelial cells that have been pretreated with α-thrombin. Some single platelets are adherent. There is no evidence of exposure of matrix or endothelial cell retraction. Platelets appear to be bound directly to endothelial cells. Original magnification × 2475. (From Venturini et al., 1990.)

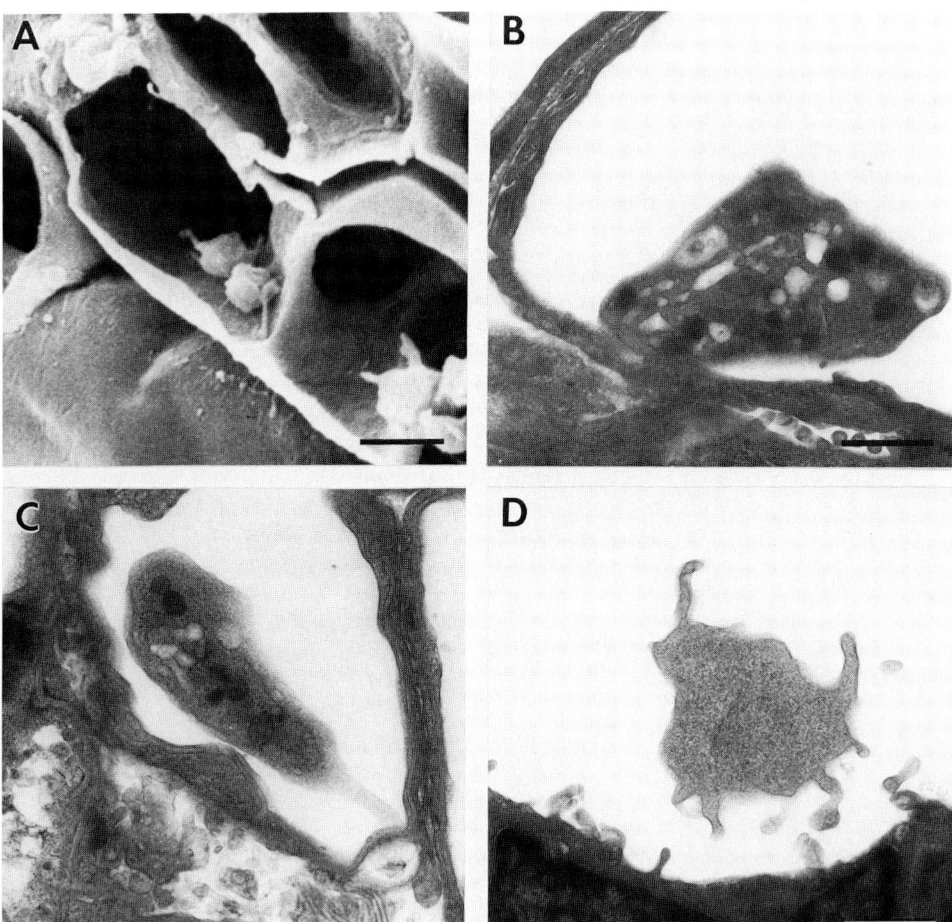

Figure 2 Electron micrographs depicting the attachment of single platelets to the pulmonary microvascular endothelium of an isolated perfused rat lung pretreated with α-thrombin. (A) A scanning electron micrograph shows two activated platelets extending pseudopodia to the endothelium. Magnification ×6000; bar = 2 μ*M*. (B–D) High-voltage electron micrographs illustrate platelets in various stages of activation adherent to endothelial cells. Magnification ×16,000; bar = 1 μ*M*. (From Venturini et al., 1989a.)

A. Thrombin Alters Endothelial Cells

Thrombin binds to and activates endothelial cells through three putative receptors: thrombomodulin (Esmon and Owen, 1981), cell-surface heparin sulfate (Machovich, 1986), and a less well-characterized receptor similar to protease nexin (Levoy-Viard et al., 1989). Thrombin binding to endothelial cells leads to hydrolysis of phosphotidyl inositol. This results in the formation of 1,4,5-triphosphate, which can elevate intracellular calcium levels, and diacylglycerol, which activates protein kinase C (Brock and Capasso, 1988).

Thrombin bound to the endothelium induces platelet adhesion (Kaplan et al., 1989). In these studies, sheep pulmonary artery endothelial cell monolayers treated for 15 min with 2 U/mL thrombin were washed free of fluid-phase thrombin. Significantly more platelets adhered to these thrombin-pretreated endothelial cells than to control monolayers. Thrombin was also circulated through isolated perfused rat lungs, and the fluid phase thrombin washed out. When platelets were circulated through these lungs, more platelets adhered than to control lungs. When the endothelial bound thrombin was treated with D-phenylalanyl-L-prolyl-l-arginine-chloromethyl ketone (PPACK), an active-site inhibitor of thrombin, this effect was abolished. Therefore, endothelial cell–bound thrombin was only capable of stimulating platelet adhesion when catalytic activity was intact.

Thrombin receptor binding alone is not sufficient for stimulation of platelet adherence to endothelium. Radiolabeled thrombin binds to both endothelial monolayers and isolated perfused lungs. This is a specific and competable event since excess unlabeled thrombin blocks binding and inhibits platelet adhesion. The catalytic activity of thrombin can be inhibited by treatment with diisopropylfluorophosphate (DIP). An enzymatically altered form of thrombin, γ-thrombin, has intact enzymatic activity but no receptor-binding activity (Fenton et al., 1988). Platelets did not adhere to endothelial cells incubated with DIP-thrombin, γ-thrombin, or a combination of both. Similarly, neither PPACK-inhibited thrombin nor hirudin-inhibited thrombin induced platelet adhesion. This indicates that the receptor binding and catalytic activity of thrombin must be proximate for induction of platelet adhesion.

In addition to binding to endothelial cells, thrombin activates intracellular signaling mechanisms. Thrombin is unique in that its influence upon cells is dependent on receptor binding and enzymatic cleavage. Thrombin stimulates the release from endothelial cells of several potent modulators of platelet reactivity, such as prostacyclin (Weksler et al., 1978), platelet activating factor (Prescott et al., 1986), nitric oxide (Rapaport et al., 1984), and adenine nucleotides (Pearson and Gordon, 1979). Thrombin binding induces changes in the endothelial cytoskeletal structure (Galdal et al., 1982).

We have examined the effect of thrombin on endothelial cell integrity by transmission, scanning, and high-voltage transmission electron microscopy. We saw no evidence of endothelial cell matrix exposure or cellular retraction in thrombin-treated sheep pulmonary artery endothelial cell monolayers (Kaplan et al., 1989) or isolated perfused rat lungs (Venturini et al., 1989b). Platelet adhesion occurred directly on intact endothelial cells when examined in cross section (Fig. 1). Platelets were more often associated with the luminal margins of the cell rather than the central area.

Laposata and co-workers (1983) reported that endothelial monolayers treated with thrombin retract and expose gaps of extracellular matrix. Most reports of thrombin causing endothelial retraction and exposure of matrix have been in cultured human umbilican vein endothelium (Galdal et al., 1982, 1983) and human umbilical veins (Chen et al., 1979). These fetal cells may not be typical of human endothelial cell physiology. Exposure of matrix upon stimulation of pulmonary endothelium has been demonstrated only at high thrombin doses (Garcia et al., 1986).

The physical connector between platelets and endothelial cells has not been thoroughly investigated. GMP-140 or PADGEM is present in the intracellular membranes of platelets and endothelial cells, and is translocated to the surface membrane after treatment with thrombin (McEver and Martin, 1984; Steinberg et al., 1985; Hattori et al., 1989). GMP-140 mediates neutrophil adhesion to endothelium and platelet adhesion to neutrophils (McEver, 1991). The role of GMP-140 has not been addressed in terms of thrombin induction of platelet adhesion. Other cell adhesion molecules, such as PECAM (Newman et al., 1990), may also be considered as candidate mediators of platelet–endothelial interactions. There is no evidence that thrombin acts as a bridge between platelets. It seems more likely that endothelial-bound thrombin stimulates platelets proximal to the endothelial cell, and these stimulated platelets adhere through other receptors.

B. Thrombin Stimulates Platelets to Adhere to Endothelium

Thrombin is a strong agonist of platelet aggregation and elicits platelet granule release, arachidonic acid metabolism, shape change, and aggregation. Thrombin binds to platelets, as it does to endothelial cells, in a saturable and reversible manner (Martin et al., 1976). Thrombin stimulates platelet intracellular guanine regulatory (G) proteins (Brass, 1984), which leads to the hydrolysis of phosphotidyl inositol 4,5-bisphosphate by phospholipase C (Rittenhouse-Simmons, 1979). This results in the formation of 1,4,5-triphosphate (IP_3), which can elevate intracellular calcium levels (O'Rourke et al., 1985) and diacylglycerol (DAG), which activates protein kinase C (Ganong et al., 1986). Via these mechanisms, platelet stimulation by thrombin leads to the phosphorylation of two specific proteins: A 20-kD protein identical to the myosin light chain and a 47-kD protein (for a review, see Seiss, 1989). The inhibition of platelet function is achieved through the activation of adenylate and guanylate cyclases, which phosphorylate a spectrum of other platelet proteins.

Protein kinase C activation has been demonstrated to promote tumor cell adhesion to the endothelium (Herbert and Maffrand, 1991). We investigated platelet protein kinase C activation as the mechanism by which thrombin stimulates platelet adhesion to the endothelium (Venturini et al., 1991a). Platelet adhesion to thrombin-pretreated endothelial cell monolayers was inhibited when platelets were pretreated with the hydroxyquinone, H7, an inhibitor of protein kinase C activation. Phorbol esters are substances known to stimulate platelet protein kinase C. Platelets treated with β-phorbol dibutyrate (PDB) adhered to endothelial monolayers in the absence of thrombin. Platelet adhesion did not occur when platelets were treated with α-phorbol didecanoate (PDD), an inactive phorbol ester. In addition, platelets treated with exogenous phospholipase C also adhered to the endothelium in the absence of thrombin. Adherence of platelets treated with H7 to block protein kinase C activation was reduced when the platelets were pretreated with either PDB or phospholipase C.

These data indicate that protein kinase C activation leads to platelet adhesion to endothelium. DAG stimulates protein kinase C activity. However, platelets treated with a synthetic analog of DAG, dioctanoyl glycerol, did not adhere to monolayers. When endothelial cells were pretreated with aspirin to inhibit cyclooxygenase activity, dioctanoyl glycerol–treated platelets did adhere to monolayers. This indicates that a cyclooxygenase product, perhaps prostacyclin, may counteract the cell signaling mechanism induced by DAG in platelets and therefore downregulate adhesion.

C. Thrombin Induces Factors That Alter Platelet Reactivity

Thrombin binds to endothelial cells and elicits the synthesis and/or release of several factors. We have investigated the ability of some of these factors to alter platelet adhesion to the endothelium. Neither arachidonic acid, platelet activating factor, adenosine diphosphate, nor calcium ionophore induced platelet adhesion to the endothelium (Kaplan et al., 1989).

Endothelial cells produce 13-hydroxyoctadecadienoic acid (13-HODE) as a product of lipoxygenase cleavage of linoleic acid. It is present in the endothelial cell but is not released into the media (Buchanan et al., 1985a). It has been reported to act as a chemorepellant and inhibit the adhesion of platelets to the endothelium. Levels of 13-HODE are significantly reduced by thrombin (Buchanan et al., 1985b). In addition, 13-HODE may be a component of the subendothelium and may contribute to the prevention of platelet adhesion to the subendothelium (Buchanan et al., 1987). Feeding New Zealand White rabbits a diet rich in black currant seed oil inhibited platelet adhesion to denuded vessel walls by increasing availability of linoleic acid for 13-HODE synthesis and inhibiting vessel wall thrombogenicity (Bertomeu et al., 1991). The effect of 13-HODE on thrombin-induced platelet adhesion to endothelium is unclear. The addition of exogenous 13-HODE inhibited thrombin-induced platelet adhesion to sheep pulmonary artery endothelium (Tloti et al., 1991), but this may have been due to the antiaggregatory effects of 13-HODE. The effect of modulation of intracellular 13-HODE levels on platelet adhesion to the endothelium requires further research.

Thrombin caused a significant and time-dependent release of prostacyclin from endothelial cells, as determined by radioimmunoassay, which was maximal after 5 min (Czervionke et al., 1979). Aspirin inhibited prostacyclin production by inhibition of the cyclooxygenase enzyme. However, in the absence of thrombin, aspirin treatment alone did not increase platelet adhesion to human umbilical vein endothelium (Czervionke et al., 1978). Aspirin did increase baseline platelet adhesion to sheep pulmonary artery endothelium (Kaplan et al., 1989). Addition of exogenous prostacyclin to incubations of platelets, thrombin, and endothelial monolayers decreased adhesion (Fry et al., 1980). Aspirin pretreatment of endothelial cells augmented thrombin-induced platelet adhesion in some models (Czervionke et al., 1979; Kaplan et al., 1989) but not in others (Curwen et al., 1980; Johnson and Helgeson, 1988; Venturini et al., 1989a).

Thrombin induces the release of endothelium-derived relaxing factor (EDRF) from the endothelium (Rapaport et al., 1984). EDRF is a labile substance that relaxes smooth muscle cells (Furchgott, 1984) and inhibits platelet aggregation (Azuma et al., 1986; Radomski et al., 1987a) and adhesion (Radomski et al., 1987b) by stimulating a soluble guanylate cyclase. The pharmacological properties of EDRF and nitric oxide are identical (for a review, see Moncada et al., 1988, 1991).

Nitric oxide is produced in the endothelium from the terminal guanido nitrogen of L-arginine (Palmer et al., 1988a; Schmitt et al., 1988). This reaction is enantiomer specific, as D-arginine is not an effective substrate. N^G-monomethyl-L-arginine (L-NMMA) inhibits the synthesis of nitric oxide in a dose-dependent manner (Palmer et al., 1988b). Radomski et al. (1990) have demonstrated that platelets can also be stimulated to release nitric oxide.

Thrombin-induced release of nitric oxide is linked to an increase in intracellular calcium (Loeb et al., 1988). The release of nitric oxide and prostacyclin may be coupled (De Nucci et al., 1988). Bradykinin-induced nitric oxide inhibits thrombin-induced platelet adhesion to cultured endothelium (Sneddon and Vane, 1988; Radomski et al., 1987b,c).

We have investigated the role of thrombin-induced nitric oxide in platelet adhesion to endothelium, in both an in vitro model and under flow conditions ex vivo. Hemoglobin binds and inactivates nitric oxide (Martin et al., 1985) and superoxide dismutase extends its short half-life (Gryglewski et al., 1986). Thrombin-induced platelet adhesion to endothelium was augmented in the presence of hemoglobin in both the in vitro model and the isolated perfused lung (Venturini et al., 1989a). Conversely, adhesion decreased in the presence of superoxide dismutase. Further, when endothelial cell monolayers were pretreated with l-N^G-monomethylarginine (L-NMMA), an inhibitor of nitric oxide synthase, platelet adhesion increased significantly. The enantiomer, D-NMMA, had no effect. These data illustrate that nitric oxide is a potent inhibitor of platelet adhesion to the endothelium in both models.

Nitric oxide (Hawkins et al., 1988) and prostacyclin (Moncada and Vane, 1979) are both potent antiaggregatory agents but work through different intracellular mechanisms. Nitric oxide diffuses into cells and directly stimulates soluble guanylate cyclase (Hawkins et al., 1988). Prostacyclin, on the other hand, binds to platelet receptors and stimulates adenylate cyclase (Lapetina et al., 1986).

D. Regulation of Platelet Adhesion Versus Aggregation

Most models of platelet adhesion to the endothelium vary in the amount of platelet aggregation that occurs, which complicates evaluation of the adhesion event. This is an important consideration in the assessment of the effects of mediators on adhesion, since adhesion and aggregation may be regulated in different ways. We have developed a model of platelet adhesion that consists of platelet adhesion to the endothelium in the absence of aggregation. Single platelets adhere to the vasculature of thrombin-treated isolated perfused lungs.

Isolated rat lungs were perfused with a Hanks balanced salt solution containing 0.5% albumin as a oncotic agent (Venturini et al., 1989b). The lungs were respirated dynamically during the experiment to provide oxygenation, and temperature was maintained at 37°C. The experiments lasted 20 min, during which time no gross edema occurred. Thrombin (2 U/mL) was perfused through the lungs, followed by a buffer rinse to remove fluid-phase thrombin. Radiolabeled platelets were then perfused through the lungs and nonadherent platelets were removed by a 2-min washout with buffer. Adherence was measured by assessing the amount of radioactivity retained within the lungs. Thrombin significantly increased platelet adhesion to these lungs.

Scanning and high-voltage transmission electron microscopy revealed that only single platelets were adherent to thrombin-pretreated lungs. In the absence of thrombin, no platelets were seen. We examined the microvasculature for aggregates lodged in small vessels, but none were observed. We saw platelets in various stages of activation adherent directly to the pulmonary microvascular endothelium (Venturini et al., 1990). Some adherent platelets still contained granules. There was no evidence of endothelial injury, desquamation, or denudation (Fig. 2).

Additional lungs were treated with thrombin, followed by circulation of PPACK, an active-site inhibitor of thrombin. This completely blocked the ability of thrombin to induce platelet adherence. Thrombin binding to the lungs is a specific, competable event, as binding of radiolabeled thrombin was inhibited by recirculation with excess unlabeled thrombin. As with thrombin-induced platelet adhesion to endothelial monolayers, catalytically inactivated and receptor binding–inhibited forms of thrombin did not induce platelet adhesion. This indicates that platelet adherence to the isolated lung is mediated by catalytically active thrombin retained at specific sites on the lung.

In contrast to the isolated lung model where single platelets were seen to adhere, the in vitro monolayer model of platelet adhesion involved the adhesion of large dense aggregates to the endothelium. Platelets were adherent to endothelial cells, but most interactions were platelet to platelet and most adherence was as aggregates. We chose to use these two models of adhesion to compare differentially the effects of modulators of platelet reactivity on single-platelet adhesion and aggregation.

Nitric oxide has been shown to inhibit single-platelet adhesion to the endothelium (Venturini et al., 1989a, 1990). L-NMMA and hemoglobin, inhibitors of nitric oxide, increased platelet adhesion, and superoxide dismutase, which increases the half-life of nitric oxide, decreased platelet adhesion. We ascertained that the effect of nitric oxide was not entirely antiaggregatory. Modulation of nitric oxide activity affected single-platelet adhesion to the isolated perfused rat lung as well as aggregate adhesion to monolayers.

The antiadherent properties of prostacyclin are less clear. Aspirin pretreatment of endothelial monolayers inhibited prostacyclin production and increased thrombin-induced platelet aggregate adhesion to the endothelium. However, when rats were given an oral gavage of aspirin before the removal of lungs for perfusion, the level of thrombin-induced platelet adhesion did not change. In addition, when platelets were treated with a stable prostacyclin analog, Iloprost, before recirculation through thrombin-pretreated lungs, platelet adhesion did not decrease. This dose of Iloprost was sufficient to inhibit in vitro platelet aggregation, yet had no effect on single-platelet adhesion to the lungs.

Since the major difference between these two models is the presence of platelet–platelet interactions, we postulated that prostacyclin preferentially inhibited platelet interactions but was not effective in the inhibition of platelet adhesion to the endothelium. On the other hand, nitric oxide, which is a potent antiaggregating agent, was also an effective antiadhesive agent.

We further tested this hypothesis by examining the intracellular mechanisms involved in the inhibition of platelet activity (Venturini et al.,

1991b). Nitric oxide is a potent stimulator of guanylate cyclase, while prostacylin activates adenylate cyclase. We treated platelets with cell-permeable stable analogs of the products of these cyclases to mimic activation of these enzymes. Platelets treated with 8-bromo cyclic guanosine monophosphate (cGMP) or 8-bromo cyclic adenosine monophosphate (cAMP) did not adhere as well as control platelets to thrombin-pretreated endothelial monolayers. When single-platelet adhesion to the endothelium of the isolated lung was examined, fewer platelets treated with 8-bromo cGMP adhered than did untreated platelets. However, platelet treatment with 8-bromo cAMP did not significantly alter adhesion when compared to control platelets. This indicates that both cGMP and cAMP inhibit aggregation, but only platelets treated with cGMP were inhibited from adhering to the endothelium.

In an in vitro endothelial monolayer system, we showed that platelet aggregate adhesion was modulated by prostacyclin (Kaplan et al., 1989). Adherence of single platelets to the ex vivo pulmonary microvessel endothelium was not affected by aspirin (Venturini et al., 1989a) or by Iloprost or 8-bromo cAMP (Venturini et al., 1991b). Superoxide dismutase and 8-bromo cGMP inhibited both platelet aggregate adhesion and single-platelet adhesion, while hemoglobin and L-NMMA enhanced both types of platelet adhesion (Venturini et al., 1989b, 1991b). Whether cAMP has no influence on platelet adhesion or is simply quantitatively less effective than cGMP cannot be concluded with the current data.

These data indicate that nitric oxide regulates platelet reactivity with the endothelium in a different manner than prostacyclin. This does not preclude the well-demonstrated effect of nitric oxide on platelet aggregation, but points to nitric oxide as an active agent in maintaining the endothelium as a nonthrombogenic surface.

IV. Conclusions

In this chapter we have reviewed the current state of research into thrombin-induced platelet adhesion to the endothelial cells of the lung. Thrombin binds to the pulmonary endothelium in a specific and competable manner. Endothelial cell–bound thrombin is capable of inducing platelet adhesion if both the catalytic and receptor binding activity of thrombin are intact. Platelet adhesion occurs directly to the endothelium in the absence of endothelial cell retraction or matrix exposure.

Thrombin may mediate platelet reactivity through a protein kinase C–dependent mechanism. Endothelial modulators of platelet adhesion are released by the endothelium in response to thrombin binding. Both prostacyclin and nitric oxide downregulate adhesion. Prostacyclin activity is cAMP dependent, while nitric oxide is cGMP dependent.

The processes of adhesion and aggregation must be examined separately to assess accurately the differential roles of mediators of platelet function. We have demonstrated that prostacyclin is less effective in the inhibition of adhesion than in the prevention of platelet aggregation. Nitric oxide activity is most important in the inhibition of platelet adhesion to endothelium.

The pathophysiological implications of thrombin-induced platelet adhesion are widespread. Deep vein thrombosis often leads to occlusive pulmonary embolism. Hypoxia or stasis in the venous circulation may lead to endothelial cell injury, local generation of thrombin, and platelet adhesion. Platelet aggregation might occur on the adherent platelets and result in the formation of a thrombus. The formation of microthrombi in the lung may occur in the same way through a variety of initiating factors. The expression of tissue factor by endothelial cells exposed to endotoxin might lead to the generation of thrombin and thus to platelet adhesion. In ARDS and DIC, thrombin circulating in the plasma as a result of the activation of the coagulation cascade may lead to edema, platelet adhesion, and intravascular thrombosis.

While platelets are generally thought to adhere to exposed subendothelium, and not to the endothelium, this may not strictly be the case. Consideration should be made that in the presence of several types of endothelial injury, especially when associated with thrombin generation and binding, the nonthrombogenic nature of the endothelial cell may be compromised.

Acknowledgments

The authors wish to thank Ms. Lisa K. Weston and Ms. Ginny Foster for expert technical assistance and Ms. Janet Hann for assistance with manuscript preparation. We also appreciate the kind contributions of Dr. John Fenton, II, Dr. Fred Minnear, Dr. Peter Del Vecchio, and Dr. Conly Reider. CMV is the recipient of an NIH Post Doctoral Training Grant (HL-08392). This work was supported by NIH Program Project Grant HL-32418 and a National Research Service Predoctoral Fellowship HL-07194.

References

Azuma, H., Ishikawa, M., and Sekizaki, S. (1986). Endothelium-dependent inhibition of platelet aggregation. *Br. J. Pharmacol.* **88:**411–415.

Bertomeu, M. C., Gallo, S., Lauri, D., Levine, M. N., Orr, F. W., and Buchanan, M. R. (1990). Chemotherapy enhances endothelial cell reactivity to platelets. *Clin. Exp. Metast.* **8**(6):511–518.

Bertomeu, M. C., Crozier, G. L., Hass, T. A., Fleith, M., and Buchanan, M. R. (1991). Selective effects of dietary fats on vascular 13-HODE synthesis and platelet/vessel wall interactions. *Thromb. Res.* **59:**819–830.

Bick, R. L. (1988). Disseminated intravascular coagulation and related syndromes: A clinical review. *Semin Thromb. Haemost.* **14:**299–338.

Bignold, L. P. (1980). Importance of platelets in increased vascular permeability evoked by experimental haemarthrosis in synovium of the rat. *Pathology* **12:**169–179.

Booyse, F. M., Bell, S., Sedlak, B., and Rafelson, M. E. (1975). Development of an in vitro vessel wall model for studying certain aspects of platelet–vessel wall interactions. *Artery* **1:**518–539.

Brass, L. F. (1984). Ca^{++} homeostasis in unstimulated platelets. *J. Biol. Chem.* **259:**12563–12566.

Brock, T. A., and Capasso, T. A. (1988). Thrombin and histamine activate phospholipase C in human endothelial cells via a phorbol ester–sensitive pathway. *J. Cell. Physiol.* **136:**54–62.

Buchanan, M. R., Haas, T. A., Lagarde, M., and Guichardant, M. (1985a). 13-Hydroxyoctadecadienoic acid is the vessel wall chemorepellant, LOX. *J. Biol. Chem.* **260**(30):16056–16059.

Buchanan, M. R., Butt, R. W., Van Ryn, J., Hirsh, J., and Nazir, D. J. (1985b). Endothelial cells produce a lipoxygenase derived chemo-repellant which influences platelet/endothelial cell interactions: Effect of aspirin and salicylate. *Thromb. Haemost.* **53**(3):306–311.

Buchanan, M. R., Richardson, M., Haas, T. A., Hirsh, J., and Madri, J. A. (1987). The basement membrane underlying the vascular endothelium is not thrombogenic: In vivo and in vitro studies with rabbit and human tissue. *Thromb. Haemost.* **58**(2):698–704.

Chen, S., Barmatoski, S., and Barnhart, M. I. (1979). Effect of thrombin on platelet–vessel wall interactions. *Scanning Electron Microsc.* **3:**783–792.

Curwen, K. D., Gimbrone, M. A., and Handin, R. T. (1980). In vitro studies of thromboresistance: the role of prostacyclin in platelet adhesion to cultured normal and virally transformed human endothelial cells. *Lab. Invest.* **42**(3):366–374.

Czervionke, R. L., Hoak, J. C., and Fry, G. L. (1978). Effects of aspirin on thrombin-induced adherence of platelets to cultured endothelial cells from blood vessel walls. *J. Clin. Invest.* **62:**847–856.

Czervionke, R. L., Smith, J. B., Fry, G. L., Hoak, J. C., and Haycraft, D. L. (1979). Inhibition of prostacyclin by treatment of endothelium with aspirin. *J. Clin. Invest.* **63:**1089–1092.

Dal Nogare, A. R. (1989). Southwestern internal medicine conference: Adult respiratory distress syndrome. *Am. J. Med. Sci.* **8**(6):413–430.

De Nucci, G., Gryglewski, R. J., Warner, T. M., and Vane, J. R. (1988). Receptor mediated release of endothelium-derived relaxing factor and prostacyclin from bovine aortic endothelial cells is coupled. *Proc. Natl. Acad. Sci. USA* **85:**2800–2804.

Esmon, C., and Owen, W. (1981). Identification of an endothelial cell cofactor for thrombin-catalyzed activation of protein C. *Proc. Nat. Acad. Sci. USA* **78**(4):2239–2252.

Essien, E. M., Cazenave, J. P., Moore, S., and Mustard, J. F. (1978). Effect of heparin and thrombin on platelet adherence to the surface of rabbit aorta. *Thromb. Res.* **13:**69–78.

Fenton, J. W., II, Olson, T. A., Zabinski, M. P., and Wilner, G. D. (1988). Anion-binding exosite of human a-thrombin and fibrin(ogen) recognition. *Biochemistry* **27:** 7106–7112.

Fenton, J. W., II, Ofosu, F. A., Moon, D. G., and Maraganore, J. M. (1991). Thrombin structure and function: Why thrombin is the primary target for antithrombotics. *Blood Coag. Fibrinol.* **2:**69–75.

Fry, G. L., Czervionke, R. L., Hoak, J. C., Smith, J. B., and Haycraft, D. L. (1980). Platelet adherence to cultured vascular cells: Influence of aspirin. *Blood* **55**(2): 271–275.

Furchgott, R. F. (1984). The role of the endothelium in the responses of vascular smooth muscle to drugs. *Annu. Rev. Pharmacol. Toxicol.* **24:**174–197.

Galdal, K. S., Evensen, S. A., and Brosstad, F. (1982). Effects of thrombin on the integrity of monolayers of cultured human endothelial cells. *Thromb. Res.* **27:**575–584.

Galdal, K. S., Evenson, S. A., and Nilson, E. (1983). Thrombin-induced shape change of activated endothelial cells: Metabolic and functional observations. *Thromb. Res.* **32:**57–66.

Ganong, B. R., Loomis, C. R., Hannun, Y. A., and Bell, R. M. (1986). Specificity and mechanism of protein kinase C activation by *sn*-1,2-diacylglycerols. *Proc. Natl. Acad. Sci. USA* **83:**1184–1188.

Garcia, J. G. N., Siflinger-Birnboim, A., Bizios, R., Del Vecchio, P. J., Fenton, J. W., II, and Malik, A. B. (1986). Thrombin-induced increase in albumin permeability across the endothelium. *J. Cell. Physiol.* **128:**96–104.

Gladner, J. A., and Laki, K. (1956). The inhibition of thrombin by diissopropylphosphofluoridate. *Arch. Biochem. Biophys.* **233:**227–245.

Gryglewski, R. J., Palmer, R. M. J., and Moncada, S. (1986). Superoxide anion is involved in the breakdown of endothelium-derived vascular relaxing factor. *Nature* **320:**454–456.

Hattori, R., Hamilton, K. K., Fugate, R. D., McEver, R. P., and Sims, P. J. (1989). Stimulated secretion of endothelial von Willibrand factor is accompanied by rapid redistribution to the cell surface of the intracellular granule membrane protein GMP-140. *J. Biol. Chem.* **264:**7768–7771.

Hawkins, D. J., Meyick, B. O., and Murray, J. J. (1988). Activation of guanylate cyclase and inhibition of platelet aggregation by endothelium-derived relaxing factor. *Biochem. Biophys. Acta* **969:**289–296.

Herbert, J., and Maffrand, J. (1991). Tumor cell adherence to cultured capillary endothelial cells is promoted by activators of protein kinase C. *Biochem. Pharmacol.* **42**(1):163–170.

Hill, R. N., Shibel, E. M., Spragg, R. G., and Moser, K. M. (1975). Adult respiratory distress syndrome: Early predictors of mortality. *Trans. Am. Soc. Artif. Intern. Organs* **21:**199–204.

Johnson, C. M., and Helgeson, S. C. (1988). Platelet adherence to cardiac and noncardiac endothelial cells in culture: Lack of a prostacyclin effect. *J. Lab. Clin. Med.* **112**(3):372–379.

Kakkar, V. V., and Day, T. K. (1983). The vessel wall and venous thrombosis. In *Biology and Pathology of the Vessel Wall.* Edited by N. Woolf. Praeger, New York, pp. 229–242.

Kaplan, J. E., and Malik, A. B. (1991). The contribution of platelets to pulmonary embolism. In *The Platelet in Health and Disease.* Edited by C. Page. Blackwell, Oxford, pp. 210–227.

Kaplan, J. E., Moon, D. Weston, L. K., Minnear, F. L., Del Vecchio, P. J., Shepard, J. M., and Fenton, J. W., II. (1989). Platelets adhere to thrombin-treated endothelial cells in vitro. *Am. J. Physiol.* **257:**H423–H433.

Lapetina, E. G., Reep, B., Reed, N. G., and Moncada, S. (1986). Adhesion of human platelets to collagen in the presence of prostacyclin, indomethacin, and compound BW755C. *Thromb. Res.* **41:**325–335.

Laposata, M., Dovarsky, D. K., and Salkin, H. S. (1983). Thrombin-induced gap formation in confluent endothelial cell monolayers. *Blood* **62:**549–556.

Levoy-Viard, K., Jandroy-Perrus, M., Tobleni, G., and Guillen, M. C. (1989). Covalent binding of human thrombin to a human endothelial cell associated protein. *Exp. Cell Res.* **181:**1–10.

Loeb, A. L., Izzo, N. J., Johnson, R. M., Garrison, J. C., and Peach, M. J. (1988). Endothelium-derived relaxing factor associated with increased endothelial cell inositol triphosphate and intracellular calcium. *Am. J. Cardiol.* **62:**36G–40G.

Lough, J., and Moore, M. B. (1975). Endothelial injury induced by thrombin or thrombi. *Lab. Invest.* **33**(2):130–135.

Machovich, R. (1986). Choices among the possible reaction routes catalyzed by thrombin. *Ann. N.Y. Acad. Sci.* **485:**170–183.

Malone, P. C. (1977). A hypothesis concerning aetiology of venous thrombosis. *Med. Hypotheses* **3:**189–201.

Marder, V. J., Martin, S. E., Francis, C. W., and Colman, R. W. (1987). Consumptive thrombohemorrhagic disorders. In *Hemostasis and Thrombosis*, 2nd ed. Edited by R. W. Colman, J. Hirsh, V. J. Marder, and E. W. Salzman. J. B. Lippincott, Philadelphia, pp. 975–1015.

Martin, B. W., Wasiewski, W. W., Fenton, J. W., II, and Detwiller, T. C. (1976). Equilibrium binding of thrombin to platelets. *Biochemistry* **15:**4886–4889.

Martin, W., Villani, G. M., Jothianadan, D., and Furchgott, R. F. (1985). Selective blockade of endothelium-dependent and glycerol nitrate-induced relaxation by haemoglobin and by methylene blue in rabbit aorta. *J. Pharmacol. Ther.* **232:** 708–716.

McEver, R. M. (1991). GMP-140, a receptor that mediates interactions of leucocytes with activated platelets and endothelium. *Trends Cardiovasc. Sci,* **1**(4):152–156.

McEver, R. M., and Martin, M. N. (1984). A monoclonal antibody to activated platelets. *J. Biol. Chem.* **259:**9799–9804.

Moncada, S., and Vane, J. R. (1979). Pharmacology and endogenous role of prostaglandin endoperoxides, thromboxane, and prostacyclin. *Pharmacol. Rev.* **30:**293–331.

Moncada, S., Radomski, M., and Palmer, R. M. J. (1988). Endothelium-derived relaxing factor: Identification as nitric oxide and role in the control of vascular tone and platelet function. *Biochem. Pharmacol.* **37:**2495–2501.

Moncada, S., Palmer, R. M. J., and Higgs, E. A. (1991). Nitric oxide: Physiology, pathophysiology, and pharmacology. *Pharmacol. Rev.* **43**(2):109–142.

Mondhiry, A. L., and McGarvey, V. (1987). Tumor interaction with vascular endothelium. *Haemostasis* **17:**245–253.

Moser, K. M. (1991). Pulmonary Thromboembolism. In *Harrison's Principles of Internal Medicine.* Edited by Wilson, J. D., Braunwald, E., Isselbach, K. J., Petersdorf, R. G., Martin, J. B., Fauci, A. S., Root, R. K. McGraw-Hill, New York, pp. 1090–1092.

Mustard, J. F., Movat, H. Z., Macmorine, D. R. L., and Senyi, A. (1965). Release of permeability factors from the blood platelet. *Proc. Soc. Exp. Biol. Med.* **199:** 988–991.

Nachman, R. L. (1978). The platelet as an inflammatory cell. In *Platelets: A Multidisciplinary Approach.* Edited by G. de Gaetano and S. Garattini. Raven Press, New York, pp. 199–203.

Newman, P. J., Berndt, M. C., Gorski, J., White, G. C., II, Lyman, S., Paddock, C., and Muller, W. A. (1990). PECAM-1 (CD31) cloning and relation to adhesion molecules of the immunoglobulin gene superfamily. *Science* **247:**1219–1222.

Orell, S. R. (1971). Lung pathology in respiratory distress following shock in the adult. *Acta Pathol. Microbiol. Scand.* **79:**65–76.

O'Rourke, F. A., Halenda, S. P., Zavoico, G. B., and Feinstein, M. B. (1985). Inositol 1,4,5-triphosphate releases calcium from a calcium-transporting membrane vesicle fraction derived from human platelets. *J. Biol. Chem.* **260:**956–962.

Palmer, R. M. J., Ashton, D. S., and Moncada, S. (1988a). Vascular endothelial cells synthesize nitric oxide from L-arginine. *Nature* **333:**664–666.

Palmer, R. M. J., Rees, D. D., Ashton, D. S., and Moncada, S. (1988b). L-Arginine is the physiological precursor for the formation of nitric oxide in endothelium-dependent relaxation. *Biochem. Biophys. Res. Commun.* **153:**1251–1256.

Pearson, J. D., and Gordon, J. L. (1979). Vascular endothelial and smooth muscle cells in culture selectively release adenine nucleotides. *Nature* **21:**384–387.

Prescott, S. M., Zimmerman, G. A., and McIntyre, T. M. (1986). Human endothelial cells in culture produce platelet activating factor (1-akyl-2-acetyl-*sn*-glycero-3-phosphocholine) when stimulated with thrombin. *Proc. Natl. Acad. Sci. USA* **81:** 3534–3538.

Radomski, M., Palmer, R. M. J., and Moncada, S. (1987a). Comparative pharmacology of endothelium-derived relaxing factor, nitric oxide and prostacyclin in platelets. *Br. J. Pharmacol.* **92:**181–187.

Radomski, M., Palmer, R. M. J., and Moncada, S. (1987b). The role of nitric oxide and cGMP in platelet adhesion to vascular endothelium. *Biochem. Biophys. Res. Commun.* **148:**1482–1489.

Radomski, M., Palmer, R. M. J., and Moncada, S. (1987c). Endogenous nitric oxide inhibits platelet adhesion to vascular endothelium. *Lancet,* Nov. 7:1057–1058.

Radomski, M. W., Palmer, R. M. J., and Moncada, S. (1990). An L-arginine/nitric oxide pathway present in human platelets regulates aggregation. *Proc. Natl. Acad. Sci. USA* **87:**5193–5197.

Rafelson, M. E., Hoveke, T. P., and Booyse, F. M. (1973). The molecular biology of platelet–platelet interactions and platelet–endothelial cell interactions. *Semin. Haematol.* **VI**(3):367–381.

Rapaport, R. M., Drazin, M. B., and Murad, F. (1984). Mechanisms of adenosine-, thrombin- and trypsin-induced relaxation of rat thoracic aorta. *Circ. Res.* **55:**468–479.

Rittenhouse-Simmons, S. (1979). Production of diglyceride from phosphatidylinositol in activated human platelets. *J. Clin. Invest.* **63:**580–587.

Schmidt, H. H. H. W., Nau, H., Wittfohl, W., Gerlach, J., Prescher, K. E., Klein, M. M., Niroomand, F., Böhme, E. (1988). Arginine is a physiological precursor of endothelium-derived nitric oxide. *Eur. J. Pharmacol.* **154:**213–216.

Seiss, W. (1989). Molecular mechanisms of platelet activation. *Physiol. Rev.* **69**(1): 58–178.

Shatos, M. A., Doherty, J. M., and Hoak, J. C. (1991). Alterations in human vascular endothelial cell function by oxygen radicals. *Atheroscler. Thromb.* **11:**594–601.

Sneddon, J. M., and Vane, J. R. (1988). Endothelium-derived relaxing factor reduces platelet adhesion to bovine endothelial cells. *Proc. Natl. Acad. Sci. USA* **85:** 2800–2804.

Steinberg, P. E., McEver, R. M., Shuman, M. A., Jaques, Y. V., and Bainton, D. F. (1985). A platelet alpha granule membrane protein (GMP-140) is expressed on the plasma membrane after activation. *J. Clin. Biol.* **101:**880–886.

Tanowitz, H. B., Burns, E. R., Sinha, A. K., Kahn, N. N., Morris, S. A., Factor, S. M., Hatcher, V. B., Bilezikian, J. P., Baum, S. G., and Wittner, M. (1990). Enhanced platelet adherence and aggregation in Chagas' disease: A potential pathogenic mechanism for cardiomyopathy. *Am. J. Trop. Med.* **43**(3):274–281.

Tloti, M. A., Moon, D. G., Weston, L. K., and Kaplan, J. E. (1991). Effect of 13-hydroxyoctadeca-9,11-dienoic acid (13-HODE) on thrombin-induced platelet adhesion to endothelial cells in vitro. *Thromb. Res.* **62:**305–317.

Turitto, V. T., and Baumgartner, H. R. (1987). Platelet surface interactions. In *Haemostasis and Thrombosis*, 2nd ed. Edited by R. W. Colman, J. Hirsh, V. J. Marder, and E. W. Salzman. J. B. Lippincott, Philadelphia, pp. 555–571.

Venturini, C. M., and Kaplan, J. E. (1992). Thrombin-induced platelet adhesion to endothelium. *Semin. Haemost. Thromb.* **18**(2):275–283.

Venturini, C. M., Fenton, J. W., II, Minnear, F. L., and Kaplan, J. E. (1989a). Rat platelets adhere to human thrombin treated rat lungs under flow conditions. *Thromb. Haemost.* **62**(3):1006–1010.

Venturini, C. M., Del Vecchio, P. J., and Kaplan, J. E. (1989b). Thrombin-induced platelet adhesion to endothelium is modified by endothelium derived relaxing factor (EDRF). *Biochem. Biophys. Res. Commun.* **159**(1):349–354.

Venturini, C. M., Minnear, F. L., Del Vecchio, P. J., Fenton, J. W., II, and Kaplan, J. E. (1990). Thrombin-induced platelet adhesion to endothelial cells in culture and under flow conditions: Role of endothelium-derived nitric oxide and prostacyclin. In *Endothelium-Derived Vasoactive Factors.* Edited by G. Rubanyi. S. Karger, Basel, pp. 315–324.

Venturini, C. M., Weston, L. K., and Kaplan, J. E. (1991a). Thrombin-induced platelet adhesion is dependent on protein kinase C activation (submitted).

Venturini, C. M., Weston, L. K., and Kaplan, J. E. (1991b). Platelet intracellular cGMP, but not cAMP, inhibits thrombin-induced platelet adhesion to endothelium (submitted).

Vercellotti, G. M. (1990). Proinflammatory and procoagulent effects of herpes simplex infection on human endothelium. *Blood Cells* **16:**209–216.

Walz, D. A., Anderson, G. F., Ciaglowski, R. E., Aiken, M., and Fenton, J. W., II. (1986). Thrombin elicited contractile responses of aortic smooth muscle. *Proc. Soc. Exp. Biol. Med.* **180:**518–526.

Weksler, B. B., Ley, C. W., and Jaffe, E. A. (1978). Stimulation of endothelial cell prostacyclin production by thrombin, trypsin, and the ionophore A23187. *J. Clin. Invest.* **62:**923–930.

AUTHOR INDEX

Italic numbers give the page on which the complete reference is listed.

A

Abboud, H. E., 50, *59*
Aboud, M., 268, *304*
Abraham, W. M., 71, 73, 74, *88*
Ackerman, S. J., 265, 266, 273, 286, 287, *290*, *293*, *294*, *297*, *301*, *305*, *307*
Acki, S., 275, *303*
Adams, D. O., 238, *256*
Adamski, S. W., 125, *131*
Adamson, I. Y. R., 122, *130*, 175, *186*
Adelstein, R. S., 107, 108, *109*, *110*, 247, *257*, 272–73, *299*
Adkinson, N. F., 71, *89*, 268, *299*
Adkinson, N. F., Jr., 47, *57*, 103, *109*
Adler, K. B., 175, *186–87*
Adminson, N. F., 47, *56*
Adolphson, C. R., 264, *295*
Aerts, R. J., 50, *61*
Ager, A., 46, *53*
Agius, R. M., 267, *290*
Aglietta, M., 29, *54*
Agosti, J. M., 192, *206*, 265, 266, 282, *290*, *297*
Agrawal, B. K., 275, 287, *305*
Aiken, M., 311, *327*
Akiba, S., 11, *53*
Aktories, R., 6, *53*
Albeida, S. M., 121, *130*
Albelda, S. M., 201, *202*
Alber, G., 270, *300*
Albert, J., *96*, 194, *209*
Alderman, I. M., 192, *208*
Alexander, H. R., 192, *202*
Alexander, J., 75, *93*, 125, *130*, *134*
Ali, H., 269, 270, *290*, *299*, *306*
Alink, G. M., 140, *172*
Allakhverdov, B. L., 119, *134*
Allan, D., *55*
Allen, R. A., 128, *133*, 269, *301*
Allende, J. E., 5, *53*
Allison, R. C., 76, 79, 81, 82, 85, *87*, 196, *203*, 288, *301*
Alpert, S. E., 139, *170*
Altenburg, B. C., 177, *186*
Altman, L. C., 282, 286, *290*
Anagnostopoulos, T., 118, *130*
Anderson, A. O., 217, *225*
Anderson, D. C., 191, *208–9*
Anderson, G. F., 311, *327*
Anderson, J., *61*
Anderson, J. M., 120, *135*
Anderson, P., 124, *134*, 167, *172*
Anderson, T., 73, *89*
Anderson, W. B., 20, 22, *59*
Andreani, J., 85, *92*
Andreasen, P., 180, *189*
Andreoli, S. P., 46, *53*
Andries, L. J., 286, *304*
Anisowicz, A., 217, *224*
Anthes, J. C., 19, 20, 21, 22, *53*, *54*

Antoni, F., *110*
Antonov, A. S., 42, *53*, 74, *87*
Anwar, A. R. E., 275, 276, *290*
Appella, E., 192, 197, *207*, 217, *225*
Arai, N., 268, 276, *295*
Archer, R. K., 265, *290*
Archer, S. L., 239, 240, *256*
Arfors, K. E., 99, *111*
Arfos, K. E., *88*
Arndt, D., 265, *301*
Asayama, K., 192, 197, *203*
Aschner, J., 9, 18, 30, 31, 32, 33, 38, 40, 41, *53*, *57*
Aschner, M., 30, 31, 40, 41, *53*
Ashton, D., 138, 140, *170*
Ashton, D. S., 317, *325*
Auger, K. R., 194, *207*
Auron, P. E., 195, 200, *204*
Aursudkij, B., 288, *293*
Aust, S. D., 161, *169*
Austen, K. F., 20, *59*, 266, 268, 272, 275, *292*, *296*, *297*, *298*, *301*, *306*
Autor, A. P., 139, 166, *171*
Auwerx, J., 185, *188*
Avraham, K. B., 193, *210*
Awbrey, B. J., 29, 30, *53*
Axelrod, J., 17, 38, *54*, *58–59*, 270, 272, *292*, *297*
Ayars, G. H., 282, 286, *290*
Azoulay-Dupuis, E., 200, *207*
Azuma, H., 317, *321*

B

Babior, B. M., 138, *168*, 267, *305*
Bach, D. S., 266, *306*
Bach, M. K., *87*
Bachofen, M., 263, *291*
Bachwich, P. R., 194, 200, *203*
Bacon, K. B., *87*
Badwey, J. A., 73, 84, *87*
Baer, H., 268, *306*
Baeza, M. L., 268, 276, *295*
Baggiolini, M., 74, *96*, 217, 218, *224*, *225*
Baglioni, C., 200, *203*
Baier, H., 249, *261*
Bainton, D. F., 264, 265, *291*, 315, *326*
Baird, B., 269, *300–301*
Baker, C. B., 282, 286, *290*
Baker, J. B., 223, *224*
Balasubramanian, K. A., 138, 140, *168*, *170*
Balazovich, K., 73, *88*
Baldwin, J. M., *55*
Baldwin, S. J., 253, 255, *259*
Baldwin, S. R., 138, *169*
Balşinde, J., 21, *53*
Bang, N. U., 29, *62–63*
Banhegyi, G., *110*
Bank, I., 194, *207*
Bar, R. S., 141, *171*
Barbacid, M., 4, *53*
Barczuk, L., 192, *209*
Bardwell, L., 217, *224*
Barenberg, D., 120, *133*
Barie, P. S., 249, *256*
Barmann, M., 6, *53*
Barmatoski, S., 315, *322*
Barnard, J. W., 76, 79, 81, *93*, 239, 253, 255, *256*, *259*
Barnes, P. J., 71, 72, *90*, 267, 275, 282, 287, 288, 289, *293*, *294*, *298*, *307*
Barnett, C. J. K., 288, *301*
Barnhart, M. I., 315, *322*
Barron, C. B., 68, *88*
Barry, B. E., 46, *55*, 122, *130*, 137, 138, *169*, 175, 176, *187*
Bar-Saci, D., 8, *55*
Bartha, K., 8, *53*
Barza, M., 192, *210*
Bass, A., 70, 74, 84, *93*
Bass, D. A., 73, 84, *87*, 264, 266, *291*
Bassenoce, E., 72, *95*
Bates, M. E., 282, *307*

Bauer, K. D., 73, 74, *90*, *91*
Bauer, S., *59*
Baum, S. G., 311, *326*
Baumann, H., 180, *186*
Baumgartner, H. R., 309, *326*
Baumgartner, W. A., 249, *261*
Bawdey, J. A., 167, *169*
Beatty, P. G., 191, *208*, 216, *225*
Beaty, G., 127, *133*
Beauchamp, G., 238, *261*
Beaven, M. A., 269, 270, 272–73, *290*, *291*, *292*, *299*, *306*
Bechtol, K. B., 223, *224*
Becker, C. G., 99, *109*, 113, 116, *130*
Becker, E. L., 70, 73, *96*, *97*
Beckman, J. S., *94*, 124, *134*, 192, 194, 195, *208*
Beeson, P. B., 264, 266, *291*
Begley, C. G., 274, 275, *299*
Belin, D., 221, *224*
Bell, R. M., 68, 69, *87*, 315, *323*
Bell, S., 311, *322*
Bendayaiv, M., 75, *93*
Bendayan, M., 125, *134*
Benedetti, E. L., 118, *130*
Bennett, C. F., 7, *55*, 71, *92*
Bentzel, C. J., 118, *130*
Benveniste, J., 70, 73, *91*
Berg, J. T., 196, *203*
Berger, E. M., 76, 79, 81, 82, *90*, 138, *173*
Bergman, M. J., 229, *259*
Bergmann, J. S., 30, 40, *54*
Berkon, A. M., 249, *261*
Berkow, R. L., *94*, 124, *134*, 192, 194, 195, *203*, *208*
Berkowitz, B. A., 232, *257*
Berliner, J. A., 121, *133*
Berndt, M. C., 315, *325*
Bernheim, H. A., 194, 195, 200, *204*
Berridge, M. J., 7, *53*, 241, *256*, 270, 271, *291*
Berry, L. C., Jr., 191, 192, *203*
Bertini, R., 195, *203*
Bertomeu, M. C., 311, 317, *321*, *322*
Besemer, J., 268, 276, *305*
Bessou, G., 70, 73, *91*
Bettleheim, P., 268, 276, *305*
Beuge, J. A., 161, *169*
Beutler, B., *96*, 194, 195, 200, *203*, *204*, *209*
Bevilacqua, M. P., 191, *203*, 216, *224*
Beyer, W. F., 198, *203*
Beyoert, R., *209*
Bianchi, M., 195, 200, *203*, *205*
Bick, R. L., 311, *322*
Bierman, A. J., 50, *61*
Bierman, M., 285, *293–94*
Bigay, J., 5, *53*
Bignold, L. P., 310, *322*
Bilah, M. M., 20, *53*
Bilezikian, J. P., 311, *326*
Billadello, J. J., 183, 185, *189*
Billah, M. M., 19, 21, 22, 51, *54*, *61*
Birdwell, C. R., 29, *57*
Birinyi, L. K., 194, *207*
Birnbaumer, L., 67, *88*
Birnboim, A. S., 40, 41, 43, 46, *56*
Birnby, L., 122, 123, 124, *134*
Birrel, G. B., 74, *88*
Bishai, I., 200, *204*
Bishop, C. T., 137, 155, *169*
Bizios, R., 40, 41, 43, 46, *56*, 122, *131*, 315, *323*
Bjork, J., *88*
Black, J. M., 167, *169*
Blackmore, P. F., *54*
Bletry, O., 266, *301*
Block, E. R., 137, 138, 143, 144, 145, 146, 150, 151, 153, 154, 156, 157, 158, 159, 160, 161, 162, 164, 165, 166, 167, *169*, *170*, *171*, *172*, 193, *203*
Block, L. H., 71, 73, 74, *88*
Blondi, A., 275, *305*
Bloom, W., 265, *291*
Bloomquist, M. A., 288, *303*
Blumenstock, F. A., 42, 43, *61*, 69, 70, 75, *91*
Bocckino, S. B., 20, *54*, *56*

Boeynaems, J. M., 8, 17, 18, *55*, *63*
Boggin, C., 249, *261*
Bohl, B. P., 84, 85, *94*
Böhme, E., *326*
Bokoch, G. M., 128, *133*, 269, *301*
Bolton, T. B., 240, *256*
Bolyraems, J. M., 10, *63*
Bomalaski, J. S., 75, *88*
Bond, E., 70, 74, 84, *93*
Bone, R. C., 102, 108, *110*
Bonser, R. W., 51, *54*
Bonventre, J. V., 140, *171*
Boonrut, A., 287, 288, 289, *293*
Booyse, F. M., 311, *322*, *326*
Borenfreund, E., 177, *188*
Borg, T., 276, *295*
Borgeat, P., 73, *92*
Borges, M., 249, *261*
Bosia, A., *61*
Bossant, M. J., 70, 73, *91*
Bottaro, D., 125, *130*
Boubekar, K., 275, *303*
Bourne, H. R., 276, *291*
Bowden, D. H., 122, *130*, 175, *186*
Bowen-Pope, D. F., 29, *55*, *58*, 176, *186*, 218, *224*, 237, *260*
Bowers, T. K., 138, *172*, 263, *303*
Bowman, C. M., 238, *256*
Bowman, C. W., 252, *260*
Boxer, L. A., 138, *169*
Brain, J. D., 84, *96*
Brandt, P. W., 266, *291*
Braquet, P., 71, 73, *88*
Brass, L. F., 4, 8, *54*, 315, *322*
Bravo, R., 180, *188*
Bray, M. A., 268, 276, *304*
Breeman, C. V., 72, *92*
Brett, J., 75, *88*, 124, *130*
Breviario, F., 200, *208*
Brieland, J. K., 73, *88*
Brigham, K. L., 45, *54*, 71, 73, 84, 85, *88*, *91*, *92*, 102, *109*, 138, *169*, *171*, 191, 192, 197, *203*, *208*, 252, *256*, 287–88, *291*, *300*
Brochenauer, A. B., 42, 43, *61*
Brock, A. F., 223, *224*
Brock, T. A., 8, 9, 14, 31, 32, 38, 40, *54*, 314, *322*
Brockenauer, A. M., 69, 70, 75, *91*
Brodde, O. E., 106, *110*
Brosstad, F., 314, 315, *323*
Brown, A. M., 67, *88*
Brown, C. D., 29, *57*
Brown, D. M., 124, *131*
Brown, J. D., 249, *261*
Brown, J. H., *62*
Brown, K. D., 214, 217, *224*
Bruade, S., 249, *256*
Bruijnzeel, P. L. B., 275, *291*
Brunette, E. N., 198, 202, *204*
Brun-Pascuad, H., 200, *207*
Bruns, R. R., 114, *130*
Brutsaert, D. L., 286, *304*
Bruzdzinski, C. J., 185, *186*
Bryant, D. H., 268, 287, *291*
Bubaybo, B. A., 175, 176, *187*
Buchanan, M. R., 311, 316, 317, *321*, *322*
Buckley, B. J., 138, *169*
Buhl, R., *206*
Buhler, F. R., 8, *63*
Bulkley, G. B., 249, *261*
Bundgaard, M., 114, 115, *130*
Burch, R. M., 17, *54*
Buresh, C. M., 192, *202*
Burger, I. M., 192, 197, *208*
Burgess, D. R., 120, *130*, 221, *224*
Burhans, M. S., 198, *205*, *210*
Burhop, K. E., 122, *130*, 288, *291*
Burke, M. D., 200, *204*
Burke, T. M., 240, *257*
Burns, E. R., 311, *326*
Burns, G. F., 275, *299*
Burr, I. A., 192, 197, *210*
Burr, I. M., 192, 197, 198, *203*, *206*
Burridge, K., 114, 117, 129, *130*, *132*, 177, *186*
Busse, R., 8, *61*, 106, 107, *109*
Busse, W. W., 267, 282, *303*, *307*
Bussolino, F., 29, *54*, *61*, 200, *203*

Butt, R. W., 316, *322*
Butterfield, J. H., 273, *292*
Butterield, J., 167, *171–72*
Butterworth, A. E., 266, *290*, *292*

C

Cabot, M. C., 21, 25, *58*
Cain, P., 46, *61*
Calderesa, C. M., 249, *261*
Caldwell, P. R. B., 122, *132*, 137, *171*
Caldwell, S. A., 191, 192, 194, *210*
Callahan, K. S., 5, 6, 9, 18, 30, 31, 32, 36, 37, 38, 46, 47, *54*, *56*, *57*, *58*, 145, *170*
Calzetti, F., 51, *63*
Cambell, W. B., 16, *59*
Camp, R. D. R., *87*
Campbell, G. R., 237, *257*
Campbell, H. D., 275, *299*
Camussi, G., 29, *54*, 200, *203*
Cannon, J. G., 194, 195, 200, *204*
Cantwell, M. E., 271, *292*
Capasso, E. A., 8, 14, 31, 32, 40, *54*
Capasso, E. L., 32, 38, *54*
Capasso, T. A., 314, *322*
Capron, A., 266, 275, *292*, *298*, *301*
Capron, M., 266, 275, 286, *292*, *298*, *301*, *304*
Carlson, K. E., 4, 8, *54*
Carlson, S., 120, 122, 123, *133*
Carney, D. H., 30, 40, *54*, *57*
Carpenter, L. J., 253, *257*
Carraway, K. L., 117, *133*
Carson, M. R., 8, *54*, 107, 108, *109*
Carter, A. J., 18, *54*
Carter, D. T., 14, 17, 39, *54*
Carty, D. J., 8, *61*
Casale, T. B., 267, *292*
Casey, F. B., 268, *301*
Cassidy, S. S., 249, *258*
Cassimeris, J., 194, *207*
Castagna, M., 68, *89*
Catravas, J. D., 85, *92*
Cavender, D., 218, *225*
Cazenave, J. P., 311, *323*
Cerami, A., *96*, 194, 195, 200, *203*, *204*, *207*, *209*
Cerasoli, F., Jr., 266, 277, 281, 282, *292*, *303*
Cerijido, M., 117, 118, 127, *133*
Chabre, M., 5, *53*
Chakraborti, S., 46, 47, *55*, 201, *203*
Chakrin, L. W., 268, *301*
Chalifa, V., 20, *55*
Chambaz, E. M., 68, *93*
Chambers, K. A., 128, *131*
Chambley-Campbell, J., 237, *257*
Chan, A., 191, *211*
Chan, M. K. W., 191, *207*
Chan, P. H., 167, *169*
Chandler, D. B., 139, *171*
Chang, C. T., 285, *305*
Chang, S. -W., 191, 192, 200, *203–4*, 285, *292*
Chan-Yeung, M., 281, *298*
Chap, H., 20, *57*
Chaponnier, C., 117, 128, *131*, *132*
Charo, I. F., *224*
Charon, J., 266, *301*
Chatterjee, M., 241, *257*
Chattopadhyay, J., 20, *55*
Chaudhari, P., 177, 180, 181, 182, 183, 184, *187*
Checknyova, E. G., 5, 8, 9, *65*
Cheeseman, K. H., 140, *168*
Cheever, A. W., 266, *301*
Cheknyova, E. G., 68, *96*
Chen, A. B., 192, *208*
Chen, M. J., 75, *88*
Chen, S., 315, *322*
Chen, S. F., 167, *169*
Chen, Z. G., 275, *305*
Cheng, J. R., 232, *260*
Chensue, S. W., 194, 200, *203*, *206*, 217, 221, 222, *225*
Chess, L., 194, *207*

Cheung, H., 252, *261*
Chi, E. Y., 273, 276, *292*, *296*
Choppa, J., 71, 85, *88*
Christensen, O., *130*
Christman, C. W., 240, 249, *261*
Christopher, M. M., 167, *171–72*
Christophers, E., 217, *225*
Chrzanowski, R., 85, *92*
Chung, K. F., 275, 282, 287, 288, 289, *293*, *298*, *307*
Church, M. K., 267, 268, *290*, *292*
Chvapil, M., 175, 176, *186*
Ciaglowski, R. E., 311, *327*
Cirillo, R., 272, *299*
Citi, S., 120, *135*
Clancy, R. M., 84, 85, *94*
Clark, J. C., 198, *210*
Clark, J. M., 139, *169*
Clark, K. J., 68, *89*
Clark, M. A., 75, *88*
Clark, R. A., 267, *301*
Clark, R. B., 50, *55*
Clark, S. C., 274, 275, *299*
Clawson, C. C., 73, 84, *94*
Clement, A., 155, *169*, *171*
Clements, J. A., 139, *169*
Clerch, L. B., 192, 193, *205*, *206*
Clifford, D. P., 138, *173*
Coburn, R. F., 68, *88*
Coceani, F., 200, *204*
Cochrane, C., 138, 155, *169*, *172*
Cockcroft, S., 269, *295*, *296*
Cockrane, C. G., 84, 85, *94*
Cockroft, S., 5, 7, 8, *55*
Coener, T. M. M., 140, *172*
Coflesky, J. T., 175, 176, *186–87*, 238, *257*
Cohen, D. A., 191, *205*
Cohen, M. L., 232, *257*, 288, *303*
Cohen, N. S., 265, *292*
Cohn, Z. A., 287, *307*
Colbran, R. J., 108, *110*
Colden-Stanfield, M., 8, *55*
Colditz, I. G., 191, *207*
Cole, J. S., 79, 80, 82–84, *93*
Collado-Escobar, D. M., 270, *290*
Collart, M. A., 221, *224*
Colman, R. W., 311, *324*
Colombo, M., 272, *299*
Columbo, M., 268, *301*
Condit, J. R., 108, *109*
Conlon, K., 202, *209*
Connolly, R. J., 195, *208*
Connolly, T. M., 18, *55*
Consigny, P. M., 72, *88*
Cook, H. W., 201, *205*
Cook, J. A., 138, *170*, 200, *210*
Cooper, J. A., 122, *130*
Corcia, A., 269, *301*
Costello, J. L., 84, *89*
Cotgreave, I., 73, 74, *95*
Cotran, R. A., 191, *203*
Counts, R. B., 29, *61*
Cousant, S., 70, 74, 84, *93*
Cox, C. C., 38, *64*
Craddock, P. R., 138, *172*, 263, *303*
Cragoe, E. J., 10, 12, 18, *59*
Crapo, J. D., 73, *89*, 122, 123, *130*, *131*, 137, 138, 140, 155, 166, *169*, *170*, *173*, 175, 176, *187*, 195, 198, 199, *204*, *206*, *208*, 237, *257*
Crapo, S. D., 46, *55*
Crase, D., 192, *208*
Crea, A. E. G., 275, *296*
Creekmore, S., 202, *209*
Crews, F. T., 270, 272, *292*, *296*
Crist, K. A., 138, 140, 166, *172*
Cromwell, O., 275, *306*
Crone, C., *130*
Cronkite, E. P., 265, *304*
Crooke, S. T., 7, *55*, 70, 75, *88*, *96*
Croset, M., 167, *169*
Cross, C. E., 45, *55*, 137, 138, *170*
Crouch, E. C., 238, *259*
Crouch, E. P., 238, *261*
Crouch, M. D., *55*
Crouch, M. F., 17, *55*
Crozier, G. L., 317, *322*
Crystal, R. G., *206*

Cuatrecasas, P., 11, 51, *61*, *64*
Cunha-Melo, J. R., 269, 270, *290*, *291*, *292*, *299*
Cunningham, D. D., 30, 40, *57*
Cunningham, M. K., *94*, 124, *134*, 192, 194, 195, *208*
Curnutte, J. T., 167, *169*
Curran, T., 184, 185, *187*
Curwen, K. D., 311, 317, *322*
Cuss, F. M., 71, *90*
Cutaia, M., 229, *257*
Cybulsky, M. I., 191, *207*
Czar, G. T., 71, 85, *88*
Czerski, D., *206*
Czervionke, R. L., 311, 317, *322*, *323*
Czuk, C. I., 266, 267, *305*

D

Dafai, N., 176, 177, *188*
Dahlén, S. E., 288, *292*
Dahms, T. E., 82, 84, 85, *95*
Dailey, P. O., 249, *259*
Dal Nogare, A. R., 310, *322*
Dame, C., 71, *92*
Dandona, P., 17, *59*
Daniel, L. W., 70, *93*
Danilov, S. M., 8, *63*
Danilov, Y. N., 74, *88*
Danis, E. H., 138, *173*
Dano, K., 180, *188*
Danon, D., 285, *304*
Darbonne, W. C., 223, *224*
DaSilva, C., 68, *89*
David, J. R., 266, 275, *292*, *293*
Davidson, R., 275, *296*
Davier, P., 249, *261*
Davies, P., 79, 80, 82–84, *93*
Davies, P. F., 8, 9, 14, *54*
Davis, B. H., 106, *109*
Davis, H., 247
Davis, H. W., 38, 43, *57*
Davitz, M. A., 21, *55*
Day, T. K., 310, *324*
Dayer, J. M., 200, *204*
Dean, N. M., 270, *292*
Deanin, G. G., 269, *301*, *306*
DeBrabender, M., 99, *109*
Debs, R. J., 198, 202, *204*
Dechatelet, L. R., 70, 74, 84, *93*
DeClerck, F., 99, *109*
de Crombrugghe, B., 184, *188*
De Groot, P. G., 74, *94*
Deimann, W., 265, *307*
Dejana, E., *61*, 200, *208*
DeKossodo, S., 221, *224*
deLaat, S. W., 50, *61*
de Lanerolle, P., 107, 108, *109*, *110*
DelCarmine, R., 18, *58*
de Leeuw, A. J., 266, 267, *298*
Della Bianca, V., 51, *63*
Del Maestro, R. F., *88*
Delmonte, S. M., 249, *261*
Del Vecchio, P. J., 31, 40, 41, 43, 46, *56*, *61–62*, 75, *88*, 122, *130*, *131*, 138, *173*, 311, 312, 314, 315, 316, 317, 318, 319, 320, *323*, *324*, *326*
DeMaster, E. G., 239, 240, *256*
Demling, R. H., 73, *88*, 288, *293*
Demolle, D., 8, 17, 18, *55*, *63*
de Monchy, J. G. R., 266, 267, *298*
Deneke, S. M., 137, *171*, 237, *257*
Dennery, P. A., 139, *170*
Denning, G. M., 164, *170*
Dennis, P. A., 8, 9, 14, *54*
Dent, G., 275, 282, *298*
De Nucci, G., 317, *322*
Derian, C. K., 8, *55*
Derse, C. P., 268, 276, *303*
De Simone, C., 266, *293*
Dessein, A. J., 275, *293*
Deterrs, P., 5, *53*
Detwiller, T. C., 315, *324*
Devall, L. J., 138, *169*
De Vries, A., 285, *293*
Deykin, D., 17, 36, *58*

Di Carleto, P. E., 218, *224*
DiCorleto, P. E., 29, *55*, 73–74, *89*
Didier, A., 264, *293*
Diehl, T. S., 8, 9, 14, *54*
Diez, E., 21, *53*
Di Napoli, A. M., 276, *301*
Dinarello, C. A., 191, 192, 194, 195, 200, *204*, *205*, *206*, *207*, *208*, *210*
Dinh, T. T., 271, *295*
Diplock, A., 138, 140, *170*
Dobbins, D. E., 125, *131*
Dodson, R. W., 192, *203*
Doherty, D. E., 71, 85, *89*
Doherty, J. M., 311, *326*
Dominguez, J., 5, 6, 9, 10, 12, 13, 14, 17, 18, 20, 31, 32, 33, 37, 38, 39, 40, *56*, *57*
Domino, S. E., 20, *56*
Donati, M. B., *61*
Donelli, G., 266, *293*
Dong, L., *91*
Dorinsky, P. M., 84, *89*, *92*
Dormandy, T. L., 140, 166, *170*
Douches, D., 192, *208*
Douches, S., 192, *208*
Dougall, W. C., 192, 197, *210*
Douglas, H. J., 137, *171*
Douglas, W. W., 272, *305*
Dovarsky, D. K., 315, *324*
Downey, G. P., 71, 85, *89*
Drazin, M. B., 314, 317, *326*
Drenckhahn, D., 113, 116, 117, *130*, *131*
Dreuth, J. P., 72, *92*
Driedger, A. A., 252, *261*
Duane, P., 47, 48, *65*
Dukes, R. E., 38, 43, 48, *56*, *57*, *64*
Dunham, P., 124, *134*, 167, *172*
Dunn, C. J., 278, 281, *293*
Dunn, M. M., 73, 74, *90*, *91*
Dunnette, S., 266, 286, *294*, *305*
Durham, S., 281, 282, *303*
Durr, R. A., 175, 176, *187*
Durstin, M., 70, *97*
Dustin, M. L., 214–16, *225*
Dvorak, A. M., 265, 267, 268, *293*, *294*
Dvorak, H. F., 267, 268, *294*
Dyer, E. L., 84, *89*
Dyson, P. G., 275, *299*

E

Eady, R. P., 288, *293*
Eaton, J. W., 167, *171–72*, 239, 240, *256*
Ebster, R. O., 71, 85, *88*
Eckel, S., 20, *53*
Eddinger, T. J., 236, *257*
Edelman, A., 118, *130*
Edelman, N. H., 229, 238, *261*
Edwards, D. A., 143, 158, *169*
Edwards, P. A., 121, *133*
Egan, R. W., 20, *53*
Eguchi, M., 275, *307*
Eisert, W. G., 18, *54*
Elias, J. A., 201, *202*
Elias, P. P., 275, *301*
Eller, T., 200, *210*
Elliot, G. A., 278, 281, *293*
Elliott, S. J., 46, *56*
Ellis, E. F., 201, *206*
Elner, S. G., 218, *224*
Elner, V. M., 218, *224*
Elwell, J. H., 196, *210*
Elwood, L., 202, *209*
Emeux, C., 8, *63*
Endres, S., 200, *204*
English, D., 4, 5, 6, 9, 10, 14, 17, 18, 30, 31, 32, 33, 36, 37, 38, 48, *56*, *63*, *64*, 72, 84, *91*, *93*, 138, *171*
Enokihara, H., 275, *293*
Eppella, E., 222, *225*
Erdmann, W., 200, *206*
Erneux, B. C., 10, *63*
Eskandari, M., 221, *225*

Eskins, S. G., 46, *56*
Esmon, C., 29, *56*, 314, *323*
Esrin, S. G., 8, *55*
Essien, E. M., 311, *323*
Evans, J., 175, 176, *186–87*, 238, *257*
Evans, P., 275, *307*
Evans, T. M., 287, 288, 289, *293*
Evans, T. W., 288, 289, *293*
Evensen, S. A., 29, *56*, 314, 315, *323*
Evenson, S. A., 315, *323*
Ewel, C., 202, *209*
Ewenstein, B. M., 76, *94*
Exton, J. F., *54*
Exton, J. H., 7, 19, 20, 22, *54*, *56*, *64*, 128, *131*

F

Fabisiak, J. P., 176, *187*
Factor, S. M., 311, *326*
Fahey, T., *96*
Fahey, T. J., III, 194, *209*
Fahimi, H. D., 265, *307*
Fain, J. N., 67, *89*
Fairhurst, S., 139, 140, *170*
Fairman, R. P., 285, *293–94*
Fallman, M., 73, *89*
Falzon, M., 200, *204*
Fan, T. P. D., 8, *61*
Fan, X., 68, *89*
Fanburg, B. L., 137, *171*, 237, *257*
Fantone, J. C., 73, *88*
Farago, A., *110*
Farquhar, M. G., 118, *131*
Farrukh, I. S., 47, *56*, 71, *89*, 100, 102, 103, 104, *109*
Fauci, A. S., 265, 267, *290*, *296*
Fawcett, D. W., 265, *291*
Fay, F. S., 108, *110*
Feddersen, C. O., 192, 200, *203*
Fein, A. M., 252, *259*, 263, *298*
Feinstein, M. B., *65*, 315, *325*
Feldman, A. M., 11, *62*
Feldman, D. R., 21, 25, *61*, 68, 70, *92*
Feldman, J. O., 285, *293*
Fendly, B. M., 192, *207*
Fenton, B., 202, *209*
Fenton, J. W., 5, 6, 9, 18, 21, 23, 24, 25, 30, 31, 32, 33, 34, 35, 36, 37, 38, 40, 41, *53*, *54*, *56*, *57*
Fenton, J. W., II, 30, 40, 41, 43, 46, *56*, 122, *131*, 311, 312, 313, 314, 315, 316, 317, 318, 319, 320, *323*, *324*, *326*, *327*
Ferro, T. J., 42, 43, 46, *56*, *59*, *61*, 69, 70, 73, 74, 75, 81, 82, 83, *90*, *91*, 124, 129, *132*, 192, 194, *206*
Feuerstein, G., 8, 17, *56*
Fewtrell, C., 269, *300*
Fick, R. B., Jr., 281, *294*
Fiers, W., 124, *135*, 192, 194, *206*, *209*, 275, *301*
Figard, P. H., 164, *170*
Fine, J. M., 192, 201, *205*
Finkelstein, J. N., 176, *188*
Finn, A., 268, 276, *295*
Fishman, A. P., 99, *110*, 121, *130*, 228, *257*
Fleisch, J. H., 288, *303*
Fleith, M., 317, *322*
Flemming, J. S., 249, *256*
Fluharty, S. J., 71, *92*
Flynn, J. T., 281, *294*
Fobinson, F. R., 237, *258*
Fogelman, A. M., 121, *133*
Folch, J., 164, *170*
Foley, J. J., 70, *96*
Foot, E. C., 265, *294*
Ford-Hutchinson, A. W., 71, *89*
Foreman, J. C., 268, 270, 271, *292*, *294*, *301*, *303*
Formisano, S., 272, *299*
Forsberg, E. J., 8, 17, *56*
Forte, J. G., 127, *134*
Foscue, H. A., 122, *130*, 137, *169*, 175, 176, *187*
Foster, C., 241, *257*

Fosue, H. A., 46, *55*
Fournier, A., 68, *89*
Fox, R., 73, *88*
Fox, R. B., 124, *131*
Foy, T., 102, *109*
Fraker, D. L., 192, *202*
France, M., 200, *205*
France, M. L., 199, *205*
Francis, C. W., 311, *324*
Frank, J. A., 121, *133*
Frank, L., 138, 139, 166, *172*, 191, 192, 193, 195, 201, *204*, *205*, *206*
Frank, M. M., *258*, 266, *301*
Franke, R. P., 117, *131*
Frankel, H. M., 229, *258*
Franza, B. R., 180, 184, 185, *187*
Fredholm, B. B., 106, *111*
Freeland, H. S., 47, *56*
Freeman, A. R., 266, *291*
Freeman, B. A., 73, *89*, *94*, 123, 124, *131*, *134*, 137, 138, 140, 155, 166, *169*, *170*, *173*, 175, *187*, 192, 194, 195, *204*, *208*
Fridovich, I., 138, *170*, 198, *203*, 239, 241
Fried, R., 228, *257*
Friedman, B., 268, 276, *303*
Friedman, M. M., 267, 287, *294*
Friedman, R. S., 214, *224–25*
Friedrich, P., 229, *257*
Friend, D. S., 119, *133*
Frigas, E., 286, *295*
Fry, G. L., 311, 317, *322*, *323*
Frzeskowizk, M., 51, *63*
Fuchs, H. J., 198, 202, *204*
Fugate, R. D., 315, *323*
Fujii, T., 11, *53*
Fujimoto, K., 277, 279, *294*
Fujiwara, K., 116, 117, *135*
Fukuda, T., 266, 275, *294*, *307*
Fulkerson, W. J., 138, *171*
Fulmer, J. D., 139, *171*
Fulton, A. B., 159, *170*
Fung, W. -J. C., 21, *58*
Furchgott, R. F., *89*, 317, *323*, *324*
Furusawa, S., 275, *293*

G

Gabbiani, F., 116, *131*
Gabbiani, G., 114, 116, 117, 119, 125, *131*, *133*, *134*
Gadek, J. E., 84, *89*, 266, *301*
Gajdusek, C. M., 201, *205*
Galdal, K. S., 29, *56*, 314, 315, *323*
Galli, S. J., 264, 267–68, *294*, *295*
Gallin, J. I., 8, 40, *63*, 124, *134*
Gallo, S., 311, *321*
Gamble, J. R., 192, *206*, 275, *294*, *299*
Gandini, G., 51, *63*
Ganong, B. R., 315, *323*
Garbarino, G., *61*
Garbers, D. L., 20, *56*
Garcia, J. G. N., 4, 5, 6, 9, 10, 12, 13, 14, 17, 18, 20–27, 29–43, 46, 48, *54*, *56*, *57*, *62–63*, *64*, 122, *130*, *131*, 288, *291*, 315, *323*
Garcia, P. L., 38, *56*
Garcia-Barreno, P., 8, *61*
Garcia-Sainz, J. A., 108, *109*
Garland, L. G., 51, *54*
Garrels, J. I., 180, *187*
Garrison, J. C., 317, *324*
Gartner, I., 266, *301*
Gartner, S. L., 75, *89*
Garzo, T., *110*
Gasson, J. C., 275, *301*
Gay, J. C., 71, 73, 74, *89*
Gearing, A. J. H., 275, *296*
Gee, M. H., 281, *294*
Geiger, B., 114, 117, *131*
Geiger, K., 282, *307*
Gelas, P., 20, *57*
Gelehrter, T. D., 29, *57*, 180, 181, 182, 183, 184, 185, *186*, *187*, *189*
Gelfand, J. A., 195, *208*

Gelfland, J. A., 266, *301*
Genovese, A., 272, *299*
Gensheimer, H. P., 268, *299*
George, J. N., *89–90*
Georgilis, K., 200, *204*
Gerad, C., 73, 84, *87*
Gerlach, H., 75, *88*, 124, *130*
Gerlach, J., *326*
Gharaee-Kermani, M., 184, *188*
Ghezzi, P., 191, 192, 194, 195, 200, 201, *203*, *205*, *208*, *210*
Ghigo, D., *61*
Ghio, A. J., 103, *109*
Ghorbani, R., 200, *204*
Giegh, G. T., 99, *111*
Giembycz, M. A., 267, 275, *294*
Gilfillan, A. M., 268, 269, 270, 271, 272, *294*, *298*
Gilis, C. N., 79, 80, 82–84, *93*
Gill, C. A., 288, *306*
Gillespie, E., 268, 271, 276, *303*
Gillespie, M. N., 191, *205*
Gillespie, R. F., 192, *208*
Gillis, C. N., 83, *92*
Gillis, N. C., 85, *90*
Gillis, S., 192, *208*, 268, 276, *303*
Gilman, A. G., 3, 4, 7, 10, *57*, *59*, 67, *90*, 269, *295*
Gilmore, V., 99, *110*
Gimbrone, M. A., 116, 117, *135*, 191, *203*, 216, 223, *224*, 311, 317, *322*
Gimbrone, M. A., Jr., 18, *65*, 70, *97*
Gladner, J. A., 311, *323*
Glauser, F. L., 285, *293–94*
Gleich, G. J., 264, 265, 266, 273, 282, 286, 287, *290*, *292*, *294*, *295*, *297*, *300*, *301*, *305*, *307*
Glenn, K. C., 30, 40, *57*
Glovsky, M. M., 268, *295*
Godard, P. H., 275, *296*
Godfrey, P. P., 73, 74, *96*
Godman, G., 75, *88*, 124, *130*
Goeddel, D. V., 192, 196, *210*
Goetzel, E. J., 20, *59*
Goetzl, E. J., 266, 267, 275, 287, *292*, *295*, *297–98*, *300*, *305*
Goldberg, A. L., *206*
Goldblum, S. E., 191, *205*
Goldsmith, J. C., 46, *64*, 74, 75, *95*, 124, *134*
Goldsmith, J. G., 16, *57*
Goldstein, I. M., *224*
Goldstein, K. E., 21, 25, *61*, 68, 70, *92*
Goligorsky, M. S., 31, 41, *57*, *61–62*
Gomez-Cambronero, J., 70, *97*
Gomperts, B. D., 5, 7, *55*, 269, 270, *294*, *295*, *296*
Gonder, J. C., 200, *205*
Goodman, E., 124, *134*, 167, *172*
Goodwin, J. D., 72, *94*
Gordon, A. S., 265, *292*
Gordon, E. A., 30, 40, *54*
Gordon, J. L., 46, *53*, 314, *325*
Gordon, J. R., 268, *295*
Gordon, T., 192, 201, *205*
Goresky, C. A., 75, *93*
Goretsky, C. A., 125, *134*
Gorman, R. R., 275, 287, *295*
Gorski, J., 315, *325*
Gospodarowicz, D., 29, *57*
Gosset, P., 266, *301*
Gotlieb, A. I., 114, 116, 117, 121, 125, *131*, *132*, *135*
Goto, M., 268, 276, *300*
Goto, T., 192, 194, *208*
Gougerot-Pocidalo, M. A., 200, *207*
Goveley, M. F., 267, 282, *303*
Grafe, M., 117, *131*
Graham, D., 192, *207*
Grandordy, B. M., 71, *90*
Granger, D. N., 239, 249, 250, *257*, *258*
Green, D. W., 198, *205*
Green, R., 249, *261*
Greenberg, B., 72, *90*
Greenberg, M. L., 265, *304*
Greengard, P., 74, *91*, *92*, 272, *305*
Greenwood, B., 288, *293*
Grega, G. J., 113, 125, *131*
Griendling, K. K., 8, 9, 14, *54*

Griffin, G. L., 238, *259*
Griffin, P. R., 217, *225*
Griffith, O. H., 74, *88*
Griffith, S. L., 229, *257*
Grigorian, G. Y., 8, *63*, 68, *96*
Grisham, M. B., 76, 79, 81, 82, *87*
Grizzle, W. E., 139, *171*
Groner, Y., 193, *210*
Groschel-Stewart, U., 113, *131*
Groscurth, P., 71, 73, 74, *88*
Grover, B. M., 228, *259*
Grover, R. F., 228, *260*
Grover, W. H., 266, *295*
Gruchalla, R. S., 271, *295*
Grulich, J., 8, 17, 30, 31, 36, *58*
Grum, C. M., 138, *169*
Grunstein, M. M., 71, 72, *94*
Gryglewski, R. J., 240, *257*, 317, 318, *322*, *323*
Guarnieri, C., 249, *261*
Guichardant, M., 316, *322*
Guillen, M. C., 314, *324*
Guinan, E. C., 124, *135*, 192, 194, *209*
Gumbay, R. S., 71, 85, *89*
Gumbiner, B., 117, 118, 127, *131*
Gundel, R. H., 279, 281, *306*
Guntner, G. H., 239, *258–59*
Guo, Y. L., 103, *109*
Gurtner, G. H., 46, 47, *55*, *56*, *57*, 71, *89*, 100, 101, 102, 103, 104, 105, 106, 107, *109*, *110*, *111*, 201, *203*
Guthrie, D. F., 270, *291*
Guthrie, L. A., 191–92, *205*, *208*

H

Haak-Frendscho, M., 268, 276, *295*
Haas, T. A., 316, *322*
Haberland, M. E., 121, *133*
Habermann, E., 6, *53*
Habermehl, G. G., 197, *207*
Habliston, D. L., 74, *88*
Hacker, A. D., 201, *209*
Haddas, R. A., 50, *63*
Haddy, F. J., 113, *131*
Hahn, W. C., 180, *188*
Hainau, B., 118, *130*
Haines, K. A., 73, *93–94*
Hakim, J., 200, *207*
Hakim, T. S., 249, *256*
Halenda, S. P., *65*, 315, *325*
Hälgren, R., 276, *295*, *300*
Hallam, T. J., 8, 14, 17, 31, 39, *54*, *57*
Halldorsson, H., 8, 12, 14, 17, 18, 32, 36, 37, *57*, *61*
Halsey, W. A., 84, 85, *94*
Halushka, P. V., 138, *170*, 200, *210*
Hamaguchi, H., 275, *293*
Hamamoto, S. T., 127, *134*
Hamasaki, Y., 288, *300*
Hamelink, M. L., 275, *291*
Hamilton, J. H., 221, *224*
Hamilton, J. T., 229, *259*
Hamilton, K. K., 315, *323*
Hamilton, T. A., 238, *256*
Hammersen, F., 116, *131*
Hammond, B., 239, 245, *257*
Hampel, G., 8, 17, 30, 31, 36, *58*
Handin, R. T., 311, 317, *322*
Handley, D., 194, *207*
Hanley-Hyde, J., 268, *301*
Hannun, Y. A., 315, *323*
Hansen, H. S., 271, *297*
Hansen, S., 192, *208*
Hansen, T. N., 199, 200, *205*
Harada, N., 275, *307*
Harada, R. N., 238, *256*
Haranaka, K., 192, 194, *208*
Harbeck, R. J., 84, *95*
Hardy, S. J., 68, *89*
Hardy, T. M., 268, *301*
Hare, G. M. T., 72, *95*
Hariri, R. J., *96*, 194, *209*
Harker, L. A., 29, 46, *58*, *61*, 138, 145, *170*, 201, *205*, 263, *295*

Harlan, J. M., 29, 46, 47, *57*, *58*, *61*, 138, 145, *170*, 191, 192, 201, *205*, *206*, *208*, 216, *225*, 238, 252, *257*, 263, 275, *294*, *295*, *299*
Harley, J. B., 265, 267, *290*, *296*
Harris, T. R., 102, *109*
Hart, C. M., 143, 144, 145, 146, 150, 151, 153, 154, 156, 157, 158, 159, 160, 161, 162, 164, 165, 166, *170*
Hart, P. H., 221, *224*
Hartman, C. T., Jr., 268, *295*
Hartwig, J. H., 128, *131*
Haselton, F. R., 121, *130*
Hasimoto, T., 265, *307*
Haslett, C., 192, *208*
Hass, M. A., 192, 193, *205*, *206*
Hass, P. E., 223, *224*
Hass, T. A., 317, *322*
Hasty, D., 100, 102, 103, 104, *109*
Hatcher, V. B., 311, *326*
Hathaway, D. R., 247, *257*
Hatta, K., 127, *132*
Hattori, H., 38, *62*
Hattori, R., 315, *323*
Hattori, T., 18, *58*
Hattori, Y., 272, *296*
Hauser, G. J., 196, *205*
Hauser, M. J., 249, *261*
Havill, A. M., 85, *90*
Hawkins, D. J., 72, *92*, 318, *323*
Haycraft, D. L., 317, *322*, *323*
Haynes, M., 249, *258*
Haynes, N., 279, 281, *306*
Hazinski, T. A., 199, 200, *205*
Heath, D., 228, *258*
Hebert, C. A., 223, *224*
Hecht, G., 120, 122, 123, 125, *131–32*
Hechtman, H. B., 73, *88*, 125, *130*, *133*, *135*
Hedberg, K. K., 74, *88*
Hedman, K., 180, *188*
Heffner, J. E., 45, 46, *58*, 138, *170*
Hefner, J. E., 73, *90*
Heiman, A. S., 272, *296*
Heinle, H., 249, *258*
Heintzelman, M. B., 120, *135*
Held, W. A., 180, *186*
Helgeson, S. C., 317, *324*
Heller, M., 20, *58*
Hemler, M. E., 201, *205*
Hemmings, H. C., *92*
Henderson, W. R., *91*, 263, 267, 273, 274, 276, *292*, *296*, *298*
Hennig, B., 159, *170*
Henson, J. E., 71, 85, *89*, 285, *292*
Henson, P. M., 71, 85, *89*, 191–92, 200, *203*, *205*, *208*, 263, 278, 279, *296*, *297*
Herbert, J., 316, *323*
Herbert, T. J., 128, *132*
Herbosa, G. J., 30, 40, *54*
Herman, I. M., 99, *111*
Hernandez, E. M., 76, 79, 81, 82, 85, *87*
Hernson, 245
Herrero, C., *61*
Hesketh, T. R., 270, *291*
Hess, M. L., 201, *206*, 239, 245, *257*
Hestdal, K., 202, *209*
Heusser, C. H., 268, *306*
Heyworth, P. G., 73, 84, *87*
Hidaka, H., *90*, 247, *258*, *260*
Higgins, P. J., 122, *133*, 176, 177, 178, 179, 180, 181, 182, 183, 184, 185, *187*, *188*, *189*
Higgs, E. A., 167, *170*, 317, *325*
Hill, J. M., 73, *96*
Hill, R. N., 310, *323–24*
Hinshaw, D. B., 155, *172*
Hinson, I., 71, 85, *88*
Hirano, S., 127, *132*
Hirata, F., 18, *58*, 270, 272, *292*, *297*
Hirata, K., 266, 267, *296*
Hirsh, J., 316, *322*
Hislop, A., 229, *258*
Ho, S., 118, *130*
Ho, Y. -S., 198, *206*
Hoak, J. C., 29, 30, *53*, *61*, 311, 317, *322*, *323*, *326*

Hocking, D., 46, *59*, 73, 74, 82, 83, *90*, 124, *132*
Hocking, D. C., 75, 124, 129, *132*
Hocking, D. L., 69, 75, 81, 82, *90*
Hoffman, M. D., 73, 84, *96*
Hoffman, M. E., 155, *171*
Hoffman, R., 4, *63*
Hoffstein, S. T., 214, *224–25*
Hohman, R. J., 270, *299*
Hoidal, J. R., 100, 102, 103, 104, *109*, 124, *131*, 264, *296*
Hokin, L. E., 7, *58*
Hokin, M. R., 7, *58*
Holgate, S. T., 267, 268, 272, *290*, *292*, *296*, *298*
Holm, B. A., 176, 177, *188*
Holmes, B. M., 73, 84, *94*
Holowka, D., 269, *300–301*
Holroyd, K. J., *206*
Holtzman, H., 252, *259*, 263, *298*
Holwka, D., 269, *300*
Hom, J., 21, *55*
Homer, L. D., 75, *89*
Honda, Z., 271, *300*
Honeyman, T. W., 50, *55*
Hong, S. L., 16, 17, 36, *58*
Honjo, T., 275, *293*
Hook, W. A., 268, *296*
Hopkins, C., 100, 102, 103, 104, *109*
Hopkins, W. E., 183, 185, *189*
Horecker, B. L., 74, *93*
Horie, S., 29, *58*
Horowitz, S., 176, 177, *188*
Horton, A. A., 139, 140, *170*
Horvath, C. J., 192, 194, *206*
Hough, G. P., 121, *133*
Houha, V., 266, *292*
Housset, B., 137, *172*
Hoveke, T. P., 311, *326*
Howard, T. H., 192, *203*
Howarth, P. H., 267, *290*
Howell, C. J., 275, *296*
Howell, T. W., 269, *295*, *296*
Hrbolich, J. K., 18, *65*, 70, *97*
Hsueh, W., *209*
Huang, C., 21, 25, *58*
Huang, C. K., 73, *96*
Huang, K-S., 21, *58*
Huang, X., 68, *89*
Hubscher, U., 155, *169*
Hudson, G., 265, *296*
Hudspeth, A. J., 127, *132*
Hughes, P. J., 268, *292*
Hugli, T. E., 268, *297*
Hui, S. W., 118, *130*
Hull, M. T., 239, 253, 255, *256*, *259*
Hulmes, J. D., 21, *58*
Hunninghake, G. W., 46, *64*, 74, 75, *95*, 124, *134*, 281, *294*
Hunt, D. F., 217, *225*
Hurley, J. V., 113, *132*
Husak, M., 167, *171–72*
Hutchin, G. M., 249, *261*
Hutchison, A. A., 200, *209*
Huval, W., 73, *88*
Hwang, O., 240, *259*
Hyde, D. M., 276, 277, *301*
Hyers, T. M., 102, 108, *110*
Hyslop, P. A., 155, 160, *170*, *172*

I

Ibarra, G., 117, 118, *133*
Iida, K., *132*
Ikebuchi, H., 272, *305*
Ikejima, T., 195, *208*
Inagaki, M., *90*, 247, *258*
Inagami, T., 72, *95*
Inauen, W., *258*
Ingelman-Sunberg, M., 73, 74, *95*
Innis, S. M., 138, 139, 166, *172*
Iozzo, R. V., 265, *296–97*
Iqbal, J., 192, 193, 198, *205*, *206*
Irvine, R. F., 7, 8, 17, *53*, *63*, *256*
Ischiropoulos, H., 192, 195, 200, *206*
Ishii, H., 29, *58*
Ishikawa, M., 317, *321*

Ishikawa, T., 247, *260*
Ishikawa, Y., 84, *91*
Ishizaka, A., *95*, 195, *209*
Ishizaka, K., 271, 272, *297*, *306*
Ishizaka, T., 269, 270, 271, 272, *297*, *303*, *306*
Ishizuka, T., 271, *300*
Issaad, C., 72, 74, *90*
Ito, K., 240, *261*
Iyengar, 8, *61*
Izzo, N. J., 317, *324*

J

Jackson, D. M., 288, *293*
Jackson, J. H., 76, 79, 81, 82, *90*, 199, *210*
Jackson, R. C., 270, 271, *298*
Jackson, S. K., 191, *207*
Jacob, H. S., 138, *172*, 263, 275, 282, 283, 287, *303*, *304*
Jacob, R., 8, *58*
Jacobsen, S., 271, *297*
Jacobson, D. P., *93*
Jaffe, E. A., 8, 16, 17, 30, 31, 36, *58*, *65*, 314, *327*
Jaffe, H. A., *206*
Jaffe, H. S., *206*
Jaffer, F. E., 50, *59*
Jafri, 101, 107
Jagarlaupaudi, S., 167, *171–72*
Jakab, G. J., 107, *110*
Jaken, S., 68, 75, *90*, *91*, 129, *132*
Jakobs, K. H., 6, *53*, *59*
Jalink, K., 50, *58*
Jamieson, G. A., Jr., *61–62*
Janco, R. L., 192, 197, *203*
Jandroy-Perrus, M., 314, *324*
Janik, J., 202, *209*
Janmey, P. A., 128, *132*
Jaques, Y. V., 315, *326*
Jay, J., 264, *293*
Jay, M., 191, *205*
Jayaram, H. N., 4, *63*
Jean-Mairet, Y., 137, *172*
Jelsema, C. L., 38, *58–59*
Jenkins, L. W., 201, *206*
Jensen, B., 271, *297*
Jensen, J. C., 192, *202*
Jeremy, J. Y., 17, *59*
Jesmols, G., 192, 194, *206*
Jiang, M. J., 71, *90*
Jin, N., 240, 241, 242, 243, 244, 245, 246, 248, 249, 250, 253, 254, 255, 256, *258*, *259*, *260*
Johns, J. A., 72, *95*
Johnson, 245
Johnson, A., 46, *56*, *59*, 69, 73, 74, 75, 76, 79, 80, 81, 82, 83, 85, *90*, 100, 102, *110*, 124, 129, *132*
Johnson, A. R., 16, *59*, 268, *297*
Johnson, C. M., 317, *324*
Johnson, D. R., 76, *94*
Johnson, G. R., 274, *299*
Johnson, K. J., 84, 85, *90*, 263, 281, *305*
Johnson, K. L., 253, *257*
Johnson, K. W., 106, *109*
Johnson, R. J., 249, *259*
Johnson, R. L., 249, *258*
Johnson, R. M., 317, *324*
Johnston, C. J., 176, *188*
Johnston, R. B., Jr., 191–92, *205*, *208*
Joly, F., 70, 73, *91*
Jondal, M., 106, *111*
Jones, P. C., 238, *257*
Jones, R., 175, 176, *188*, 228, 237, 238, *258*
Jones, R. C., 176, *186*
Jong, E. C., 273, 274, *296*
Jordan, C. C., 268, *294*
Jorg, A., 265, 266, 273, *296*, *297*
Jorgensen, J. L., 180, *188*
Jornot, L., 46, *59*, 155, *171*
Joseph, M. L., 29, *61*
Jothianadan, D., 317, *324*
Jubiz, W., 46, *56*
Juliano, R. L., 74, *88*

Junod, A. F., 46, *59*, 137, 138, 155, *169*, *171*, *172*
Juttner, C. A., 275, *299*

K

Kachar, B., 127, *132*
Kaduce, T. L., 141, 164, *170*, *171*
Kaever, V., 70, 73, *93*
Kagey-Sobotka, A., 268, 276, *299*, *301*
Kahn, N. N., 311, *326*
Kaibuchi, K., 271, *297*
Kajita, T., 267, *297*
Kajitani, H., 275, *293*
Kajiyama, Y., 18, 38, *59*
Kakkar, V. V., 11, *61*, 310, *324*
Kaliner, M. A., 264, 267, 268, 287, *293*, *294*, *303*, *306*
Kalunig, J. E., 138, 140, 166, *172*
Kamp, D. W., 73, 74, *90*, *91*
Kanfer, J. N., 20, *61*, *64*
Kang, Y. H., 75, *89*
Kanzaki, T., 18, *59*
Kapanci, Y., 122, *132*, 237, *258*
Kaplan, A. P., 268, 276, *295*
Kaplan, E., 312, 313, 317, 318, 319, 320, *326*
Kaplan, H. P., 122, *132*, 237, *258*
Kaplan, J. E., 288, *291*, 309–12, 314–20, *324*, *326*, *327*
Karnovsky, M. J., 114, *132*
Karnovsky, M. L., 73, 84, *87*, 167, *169*
Karnovsky, M. U., 120, *134*
Kasahara, K., 221, *225*
Kasahara, T., *92*
Katada, T., *59*
Katakami, Y., 271, *297*
Katchalski, E., 285, *293*
Kater, L. A., 20, *59*, 266, *297*
Kato, Y., *96*
Katusic, Z. S., 72, *91*, 240, *258*
Katz, S. A., 138, *170*
Kauffman, H. F., 266, 267, *298*
Kaufman, E. N., 192, *210*
Kaufmann, S., 68, *91*
Kawai, T., *92*
Kawakami, A., 127, *132*
Kawamoto, S., *90*, 247, *258*
Kay, A. B., 268, 275, 276, 287, *290*, *291*, *297*, *300*, *306*
Kayes, S. G., 76, 79, 81, *93*, 277, 279, *294*
Kazama, M., 29, *58*
Kehrer, J. P., 139, 166, *171*
Keller, J., 202, *209*
Keller, T. C. S., 120, *132*
Kelley, J., 176, *187*
Kelley, T., 114, 117, 129, *130*
Kelley, V. E., 200, *204*
Kelly, B., 239, 240, *256*
Kennedy, J. L., 139, *171*
Kennedy, K. A., 199, 200, *205*
Kennedy, T. P., 100, 102, 103, 104, *109*
Kennerly, D. A., 271, *295*, *297*
Kent, R. S., 5, 8–10, 46, 47, *61*, *65*
Kenyon, J. L., 240, *261*
Keramidas, M., 68, *93*
Kern, J. A., 201, *202*
Kernen, P., 74, *96*
Kerr, J. S., 229, *258*
Kerstein, M. D., 102, 108, *110*
Kester, M., 22, *59*
Ketai, L. H., 138, *169*
Kettelhut, I. C., *206*
Khalil, R. A., 71, *91*
Kiauck, T., 75, *90*
Kieffer, N., *89–90*
Kierszenbaum, F., 286, 287, *297*
Kijne, A. M., 275, *291*
Kikkawa, Y., 192, 195, 200, *206*
Kikuchi, A., 5, 38, *65*
Kiley, S. C., *91*
Killen, P. D., 138, *170*
Kim, D. W., 116, 117, *132*
Kim, S., 5, 38, *65*
Kimani, G., 278, 279, *297*
Kimbel, P., 252, *259*, 263, *298*

King, W. G., 18, *59*
Kings, M. A., 275, *303*
Kinsella, J. E., 167, *169*
Kirkin, A. H., 119, *134*
Kiss, Z., 20, 22, *59*
Kissinger, M., 192, *209*
Kistler, G. S., 122, *132*, 137, *171*
Kitazono, T., 10, 12, 18, *59*
Kjeld, M., 8, 12, 14, 17, 18, 32, 36, 37, *57*, *61*
Klalid, R. A., 72, *92*
Klauck, T., 129, *132*
Klebanoff, S. J., 192, *206*, 265, 266, 267, 273, 274, 275, 276, *292*, *294*, *296*, *297*, *299*
Klein, J., 200, *206*
Klein, M. M., *326*
Klempner, M. S., 200, *204*
Klickstein, L. B., 287, *297–98*
Kloprogge, E., 266, 267, *298*
Kluft, C., 180, *189*
Knap, A., *91*
Knauss, T. C., 50, *59*
Knoblanch, A., 47, *57*
Knudsen, P. J., 200, *206*
Knutson, V. P., 121, *133*
Kobayashi, E., 76, *91*
Kobayashi, M., 20, *61*
Kobayashi, T., 198, *206*, 285, *305*
Kobayashi, Y., 192, 197, *207*
Koch, L. E., 117, *132*
Kohmura, Y., 271, *300*
Kohr, W. J., 223, *224*
Koizumi, M., 201, *206*
Kok, P. T. M., 275, *291*
Konings, A. W. T., 140, *172*
Konopka, R., 71, 85, *88*
Kontos, H. A., 201, *206*, 239, 240, 245, 249, *257*, *261*
Koopman, W. R., Jr., 270, 271, *298*
Kopp, W., 202, *209*
Korchak, H. M., 73, *93–94*
Kotikoff, M. I., 71, *92*
Kowalski, M. L., 264, *293*, *303*
Koyama, I., 239, *258–59*
Koyama, S., 285, *305*
Kramer, C. M., 139, *170*
Kramer, S., *206*
Krausz, T., 249, *256*
Krishnamurthi, S., 11, *61*
Kroegel, C., 267, 275, 282, *294*, *298*, *307*
Kroll, M. H., 50, *61*
Kronke, M., 75, *94*
Kruijer, W., 50, *61*
Kulcycki, A., 272, *305*
Kumae, T., 192, 195, 200, *206*
Kunicki, T. J., *89–90*
Kunkel, R., 238, *261*, 263, 281, *305*
Kunkel, R. G., 195, *208*, 253, *257*
Kunkel, S. L., 194, 195, 200, *203*, *206*, *207*, *208*, 217, 218, 221, 222, *224*, *225*
Kunze, D. N., 8, *55*
Kuratsu, J. I., 222, *225*
Kuriyama, H., 191, *211*
Kuroda, M., 84, *91*
Kusama, S., 285, *305*

L

LaBrecque, J. F., 71, 85, *89*
Lacal, J. C., *61*
Lacey, C., 116, *131*
Lafuze, J. E., 253, 255, *259*
Lagarde, M., 316, *322*
Lagunoff, D., 41, 43, *65*, 122, 125, *135*
Lai, Y., 74, *91*
Laki, K., 311, *323*
Lam, S., 281, *298*
Lamas, A. M., 278, 279, *298*
Lambert, T. L., 5, 8–10, *61*
Lambertsen, C. J., 139, *169*
Lamkin, G. E., 74, 75, *91*
LaMont, J. T., 120, 122, 123, 125, *131–32*
Lampugnani, M. G., *61*

Landau, E. M., 8, *61*
Lands, W. E. M., 201, *205*
Lane, T. A., 74, 75, *91*
Lanefelt, F., 106, *111*
Langille, B. L., 116, 117, *132*
Langleben, D., 228, *258*
Langstein, H. N., 192, *202*
Lapetina, E. G., 11, 17, 51, *55*, *61*, *64*, 318, *324*
Laposata, M., 315, *324*
Larrick, J., 192, 194, 195, 200, *203*, *207*, *208*, *209*, 221, *225*
Larrk, J. W., *95*
Larsen, C. G., 217, *225*
Laslo, A., 31, *57*
Lassing, I., 128, *132*
Lauri, D., 311, *321*
Lauterburg, B. H., 191, *203*
Lawing, W. J., Jr., 18, *55*
Lawrence, D. A., 182, *189*
Lazar, R., 100, 102, 103, 104, *109*
Lazarides, E., 117, *132*
Lazo, J. C., 247, *259*
Lazo, J. S., 12, *62*, 71, *92*
Leach, K., 75, *90*, 129, *132*
Leach, K. L., 68, *91*
Leadon, S. A., 191, *211*
Leaf, A., 140, *171*
Leake, E. S., 70, 74, 84, *93*
Lechner, K., 268, 276, *305*
Lee, C. T., 252, *259*
Lee, C. Y., 198, *209*
Lee, S. L., 137, *171*
Lee, T. C., 263, 267, *298*
Lee, T. H., 167, *171*, 275, *296*
Lees, M., 164, *170*
Leff, A. R., 71, *92*
Leiferman, K. M., 273, *292*
Lembeck, F., 287, 288, *303*
Lempereur, C., 266, *298*
Lenethal, M., 99, *110*
Lenihan, D. J., 267, *298*
Lennon, J. M., 30, 31, 40, 41, *53*
Leonard, E. J., 217, 222, *225*
Leowenherez, J. W., 249, *261*
LeRiche, J., 281, *298*
Letourneau, L., 265, *293*
Letts, L. G., 279, 281, *306*
Leung, D. W., 223, *224*
Levacher, M., 200, *207*
Levanthal, M. M., 287, *299*
Leventhal, M. M., 99, *110*, 113, *133*
Levin, E. G., *61*
Levin, J., 192, 201, *205*
Levine, E. M., 121, *130*, 201, *202*
Levine, J. D., 29, 46, *58*, *61*, 145, *170*
Levine, M. N., 311, *321*
Levoy-Viard, K., 314, *324*
Lew, D. P., 73, *89*
Lewis, M. S., 46, *61*
Lewis, R. A., 268, 272, *296*, *298*
Lewis-Molock, 198
Ley, C. W., 16, *65*, 314, *327*
Leyravaud, S., 70, 73, *91*
Li, S., 21, *58*
Libby, P., 194, *207*
Lichtenstein, L. M., *110*, 268, 271, 272, 276, *291*, *299*, *301*, *303*, *305*
Liggitt, D., 192, 198, 202, *204*, *208*
Liles, W. C., *91*, 263, *298*
Lin, H. L., *132*
Lin, J. X., 76, *97*
Lin, L., 192, *207*
Lin, P., 270, 271, 272, *298*
Lincoln, T. M., 107, *110*
Lind, S. E., 46, *64*, 74, 75, *95*, 124, 128, *132*, *134*
Lindberg, U., 128, *132*
Lindley, I., 217, 218, *224*, *225*
Lineberger, A. S., 70, 74, 84, *93*
Lippman, M., 252, *259*, 263, *298*
Liscovitch, M., 20, *55*
Liu, M. C., 268, *299*
Lloyd, T. C., 250, *258*
Lo, S. K., 288, *291*
Lo, T. N., 270, *299*
Lo, W. W. Y., 8, *61*
LoBue, J., 265, *292*
LoBuglio, A. F., 46, *65*, 137, 138, *173*
Loeb, A. L., 317, *324*

Loegering, D. A., 265, 266, 282, 286, *290*, *292*, *295*
Login, G. R., 265, *293*
Lohse, M. J., 268, *299*
Lollar, P., 29, 30, *61*
Lombardi, D., 116, *131*
Longo, D., 192, 197, 202, *207*, *209*
Lonigro, A. J., 82, 84, 85, *95*
Lonnemann, G., 200, *204*
Loomis, C. R., 315, *323*
Lopez, *61*
Lopez, A. F., 274, 275, *299*
LoPreste, G., 195, 200, *204*
Loskutoff, D. J., 182, *189*
Lough, J., 311, *324*
Love, R. N., 195, 200, *204*
Low, M. G., 21, *58*
Lowe, D. G., 223, *224*
Lowry, S. F., *96*, 194, *209*
Loyd, J. E., 84, 85, *91*, *92*, 138, *171*
Luchtel, D. L., 282, *290*
Luckhoff, A., 106, 107, *109*
Luckoff, A., 8, *61*
Ludowyke, R. I., 270, 272–73, *299*, *300*
Luini, A., 17, *54*
Luis, E. A., 223, *224*
Lukashev, M. E., 42, *53*, 74, *87*
Lum, H., 31, 41, *57*, *60–61*, 74, 75, *93*, 125, 126, *134*
Lun, H., 41, *63*
Lundberg, J. M., 287, 288, *303*
Lybert, T., 29, *56*
Lyman, S., 315, *325*
Lynch, J. J., 42, 43, *61*, 69, 70, 75, *91*
Lynch, J. P., 221, *225*
Lynn, D. L., 195, 200, *204*

M

McCabe, J., 192, *208*
McCall, C. E., 70, 73, 74, 84, *87*, *93*, *96*
McClain, C. J., 191, *205*
McCloskey, M. A., 269, *299*
McCord, J. M., 72, *93*
McCormick, J. R., 85, *92*
MacDonald, G. H., 265, *296–97*
McDonald, J. A., *92*
McDonald, R. J., 276, 277, *301*
McEver, R. M., 315, *324*, *326*
McEver, R. P., *89–90*, 315, *323*
McGarvey, V., 311, *325*
McGivney, A., 270, *292*
MacGlashan, D. W., *110*, 271, *306*
MacGlashan, D. W., Jr., 268, 276, *303*
MacGlashan, R. P., 268, *299*
MacGlashin, D. W., 269, 270, *306*
McGuire, J. C., *91*
Machman, R. L., 99, *109*
Machovich, R., *110*, 314, *324*
Macias, W. L., *56*
McIntosh, J. K., 196, *205*
McIntyre, T. M., 29, 46, *61*, *63*, 70, *94*, 314, *325*
Mackie, K., 74, *91*
McLaughlin, N. J., 17, 36, *58*
McMahon, S., 191, 192, 195, *210*
McManus, M. M., 282, *290*
Macmorine, D. R. L., 310, *325*
McMurtry, I., 73, 74, 75, 76, *94*, 253, *260*, 281, *304*
McMurtry, I. F., 47, *64*, 72, *93*, 191, 192, 194, *210*
McMurty, I., 138, *172*
McMurty, I. F., 76, 79, 81, 82, *90*, 199, *210*, 229, 240, *259*, *261*
McNally, J., 73, 74, *96*
McNiff, J. M., 121, *130*
McPhail, L. C., 68, 73, 84, *87*, *96*, 191–92, *205*
Madara, J. L., 117, 118, 119, 120, 122, 123, 125, *131–32*, *133*
Madonna, G. S., 192, *207*
Madri, J. A., 316, *322*
Maeda, M., 191, *211*
Maeyama, K., 270, *292*, *299*
Maffrand, J., 316, *323*
Magno, G., 113, *133*

Magnuson, D. K., 75, *91*
Magnusson, M. K., 14, 18, 32, 37, *61*
Maguire, J. F., 272, *298*
Maier, R. V., 75, *91*
Majdic, O., 268, 276, *305*
Majerus, P. W., 18, *55*
Majno, G., 99, *109*, *110*, 287, *299*
Malavasi, F., 29, *54*
Maldonado, J. E., 265, *295*
Malik, A. B., 9, 18, 30–33, 38, 40–43, 46, *53*, *56*, *57*, *59*, *61–62*, *63*, 69, 70, 74, 75, *91*, *93*, 100, 102, *110*, 122, 125, 126, *130*, *131*, *133*, *134*, 177, 180, *188*, 192, 194, *206*, 249, *256*, 288, *291*, 310, 315, *323*, *324*
Malis, C. D., 140, *171*
Malone, B., 267, *298*
Malone, P. C., 310, *324*
Mandell, B. F., 71, 85, *96*
Mandl, J., *110*
Mann, J., 272, *306*
Manning, D. R., 4, 8, *54*
Manogue, K. R., 194, *207*
Manohar, M., 138, 140, *168*, *170*
Mano-Hirano, Y., 192, 194, *208*
Mansour, H., 200, *207*
Mantovani, A., 200, *208*, 275, *305*
Maraganore, J. M., 311, *323*
Marble, K. T., 76, 79, 81, 82, 85, *87*
Marcus, A. J., 16, *61*
Marder, V. J., 311, *324*
Margiotta, M., 281, *294*
Marks, R. M., 217, 218, *225*
Marlin, S. D., 191, *208–9*, 214–16, *225*
Marnoy, S. I., 200, *204*
Marom, Z., 267, *292*
Marone, G., 268, 272, 276, *299*, *301*
Marquardt, D. L., 268, *299*
Marquetty, A. C., 200, *207*
Marquetty, C., 200, *207*
Marrion, J., 102, *109*
Marsh, J., 71, 85, *88*
Marsh-Salin, J., 137, *169*
Martin, B. W., 315, *324*
Martin, M. N., 315, *324*
Martin, R. J., 249, *259*
Martin, S. E., 311, *324*
Martin, T. W., 16, 20, 21, 22, 25, 51, *61*, 68, 70, *92*
Martin, W., 317, *324*
Martinez-Palomo, A., 117, 118, 127, *133*
Marzec, U., *61*
Massaro, D., 191, 192, 193, 195, 201, *204*, *205*, *206*
Mastrangeli, A., *206*
Masuda, A., 192, 197, *207*
Matalon, S., *94*, 124, *134*, 192, 194, 195, *208*
Mathan, V. I., 138, 140, *168*, *170*
Mathias, M. M., 140, *172*
Mathison, J. C., 195, *207*
Matrisian, L., 177, 184, 185, *188*
Matsubara, T., 191, 197, *207*
Matsuda, K., 18, *58*
Matsushima, K., 192, 197, *207*, 217, 223, *225*
Matsushima, S., 247, *260*
Matthews, G., 270, *301*
Matthews, N., 191, 194, *207*
Maunder, R., 102, 108, *110*
Maurer, K., 268, *299*
May, M. A., 200, *207*, 221, *225*
Mead, M., 268, *301*
Mecham, R. P., 238, *259*, *261*
Meels, H., 99, *109*
Mehta, N., 167, *171–72*
Meier, B., 197, *207*
Meier, K. E., 263, *298*
Meir, K. E., *91*
Meisheri, K. D., 108, *110*, 240, *259*
Meiss, R. A., 229, 240, 241, 242, 243, 248, 249, 253, 255, *257*, *260*
Meldrum, L., 71, *90*
Meli, D., 266, *293*
Mello Filho, A. C., 155, *171*
Melloni, E., 74, *93*
Mellstrom, B., 185, *188*
Melmon, K. L., 276, *291*

Menconi, M. J., 201, *209*
Mene, P., 22, *59*
Meneghini, R., 155, *171*
Menton, D. N., 31, *57*
Mercurio, A. M., 74, *95*
Merker, M. P., 83, *92*
Merryweather, J., *96*, 194, *209*
Messier, J. M., 74, *95*
Meszaros, G., *110*
Metcalf, D., 274, 275, *293*, *299*
Metcalfe, J. C., 270, *291*
Metcalfe, J. D., 270, *291*
Metzger, H., 270, *300*
Metzger, W. J., 281, *294*
Meulemans, A. L., 286, *304*
Meyer, B. D., 74, *97*
Meyick, B. O., 318, *323*
Meyrick, B. O., 84, 85, *91*, *92*, 138, *169*, 191, 192, 197, 198, *203*, *206*, *208*, 228, 229, 252, *256*, *259*, 287–88, *300*
Meza, I., 117, 118, 127, *133*
Michael, J. R., 11, 46, 47, *55*, *56*, *62*, 71, *89*, 100, 102, 103, 104, *109*, *110*, 201, *203*
Michaelis, K. C., 21, 22, 25, *61*
Michel, M. C., 106, *110*
Michetti, M., 74, *93*
Michie, H. R., 194, *207*
Mier, J. W., 195, 200, *204*
Milagros, S., 125, *131*
Miller, D. S., 229, *259*
Miller, J. R., 72, *92*
Miller, L., 270, *300*
Milligan, S. A., 192, 201, *205*
Milsark, I. W., *96*, 194, *209*
Milton, A. S., 200, *204*
Milton, S. G., 121, *133*
Minakami, S., 10, 12, 18, *59*
Minami, A., 192, *208*
Mineau-Hanschke, R., 125, *133*
Minnear, F. L., 100, 102, *110*, 122, *130*, 311, 312, 313, 314, 315, 316, 317, 318, 319, 320, *324*, *326*
Miossec, P., 218, *225*
Mirault, M. E., 46, *59*
Mirza, Z., 137, 155, *169*
Mishima, T., 267, *297*
Mita, H., 267, *297*
Mitchell, J., 175, *186–87*
Mitsuhashi, M., 71, *92*
Mittermayer, C., 117, *131*
Miura, Y., 275, *307*
Miyamoto, T., 268, 271, 276, *300*
Mizer, L. A., 84, *92*
Mizus, I., 100, 101, 102, 103, 105, 106, *110*
Modig, J., 276, *295*, *300*
Mohn, H., 20, *55*
Mojarad, M., 288, *300*
Moldabaeva, A. K., 8, *63*
Moldow, C. F., 47, 48, *65*, 138, *172*, 263, *303*
Mollinedo, F., 21, *53*, 185, *188*
Molony, L., 114, 117, 129, *130*
Molski, T. F., 269, 270, *303*
Molski, T. F. P., 70, 73, *92*, *97*
Monahan-Earley, R. A., 265, *293*
Moncada, A., 167, *170*
Moncada, S., 240, *257*, 317, 318, *323*, *324*, *325–26*
Mondhiry, A. L., 311, *325*
Mongar, J. L., 270, *294*
Montesano, R., 119, 125, *131*, *133*
Montgomery, A. B., 198, 202, *204*
Montgomery, M. E., 46, 47, *65*
Moolenaar, W. H., 50, *58*, *61*
Moon, D. G., 311, 314, 315, 316, 317, 320, *323*, *324*, *326*
Moore, A. S., 268, *304*
Moore, J. P., 270, *291*
Moore, M. B., 311, *324*
Moore, P. B., 117, *133*
Moore, R., 120, 122, 123, *133*
Moore, S., 311, *323*
Mooseker, M. S., 120, *132*, *135*
Moqbel, R., 275, *300*, *306*
Moreau, J., 200, *207*
Moreno, F., 8, *61*

Morgan, K. G., 71, *90*
Moriarty, T. M., 8, *61*
Morimoto, M., 76, *91*, *96*
Morisake, N., 18, *59*
Morita, E., 217, *225*
Morita, Y., 268, 270, 271, 276, *292*, *300*
Morley, J., 275, *303*
Moroni, C., 268, *306*
Morris, S. A., 311, *326*
Morris-Natsclke, S., 73, 84, *87*
Morrison, W. R., *171*
Moscat, J., 8, *61*
Moseley, P. L., 281, *294*
Moser, K. M., 71, 85, *88*, 249, *259*, 310, *323–24*, *325*
Moskowitz, M. A., 8, *55*
Mosmann, T. R., 214, 217, *224*
Motte, C. A., 73–74, *89*
Movat, H. Z., 191, *207*, 310, *325*
Moy, J. N., 273, *300*
Moyer, J. D., 270, *292*
Mrowietz, U., 217, *225*
Mucha, I., *110*
Mueller, S. N., 121, *130*
Muhm, M., 268, 276, *305*
Mukaida, N., *92*
Muldoon, L. L., *61–62*
Muller, T. H., 18, *54*
Muller, W. A., 315, *325*
Müller-Eberhard, H. J., 268, *297*
Muller-Peddinghaus, R., 8, *53*
Mulroney, C. M., 278, 279, *298*
Mulsch, A., 106, 107, *109*
Munoz, N. M., 71, *92*
Murad, F., 314, 317, *326*
Murakami, K., 84, *91*
Murayama, T., 10, 18, 38, 50, *59*, *62*
Murphy, R. A., 72, *94*
Murphy, R. C., 192, *203–4*
Murphy, T. M., 71, *92*
Murray, A. W., 68, *89*
Murray, J. J., 318, *323*
Murray, R. K., 71, *92*
Mustard, J. F., 310, 311, *323*, *325*
Myers, C. L., 12, *62*, 71, *92*, 247, *259*

N

Naccache, P. H., 73, *92*, *96*
Nachman, R. L., 113, 116, *130*, 310, *325*
Nadziejko, C. E., 192, 195, 200, *206*
Nagao, S., 271, *300*
Nagashima, S., 275, *293*
Nagata, K., 271, *300*
Nagaya, K., 287, *305*
Nairn, A. C., 74, *91*, *92*
Naka, M., 247, *260*
Naka, N., 247, *260*
Nakahara, K., 288, *300*
Nakamo, H., 76, *91*
Nakamura, S. A., 192, *208*
Nakamura, T., 270, *300*
Nakashima, S., 38, *62*
Nalini, S., 140, *168*
Nanago, M., 287, *305*
Narasimhan, V., 269, *300–301*
Nariuchi, H., 192, 194, *208*
Narranjo, J. R., 185, *188*
Narumiya, S., 6, *62*
Nash, T. E., 266, *301*
Natarajan, V., 5, 12, 13, 14, 17, 18, 20, 21, 22, 23, 24, 25, 26, 27, 32, 33, 34, 35, 38, 39, 40, 48, *55*, *56*, *57*, *62*, *63*, *64*, 68, *96*
Nau, H., *326*
Nauseef, W. M., 267, *301*
Navab, M., 121, *133*
Navarro, L. T., 8, *55*
Nawroth, P., 75, *88*, 124, *130*, 194, *207*
Nazir, D. J., 316, *322*
Neale, M. L., 191, *207*
Neda, H., 191, *211*
Needham, L. A., 17, 31, *57*
Needleman, S. N., 16, *57*
Neher, E., 270, *301*
Nelson, D. P., 239, 240, *256*
Nelson, R. D., 275, 282, 283, 287, *304*
Nelson, S., 107, *110*
Neta, R., 192, *208*, *210*
Neubauer, J. A., 229, *258*

Newman, J. H., 84, 85, *91*, *92*, 138, *171*, 198, *206*
Newman, K. B., 11, *62*
Newman, P. J., 315, *325*
Newman, R. J., *89–90*
Newman, S. B., 120, *134*
Neyfakh, A. A., 180, *188*
Nguyen, D., 221, *225*
Nick, H. S., 192, 197, *210*
Nicola, N. A., 274, 275, *293*, *299*
Niedel, J. E., 43, *65*
Nielsen, L. S., 180, *188*
Niitsu, Y., 191, *211*
Nilsen, E., 29, *56*
Nilsen-Hamilton, M., 180, *189*
Nilson, E., 315, *323*
Nimeh, N. F., 46, *65*, 137, 138, *173*
Ninio, E., 70, 73, *91*
Nirromand, F., *326*
Nishikawa, M., 107, *110*
Nishimura, J., 72, *92*
Nishizuka, Y., 11, *62*, *64*, 67, 68, 69, 71, *92*, *93*, *95*, 271, *297*
Nolop, K. B., 249, *256*
Noma, T., 275, *293*
Nomoto, H., *96*
Nomura, Y., 18, 38, *59*
Nordan, R. P., 268, *301*
Nordby, E. C., 185, *186*
Nordoy, A., 164, *172*
Normansell, D. E., 266, *295*
Norton, J. A., 192, *202*
Nose, A., 127, *132*
Notsu, Y., 18, *58*
Notter, R. H., 176, 177, *188*
Nozawa, Y., 18, 38, *62*
Nozowa, Y., 271, *300*
Nupenko, E. V., 5, 6, 8, 9, 10, 11, *65*
Nusse, O., 269, *295*

O

Oates, J. A., 272, *298*
Oberley, L. W., 196, 198, *209*, *210*
Obin, M. S., 223, *224*
O'Brien, R. F., 43, *64*, 102, *110*
Ochs, H. D., 191, *208*, 216, *225*, 263, *295*
O'Connell, T. M., 180, *188*
O'Connor, J. V., 194, 195, 200, *204*
O'Donnell, M. C., 273, 287, *301*
O'Donnell, S. R., 288, *301*
O'Dwyer, S., 194, *207*
Ody, C., 138, *171*
O'Flaherty, J. T., 70, 74, 84, *93*, *96*
Ofosu, F. A., 311, *323*
Ogletree, M. L., 71, 84, 85, *88*, *91*, *92*, 138, *171*, 200, *209*
Ohashi, T., 192, *208*
Ohashi, Y., 6, *62*
Ohishi, I., 6, *53*
Ohkuda, K., 288, *300*
Ohno, I., 268, *301*
Okajima, F., 269, 270, *303*
Okano, Y., 18, 38, *62*
Oku, N., 287, *305*
Okusawa, S., 195, *208*
Olbrantz, P., 73, 84, *87*
Oliver, J. M., 269, *301*, *306*
Olofsson, T., 266, *301*
Olson, T. A., 311, 314, *323*
Olssen, E. G. J., 286, *305*
Olsson, I., 265, 266, *290*, *301*
Omann, G. M., 128, *133*, 269, *301*
Omri, G., 8, *61*
Oostveen, J. A., 278, 281, *293*
Oppenheim, J. J., 192, 197, 202, *207*, *208*, *209*, 217, 223, *225*
Oppenheimer, J. J., 192, *208*
Orci, L., 119, 125, *131*, *133*
Ordovas, J. M., 194, *207*
Orell, S. R., 310, *325*
Orellana, S., *62*
O'Rourke, F. A., 315, *325*
Orr, F. W., 311, *321*
Orr, T. S. C., 288, *293*
Orton, E. C., 72, *93*, 238, *261*
Osborn, M., 117, *135*

Ottesen, E. A., 266, *301*
Owen, P. J., 73, *88*, 288, *291*
Owen, W., 314, *323*
Owen, W. F., 275, *301*
Owen, W. F., Jr., 275, *301*
Owen, W. G., 29, 30, *53*, *56*, *61*
Ownby, C. L., 117, *133*
Ozaki, Y., 192, *208*

P

Packer, C. S., 229, 232, 240, 241, 242, 243, 244, 245, 246, 248, 249, 250, 253, 254, 255, 256, *257*, *258*, *259*, *260*
Paddock, C., 315, *325*
Padrell, E., 8, *61*
Painter, R. G., 5, 6, 9, 18, 30, 31, 32, 36, 37, 38, *56*, 128, *133*, 269, *301*
Paky, A., 47, *56*
Palade, G. E., 99, *109*, 114, 118, *130*, *131*, *135*
Palladino, M. A., Jr., 194, 195, 200, *204*
Palmer, J. B., 71, *90*
Palmer, R. M. J., 240, *257*, 317, 318, *323*, *325–26*
Pan, Y. -C. C., 21, *58*
Panchenko, M. P., 5, 6, 8, 9, 10, 11, *65*, 68, *96*
Parinandi, N. L., 48, *62*
Park, S., 71, 72, *93*, *96*
Park, W. C., 238, *259*
Parker, C. W., 268, 271, 272, 276, *297*, *299*, *304*, *305*
Parker, J., 70, *93*
Parker, J. C., 277, 279, 288, *294*, *301*
Parker, K. L., 272, *305*
Parker, P. J., 69, *95*
Parker, R., 71, 85, *88*
Parker, S. D., 100, 102, *110*, *111*
Parkinson, J. E., 29, *62–63*
Parra, S. C., 175, *189*, 201, *209*
Parwaresch, M. R., 265, *301*
Pastan, K., 43, *65*
Patarroyo, M., 73, 74, *95*
Patel, J. M., 157, 167, *171*, *172*
Paterson, N. A. M., 229, *259*
Patterson, C. E., 12, 13, 14, 17, 18, 20, 32, 33, 38–43, *57*, *63*, *64*, 239, 253, 254, 255, *256*, *259*
Patton, G., 17, 36, *58*
Patton, J. S., 192, 198, 202, *204*, *208*
Paul, W. E., 268, *301*
Payan, D. G., 71, *92*
Peach, M. J., 73, 74, 75, 76, 79, 81, *94*, 102, *110*, 121, *134*, 138, *172*, 253, *260*, 281, *304*, 317, *324*
Peachell, P. J., 287, *301*
Peachell, P. T., *110*, 268, 272, *301*, *305*
Pearce, F. L., 287, *301*
Pearson, A. M., 235, *259*
Pearson, J. D., 8, 14, 17, 31, 39, *54*, *57*, 314, *325*
Pecht, I., 269, 271, *301*, *303*
Pedenovi, M., *61*
Pele, J. P., 266, 267, *296*
Peleg, I., 272–73, *299*
Pelosin, J. M., 68, *93*
Peng, Y. -M., 175, 176, *186*
Penner, R., 269, 270, *301*
Perez, H. D., *224*
Perlman, M. B., 46, *56*
Perrelet, A., 119, 125, *133*
Perruchoud, A. P., 71, 73, 74, *88*
Perry, M., 76, 79, 80, 81, 84, *93*
Persson, C., 287, *301*
Peters, M. S., 265, 266, *294*, *301*
Peters, P. M., 192, *208*
Peters, S. P., 47, *56*
Peters, T. J., 167, *172*
Petersen, H., 155, *171*
Peters-Golden, M., 137, *169*
Peterson, C. G. B., 287, *307*
Peterson, D., 239, 240, *256*
Peterson, D. A., 167, *171–72*
Peterson, E. A., 273, *292*
Peterson, H., 155, *171*

Peterson, J. E., 192, *207*
Peterson, M. W., 285, *301*
Petreccia, D., 267, *301*
Petrone, W. F., 72, *93*
Petrun, D. M., 229, *259*
Peveri, P., 74, *96*
Pfannkuche, H. J., 70, 73, *93*
Pfeiffer, J. M., 269, *301*
Pfister, C., 5, *53*
Pfizenmaier, K., 75, *94*
Phan, S. H., 184, *188*, 200, *206*, 217, 218, 222, *225*
Philip, R., 198, 202, *204*
Phillips, D., 281, *298*
Phillips, G., 74, 75, *93*
Phillips, P., 46, *59*, 73, 74, 82, 83, *90*
Phillips, P. G., 41, *63*, 75, 122, 123, 124, 125, 126, 129, *132*, *133*, *134*, 176, 177, 179, 180, 185, *188*, *189*
Philpott, C. W., 266, *301*
Piacibello, W., 29, *54*
Piccoli, D. S., 221, *224*
Pickett, E. B., *89–90*
Pickett, W. C., 192, *203–4*, 287, *295*
Pierce, J. H., 268, *301*
Pietra, G. G., 99, *110*
Pike, M. C., 214, *225*
Pincus, S. H., 276, 282, *301*
Pinto Da Silva, P., 127, *132*
Piotrowski, W., 268, *294*, *301*
Piper, P. J., 71, *93*
Pirotton, S., 8, 10, *63*
Pitelka, D. R., 120, 127, *134*
Pitt, B. R., 12, *62*, 71, 74, 79–85, *90*, *91*, *92*, *93*, *96*, 247, *259*
Planker, M., *88*
Plaut, M., 268, 276, *299*, *301*, *303*
Plummer, K. K., 180, *188*
Pober, J. S., 76, *94*, 124, *135*, 191, 192, 194, *203*, *209*
Pocidalo, J. J., 200, *207*
Pohl, U., 72, *95*
Pohlman, T. H., 75, *91*, 191, 201, *208*, 216, *225*
Poinani, G. J., 229, 238, *261*
Polgar, P., 201, *209*
Pollanen, J., 180, *188*
Pollard, H. B., 8, 17, *56*
Pollard, T. D., 99, *111*
Pollock, W. K., 8, 17, *63*
Pontremoli, S., 74, *93*
Popov, V. I., 119, *134*
Porcelli, R. S., 229, *259*
Porzio, M. A., 235, *259*
Pothoulakis, C., 120, 122, 123, 125, *131–32*
Potter, G. K., 268, *304*
Povlishock, J. T., 201, *206*, 240, 249, *261*
Powers, E. A., 68, *91*
Prasad, V. R., 76, 79, 81, 82, *87*, 196, *203*
Prescher, K. E., *326*
Prescott, S. M., 29, 46, *61*, *63*, 70, *94*, 314, *325*
Price, J., *56*
Primack, S., 71, *92*
Prin, L., 266, *301*
Proctor, R. A., 200, *205*
Proud, D., 268, *299*
Prydz, H., 29, *56*
Pujol, J. L., 275, *296*
Putney, J. W., Jr., 50, *63*
Putney, S. D., 195, 200, *204*

Q

Qiao, B. Y., 71, 73, 74, *88*
Quible, D. J., 176, 177, *188*
Quinton, P. M., 266, *301*

R

Radeke, H. H., 197, *207*
Radomski, M., 317, *325–26*

Rafelson, M. E., 311, *322*, *326*
Rafferty, U. M., 180, *189*
Raffestin, B., 72, *93*
Raffin, T. A., *95*, 195, *209*
Raines, E., 237, *260*
Rambaldi, A., 275, *305*
Randall, R. W., 51, *54*
Rando, R. R., 68, *93*
Rapaport, R. M., 314, 317, *326*
Rasio, E. A., 75, *93*, 125, *134*
Rasmussen, H., 71, 72, *93*, *96*
Rasp, E., 8, *63*
Rastogi, B. K., 164, *172*
Raymond, R. M., 99, *111*
Record, M., 20, *57*
Reddy, P. V., 20, 21, *62*, *63*
Redman, J. F., *93*
Reed, C. E., 266, *294*
Reed, N. G., 318, *324*
Reep, B., *61*, 318, *324*
Rees, D. D., *325*
Rees, P. K., 266, *292*
Reeves, J. T., 228, 229, 238, *259*, *260*, *261*
Regal, J. F., 268, *301*
Reibman, J., 73, *93–94*
Reid, L., 175, 176, *188*, 228, 229, 237, 238, *257*, *258*, *259*
Reid, L. M., 176, *186*, 228, 237, 238, *257*, *258*, *260*
Reid, L. M. C., 249, *261*
Reidy, M. A., 201, *205*, 263, *295*
Reik, L., 21, *58*
Reilly, P., 279, 281, *306*
Reinders, J. M., 74, *94*
Reinhold, S. L., 70, *94*
Reitz, D. A., 249, *261*
Rembold, C. M., 72, *94*
Remick, D. G., 195, 200, *207*, *208*, 217, 218, 221, 222, *225*
Repin, V. S., 42, *53*, 74, *87*
Repine, J. E., 45, 46, 47, *58*, *64*, 73, 74, 75, 76, 79, 81, 82, 84, *90*, *94*, 123, 124, *131*, *135*, 138, *170*, *172*, *173*, 191, 192, 194, 195, 199, *203*, *210*, 238, 240, 252, 253, *256*, *260*, *261*, 263, 281, *304*, *305*
Resch, K., 70, 73, *93*, 197, *207*
Resink, T. J., 8, *63*
Reuben, R. C., 195, 200, *204*
Revak, S. D., 138, *169*
Revhaug, A., 194, *207*
Revtyak, G., 16, *59*
Reyak, S. D., 84, 85, *94*
Reynolds, R. L., 249, *258*
Rheinwald, J. G., 180, *188*
Rhoades, R. A., 40, 41, 43, *63*, 229, 239–46, 248, 249, 250, 253, 254, 255, *256*, *257*, *258*, *259*, *260*
Ribbes, G., 20, *57*
Ribi, E. E., 192, *207*
Rice, C. L., 84, 85, *94*
Rich, A., 195, 200, *204*
Richa, A. B., 73, *93–94*
Richards, I. M., 278, 281, *293*
Richardson, B. A., 266, *290*
Richardson, M., 316, *322*
Richerson, H. B., 281, *294*
Rietjens, I. M. C. M., 140, *172*
Riggs, D., 85, *90*
Riley, D. J., 229, 238, *258*, *261*
Rimland, D., *110*
Rincon, J., 73, 74, *95*
Rink, T. W., 17, *63*
Riordan-Johnson, M., 185, *186*
Rippe, B., 288, *301*
Ritchie, A. J., 76, *94*
Ritchie, A. K., 8, *55*
Rittenhouse, S. E., 18, *59*
Rittenhouse-Simmons, S., 315, *326*
Rizzo, M. T., 4, *63*
Rloden, K., 72, *90*
Robbins, A. H., 194, *207*
Roberts, A. B., 184, *188*
Roberts, J. J., 272, *298*
Roberts, R., 191, 193, *204*
Robidoux, C., 266, 267, *296*
Robinson, C., 267, *290*

Robinson, E. A., 217, 222, *225*
Robinson, F. R., 122, *132*
Robinson, W., 192, *209*
Robson, A. M., 285, *305*
Roddy, L. L., 267, *298*
Rodewald, R., 120, *134*
Rodrigues, A. M., 240, *261*
Rodriguez, M., 265, *301*
Rodriguez, M. A., 180, *189*
Rodriguez-Pena, A., 69, *95*
Roepke, D. A., 240, 241, 242, 243, 248, 249, 253, 255, *260*
Roepke, J. E., 229, *260*
Rogers, D. F., 287, 288, 289, *293*
Rogers, J., 270, *291*
Rogers, M. C., 239, *258–59*
Rogers, T. S., 200, *204*
Roka, L., 138, *173*
Romanov, Y. A., 42, *53*, 74, *87*
Rosano, C. L., 138, *173*
Rosati, F., 266, *293*
Rosenbaum, W. I., 240, *260*
Rosenberg, S. A., 196, *205*
Rosengurt, E., 69, *95*
Rosenwasser, L. J., 200, *204*
Ross, R., 176, *186*, 237, *257*, *260*
Ross, R. R., 29, *58*
Rossi, F., 51, *63*
Rossi, V., 200, *205*, *208*
Rossio, J., 202, *209*
Roth, H. J., 267, *304*
Roth, R. A., 253, *257*
Rothenberg, M. E., 275, *301*
Rothlein, R., 191, *208–9*, 214–16, *225*, 279, 281, *306*
Rothrock, J. K., *56*
Rothstein, J. L., 192, *210*
Rotilio, D., *61*
Rotrosen, D., 8, 40, *63*, 124, *134*
Roubin, R., 275, *301*
Rowe, G. T., 201, *206*
Rowen, J., 276, 277, *301*
Royall, J. A., *94*, 124, *134*, 192, 194, 195, *208*
Royston, D., 249, *256*
Rubanyi, G. M., 72, *94*, 239, 249, *260*
Rubin, D. B., 73, 74, *90*, 137, *172*
Ruch, R. J., 138, 140, 166, *172*
Rudich, Z., 285, *304*
Ruff, V. A., 68, *91*
Rungger-Brandle, E., 114, 117, *134*
Ruppert, C. L., 229, *258*
Rutledge, B. K., 216, *225*
Ryan, M. P., 177, 178, 179, 180, 181, 182, 183, 184, 185, *187*, *188*, *189*
Ryan, T. J., 122, 123, 124, *134*
Ryan, U. S., 68, *96*, 184, *188*
Ryan, V. S., 72, *94*
Rybin, V. O., 5, 6, 8, 9, 10, 11, *65*

S

Sabanero, M., 117, 118, *133*
Saccardo, B., 200, *205*
Sacco, O., 74, *93*
Sacks, T., 138, *172*, 263, *303*
Sager, R., 217, *224*
Sagi-Eisenberg, R., 271, *303*
Sahn, S. A., 73, *90*
Said, S. I., 288, *300*
Saito, H., 267, 269, 270, *297*, *303*
Saito, K., 275, *293*
Saito, Y., 18, *59*
Saitoh, M., 247, *260*
Salamino, F., 74, *93*
Salkin, H. S., 315, *324*
Salmon, D. M., 50, *55*
Saltini, C., *206*
Salvidio, G., 200, *203*
Sampson, A. S., 71, *90*
Sampson, P. M., 121, *130*
Samuelson, T., 276, *300*
Samuelsson, T., 276, *295*
Sanavio, F., 29, *54*

Sanborg, R. R., 269, *303*
Sandblom, R. L., 249, *259*
Sanderson, C. J., 275, 286, *299*, *304*, *305*
Sands, M. F., 71, *92*
Sanjar, S., 275, *303*
Santana, T. A., 198, *209*
Santaren, J. F., 180, *188*
Sarau, H. M., 70, *96*
Saria, A., 287, 288, *303*
Sasaki, Y., *90*, 247, *258*
Sass-Kuhn, S. P., 275, *300*
Sassone-Corsi, P., 185, *188*
Sato, N., 192, 194, *208*
Sato, T., 11, *53*
Satomi, N., 192, 194, *208*
Saul, W., 270, *299*
Saul, W. F., 269, 270, *290*
Sawamura, M., 271, *297*
Sawasaki, Y., 192, 194, *208*
Saxon, M. E., 119, *134*
Schaefer, E. J., 200, *204*
Schafer, A. I., 18, 50, *61*, *65*, 70, *97*
Schatte, C. L., 140, *172*
Scheid, C. R., 108, *110*
Schenkman, S., 21, *55*
Scheurich, P., 75, *94*
Schiffer, L. M., 265, *304*
Schilling, W. P., 8, 46, *55*, *56*
Schleimer, N. F., 268, *299*
Schleimer, R. P., *110*, 216, *225*, 268, 271, 276, 278, 279, *298*, *303*
Schmid, H. H. O., 20, 21, 48, *55*, *62*, *63*
Schmid, P. C., 20, 21, *62*, *63*
Schmidt, H. H. H. W., *326*
Schmitt, J. D., 73, 84, *87*
Schneeberger, E. E., 114, *134*
Schneider, A. S., 31, 41, *61–62*
Schnittler, H., 117, *131*
Schoderbek, W. E., 281, *294*
Schooley, W. R., 276, *301*
Schramm, C. M., 71, 72, *94*
Schraufshatter, A., 84, 85, *94*
Schraufstatter, I. U., 155, *172*
Schreiber, H., 192, *210*
Schroeder, J., 217, *225*
Schulman, E. S., 268, *299*
Schulz, W., 249, *258*
Schumacher, H. R., 71, 85, *96*
Schutze, S., 75, *94*
Schwartz, B. R., 46, *58*, 145, *170*, 263, *295*
Schwartz, S. M., 116, *131*, 201, *205*, 263, *295*
Sciuto, A. M., 100, 102, 103, 104, *109*
Sciuto, M., 47, *56*
Scott, D., 30, 40, *54*
Seagrave, J. C., 269, *301*
Sedar, A. W., 127, *134*
Sedgwick, J. B., 267, 282, *303*, *307*
Sedlak, B., 311, *322*
Sedov, J. R., 22, *59*
Seed, B., 216, *224*
Seiffge, D., 117, *131*
Seiss, W., 315, *326*
Sekharam, K. M., 167, *172*
Sekiguchi, K., *64*, 67, 68, 71, *95*
Sekino, H., 287, *305*
Sekizaki, S., 317, *321*
Selig, W. M., 122, *130*, 266, 277, 281, 282, 288, *291*, *292*, *303*
Selle, S., 197, *207*
Selvaraj, P. M., 72, *94*
Senoir, R. M., 238, *259*
Senyi, A., 310, *325*
Senyk, G., 192, *207*
Serhan, C., 124, *134*, 167, *172*
Sertl, K., 264, *303*
Sessler, C. N., 285, *293–94*
Severson, S. P., 47, 48, *65*
Sha'afi, R., *65*, 271, *306*
Shaafi, R. I., 70, 73, *92*, *96*, *97*
Sha'afri, R. I., 269, 270, *303*
Shabanowitz, J., 217, *225*
Shanley, P. F., 193, *210*
Shannon, M. F., 275, *299*
Shapiro, D. L., 176, 177, *188*
Shapleigh, C., 287, *297–98*

Sharfman, W., 202, *209*
Shasby, D. M., 8, 46, 47, 48, *54*, *64*, 73, 74, 75, 76, 79, 81, *94*, *95*, 102, 107, 108, *109*, *110*, 121, 124, 128, *134*, 138, 159, *170*, *172*, 240, 253, *260*, *261*, 281, 285, *301*, *304*
Shasby, S. S., 8, 46, 47, 48, *54*, *64*, 73, 74, 75, 76, 79, 81, *94*, *95*, 102, 107, 108, *109*, *110*, 121, 124, 128, *134*, 138, *172*, 253, *260*, 281, *304*
Shatos, M. A., 311, *326*
Shaw, K., 7, *64*
Shaw, L. M., 74, *95*
Shay, A. M., 286, *304*
Shea, S. M., 113, *133*, 287, *299*
Shearman, M. S., *64*, 67, 68, 71, *95*
Shelburne, J., 46, *55*, 122, *130*, 137, *169*, 175, 176, *187*
Shelburne, J. D., 175, *189*, 201, *209*
Shelburne, J. S., 137, *169*
Shelley, R. I., 271, *303*
Shellito, J. E., 198, 202, *204*
Shen, T. Y., 71, 73, *88*
Shenolikar, S., 67, *95*
Shepard, J. M., 311, 314, 315, 316, 317, 320, *324*
Shephard, H. M., 192, *210*
Sheppard, B. C., 192, *202*
Sheppard, D., 192, 201, *205*
Shepro, D., 75, *93*, 125, *130*, *133*, *134*, *135*
Sher, A., 266, *292*
Sherwin, S., *206*
Shibata, S., 232, *260*
Shibel, E. M., 310, *323–24*
Shida, T., 267, *297*
Shiki, Y., 192, 197, 198, *206*, *208*
Shimuzu, M., 202, *209*
Shioya, T., 71, *92*
Shipman, L. J., 73, 74, *96*
Shirato, L., 38, *62*
Shires, G. T., *96*, 194, *209*
Shishido, H., 275, *293*
Shohami, E., 8, 17, *56*
Showaiter, S. D., 217, *225*
Showell, H. J., 217, 218, 222, *225*
Shuman, M. A., 315, *326*
Shwabe, U., 268, *299*
Sibbald, W. J., 252, *261*
Sieckmann, D. G., 75, *89*
Siegart, W., 272, *305*
Siegel, M. I., 20, *53*
Sies, H., 47, *57*, 197, *207*
Siess, W., 11, *64*
Siflinger-Birnboim, A., 122, *131*, 315, *323*
Silberstein, D. R., 275, *301*
Silberstein, D. S., 275, *301*
Silverman, H. J., 102, 108, *110*
Simionescu, M., 114, *135*
Simionescu, N., 114, *135*
Simon, M. L., 137, *173*
Simon, R. H., 138, *169*
Simons, K., 127, *131*
Simonson, M. S., 22, *59*
Simpson, R. J., 167, *172*
Sims, P. J., 315, *323*
Sinha, A. K., 311, *326*
Siraganian, R. P., 264, 267, 268, 269, 270, 272, *292*, *296*, *304*, *306*
Sirois, P., 266, 267, *296*
Sitt, E. S., 71, 73, 74, *89*
Sjostrom, K., 199, *208*
Skar, L. A., 269, *301*
Skeel, A., 217, *225*
Sklar, L. A., 128, *133*, 155, 160, *170*, *172*
Skofitsch, G., 287, 288, *303*
Skoglund, G., 73, 74, *95*
Skoza, L., 200, *206*
Skutelsky, E., 285, *304*
Slaso, J., 74, *91*
Slater, J., 264, *303*
Slater, T. F., 140, *168*
Slivka, A., 46, *65*, 137, 138, *173*
Sloane-Stanley, G. H., 164, *170*
Slotman, G., 102, 108, *110*
Slungaard, A., 275, 282, 283, 287, *304*

Smedley, L. A., 192, *208*
Smirnov, V. N., 42, *53*, 74, *87*
Smith, A. D., 153, *173*
Smith, C. D., 38, *64*
Smith, C. W., 191, *208–9*
Smith, D., 275, *303*
Smith, G. A., 270, *291*
Smith, J., II, 202, *209*
Smith, J. A., 7, *64*
Smith, J. B., 317, *322*, *323*
Smith, J. R., 75, *88*
Smith, K. A., 106, *109*
Smith, L. M., *171*
Smith, M. E., 117, *132*
Smith, M. K., 108, *110*
Smith, P., 228, *258*
Smith, P. S., 47, *57*
Smith, W. W., 192, *208*
Smolen, J. E., 269, *303*
Snadhaus, R. A., 192, *208*
Snapper, J. R., 84, *89*, 200, *209*
Snapper, J. S., 71, 85, *88*
Sneddon, J. M., 317, *326*
Snyderman, R., 38, *64*, 68, *96*, 214, *225*
Soberman, R. J., 275, *301*
Soderling, T. R., 108, *110*
Soiecerman, S., *89-90*
Solski, P. A., *62*
Sonowane, B. R., 200, *209*
Sorici, F., 266, *293*
Sosenko, I. R. S., 138, 139, 166, *172*
Souhrada, J. F., 71, 72, *95*
Souhrada, M., 71, 72, *95*
Souvignet, C., 68, *93*
Spannhake, E. W., 47, *56*
Sparatore, B., 74, *93*
Sparks, L. H., 192, *206*
Spector, A. A., 141, 153, 159, 164, 167, *170*, *171*, *173*
Spector, W., 116, *131*
Spengler, M., 200, *207*, 221, *225*
Spengler, R., 200, *207*, 221, *225*
Spitz, D. R., 198, *209*
Spolarics, Z., *110*
Sporn, M. B., 184, *188*
Spragg, G. R., 138, *169*
Spragg, R. G., 155, *172*, 310, *323–24*
Sprague, R. S., 82, 84, 85, *95*
Spragy, R. G., 249, *259*
Sprengers, E. D., 180, *189*
Spriggs, D. R., 194, *207*
Springer, T. A., 214–16, *225*
Sprung, C. L., 249, *261*
Spry, C. J. F., 264, 265, 266, 286, *304*, *305*
Stabel, S., 69, *95*
Stalcup, S. A., 137, 138, *169*
Standefer, J. C., 269, *306*
Standiford, T. J., 221, *225*
Stanley, A. M., 266, *301*
Stanness, K. A., 191, *208*, 216, *225*
Stark, J. M., 191, *207*
Stasek, J. E., 12, 13, 14, 17, 18, 20, 27, 32, 33, 38, 39, 40, 42, 43, *57*, *64*
Staub, N. C., 288, *300*
Stechschulte, D. J., 275, *297*
Steffen, M., 268, *304*
Stein, O., 285, *293*
Stein, Y., 285, *293*
Steinberg, J., 30, 40, *54*
Steinberg, P. E., 315, *326*
Steinberg, S., 75, *88*, 124, *130*
Steiner, S. H., 177, *186*
Steinhilber, D., 267, *304*
Steinmuller, D., 286, *295*
Steis, R., 202, *209*
Stelzner, T. J., 43, *64*, 102, *110*
Stendahl, O., 73, *89*
Stengelin, S., 216, *224*
Stenmark, K. R., 238, *259*, *261*
Stephens, K. E., *95*, 195, *209*
Stephens, N. L., 232, *259*
Stephenson, A. H., 82, 84, 85, *95*
Sterk, A. R., 272, *297*
Stern, A., 46, *64*
Stern, D., 75, *88*, 124, *130*, 194, *207*
Steven, 75, *93*
Stevens, J. K., 285, *305*
Stevens, R. L., 275, *301*
Stevenson, B. R., 120, *135*

Stewart, D. J., 72, *95*
Stewart, J. M., 68, *96*
Stiernberg, J., 30, *54*
Stolpen, A. H., 124, *135*, 192, 194, *209*
Stone, P., 285, *301*
Stork, L., 192, *209*
Stossel, T. P., 114, 117, 128, *131*, *132*, *135*
Stovroff, M. C., 192, *202*
Strath, M., 286, *304*
Strieter, R. M., 217, 218, 221, 222, *224*, *225*
Striker, G. E., 138, *170*, 201, *205*
Strom, T. B., 200, *206*
Struhar, D., 84, *95*
Stryckmans, P. A., 265, *304*
Stuart, R. S., 249, *261*
Stubbs, C. D., 153, *173*
Stump, R. F., 269, *301*
Sturrock, R. F., 266, *292*
Sturton, R. G., 71, *90*
Subramanian, N., 268, 276, *304*
Suda, J., 275, *307*
Suda, T., 275, *307*
Suffys, P., *209*
Sugarman, B. J., 192, *210*
Sugiura, M., 72, *95*
Suliaman, F. A., 275, 287, *305*
Sullivan, J. M., 73, 74, 75, 76, *94*, 102, *110*, 121, *134*
Sullivan, S. G., 46, *64*
Sullivan, T. J., 268, 271, 272, 276, *297*, *299*, *304*, *305*
Summer, W. R., 47, *56*, 71, *89*, 100, 101, 102, 105, 106, 107, *110*
Summerville, J., 191, 192, 193, 195, *204*
Sun, F. F., 266, 267, *295*, *305*
Sun, X. M., *209*
Suter, S. M., 185, *186*
Sutko, J. L., 240, *261*
Suttorp, N., 137, 138, *173*
Suzuki, M., *258*
Suzuki-Nushimura, T., 287, *305*
Svensjo, E., 99, *111*, 113, *131*
Svitkina, T. M., 180, *188*
Swanson, J. E., 167, *169*
Sylvester, P., 271, *297*
Szidon, J. P., 99, *110*
Sznol, M., 202, *209*
Sznycer-Laszuk, R., 29, *57*
Sztein, M. B., 192, *208*

T

Taelman, H., 266, *301*
Taggart, B. N., 120, 127, *134*
Tahamont, M. V., 281, *294*
Tai, P. C., 286, *305*
Takahashi, I., *96*
Takai, T., 20, *64*
Takai, Y., 5, 38, *65*, 271, *297*
Takaishi, T., 269, 270, 271, *300*, *306*
Takatsu, K., 275, *307*
Takayanagi, I., 241, *261*
Takeichi, M., 127, *132*
Takenaka, A., 38, *62*
Takeshige, K., 10, 12, 18, *59*
Takishima, T., 268, *301*
Takuwa, N., 71, *96*
Takuwa, Y., 71, 72, *93*, *96*
Tamaguchi, N., 267, *297*
Tamaoki, T., 76, *91*, *96*
Tamura, N., 275, 287, *305*
Tanaka, S., 217, 222, *225*
Tanaka, Y., 185, *187*
Tanenbaum, M., 108, *109*
Tanimoto, T., 5, 38, *65*
Tank, D. W., 117, *135*
Tanowitz, H. B., 311, *326*
Tanswell, A. K., 138, *169*
Tate, G. A., 71, 85, *96*
Tate, M. D., 192, *210*
Tate, R. M., 47, *64*, 73, 74, 75, 76, *94*, 138, *172*, 240, 252, 253, *260*, *261*, 263, 281, *304*, *305*
Tatham, P. E. R., 269, *295*
Tauber, A. L., 267, *305*

Taylor, A. E., 76, 79, 80, 81, 82, 84, 85, *87*, *93*, 196, *203*, 288, *301*
Taylor, B. M., 266, 267, *305*
Taylor, G. S., 48, *64*
Taylor, K. M., 249, *256*
Taylor, L., 201, *209*
Taylor, R. G., 84, *96*
Taylor, S. J., 7, *64*
Terao, T., 272, *305*
Terce, F., 20, *57*
Terpstra, A. J., 180, *188*
Tertoolen, L. G. J., 50, *61*
Teshima, R., 272, *305*
Tetsuhiro, H., 241, *261*
Tetta, C., 29, *54*
Thalacker, F. W., 180, *189*
Thaw, H. H., *88*
Thelen, M., 74, *96*
Theoharides, T. C., 272, *305*
Thet, L. A., 175, 176, *187*, *189*, 201, *209*
Thomas, L. L., 273, 287, *300*, *301*, *307*
Thomopoulos, P., 72, 74, *90*
Thompson, J. E., 192, 201, *205*
Thompson, N. T., 51, *54*
Thompson, P. J., 29, *58*
Thorgeirsson, G., 8, 12, 14, 17, 18, 32, 36, 37, *57*, *61*
Thornton, A. J., 217, 218, *225*
Thrall, R. S., 84, *96*
Tierney, D. F., 201, *209*
Till, G. O., 238, *261*, 263, 281, *305*
Tilly, B. C., 50, *61*
Tkachuk, V. A., 5, 6, 8, 9, 10, 11, 42, *53*, *65*, 68, 74, *87*, *96*
Tloti, M. A., 317, *326*
To, L. B., 275, *299*
Tobleni, G., 314, *324*
Tocker, J., 266, 277, 281, 282, *292*, *303*
Toepfer, W., 138, *173*
Tolley, E., 100, 102, 103, 104, *109*
Tolson, J. K., 143, 144, 145, 146, 150, 151, 153, 154, 156, 157, 158, 159, 160, 161, 162, 164, 165, 166, *170*
Toman, C., 191, *208–9*
Tomashefski, J. F., Jr., 249, *261*
Tominaga, A., 275, *307*
Tomita, F., *96*
Tonnel, A. B., 266, *301*
Tonnesen, M. G., 192, *208*, 278, 279, *297*
Topolosky, M. K., 175, *187*
Toth, K. M., 138, *173*
Toung, T. J. K., 239, *258–59*
Touqui, L., 71, 73, *88*
Townley, R. G., 275, 287, *305*
Townsley, M. I., 76, 79, 81, 82, 85, *87*
Toy, K., 192, *207*
Toyofuku, T., 285, *305*
Tozzi, C. A., 229, 238, *258*, *261*
Tracey, K. J., *96*, 194, *209*
Travis, W. D., 196, *205*
Traynor, A. E., 128, *133*, 269, *301*
Traystman, R. J., 100, 102, *110*, *111*, 239, *258–59*
Trelstad, R. L., *258*
Tricot, G., 4, *63*
Triggiani, M., 272, *299*
Trotta, R. J., 46, *64*
Trouwborst, A., 200, *206*
Tsan, M. -F., 41, 46, *59*, *63*, 73, 74, 75, 82, 83, *90*, *93*, 122, 123, 124, 125, 126, *132*, *133*, *134*, 138, *173*, 176, 177, 179, 180, 185, *188*, *189*, 194, 198, *209*
Tscharner, V. V., 74, *96*
Tsujimoto, M., 192, *210*
Tsuyamam, S., 6, *53*
Tuchweber, B., 125, *131*
Turitto, V. T., 309, *326*
Turnbull, L. W., 268, 287, *291*
Turrens, J. F., 138, *169*, *173*
Twarog, B. M., 237
Tzeng, C., 17, 36, *58*

U

Uchida, M. K., 287, *305*

Ueda, G., 285, *305*
Ui, M., 10, 50, *62*, 269, 270, *300*, *303*
Ulevitch, R. J., 195, *207*
Ullberg, M., 106, *111*
Undem, B. J., 272, *305*
Urba, W., 202, *209*
Urban, J. L., 192, *210*
Ursprung, J. J., 102, 108, *110*
Utley, J., 249, *259*

V

Vadas, M. A., 274, 275, *293*, *294*, *299*
Vads, M. A., 192, *206*
Vaheri, A., 180, *188*
Valent, P., 268, 276, *305*
Vanbenthuysen, K. M., 73, 74, 75, 76, *94*, 138, *172*, 240, 253, *260*, *261*, 281, *304*
van Breemen, C., 71, *91*, 108, *110*, 240, *259*
Van Corven, E. J., 50, *58*
Vande, V., 99, *109*
Van Den Bosch, H., 16, *64*
Vandeplassche, G., 249, *261*
Vanderjagt, D., 269, *306*
van der Meer, J. W. M., 192, 200, *204*, *210*
van der Zee, H., 288, *291*
Van De Walle, C. M., 50, *63*
Vane, J. R., 167, *170*, 317, 318, *322*, *325*, *326*
Vanhoutte, P. M., 72, *91*, *94*, 240, *258*
van Mourik, J. A., 74, *94*, 182, *189*
VanRooijen, L. A. A., 8, *53*
Van Roy, R., *209*
Van Ryn, J., 316, *322*
van Tilburg, C. A. M., 140, *172*
Vargaftig, B. B., 71, 73, *88*
Varin-Blank, N., 270, *300*
Vassalli, D., 221, *224*
Vassalli, J., 221, *224*
Vassalli, P., 117, *131*
Vavrek, R. J., 68, *96*
Vedia, L. M. Y., *61*
Vehaskari, V. M., 285, *305*
Venge, P., 265, 275, 276, 282, 287, *290*, *295*, *298*, *307*
Venthuysen, K. M., 47, *64*
Ventura, C., 249, *261*
Ventura, M. A., 72, 74, *90*
Venturini, C. M., 309, 312, 313, 315–20, *326*, *327*
Venzon, D., 192, *202*
Vercellotti, G. M., 47, 48, *65*, 275, 282, 283, 287, *304*, 311, *327*
Verhagen, J., 275, *291*
Verlaan, I., 50, *61*
Vervoorn, R. C., 74, *94*
Verwe, C. L., 74, *94*
Via, D. P., 177, *186*
Vilcek, J., 76, *97*, 192, *210*
Villa, P., 200, *205*
Villani, G. M., 317, *324*
Villereal, M. L., *61–62*
Visner, G. A., 192, 197, *210*
Vitti, G. F., 221, *224*
Voelkel, N. F., 191, 192, 200, *203–4*, 238, *259*, *261*, 285, *292*
Vogel, S. N., 192, *207*, *210*
Vosshall, L. B., 73, *93–94*
Voyno-Yasenetskaya, T. A., 5, 6, 8, 9, 10, 11, *65*, 68, *96*
Vrtis, R. F., 267, 282, *303*

W

Wagenvoort, A., 237, *261*
Wagenvoort, C. A., 237, *261*
Wagner, J. R., 21, 25, *61*, 68, 70, *92*
Wagner, W. W., Jr., 239, *256*
Wahl, S. M., 268, *296*
Waite, M., 70, *93*

Wakefield, L. M., 184, *188*
Waldmann, R., 107, *111*
Walker, E. C., 192, *202*
Walker, G., 275, 282, 283, 287, *304*
Wallace, M. A., 67, *89*
Walle, A. J., 265, *301*
Walman, A. T., 100, 102, *110*, *111*
Wals, A., 74, *96*
Walter, U., 107, *111*
Waltersdorf, A. M., 265, 266, *297*
Waltersdorph, A. M., 192, *206*, 275, *299*
Walz, A., 217, *224*
Walz, D. A., 311, *327*
Wancewicz, E. V., 74, 75, *91*
Wang, D., 192, *203*
Wang, E. A., 274, *299*
Wang, J. M., 275, *305*
Ward, P. A., 84, 85, *90*, 217, 218, *225*, 238, *261*, 263, 281, *305*
Wardlaw, A. J., 275, *306*
Warner, A. E., 84, *96*
Warner, B. B., 198, *210*
Warner, J. A., 269, 270, 271, *306*
Warner, T. M., 317, *322*
Warram, B. L., 217, 222, *225*
Warren, D. J., 286, *304*
Warshawski, F. J., 252, *261*
Wasiewski, W. W., 315, *324*
Wasserman, M. A., 288, *306*
Wasserman, S. I., 267, *298*
Wassom, D. L., 286, *295*
Wasson, D. C., 266, *292*
Watanabe, K., 8, 17, 30, 31, 36, *58*
Watanabe, N., 191, *211*
Watanabe, Y., *59*
Watras, J., 106, *111*
Watson, C., 268, *301*
Watson, L. P., 75, *89*
Watson, P., 73, 74, *96*
Webb, C., 195, 200, *204*
Webb, W. W., 117, *135*
Weber, G., 4, *63*
Weber, K., 117, *135*
Weber, P. C., 140, *171*, 200, *204*
Wegner, C. D., 279, 281, *306*
Wehland, J., 117, *135*
Wei, E. P., 201, *206*, 240, 249, *261*
Weibel, E. R., 122, *132*, 137, *171*, 237, *258*, 263, *291*
Weichman, B. M., 288, *306*
Weil, J. V., 43, *64*
Weiland, T., 125, *135*
Weiler, D., 273, *292*
Weill, J. V., 102, *110*
Weinbaum, G., 252, *259*, 263, *298*
Weir, E. K., 239, 240, *256*
Weisbrode, S. E., 84, *92*
Weismann, G., 167, *172*
Weiss, S. J., 46, 50, *63*, *65*, 137, 138, *173*
Weissman, G., 124, *134*, 192, *210*
Weissmann, G., 73, *93–94*, 214, *224–25*
Weksler, B. B., 8, 16, 17, 30, 31, 36, *58*, *65*, 314, *327*
Weller, P. F., 265, 266, *293*, *306*
Weller, P. H., 267, *295*
Welles, S. L., 125, *135*
Wells, E., 272, 288, *293*, *306*
Wells, J. N., 72, *92*
Wells, N., 202, *209*
Welton, A., 281, 282, *303*
Welton, A. F., 268, 269, 270, 271, *294*
Weng, W., 83, *96*
Wert, M. D., 139, *171*
Werth, D. K., 43, *65*
Wescott, J. Y., 285, *292*
Westcott, J. Y., 192, *203–4*
Westerhausen, D. R., 183, 185, *189*
Weston, K. K., 316, 319–20, *327*
Weston, L. K., 311, 314, 315, 316, 317, 320, *324*, *326*
Westwick, J., 221, *225*, 275, 282, *298*
Whatley, R. E., 46, *61*
Wheeler, M. E., 191, *203*
Wheeler-Jones, C. P. D., 11, *61*
White, C. W., 76, 79, 81, 82, *90*, 123, *135*, 138, *173*, 191, 192, 193, 194, 195, 198, 199, 201, *210*

White, G. C., II, 315, *325*
White, G. E., 116, 117, *135*
White, J. E., 176, 177, 179, 180, 185, *189*, 198, *209*
White, J. G., 73, 84, *94*
White, J. R., 73, *96*, 271, *306*
White, M. V., 268, *306*
Whitehouse, L. A., 238, *259*
Whitney, P., 198, *206*
Whitty, G. A., 221, *224*
Whorton, A. R., 5, 8–10, 46, 47, *61*, 65
Wiggan, G. A., 268, 269, 270, 271, 272, *294*, *298*
Wiggins, R., 217, 222, *225*
Wiliamson, D. J., 275, *299*
Will, J. A., 200, *205*
Williams, D. R., 228, *258*
Williams, S. K., 121, *130*
Williamson, D. J., 274, *299*
Willmore, D. W., 194, *207*
Wilner, G. D., 311, 314, *323*
Wilson, B. S., 269, *306*
Wilson, J., 73, 84, *87*
Wilson, J. M., 192, 197, *210*
Wilson, P. B., 20, *54*
Winkler, H. H., 266, *295*
Winkler, J. D., 70, *96*
Winslow, C. M., 272, *306*
Winter, M., *95*
Wise, W. C., 200, *210*
Wispé, J. R., 198, *205*, *210*
Witmer, C. M., 200, *209*
Wittfohl, W., *326*
Wittner, M., 311, *326*
Wodnar-Filipowicz, A., 268, *306*
Wojcikieqicz, R. J. H., 67, *89*
Wolber, F., 184, *188*
Woldemussie, E., 269, 270, *306*
Wolff, S. M., 192, 194, 195, 200, *204*, *207*, *210*
Wolfson, E., 195, *207*
Wolfson, M., 68, *96*
Wolin, M. S., 240, *257*, *261*
Wolpe, S., *96*, 194, *209*
Wong, A. J., 99, *111*
Wong, C., 73, *88*
Wong, G., 275, *299*
Wong, G. G., 274, *299*
Wong, G. H. W., 192, 196, *210*
Wong, K., 72, *93*
Wong, M. K. K., 114, 116, 117, 121, 125, *131*, *132*, *135*
Wood, P. A., 177, *189*
Woodcock-Mitchell, J., 175, *186–87*
Woodruff, R. D., 84, *96*
Woods, J., 275, *301*
Woodward, D. F., 288, *306*
Worthen, G. S., 71, 85, *89*, 192, *208*
Wreggett, K. A., 8, 17, *63*
Wrenn, D. S., 238, *259*
Wright, C. D., 73, 84, *96*
Wright, D. G., 138, *170*
Wright, S. D., 74, *97*
Wright, T. N., 265, *296–97*
Wu, E. S., 117, *135*
Wykle, R. L., 73, 84, *87*
Wysolmerski, R., 122, 125, *135*
Wysolmerski, R. B., 16, 41, 43, *61*, *65*

Y

Yaffe, S. J., 200, *209*
Yaghi, A., 229, *259*
Yagisawa, H., *92*
Yam, J., 191, 193, *204*
Yamada, K., 18, 38, *62*
Yamaguchi, T., 275, *307*
Yamamoto, K., 5, 38, *65*
Yamauchi, K., 268, *301*
Yamauchi, N., 191, *211*
Yamazaki, M., 70, *97*
Yancey, K. B., 269, 270, *306*
Yang, Y. C., 275, *299*
Yano, K., 18, 38, *62*

Yano, S., 200, *206*
Yip, Y. K., 76, *97*, 223, *224*
Yokota, S., 192, *210*, 265, *307*
Yoneda, K., 191, *205*
Yorek, M., 46, 47, 48, *64*, *95*, 124, 128, *134*
Yorek, M. A., 153, 167, *173*
Yoshida, S., 18, *59*
Yoshimura, T., 217, 222, *225*
Yoshino, Y., 287, *305*
Younes, M., 197, *207*
Young, I. G., 275, *299*
Young, J., 46, *65*, 137, 138, *173*
Young, J. D., 287, *307*
Young, S., 69, *95*
Young, S. L., 138, 140, 166, *169*, *170*
Yu, A. C. H., 167, *169*
Yu, J. M., 240, *261*
Yu, S. Y., 229, *258*
Yuen, C., *224*
Yui, Y., 267, *297*
Yukawa, T., 275, 282, *298*, *307*
Yung, Y. P., 268, *304*

Z

Zabinski, M. P., 311, 314, *323*
Zapol, W. M., 175, 176, *188*, 228, 237, 238, 249, *258*, *261*
Zavala, D. C., 281, *294*
Zavoico, G. B., 18, *65*, 70, *97*, 315, *325*
Zeheb, R., 180, 181, 182, 183, 184, *187*, *189*
Zentella, A., *96*, 194, *209*
Zetter, B. R., 29, *57*
Zhang, Y., 76, *97*
Zheutlin, L. M., 273, 287, *307*
Ziff, M., 191, 197, *207*, 218, *225*
Zimmerman, G. A., 29, 46, *61*, *63*, 70, *94*, 314, *325*
Zimmerman, R. J., 191, *211*
Zoratti, E. M., 282, *307*
Zovoico, G. B., 50, *61*
Zucker-Franklin, D., 265, *307*
Zumbe, A., 117, *131*
Zurawski, G., 214, 217, *224*
Zurawski, S. M., 214, 217, *224*
Zurier, R. B., 71, 85, *96*

SUBJECT INDEX

A

Actin microfilament system
in endothelial cells, 116
Activators of protein kinase C, 69
Acute lung injury
effects of cyclic adenosine monophosphate (cAMP), 100
Adhesion versus aggregation, regulation of in platelets, 318
Aggregation versus adhesion, regulation of in platelets, 318
Arachidonate metabolites
cytokine-induced oxidant tolerance, 200

B

Bacterial toxin substrates in endothelium, 5
Basophils
activation, 271
adenylate cyclase, 272
diacylglycerol production and protein kinase C, 271
G proteins, 269
inositol triphosphate and intracellular calcium, 270

[Basophils]
location, morphology, and function, 267
lung microvascular injury, 287
mediators that effect eosinophils, 274
protein phosphorylation, 272

C

Calcium
activity, protein kinase C, and G protein regulation of thrombin-stimulated, 32
mobilization, 7
mobilization, and thrombin-induced phospholipase C activity, 31
mobilization, protein kinase C regulation of, 14
protein kinase C regulation of, in endothelium, 17
regulation of phospholipase A_2 in endothelium, 16
regulation of phospholipase D activity, 25
regulation of thrombin-induced barrier dysfunction, 41
Cell movement, 214

Cellular activation
role of guanine nucleotide regulatory proteins in, 3
Cellular effects of protein kinase C, 69
Cellular gene expression
analysis of hyperoxia-associated changes in, 176
Chronic hypoxia
pulmonary hypertension, 228
Control of extracellular matrix-regulating gene expression
by growth factors, 183
by hyperoxic stress, 183
Copper-zinc superoxide dismutase
role in endotoxin-induced tolerance to hyperoxia, 193
Cyclic adenosine monophosphate (cAMP)
effect on acute lung injury, 100
immune system, 106
mechanisms of action on vascular permeability, 107
mechanisms of action on vasomotor tone, 107
mediator production—animal experiments, 103
mediator production—cell culture, 106
permeability of endothelial cell monolayers, 102
temporal nature of protective effects, 101
therapeutic strategy in acute lung injury, 108
Cytokines
effect of on oxidant production, 199
effect of protein kinase C on biological response to, 75
-induced tolerance to oxidants, role of manganese superoxide dismutase in, 196
interleukin-8/neutrophil activating protein, 218
monocyte chemotactic protein, 217
Cytoskeleton
functional links with tight junctions in endothelium, 121
functional links with tight junctions in epithelium, 118
Diacylglyceral production and PKC activation, 271

E

Endothelial cell(s)
actin microfilament system, 116
activation, 1
bacterial toxin substrates in, 5
barrier dysfunction, regulation of thrombin-induced, 40
cytoskeleton, 121
dysfunction, 1
effects of cyclic adenosine monophosphate (cAMP) on permeability of monolayers, 102, 107
effects of cyclic guanosine monophosphate (cGMP) on permeability of monolayers, 107
effects of thrombin, 314
functional links between the cytoskeleton and tight junctions, 121
interleukin-8 gene expression, 218
monocyte chemotactic protein gene expression, 222
permeability of monolayers, 102, 107
phosphatidic acid directly activates protein kinase C in, 27
phosphoinositol-phospholipase C, protein regulation of, 8
phosphoinositol-phospholipase C and calcium mobilization in, 8
phospholipase C and calcium regulation of phospholipase A_2 in, 16

[Endothelial cell(s)]
phospholipase D activity in, 21
platelet adhesion, 311
prostacyclin synthesis, thrombin-induced, protein kinase C regulation of, 38
protein kinase C and the control of vascular permeability, 74
protein kinase C activation in cultured, 12
protein kinase C regulation of calcium in, 17
protein kinase C regulation of phospholipase A_2 in, 17
protein kinase C regulation of phospholipase D in, 23
protein regulation of phosphoinositol-phospholipase C in, 8
signaling, thrombin-receptor dynamics in, 29
tight junctions, structure of, 114
use of modified thrombins in, 30
Endotoxin-induced tolerance to hyperoxia
copper-zinc superoxide dismutase, 193
Eosinophils
activation, 271
adenylate cyclase, 272
basophils, 273
diacylglycerol production and protein kinase C, 271
G proteins, 269
inositol triphosphate and intracellular calcium, 270
location, morphology, and function, 264
lung microvascular injury, 276
mediators effecting mast cells and basophils, 272
Epithelium
functional links between the cytoskeleton and tight junctions, 118
Extracellular matrix-regulating gene expression
by growth factors, 183
by hyperoxic stress, 183

F

Fatty acids
antioxidant enzyme activity, 153
biophysical properties of pulmonary artery endothelial cell membranes, 157
extracellular hydrogen peroxide concentration, 159
lipid composition and reactivity, 162
mechanisms of modulation of oxidant injury, 153
oxidant-induced lipid peroxidation, 160
oxidant-induced pulmonary artery endothelial cell injury, 142
Functional links between the cytoskeleton and tight junctions
endothelium, 121
epithelium, 118

G

G protein
regulation of thrombin-stimulated phospholipase C and calcium activities, and protein kinase C, 32
regulation of thrombin-stimulated prostacyclin synthesis, 37
in signal transduction in eosinophils, mast cells, and basophils, 269
Gene expression
endothelial interleukin-8, 218
endothelial monocyte chemotactic protein, 222
extracellular matrix-regulating gene

[Gene expression]
expression, regulation by growth factors, 183
extracellular matrix-regulating gene expression, regulation by hyperoxic stress, 183
Growth factors
potential molecular mechanisms underlying control of extracellular matrix-regulating gene expression by, 183
Guanine nucleotide regulatory proteins
in cellular activation, 3
Guanosine triphosphate-binding protein(s)
in regulation of phospholipase D activation, 25

H

Hydrogen peroxide
modification of extracellular, 159
Hyperoxia
-associated changes in cellular gene expression, 176
potential molecular mechanisms underlying control of extracellular matrix-regulating gene expression by, 183
pulmonary hypertension, 257
pulmonary tissue response to, 175
tolerance to, role of endotoxin-induced copper-zinc superoxide dismutase, 193

I

Immune system
cyclic adenosine monophosphate (cAMP), 106
Inflammatory cells
effect of protein kinase C, 73
Inflammatory mediators
cytokin-induced oxidant tolerance, 200
Inhibitors of protein kinase C, 69
Injury
ischemia-reperfusion, 249
neutrophil, 252
reactive oxygen species, 238
Interleukin-8
gene expression by endothelial cells, 218
Ischemia-reperfusion
injury, 249
Isolated lung
effect of pulmonary protein kinase C activation in, 76

L

Lipid peroxidation, 160
Lung microvascular injury
basophils, 287
eosinophils, 276
mast cells, 287

M

Manganese superoxide dismutase
role of in cytokine-induced tolerance to oxidants, 196
Mast cell
activation, 271
adenylate cyclase, 272
diacylglycerol production and protein kinase C, 271
G proteins, 269
inositol triphosphate and intracellular calcium, 270
location, morphology, and function, 267
lung microvascular injury, 287
mediators effecting eosinophils, 274

[Mast cell]
protein phosphorylation, 272
Mediator production
animal experiments, 103
cell culture, 106
Mediators
basophils, 274
eosinophils, 273
mast cell, 274
Monocyte chemotactic protein
expression by endothelial cells, 222
Monokine(s)
effect of on oxidant production, 199
effect of protein kinase C on
biological response to, 75
-induced tolerance to oxidants, role
of manganese superoxide
dismutase in, 196
interleukin-8/neutrophil activating
protein, 218
monocyte chemotactic protein, 217
Morphology
basophils, 267
eosinophils, 264
mast cell, 267

N

Neutrophil
injury, 252

O

Oxidant
-induced activation of phospholipase
and modulation of signal
transduction, 45
injury, 238
-mediated activation of
phospholipase C, 47
-mediated activation of
phospholipase D, 48

[Oxidant]
-mediated modulation of
phospholipase A_2 and altered
prostaglandin synthesis, 46
permeability effects of, 122
Oxidant-induced pulmonary artery
endothelial cell injury
antioxidant enzyme activity, 153
effects of supplemental fatty acids,
142
mechanisms of fatty acid-induced
modulation of injury, 153

P

p52
as plasminogen activator inhibitor
type 1, 180
Permeability
effect of oxidants on, 122
of endothelial monolayers, 102, 107
Phosphatidic acid
direct activation of endothelial cell
protein kinase C, 27
Phosphoinositoi
-phospholipase C and calcium
mobilization in endothelium, 8
-phospholipase C, protein regulation
of in endothelial cell, 8
Phospholipase A_2
activity in endothelium, 16
in endothelium, 16
oxidant-induced activation of, and
modulation of signal
transduction, 45
protein kinase C regulation of, in
endothelium, 17
phospholipase C and calcium
regulation of, in endothelium, 16
and signal transduction, 16
Phospholipase C
activation, protein kinase C
regulation of, 14

[Phospholipase C]
activity, regulation of, 7
activity, thrombin-induced, and calcium mobilization, 31
and calcium regulation of phospholipase A_2 in endothelium, 16
oxidant-mediated activation of, 47
protein kinase C and G protein regulation of thrombin-stimulated, 32
protein regulation of endothelial cell phosphoinositol-phospholipase C, 8
regulation of phospholipase A_2 in endothelium, 16
Phospholipase D
calcium regulation of, 25
guanosine triphosphate-binding protein(s), in regulation of, 25
in endothelium, 21
oxidant-mediated activation of, 48
protein kinase C regulation of endothelial cell, 23
regulation of thrombin-induced, 33
signal transduction, 19
Plasminogen activator inhibitor type 1
as p52, 180
Platelet
adhesion versus aggregation, regulation of, 318
reactivity, effect of thrombin, 316
Prostacyclin synthesis
G protein regulation of, thrombin-stimulated, 37
protein kinase C regulation of thrombin-induced, endothelial cell, 38
regulation of thrombin-induced, 36
Prostaglandin synthesis
altered, and oxidant-mediated modulation of phospholipase A_2, 46
Protein kinase C
activation in cultured endothelium, 12
[Protein kinase C]
activators and inhibitors of, 69
and the biological response to monokines, 75
diacylglycerol production and activation of, 271
effects at the cellular level, 69
effects of pulmonary protein kinase C activation, 76
effects on smooth muscle contraction and pulmonary vasoreactivity, 71
endothelial protein kinase C activation and the control of vascular permeability, 74
G protein regulation of thrombin-stimulated phospholipase C and calcium activities, 32
generation of soluble mediators by, 69
in inflammatory cells, 73
mechanisms of stimulus-response coupling mediated by, 67
phosphatidic acid directly activates endothelial cell, 27
pulmonary protein kinase C activation in the isolated lung, 76
pulmonary protein kinase C activation *in vivo,* 84
regulation of endothelial cell phospholipase D activity, 23
regulation of phospholipase A_2 in endothelium, 17
regulation of phospholipase C activation and calcium mobilization, 14
regulation of thrombin-induced barrier dysfunction, 41
regulation of thrombin-induced endothelial cell prostacyclin synthesis, 38
and signal transduction, 11
Protein regulation
of endothelial cell phosphoinositol-phospholipase C, 8

[Protein regulation]
of thrombin-induced barrier dysfunction, 43
Pulmonary artery endothelial cell membranes
biophysical properties of, 157
composition and reactivity, 162
Pulmonary hypertension
chronic hypoxia, 228
hyperoxia induced, 257
Pulmonary protein kinase C activation
effects of, 76
in vivo, 84
Pulmonary thrombosis, 310
Pulmonary tissue response to hyperoxia, 175
Pulmonary vasoreactivity
effect of protein kinase C, 71

R

Regulation
of phospholipase C activity and calcium mobilization, 7
of phospholipase D activation, guanosine triphosphate-binding protein(s) in, 25
of platelet adhesion versus aggregation, 318
of thrombin-induced endothelial cell barrier dysfunction, 40
of thrombin-induced phospholipase D activity, 33
of thrombin-induced prostacyclin synthesis, 36

S

Signal transduction
activation, 271
adenylate cyclase, 272
[Signal transduction]
diacylglycerol production and protein kinase C, 271
G proteins, 269
inositol triphosphate and intracellular calcium, 270
phospholipase A_2 and, 16
phospholipase D and, 19
protein kinase C and, 11, 67
protein phosphorylation, 272
Signaling
use of modified thrombins in endothelial cell, 30
Smooth muscle contraction
effect of protein kinase C, 71
Soluble mediators
generated by protein kinase C, 69
Stimulus-response coupling
mediated by protein kinase C, 67

T

Therapeutic strategy
cyclic adenosine monophosphate (cAMP), 108
Thrombin
effects on endothelial cells, 314
-induced barrier dysfunction, calcium regulation of, 41
-induced barrier dysfunction, protein kinase C regulation of, 41
-induced barrier dysfunction, protein regulation of, 43
-induced endothelial cell barrier dysfunction, regulation of, 40
-induced endothelial cell prostacyclin synthesis, protein kinase C regulation of, 38
-induced phospholipase C activity and calcium mobilization, 31
-induced phospholipase D activity, regulation of, 33

[Thrombin]
-induced prostacyclin synthesis, regulation of, 36
platelet adherence to pulmonary endothelium, 311
platelet adhesion versus aggregation, 318
platelet reactivity, 316
-receptor dynamics in endothelium, 29
receptor occupancy transmembrane signaling after, 29
-stimulated phospholipase C and calcium activities, and protein kinase C and G protein regulation of, 32
-stimulated prostacyclin synthesis, G protein regulation of, 37
Tight junctions
functional links with cytoskeleton in endothelium, 121
functional links with cytoskeleton in epithelium, 118
structure of endothelial, 114
Tolerance to hyperoxia
role of endotoxin-induced
[Tolerance to hyperoxia]
copper-zinc superoxide dismutase, 193
Transmembrane signaling
after thrombin receptor occupancy, 29

U

Use of modified thrombins
in endothelial cell signaling, 30

V

Vasomotor tone
effects of cyclic adenosine monophosphate (cAMP), 107
effects of cyclic guanosine monophosphate (cGMP), 107
Vascular permeability
effects of endothelial cell protein kinase C activation, 74